Pharmacology for the Physical Therapist

Second Edition

Erin E. Jobst, PT, PhD

Professor
Physical Therapy Program
School of Physical Therapy & Athletic Training
College of Health Professions
Pacific University
Hillsboro, Oregon

Peter C. Panus, PhD, PT

Professor Emeritus
Department of Pharmaceutical Sciences
Gatton College of Pharmacy
East Tennessee State University
Johnson City, Tennessee

Marieke Kruidering-Hall, PhD

Professor
Department of Cellular and Molecular Pharmacology
University of California, San Francisco
San Francisco, California

New York   Chicago   San Francisco   Athens   London   Madrid   Mexico City
Milan   New Delhi   Singapore   Sydney   Toronto

Pharmacology for the Physical Therapist, Second Edition

Copyright © 2020, 2009 by McGraw-Hill Education. All rights reserved. Printed in the United States of America. Except as permitted under the United States Copyright Act of 1976, no part of this publication may be reproduced or distributed in any form or by any means, or stored in a database or retrieval system, without the prior written permission of the publisher.

1 2 3 4 5 6 7 8 9   LWI   24 23 22 21 20 19

ISBN 978-1-259-86222-9
MHID 1-259-86222-4

Notice

Medicine is an ever-changing science. As new research and clinical experience broaden our knowledge, changes in treatment and drug therapy are required. The authors and the publisher of this work have checked with sources believed to be reliable in their efforts to provide information that is complete and generally in accord with the standards accepted at the time of publication. However, in view of the possibility of human error or changes in medical sciences, neither the authors nor the publisher nor any other party who has been involved in the preparation or publication of this work warrants that the information contained herein is in every respect accurate or complete, and they disclaim all responsibility for any errors or omissions or for the results obtained from use of the information contained in this work. Readers are encouraged to confirm the information contained herein with other sources. For example and in particular, readers are advised to check the product information sheet included in the package of each drug they plan to administer to be certain that the information contained in this work is accurate and that changes have not been made in the recommended dose or in the contraindications for administration. This recommendation is of particular importance in connection with new or infrequently used drugs.

This book was set in Minion Pro by Cenveo® Publisher Services.
The editors were Michael Weitz and Peter J. Boyle.
The production supervisor was Richard Ruzycka.
Project management was provided by Sarika Gupta, Cenveo Publisher Services.
The cover designer was W2 Design.

This book is printed on acid-free paper.

Cataloging-in-publication data for this book is on file at the Library of Congress.

McGraw-Hill Education books are available at special quantity discounts to use as premiums and sales promotions, or for use in corporate training programs. To contact a representative, please visit the Contact Us pages at www.mhprofessional.com.

Contents

Preface

According to the Patient-Centered Primary Care Collaborative, medications are involved in approximately 80% of all treatments and impact *every* aspect of a patient's life. Understanding how the effects of drugs may influence the outcome measures and interventions provided by physical therapists provided the impetus for the first edition of this textbook more than 10 years ago. For example, therapists perform comprehensive assessments of the visual, vestibular, and proprioceptive inputs that control balance to predict an individual's risk of falling. However, this prediction will fall short if the therapist fails to inquire what medications the patient is taking, as many medications—both prescription and over-the-counter—negatively affect balance.

The goal of this book is to provide a comprehensive—yet *focused*—foundation in pharmacology to help rehabilitation professionals understand how medication use may alter the clinical presentation of our patients as well as their responses to therapeutic interventions. In this second edition, two licensed physical therapists (Drs. Jobst and Panus) with extensive training in pharmacology worked closely with Dr. Marieke Kruidering-Hall, a pharmacologist previously involved in medical pharmacology texts.

The information follows the sequence of traditional pharmacology textbooks and integrated organ systems-based curricula. The initial section is a synopsis of the nature of drugs, basic principles of pharmacodynamics and pharmacokinetics, and an overview of the drug development and approval process in the United States. Subsequent chapters include drugs that affect the autonomic and central nervous systems; cardiovascular and pulmonary systems; and the endocrine, gastrointestinal, and musculoskeletal systems. A chemotherapeutic section includes chapters covering anti-microbial drugs, cancer chemotherapy agents, and drugs that modify the immune system.

Each chapter follows a similar outline. A *Case Study* that illustrates how the patient's medications can affect the physical therapy encounter opens the chapter, while the explanation of how the therapy might need to be adjusted closes the chapter. An introductory *Rehabilitation Focus* section highlights the importance of the drugs in the rehabilitation setting. Next, a brief synopsis of relevant pathophysiology is followed by a discussion on the drug classes. Within each drug class, common prototypes, important chemistry, relevant pharmacokinetics, and mechanism(s) of action, as well as physiologic effects, clinical uses, and potential adverse effects are presented. At the end of each chapter, the *Rehabilitation Relevance* section provides a quickly accessible bullet-pointed summary of the adverse drug reactions for the therapist working with patients using these drug classes. End-of-chapter *Questions* are provided to quiz the reader's recall and comprehension.

An accurate medical history is required to provide a correct clinical diagnosis and effective treatment regimen. An essential component of the medical history is the patient's current medication list. The drugs an individual takes have the potential to significantly influence *both* medical and functional outcomes. Rehabilitation therapists often have the privilege of spending more time with patients than other healthcare providers. This privilege comes with the responsibility of understanding patients' responses to medications, recognizing the potential for interactions between responses to medications and therapy interventions, and communicating with key members of the healthcare team and/or the patient when questions or concerns arise regarding potential adverse drug reactions and medication nonadherence. We hope this textbook will assist all healthcare professionals—especially those in physical therapy—in that process.

Acknowledgments

First, I acknowledge my sincere gratitude to Peter C. Panus. Had I not answered a specific phone call more than ten years ago, I would not have had the opportunity to co-author this textbook and work with such talented colleagues. Second, I would like to thank each of the hundreds of physical therapy students who have taught me how to be a better teacher—both in the classroom and hopefully, on the written page. A very special note of appreciation is due to Dr. Bert Katzung, whose early interest in helping me become a better writer has made a lasting impression. Finally, I would like to thank my husband, Kenneth Tovar, for his consistent encouragement. Nothing productive could have occurred without his patient love and support. To all the individuals that I have undoubtedly forgotten to mention, I express my sincere appreciation.

—*Erin E. Jobst*

I would first like to express my appreciation to McGraw-Hill for continuing to support the publication of the first and second editions of this textbook. Along with the other authors of this book, I too would like to thank Dr. Bert Katzung, who took a chance that an unknown in both pharmacology education and physical therapy would be able to develop a textbook for physical therapy education. Although not listed as authors in this edition, the input and style of both Dr. Susan B. Masters and Dr. Anthony J. Trevor are also apparent in this edition as well as the first. Finally, I would like to thank my wife, Dr. Leslie W. Panus, who supported me during the writing of this edition and helped proof the final version of these chapters.

—*Peter C. Panus*

I would like to express my gratitude to Dr. Erin Jobst and Dr. Peter Panus for inviting me to join the team. It's been my honor to serve as part of the UCSF Cellular and Molecular Pharmacology department. I am deeply grateful to my pharmacology mentors, Dr. Susan B. Masters, Dr. Anthony J. Trevor, and above all Dr. Bert G. Katzung. They shared with me their passion for pharmacology and for teaching. They inspire me every day to do my best in the classroom and in our textbooks. I thank the numerous students for their insightful questions, which pushed me to become a better educator. Finally, I thank my husband Carl T. Hall for his support and advice.

—*Marieke Kruidering-Hall*

Introduction

Pharmacology is the study of substances that interact with living systems through chemical processes, especially by binding to regulatory molecules and activating or inhibiting normal body processes. In this book, these substances will usually be referred to as *drugs*. Medical pharmacology, or pharmacotherapeutics, is the use of drugs to achieve a beneficial therapeutic effect on some process within the patient or to promote toxic effects on the regulatory processes in organisms that are infecting the patient. Pharmacotherapeutics may be further subdivided into pharmacodynamics and pharmacokinetics. Pharmacodynamics (Chapter 2) evaluates the effect of the substance on biologic processes—or, the "effect of the *drug* on the *body*." Pharmacokinetics (Chapter 3) examines the absorption, distribution, and elimination of substances—or, the "effect of the *body* on the *drug*." Toxicology is the branch of pharmacology that deals with the undesirable effects of chemicals on individual cells and humans (medical toxicology) all the way up to their negative effects on complex ecosystems (environmental toxicology).

Humans have been using substances for their medicinal value throughout history. The earliest written records from China and Egypt list many remedies derived from plants and animals, including a few still recognized today as useful drugs. Most, however, were of limited clinical value or were actually harmful. Near the end of the 17th century, observation and experimentation began to replace theorizing in physiology and medicine. In the late 18th and early 19th centuries, experimental animal physiology and advances in chemistry further increased understanding of how chemical substances had their effects at the organ and tissue levels. Eventually, these discoveries led to the concept of drug selectivity in which a drug's action is related to its structure because of how it *specifically* binds to

a receptor. Also recognized at this time was that drugs could be grouped together into pharmacologic classes based on their chemical structure or physiologic effect. About 60 years ago, a major expansion of research efforts in all areas of biology began. This expansion coincided with the systematic development of controlled clinical trials that allow accurate evaluation of the therapeutic value of drugs. As new concepts and techniques have been introduced, information has accumulated about the action of drugs on their specific receptors. Many fundamentally new classes of drugs as well as new members of old classes have been introduced. Though still in its infancy, the field of pharmacogenomics will likely herald a new era of pharmaceutical intervention in which the knowledge of an individual's response to drugs based on his or her genes will enable tailoring of medications and dosages to allow more effective medications with ever-safer profiles.

The extension of scientific principles into everyday pharmacotherapeutics is still ongoing. Unfortunately, the drug-consuming public is also exposed to vast amounts of inaccurate, incomplete, or unscientific information regarding the pharmacologic effects of drugs. This has resulted in the faddish use of innumerable expensive, ineffective, and sometimes harmful remedies and the growth of a huge "alternative healthcare" industry. A lack of understanding of basic scientific principles, the investigative process, and statistics has led to rejection of medical pharmacology by a segment of the public, and a common tendency to assume that all adverse drug effects are the result of malpractice. Two general principles should form the basis of understanding for the evidence-based use of drugs. First, *all* substances may, under certain circumstances, be toxic. Second, *all* therapies promoted as health enhancing should meet the same standards of evidence of efficacy and safety. There should be no artificial separation between evidence-based medicine and "alternative" or "complementary" medicine.

To learn every pertinent fact about every drug would be impractical for the physical therapist. Fortunately, this is also unnecessary because almost all of the several thousand drugs currently available may be arranged in about 70 pharmacologic classes. Many of the drugs within each class are very similar in pharmacodynamic actions and often in their pharmacokinetic properties as well. For most pharmacologic classes, one or more prototypic drugs may be identified that typify the key characteristics of the class. This permits classification of other important drugs in the class as variants of the prototype, so that only the prototype must be learned in detail; for the remaining drugs, only the differences from the prototype need to be learned.

THE NATURE OF DRUGS

In the most general sense, a drug may be defined as any substance that brings about a change in biologic processes through its chemical actions. Commonly used drugs include inorganic ions, nonpeptide organic molecules, small peptides and proteins, nucleic acids, lipids, and carbohydrates. Although proteins (eg, insulin) have been used as drugs for decades, recently the term "biologicals" has come to represent proteins that are commercially produced in prokaryotic or eukaryotic cell lines using recombinant DNA technology (eg, recombinant human insulin, or rh insulin). Poisons have almost exclusively detrimental effects, but they may also be used clinically as drugs. For example, foxglove (*Digitalis purpurea*) is a plant found in many flower gardens that is considered toxic when consumed. However, an extract from the leaves of the plant yields digoxin, a therapeutic cardiac glycoside (Chapter 9). Toxins are usually defined as poisons of biologic origin that are synthesized by plants or animals. Rarely, toxins may also be used as drugs. The most obvious example is botulinum toxin. Botulinum toxin is a potent exotoxin produced by the bacterium *Clostridium botulinum* as a result of inappropriate food canning for preservation. Now, botulinum toxin is used clinically for many conditions as a selectively injected skeletal muscle relaxant. Finally, though not traditionally thought of as drugs, pieces of genetic material can be manipulated to alter intracellular targets. The discovery that small segments of RNA may selectively interfere with protein synthesis has led to the clinical application of small interfering RNAs (siRNAs) and microRNAs (miRNAs). Similarly, short nucleotide chains called antisense oligonucleotides that are complementary to RNA or DNA can interfere with gene expression and RNA transcription.

A drug is often administered at a location distant from its intended site of action. For example, a tablet or capsule is taken orally to relieve a headache. Therefore, a clinically applicable drug must have the necessary properties to be transported from its site of administration to its site of action. The drug should also be inactivated or excreted from the body at a reasonable rate so that its actions will be of a desired duration. In the majority of cases, the drug interacts with a specific molecule called a receptor that plays a regulatory role. In order to interact chemically with its receptor, a drug molecule must have the appropriate size, electrical charge, shape, and atomic composition.

At room temperature, a drug may be a solid, liquid, or gas. These physical factors often determine the best route of administration. Many drugs are weak acids or weak bases. Drugs vary in size from a small ion (eg, lithium cation) to a large protein (eg, tissue-plasminogen activator). In order to have a good "fit" to only one type of receptor, a drug molecule must be sufficiently unique in shape and charge and other physical properties to prevent binding to other receptors. In contrast, drugs that are too large will not diffuse readily between compartments of the body.

Rational Drug Design

Rational design of drugs implies the ability to predict and then construct the appropriate molecular structure of a drug on the basis of information about its biologic receptor. Until recently, no receptor was known in sufficient detail to permit such drug design. Instead, drugs were developed through random testing of chemicals or modification of drugs already known to have some effect. However, during the past three decades, many receptors have been isolated and characterized. A few drugs now in use were developed through molecular design based on knowledge of the three-dimensional structure of the receptor site. As more receptor structures are systematically identified, rational drug design will become more frequent.

NEW DRUG DEVELOPMENT

Preclinical Development

By federal law, the safety and efficacy of drugs must be determined *before* they are marketed in the United States. The development of new drugs is a multistep process requiring molecular, cellular, animal, and human clinical trials prior to governmental approval and marketing (Figure 1-1). New drugs may be developed in different ways. They may be developed through investigation of chemical structure or biologic mechanisms, or based on the actions of known drugs. Alternatively, drugs may be developed from screening a large number of biologically derived or synthesized substances. Regardless of the source or the key idea leading to a candidate drug molecule, testing a new drug involves a sequence of experimentation and characterization called drug screening. A variety of biologic assays at the molecular, cellular, organ, and whole animal levels are used to define the activity and selectivity of the drug. The molecule is studied for a broad array of actions to establish its mechanism of action and selectivity. These assays, especially at the whole animal level, may demonstrate unsuspected toxic effects and occasionally disclose a previously unsuspected therapeutic action. Research efforts may result in a candidate molecule, called a lead compound, which is then investigated further. At this juncture, the company or university that performed the preclinical

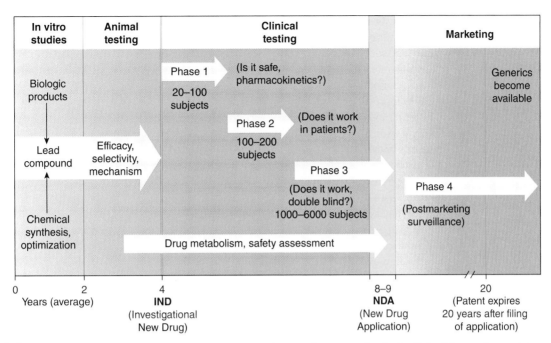

FIGURE 1-1 **The development and testing process required to bring a drug to market in the United States.** Some of the requirements may be different for drugs used in life-threatening diseases.

research may file a patent application for an effective novel compound or for a new and nonobvious therapeutic use for a previously known drug.

As part of the preclinical investigative process, lead compounds are evaluated for clinical potential. Table 1-1 lists several toxicity tests conducted during this phase. The precise sequence of tests is determined following deliberation by the Food and Drug Administration (FDA) and the applying entity. The goal of these investigations is to be able to estimate the risk associated with exposure to the drug under specified conditions. It is important to realize that no drug can be certified as completely free of risk since every drug is toxic at some dosage. In addition to the safety tests shown in Table 1-1, several quantitative estimates conducted during these preclinical investigations are required and are discussed in Chapter 3.

Due to the urgent need in treating life-threatening diseases, certain drugs require less preclinical evidence of safety. For example, some anticancer or anti-infective drugs are investigated and approved on an accelerated schedule.

Clinical Evaluation in Humans

Less than one-third of the drugs that are tested in clinical trials reach the marketplace. Federal law requires that the study of new drugs in humans be conducted in accordance with stringent guidelines. The FDA is the administrative body that oversees the drug evaluation process and grants approval for marketing of new drugs in the United States. The FDA's authority to regulate drug marketing is derived from federal legislation. To receive approval by the FDA for marketing, a drug

TABLE 1-1 **Safety tests conducted in animals.**

Type of Test	Comment
Acute toxicity	Usually two species and two routes. Determine doses at which there is no toxicity and maximum tolerated dose. In some cases, determine the acute dose that is lethal in approximately 50% of animals.
Subacute toxicity	Three doses and two species with physiologic and biochemical effects examined. Duration is dependent on length of clinical use. The longer the intended clinical use, the longer the duration of testing.
Chronic toxicity	Rodent and one additional nonrodent species for ≥ 6 months. Required if clinical application for the drug is anticipated to be chronic.
Carcinogenic potential	Two-year duration and in at least two animal species. Conducted when drug is intended for prolonged clinical use.
Reproductive performance effect	To test effects on animal mating behavior, reproduction, parturition, progeny, birth defects, and postnatal development. Conducted in two species (usually one rodent and rabbits).
Mutagenic potential	Examines genetic stability and the potential for mutations in prokaryotic and eukaryotic organisms.

must be demonstrated to be "safe and efficacious" through experimental investigation. Unfortunately, "safe" means different things to the patient, the physician, and society. A complete absence of risk is impossible to demonstrate, but this fact is not well understood by the average member of the public, who assumes that any drug sold with FDA approval must be free of serious "side effects." Obviously, it is impossible to certify that a drug is absolutely safe for every person at every dosage. Experimental investigation can identify most of the hazards likely to be associated with use of a new drug and place some statistical limits on the frequency of occurrence of such events in the population under study. As a result, an operational and pragmatic definition of "safety" can usually be reached that is based on the nature and incidence of drug-associated hazards compared with the hazard of nontherapy for the target disease. However, the frequent mismatch between unrealistic expectation of "safety" and scientific determination of adverse event probability continues to be a major cause of litigation and dissatisfaction with medical care.

Clinical Trials

The new drug approval process involves a systematic series of investigations. Once a lead compound is judged ready to be studied in humans, the originating university or company files a Notice of Claimed Investigational Exemption for a New Drug (IND) and the FDA must approve the proposed clinical studies before any testing can occur in humans (Figure 1-1).

In phase 1, the dose-dependent effects of the drug are established in a small number (20-100) of healthy volunteers. Phase 1 trials are done to determine whether humans and animals show significantly different responses to the drug, and to establish the probable limits of the safe clinical dosage range. Note that *efficacy* cannot be determined in phase 1 because the volunteer subjects do not have the target disease for which the drug is being evaluated. Pharmacokinetic parameters (Chapter 3) are often established in phase 1.

In phase 2, the drug is administered for the first time to determine its efficacy in patients with the target disease. A small number of patients (100-200) are studied in great detail to evaluate the drug's therapeutic benefits and a broader range of its toxicities. If the drug is expected to have significant toxicities, as is often the case in cancer and anti-infective therapy, volunteer patients with the disease are used. This design is designated as a phase 1/2 study.

In phase 3, the drug is evaluated in a much larger sample size to establish safety and efficacy under conditions of its proposed use. Phase 3 clinical trials can be difficult to design and execute, and are usually very expensive because of the large numbers of patients involved and the amount of data that must be systematically collected and analyzed.

During phases 2 and 3, the clinical efficacy of the investigational new drug is typically compared to a placebo or an alternative drug (ie, current standard therapy for the clinical condition). Phase 2 trials utilize single blinding or double blinding, in which the patient or the patient and the treating physician are unaware of whether the experimental drug is being administered. In double-blind trials, a third party not involved in the experimental procedure is responsible for holding the code that identifies each drug sample; this code is only broken when all clinical data have been collected. All phase 3 clinical trials are double blind. Often, 4-6 years of clinical testing are needed to accumulate enough data. Chronic safety testing in animals is usually done concurrently with clinical trials. In all three formal phases of clinical trials, volunteers or patients must be informed of the investigational status of the drug as well as possible risks. They must be allowed to either decline or consent to participate in the research process and provide written informed consent prior to participation.

If the results from the animal and human studies meet expectations, the drug manufacturer must submit a New Drug Application (NDA)—or, for biologicals, a Biological License Application (BLA)—to the FDA prior to marketing the new drug (Figure 1-1). If the FDA approves the NDA, the drug manufacturer in conjunction with the FDA develops a "label" for the drug. This label describes the specific medical condition treated by the drug (ie, the condition for which the drug was tested in clinical trials), adverse effects of the drug, and appropriate dosages for the drug. After the drug has been approved and marketed, it may be prescribed for other medical conditions not listed on the label. Such usage is the drug's "off-label" use. In cases where an urgent need is perceived, the process of preclinical and clinical testing and FDA review may be greatly accelerated. For serious diseases, the FDA can permit extensive but controlled marketing of a new drug before phase 3 studies are completed.

Once marketing of a drug has commenced, phase 4 or postmarketing surveillance begins. This phase constitutes monitoring the safety of the new drug under actual conditions of use in large numbers of patients. While phase 4 has no fixed duration and has not been as rigidly regulated by the FDA, its importance should not be underestimated. Careful monitoring by physicians prescribing the new drug provides valuable data regarding adverse effects that occur at a low incidence rate that may not have been detected in the smaller sample sizes of the phases 1, 2, and 3 studies.

The time from the filing of a patent application to approval for marketing of a new drug can be 5 years or considerably longer. Since the lifetime of a patent is 20 years in the United States, the owner of the patent, usually a pharmaceutical company, has exclusive rights for marketing the product for only a limited time after approval of the NDA. Because the FDA review process can be lengthy, the time consumed by the review process is sometimes added to the patent life. However, the extension (up to 5 years) cannot increase the total life of the patent to more than 14 years after NDA approval. After the patent expires, any company may produce a bioequivalent that has similar content, purity, and bioavailability and market this compound as a generic drug, without paying license fees to the original patent owner. The FDA drug approval process is one of the rate-limiting factors in the time it takes for a drug to be released to the market and used by patients.

ADVERSE DRUG REACTIONS

As discussed in later chapters, all drugs interact in specific ways with living systems. In part, the specificity of these interactions dictates the range of effects on these systems. As such, some interactions result in *unintended* physiologic reactions. No drug, whether prescribed, over-the-counter, or procured in another form (eg, vitamin, herbal product, or supplement), is completely without the potential for unintended physiologic reactions. The term "side effect" is often used to indicate *any* unintended effect that a drug may have. However, some unintended reactions may go unnoticed or are not bothersome to the patient, whereas other reactions are deleterious to the patient. The latter are described as adverse drug reactions (ADRs) or adverse drug events (ADEs). Since most physical therapists are not prescribers but have more pharmacology knowledge than the typical layperson, use of the term "ADR" or "ADE" may be preferred over "side effect" for two reasons. First, physical therapists are primarily concerned with harmful unintended drug reactions that may be detrimental to rehabilitation goals. Second, preferential use of the term "ADR" or "ADE" with other healthcare professionals helps set the stage for interprofessional communication regarding patient compliance with medications and suspected ADRs that may be limiting rehabilitation progress.

Severe ADRs to marketed drugs are uncommon; life-threatening reactions probably occur in less than 2% of patients admitted to medical wards. Less dangerous toxic effects, as noted elsewhere in this book, are frequent for some pharmacologic classes. Mechanisms of these ADRs fall into two main categories. The first category is often an extension of known pharmacologic effects and thus is predictable. Predictable toxicities are generally discovered during phases 1 through 3 of testing. The second category, which might be immunologic in origin or of unknown mechanism, is frequently unexpected and often not recognized until a drug has been marketed for some years. These toxicities are therefore usually discovered after marketing (phase 4). Thus, healthcare professionals should be aware of the various types of allergic reactions to drugs.

CHAPTER 1 QUESTIONS

1. Which of the following describes the undesirable effects of chemicals on living systems?

    a. Toxicology
    b. Pharmacology
    c. Pharmacodynamics
    d. Pharmacokinetics

2. Which of the following is a chemical that is synthesized by a plant or animal and is also detrimental to biologic processes?

    a. Toxin
    b. Poison
    c. Drug
    d. Biological

3. Which of the following federal agencies oversees drug evaluation and marketing in the United States?

    a. Drug Enforcement Agency (DEA)
    b. National Institutes of Health (NIH)
    c. United States Department of Agriculture (USDA)
    d. Food and Drug Administration (FDA)

4. Which of the following must be filed prior to clinical human studies?

    a. New Drug Application (NDA)
    b. Investigation Exemption for a New Drug (IND)
    c. Label of Research (LOR)
    d. Program Project Grant (PPG)

5. The process of applying for marketing approval for a new drug is an NDA.

    a. True
    b. False

6. What is the maximum lifetime of a patent on a drug in the United States?

    a. 4 years
    b. 10 years
    c. 15 years
    d. 20 years

7. Which clinical research phase involves the largest number of human research subjects and is double blinded?

    a. Phase 1
    b. Phase 2
    c. Phase 3
    d. Phase 4

8. Once a drug receives an NDA, the manufacturer is not required to continue monitor the drug for safety.

    a. True
    b. False

9. If a drug is expected to have significant toxicity, phases 1 and 2 may be combined.

    a. True
    b. False

10. Which of the following identifies the clinical use of a drug other than what the FDA provided the NDA for?

    a. Label
    b. Off-label
    c. Prescription
    d. Tag

Pharmacodynamics

REHABILITATION FOCUS

It is estimated that medications are involved in up to 80% of all treatments and impact every aspect of a patient's life. As a result, physical therapists must recognize that drugs may alter a patient's clinical presentation, which at times may require that physical therapy interventions be modified. Knowledge of drug classes and their mechanisms of actions is key to understanding patients' responses to medications. The beneficial clinical effects of drugs occur within specific concentration ranges. These ranges are unique to the different pharmacologic classes of drugs and, for some drugs, unique to the specific individual. Concentrations *below* the effective range provide no therapeutic benefit, while concentrations *above* the range almost always result in adverse drug reactions (ADRs). As discussed in the Chapter 3, the goal of dosing regimens is to utilize knowledge of the therapeutic range for each drug to determine the frequency and dose for a specific person.

Both the therapeutic and toxic effects of the majority of drugs result from interactions with their specific molecular targets—receptors. A drug molecule is an exogenous ligand that interacts with a receptor and initiates a chain of biochemical and physiologic events leading to the drug's observed effects. Pharmacodynamics is the branch of pharmacology concerned with the interaction between drug and receptor and the subsequent results.

A drug's mechanism of action is based on whether it mimics or inhibits an endogenous ligand or has some other unrecognized effect(s). A drug may directly compete with an endogenous ligand for a specific receptor or modulate the affinity (binding strength) of the receptor for the endogenous ligand. Some drugs may permanently inactivate the receptor to which they bind or stimulate additional cellular homeostatic mechanisms, which can result in a clinical effect lasting after the drug itself is no longer present in the body.

Key principles underlying the receptor concept form the basis of understanding the actions and clinical uses of drugs. These principles also have important practical consequences for drug development. First, receptors largely determine the quantitative relationship between dose or concentration of a drug and its pharmacologic effects. The receptor's affinity for binding a drug determines the concentration of drug required to form a significant number of drug-receptor complexes. In addition, the total number of receptors may limit the maximal effect a drug may produce. Second, receptors are responsible for the *selectivity* of drug action. The molecular size, shape, and electrical charge of a drug determine whether it will bind to a particular receptor among the vast array of chemically different binding sites available within the body. Accordingly, changes in a drug's chemical structure can dramatically alter its affinity for different classes of receptors, with resulting alterations in therapeutic and toxic effects. Finally, receptor activation (by agonists) or receptor blockade (by antagonists) are the primary factors responsible for many clinical effects of drugs. Knowledge of whether a drug is an agonist, antagonist, or partial agonist makes it possible to understand the actions of a drug, an individual's physiologic responses to a drug, a drug's potential ADRs, as well as interactions with many other drugs.

DRUG-RECEPTOR BONDS

Receptors are specific molecules that drugs interact with to produce changes in cellular function, and ultimately to produce functional changes in the whole person. Most receptors are proteins. A few receptors are macromolecules such as DNA. Enzymes that are affected by drugs are also considered receptors.

In order to respond to *specific* chemical stimuli, receptors must be selective in their ligand-binding characteristics. The receptor site presents a unique three-dimensional configuration upon which the drug can bind. The complementary configuration of the drug is in part what creates the affinity of the drug for the receptor site (Figure 2-1). Drugs that bind to a limited group of receptor types may be classified as selective, whereas drugs that bind to a larger number of receptor types may be considered nonselective.

Drugs interact with receptors by means of chemical bonds. The three major types of bonds are covalent, electrostatic, and hydrophobic. Covalent bonds are strong and in many cases not reversible under biologic conditions. Electrostatic bonds are weaker, more common, and often reversible. Hydrophobic bonds are the weakest, and probably most important in the interactions of lipid-soluble drugs, and within hydrophobic "pockets" of receptors.

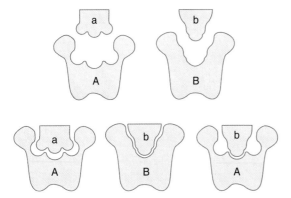

FIGURE 2-1 **Model of specificity of a drug for the receptor.** The structure of drug "a" allows binding only to receptor "A." In contrast, the structure of drug "b" allows binding to either receptor "A" or "B." Drug "a" would be considered selective to receptor "A," while drug "b" would be considered nonselective.

DOSE-RESPONSE CURVES

Graded Dose-Response Relationships

In order to initiate a sequence of cellular events that ultimately results in physiologic and clinical responses, a drug or an endogenous ligand (eg, hormone or neurotransmitter) must bind to a specific receptor. The response induced by activation of this receptor system can be measured against the concentration (dose) and displayed in a graded dose-response curve (Figure 2-2A). Plotting the data with a logarithmic dose axis usually results in a sigmoid curve, which simplifies the manipulation and interpretation of the dose-response data (Figure 2-2B).

The concentration of a drug required to achieve 50% of the maximal response is called the EC_{50}. For some ligands, the EC_{50} also estimates the drug concentration that binds 50% of available receptors. Thus, the dose-response curve relates the binding of the drug to the receptor (ie, the affinity of the drug for the receptor). A drug's efficacy is its ability to produce a measurable response, which is primarily determined by the nature of the drug and its receptor and associated effector system. The minimal effective dose is the concentration below which a drug produces no clinical benefit. At higher concentrations, the maximal efficacy of the drug (maximal effect; E_{max}) will be reached and no additional beneficial clinical response is observed.

Quantal Dose-Response Relationships

When the minimum dose required to produce an intended magnitude of response is evaluated for a *population*, a quantal dose-response relationship may be determined. When the fraction of the population that responds at each dose is plotted against the log of the dose administered, a cumulative quantal dose-response curve is obtained (Figure 2-3). From this curve, several clinically important doses can be determined. These include the median effective dose (ED_{50}) and the median toxic dose (TD_{50}). In preclinical animal studies, the median lethal dose (LD_{50}) is also calculated. Two key safety characteristics may also be determined: the therapeutic index and the therapeutic window. The therapeutic index is calculated by dividing the TD_{50} (or LD_{50}) by the ED_{50}. A very safe drug might be expected to have a very large toxic dose and a much smaller effective dose; thus, a safe drug would have a relatively high therapeutic index. Unfortunately, varying slopes for the dose-response plots sometimes make the therapeutic index a poor measure of safety. An alternative and potentially more clinically useful safety index is the therapeutic window. The therapeutic window is the dosage range between the minimum effective dose and the minimum toxic dose.

Potency

Potency is defined as the amount of drug needed to produce a given effect. Potency can be determined from either graded dose-response curves or quantal dose-response curves; however, the obtained values are not identical. In graded dose-response curves, potency is characterized by the EC_{50}

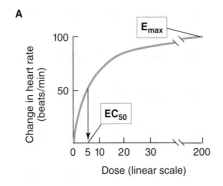

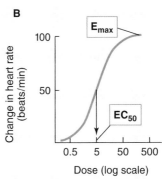

FIGURE 2-2 **Graded dose-response graphs in which drug dose or concentration is plotted against a chosen clinical effect (change in heart rate).** The EC_{50} is the dose of a drug at which the effect is half-maximal. The E_{max} is the dose of a drug at which the maximal beneficial clinical response is produced. When the dose axis is linear **(A)**, a hyperbolic curve is commonly obtained; when the dose axis is logarithmic **(B)**, a sigmoidal curve is often obtained.

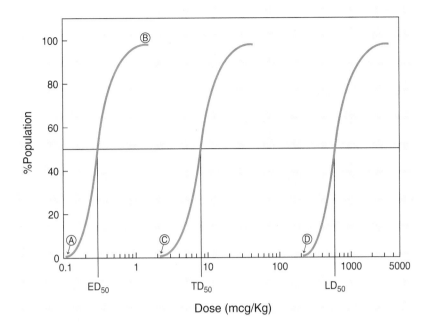

FIGURE 2-3 Quantal dose-response plot. The curves are generated from the frequency distribution of doses of a hypothetical drug required to produce a specified effect. The median effective dose (ED_{50}), median toxic dose (TD_{50}), and median lethal dose (LD_{50}) are depicted. A: minimal effective dose (MED; 0.1 mcg/kg). B: maximal effective dose (1.5 mcg/kg). C: minimal toxic dose (MTD; 2.0 mcg/kg). D: minimal lethal dose (200 mcg/kg). The therapeutic index is calculated by dividing the TD_{50} (8 mcg/kg) by the ED_{50} (0.3 mcg/kg) to obtain approximately 27. The therapeutic window is the range between the MED (A) and the MTD (C), which is 0.1-2 mcg/kg.

(Figure 2-2). The smaller the EC_{50}, the greater the potency of the drug. In quantal dose-response curves, the ED_{50}, TD_{50}, and LD_{50} measurements are identified as the potency variables (Figure 2-3).

DRUG-RECEPTOR DYNAMICS

Full Agonists, Partial Agonists, and Inverse Agonists

Figure 2-4 illustrates the modern two-state receptor theory, which considers the receptor to have at least two states: active (R_a) and inactive (R_i). In the absence of ligand, a receptor might be completely inactive or fully active. Alternatively, an equilibrium state might exist with most receptors in the inactive state and some receptors in the activated state ($R_i + R_a$). Many receptor systems exhibit some activity in the *absence* of a ligand, suggesting that some fraction of the receptor population is always in the activated state. This type of activity in the absence of ligand is called constitutive activity.

A full agonist is a drug (or endogenous ligand such as a neurotransmitter or hormone) that is capable of fully activating the effector system upon binding to the receptor. In the model system illustrated in Figure 2-4, a full agonist drug (D_a) has high affinity for the activated receptor conformation (R_a), and sufficiently high drug concentrations result in all the receptors achieving the activated state ($R_a - D_a$). In contrast, a partial agonist produces less than the full effect, even when it has saturated the receptors (R_a-D_{pa} + R_i-D_{pa}), presumably by combining with both receptor conformations,

but favoring the active state. In the presence of a full agonist, a partial agonist actually acts as an inhibitor. In this model, neutral antagonists bind with *equal* affinity to the R_i and R_a states, preventing binding by an agonist and preventing any deviation from the level of constitutive activity. In contrast, inverse agonists have a higher affinity for the inactive R_i state than for R_a and decrease or abolish any constitutive activity ($R_i - D_i$).

Full agonists demonstrate both affinity and maximal efficacy for the receptors that ultimately result in the physiologic response(s). A partial agonist binds to the receptor at the same location as the full agonist. However, the partial agonist achieves a *lower* maximal effect, even with full receptor occupancy (Figure 2-5). By definition, partial agonists have a lower maximal efficacy than full agonists, and in the presence of full agonists, they may inhibit the full agonists, decreasing their response.

A concept worth emphasizing is the distinction between a drug's potency and its efficacy. Figure 2-5 presents two full agonists (A and B) that produce equal and maximal efficacy. However, agonist B has a lower affinity for the receptor compared to A. As a result of this binding difference, agonist A is described as having a higher potency compared to B because a lower dose of A is needed to achieve the same effect. The partial agonist C demonstrates a lower maximal efficacy than either of the full agonists (A or B), yet has a higher potency than either of the full agonists. Thus, potency and efficacy are not interchangeable. In other words, one drug may have a higher potency and a lower maximal efficacy than another drug that acts at the same receptor.

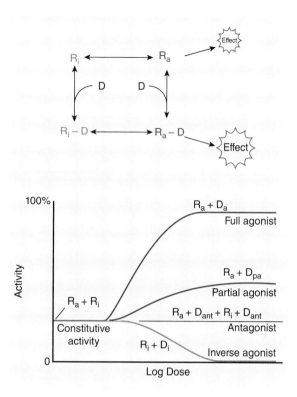

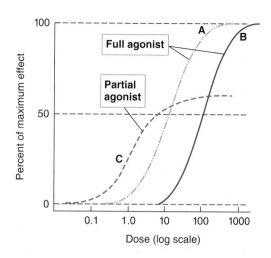

FIGURE 2-5 **Comparison of theoretical log dose-response curves for full agonists (A and B) and a partial agonist (C).** Both full agonists demonstrate the same maximal efficacy. Drug A is more potent than drug B because the EC_{50} for drug A is approximately 10, whereas the EC_{50} for drug B is approximately 100. The partial agonist demonstrates affinity and efficacy at the same receptor site as the full agonists. However, compared to the full agonists, the partial agonist produces a lower maximal effect (ie, less efficacy). The EC_{50} for partial agonist C is approximately 1. A partial agonist may be more potent (as depicted), less potent, or equally potent as the full agonist.

FIGURE 2-4 **Upper panel:** One model of drug-receptor interactions. The receptor is able to assume two conformations: R_i and R_a. In the R_i state, the receptor is inactive and produces no effect, even when combined with a drug (D) molecule. In the R_a state, the receptor activates its effectors and an effect is measured, even in the absence of drug. In the absence of a drug, the equilibrium between R_i and R_a determines the degree of constitutive activity. When D is present and binds with the R_a state of the receptor, the magnitude of the response is greater. **Lower panel:** A full agonist drug (D_a) has a much higher affinity for the R_a than for the R_i receptor conformation, and a maximal effect is produced at sufficiently high drug concentration ($R_a + D_a$). A partial agonist drug (D_{pa}) has somewhat greater affinity for the R_a than for the R_i conformation and produces less effect, even at saturating concentrations ($R_a + D_{pa}$). A neutral antagonist (D_{ant}) binds with equal affinity to both receptor conformations and prevents binding of agonist ($R_a + D_{ant} + R_i + D_{ant}$). An inverse agonist ($D_i$) binds much more avidly to the R_i receptor conformation ($R_i + D_i$), prevents conversion to the R_a state, and reduces constitutive activity.

Competitive and Noncompetitive Antagonists

Whereas full agonists demonstrate both affinity and efficacy, antagonists demonstrate affinity, but not efficacy. A competitive antagonist is a drug that binds to, or very close to, the agonist receptor site in a reversible way, but does not activate the effector system for that receptor. Competitive antagonists bind the receptor without shifting the ratio of R_a to R_i (Figure 2-4). If given in high enough concentration, the agonist can effectively displace the competitive antagonist and fully activate the receptors. In the presence of a competitive antagonist, the dose-response curve for an agonist shifts the ED_{50} to higher

doses (ie, horizontally to the right on the dose axis), but the same maximal effect (E_{max}) can still be achieved (Figure 2-6A).

In contrast, a noncompetitive antagonist causes a downward shift of the maximum response, with no shift of the curve on the dose axis. Noncompetitive antagonists bind to the agonist receptor site either covalently or with very strong electrostatic and hydrogen bonds. Once bound to the receptor, noncompetitive antagonists release slowly such that their binding may be considered irreversible or nearly irreversible. From a functional viewpoint, this may be considered noncompetitive antagonism because—unlike the situation with a competitive antagonist—the effects of a noncompetitive antagonist cannot be overcome by higher doses of the agonist. The log dose-response curve for noncompetitive antagonists results in a decrease in E_{max} and a minimal rightward shift of the ED_{50} (Figure 2-6B).

Allosteric Regulation

Some drugs bind at a different site on a receptor than that of the endogenous ligand or agonist. If a drug binds to the receptor at a different site and *potentiates* the effects of the ligand or agonist, the drug is known as an allosteric activator. If a drug binds to the receptor at a different site and *inhibits* the effects of the ligand or agonist, the drug is an allosteric inhibitor. The log dose-response curve for an allosteric inhibitor results in a minimal rightward shift of the ED_{50} and a decrease in the E_{max}. Thus, no concentration of agonist can displace the allosteric inhibitor. Figure 2-7 illustrates the effects of allosteric modulators on dose-response relationships. The allosteric activator

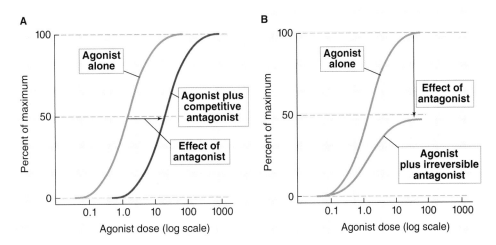

FIGURE 2-6 **Agonist dose-response curves in the presence of competitive and irreversible (noncompetitive) antagonists.** Note the use of a logarithmic scale for drug concentration. **(A)** The effect of a competitive antagonist is illustrated by the shift of the agonist curve to the right, increasing the ED_{50} for the agonist in the presence of the competitive antagonist. There is no decrease in the maximal response for the agonist (E_{max}). **(B)** An irreversible antagonist shifts the agonist curve downward, decreasing the E_{max} of the agonist. There is little to no shift to the right for the ED_{50}.

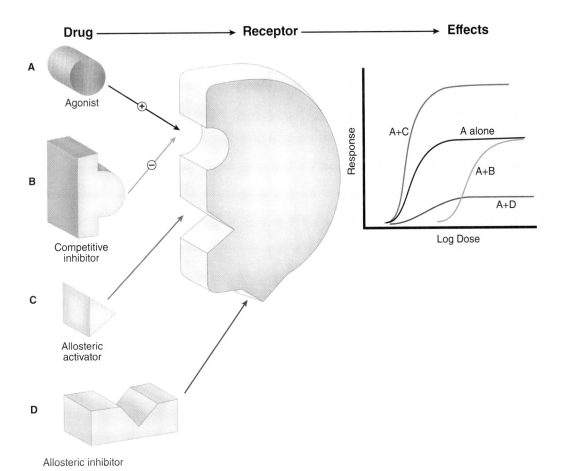

FIGURE 2-7 **Potential mechanisms of drug interaction with a receptor.** Possible effects resulting from these interactions are diagrammed in the dose-response curves. The traditional agonist (drug A)-receptor binding process results in the dose-response curve denoted "A alone." B is an antagonist that competes with the agonist for binding to the same receptor site. The dose-response curve produced by increasing doses of agonist A in the presence of a fixed concentration of competitive antagonist B is indicated by the curve "A + B." Drugs C and D act at different sites on the receptor molecule; they are *allosteric* activators or inhibitors. Allosteric activators and inhibitors can bind reversibly or irreversibly but they do not compete with the agonist for binding to the receptor site.

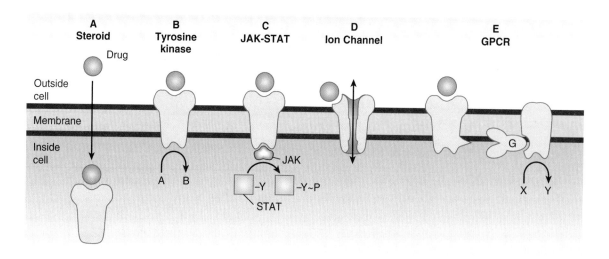

FIGURE 2-8 Signaling mechanisms for drug effects. Five major transmembrane signaling mechanisms: **(A)** transmembrane diffusion of the drug to bind to an intracellular receptor; **(B)** transmembrane enzyme receptors, whose outer domain provides the receptor function and inner domain provides the effector mechanism converting A to B; **(C)** transmembrane receptors that, after activation by an appropriate ligand, activate separate cytoplasmic tyrosine kinase molecules (Janus kinases, JAKs), which phosphorylate signal transducer and activator of transcription (STAT) proteins that regulate transcription (Y, tyrosine; P, phosphate); **(D)** transmembrane channels that are gated open or closed by binding of a drug to the receptor site; **(E)** G protein-coupled receptors (GPCR) that use a coupling protein to activate a separate effector molecule.

increases the response of the agonist (Figure 2-7, A + C), shifting the curve to the left. In contrast, the allosteric inhibitor decreases the agonist maximal response (E_{max}) with minimal rightward shift for the ED_{50} (Figure 2-7, A + D). Note the similarity in the dose-response curves between the allosteric inhibitor (Figure 2-7, A + D) and the irreversible antagonist (Figure 2-6B), even though the mechanisms of action are different. That is, an increase in agonist concentration will not reverse the inhibitory effects of an allosteric inhibitor or of an irreversible antagonist.

Physiologic and Chemical Antagonism

Antagonism is not restricted to an antagonist binding to the same receptor as the agonist. Physiologic antagonism may occur by one drug binding to a receptor that produces an effect opposite to that of a different drug binding at a different receptor. A classic example of physiologic antagonism is a drug that stimulates the parasympathetic nervous system, which antagonizes a drug that activates the sympathetic nervous system. Chemical antagonism is not receptor dependent. In this case, an antagonist interacts with another drug to remove it or prevent it from binding to the target receptor. An example of chemical antagonism is the binding of protamine sulfate to heparin to form a stable complex that is devoid of activity. This chemical antagonism is clinically utilized to rapidly reverse the anticoagulant effects of heparin (Chapter 11).

SIGNALING MECHANISMS

After an agonist binds to the receptor, some effector mechanism produces the cellular change that ultimately accomplishes a biologic effect. The receptor-effector system may be in the intracellular space, extracellular space, or across the plasma membrane. Most drug-receptor interactions involve signaling across the plasma membrane such that the agonist binds to a site on the receptor's extracellular surface, which then activates the effector mechanism inside the cell to initiate a series of intracellular changes.

Figure 2-8 shows five well-characterized mechanisms of transmembrane signaling. Each uses a different strategy to circumvent the barrier posed by the lipid bilayer of the plasma membrane. Each receptor type is made up of distinctive protein families with a specific mechanism to transduce one or many different signals. These protein families include receptors on the cell surface and within the cell, as well as enzymes and other components that generate, amplify, coordinate, and terminate postreceptor signaling within the cell.

Intracellular Receptors

Intracellular receptors bind to lipid-soluble agonists that are able to cross the phospholipid bilayer plasma membrane (Figure 2-8A). A classic example of an agent that activates intracellular receptors is the gas nitric oxide (NO). Whether endogenously released by the endothelial lining of blood vessels or liberated by a drug, NO diffuses across the plasma membrane of the endothelial cells and into smooth muscle cells to stimulate the intracellular enzyme guanylate cyclase, which produces cyclic guanosine monophosphate (cGMP), a second messenger.

Other endogenous agonists that act on intracellular receptors include the steroid hormones derived from cholesterol (adrenocorticosteroids, gonadal hormones, and vitamin D) and thyroid hormones. When these agonists bind to their intracellular receptors, the drug-receptor complex is often translocated to the nucleus to subsequently stimulate gene transcription. Because this mechanism of action involves regulating gene expression, two therapeutically important consequences should be highlighted. First, these hormones produce their effects after a characteristic lag period of 30 minutes to several hours, the timeframe required for synthesizing new proteins. Thus, therapeutically administered steroid and thyroid hormones cannot be expected to alter a pathologic state within minutes. Second, the physiologic effect from stimulation of these intracellular receptors may persist for hours or days *after* the plasma agonist concentration has been reduced to zero. The persistence of the effect is primarily due to the relatively slow turnover of most enzymes and proteins, which can remain active in cells for hours or days after they have been synthesized. Consequently, this means that the beneficial (or toxic) effects of a gene-activated system will usually decrease slowly following termination of the administered drug that stimulated the process.

Receptors on Transmembrane Proteins

Some transmembrane receptors have intracellular enzymatic activity that is allosterically regulated when an agonist binds to a site on the receptor's extracellular domain (Figure 2-8B and C). These membrane-spanning receptors consist of an extracellular binding domain and a cytoplasmic domain that may have enzymatic activity directly linked to the receptor, or a separate enzyme molecule associated with the cytoplasmic domain. These receptors include those that mediate the first steps in signaling by insulin, various growth factors (interleukin 6, interferon), and trophic hormones. For example, when insulin binds to the extracellular domain, the receptor changes its conformation, bringing together the intracellular kinase domains of two adjacent receptors that become enzymatically active and phosphorylate additional downstream signaling proteins. Activated receptors catalyze phosphorylation of tyrosine residues on different target signaling proteins, thereby allowing a single type of activated receptor to modulate a number of biochemical processes.

Receptors on Transmembrane Ion Channels

Many useful drugs act by mimicking or blocking the actions of endogenous agents that regulate the flow of ions through plasma membrane channels (Figure 2-8D). Receptors for the neurotransmitters acetylcholine, serotonin, gamma-aminobutyric acid, glycine, aspartate, and glutamate transmit their signals across the plasma membrane by increasing transmembrane conductance of the relevant ion (usually sodium, potassium, calcium, or chloride) and thereby altering the membrane potential. The ion channel opened by activation of the receptor-ion channel complex eventually closes, terminating the event. The effect lasts only as long as the drug occupies the receptor, so that dissociation of drug from the receptor automatically terminates the effect.

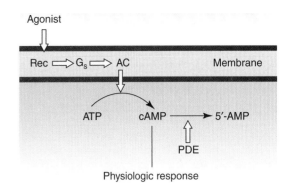

FIGURE 2-9 **The cyclic adenosine monophosphate (cAMP) second messenger pathway.** Key proteins include hormone receptors (Rec), a stimulatory G protein (G_s), catalytic adenylate cyclase (AC), and phosphodiesterases (PDE) that hydrolyze cAMP. Hydrolysis of cAMP terminates the activity of the second messenger.

G Protein-Coupled Receptors

Many extracellular ligands act by increasing the intracellular concentrations of second messengers such as cyclic adenosine monophosphate (cAMP), calcium ion, or the phosphoinositides (Figure 2-8E). In most cases, the transmembrane signaling system has three separate components. First, the extracellular ligand binds to a specific cell-surface receptor. Next, receptor binding triggers the activation of a G protein located on the cytoplasmic face of the plasma membrane. The activated G protein then changes the activity of an effector element, usually an enzyme or ion channel. This last effector then changes the concentration of the intracellular second messenger.

Termination of drug action in G protein-coupled receptor (GPCR) systems often involves the inactivation of the second messenger (as exemplified by cAMP) by a phosphodiesterase (Figure 2-9). For example, when norepinephrine and epinephrine act on G protein-coupled β-adrenergic receptors in the heart, one effect is increased heart rate. Caffeine, a universally common drug, increases heart rate. One mechanism by which caffeine increases heart rate is by inhibiting the phosphodiesterase that inactivates cAMP. Thus, caffeine does not increase heart rate by directly interacting with the extracellular domain of β-adrenergic receptors, but rather by modulating the activity of the downstream effector system to increase the duration of cAMP's actions.

RECEPTOR REGULATION

The number of receptors present in a biologic system and available for interaction with a drug is not constant. That is, the actual number of receptors available for binding the agonist varies, as does the ability of the receptor to initiate a signal as a result of the agonist binding. The variables responsible for this receptor regulation include repeated short-term or long-term activation of the receptors and other variations in the homeostasis of the cell. Changes can occur over a short duration (minutes) and a longer duration (days). Pharmacologic therapy can cause changes in receptor regulation that may have significant effects.

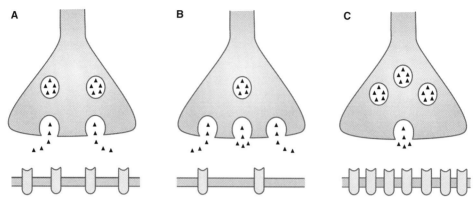

FIGURE 2-10 A generic synapse with neurotransmitter receptors located on the postsynaptic membrane under three conditions: **A**, normal number of receptors; **B**, decreased number of receptors (downregulation); **C**, increased number of receptors (upregulation). Downregulation may result from increased neurotransmitter release from the presynaptic terminal and stimulation of the receptors by an agonist over hours or days. Upregulation may result from chronic blockade of receptors by a competitive antagonist or diminished stimulation of the receptor for a similar period.

Downregulation

Frequent or continuous receptor stimulation often results in short-term diminution of the receptor response, sometimes called tachyphylaxis. Several mechanisms are responsible for this phenomenon. First, an intracellular molecule may block access of a G protein to the activated receptor molecule. Alternatively, receptors may be internalized by endocytosis after repeated stimulation, removing them from the pool of receptors available for stimulation. Finally, repetitive frequent stimulation may result in loss of some essential substrate required for intracellular downstream effects.

Long-term changes in the number of receptors or their responsiveness to stimulation involve different mechanisms (Figure 2-10). Downregulation is a decrease in the number of receptors available for binding by the agonist (Figure 2-10B). Downregulation results from exposure of the receptors to an agonist for periods of hours to days. Downregulation occurs slowly and is usually the result of degradation of receptors exceeding synthesis of new receptors. Both tachyphylaxis and downregulation can result in a decrease in the maximal response when an agonist stimulates the receptors. A likely familiar clinical example of tachyphylaxis is the rebound congestion that occurs after several days of using intranasal decongestants (such as oxymetazoline). This response is thought to be due to downregulation of α-adrenergic receptors and desensitization of the response.

Upregulation

Upregulation is an *increase* in the number of receptors available for binding and stimulation (Figure 2-10C). Prolonged lack of receptor stimulation or chronic blockade of receptors might decrease the rate of receptor degradation; if the rate of receptor synthesis is maintained, the result is a net increase in the total number of receptors available for stimulation. Due to the increase in the total number of receptors available in an upregulated system, stimulation may result in an enhanced maximal response. A clinically relevant example would be the chronic use of β-receptor antagonists, which results in upregulation of β receptors on the heart (Chapter 6).

CHAPTER 2 QUESTIONS

1. Which of the following would bind mainly to the inactive form of the receptor and decrease the constitutive activity of the receptor-mediated system?

   a. Inverse agonist
   b. Full agonist
   c. Partial agonist
   d. Neutral antagonist

2. Four drugs bind to the same receptor. The drug and dose for each drug that produces a 50% maximal response is listed below. Which drug has the greatest potency?

   a. Drug A 5 mcg/kg
   b. Drug B 2 mcg/kg
   c. Drug C 6 mcg/kg
   d. Drug D 3 mcg/kg

3. Which of the following formulas represents the therapeutic index?

   a. TD_{50} divided by the LD_{50}
   b. LD_{50} divided by the TD_{50}
   c. TD_{50} divided by the ED_{50}
   d. ED_{50} divided by the LD_{50}

4. Which of the therapeutic indices below represents the safest drug based on the therapeutic index?

   a. 5
   b. 0
   c. −3
   d. 8

5. Drug A is a full agonist at a receptor. When drug B is added, the maximal response to drug A is decreased, but there is minimal change in the dosage of drug A required to generate a 50% maximal response. Drug B binds at a different site at the same receptor for drug A. Which of the following is drug B?

   a. Allosteric inhibitor
   b. Partial agonist
   c. Competitive antagonist
   d. Irreversible antagonist

6. A drug binds to a receptor, causing the intracellular formation of cyclic adenosine monophosphate (cAMP) by the enzyme adenylate cyclase. This system is which of the following?

   a. Intracellular receptor
   b. G protein-coupled receptor
   c. Tyrosine kinase–mediated receptor
   d. Ligand-gated ion channel receptor

7. Which of the following phenomena is an increase in the number of receptors after long-term blockade by an antagonist?

   a. Tachyphylaxis
   b. Downregulation
   c. Upregulation
   d. Bradyphylaxis

8. Drug A binds to both the active and inactive forms of the receptor, favoring the active form of the receptor. What type of drug is drug A?

   a. Full agonist
   b. Competitive antagonist
   c. Allosteric inhibitor
   d. Partial agonist

9. Drug A stimulated the sympathetic nervous system. Drug B counters the effects of drug A by stimulating the parasympathetic nervous system. Which of the following processes does this represent?

   a. Physiologic antagonism
   b. Chemical antagonism
   c. Competitive antagonism
   d. Allosteric inhibition

10. Drug A binds to a receptor causing an influx of sodium ions into a cell. Which of the following receptor types does this represent?

    a. Intracellular receptor
    b. Ligand-gated ion channel
    c. G protein-coupled receptor
    d. Tyrosine kinase–mediated receptor

Pharmacokinetics and Pharmacogenomics

REHABILITATION FOCUS

Pharmacokinetics is the branch of pharmacology that is concerned with the effects of the body on both endogenous ligands and drugs. Almost all drugs (except those delivered directly to the target tissue where the proposed receptors are located) are absorbed from the site of administration and transported by the circulation to various tissues before they arrive at the target tissue. At the same time, chemical reactions in the tissues attempt to convert drugs into forms that allow for easier removal from the body. This sequence of actions represents the absorption, distribution, biotransformation, and elimination of drugs.

Chapter 2 defined the effective drug concentration as its concentration at the receptor site. However, the concentration of the drug in the blood is more readily measured. Except for topically applied agents, the effective drug concentration is usually proportional to its concentration in the plasma or whole blood. The plasma concentration is a function of the rate of input of the drug through absorption, distribution to the peripheral tissues (including the target tissue), and elimination from the body. These are all functions of time. If the rate of drug delivery is known, the remaining processes are well described by the pharmacokinetic parameters known as volume of distribution and clearance. Although these parameters are unique for a particular drug in a particular patient, average values in large populations can be used to predict drug concentrations. These parameters allow the calculation of loading and maintenance doses required for dosage regimens.

Dosage regimens depend on the pharmacodynamics (Chapter 2) and pharmacokinetics of the drug (this chapter) as well as an individual's specific comorbidities. While general guidelines for dosing regimens are available, certain comorbidities will affect drug clearance, or the rate at which active drug is removed from the body. Decreased clearance will increase how long the drug stays in the body and thus how long its effects—beneficial and adverse—will last. Renal disease or reduced cardiac output often decrease the clearance of drugs that depend on renal function. Altered clearance by liver disease is less common but can occur, especially if hepatic biotransformation of the drug is reduced. When liver blood flow is reduced, such as in heart failure, clearance for drugs that are extensively cleared from the blood by the liver also decreases. When clearance of a drug is reduced by such conditions, the dose (specific amount of medication taken at one time) and possibly the dosage (frequency of doses over a specific period of time) must be modified appropriately. During an episode of care, physical therapists often become aware of a patient's new or progressive comorbidities as well as potential drug interactions. It is important for therapists to initiate and participate in discussion with other (prescribing) healthcare professionals to determine whether these factors may affect the dosing regimen and the rehabilitation treatment program for the patient. Ongoing interprofessional communication can improve dosing regimens by providing the prescriber a clearer picture of how the medication is altering the patient's clinical presentation. In addition, clear communication between patients and healthcare providers can improve medication adherence and potentially decrease the risk and frequency of adverse drug reactions (ADRs).

PHYSICAL AND CHEMICAL NATURE OF DRUGS

Currently available drugs include inorganic ions, nonpeptide organic molecules, small peptides and proteins, nucleic acids, lipids, and carbohydrates. The majority of drugs have molecular weights between 100 and 1000, though some may be as small as molecular weight (MW) 7 for lithium to over MW 50,000 for thrombolytic enzymes. Drugs are often found in or derived from plants or animals, but many are partially or completely synthetic. Although it is a popular misconception that natural drugs or herbs are safer than synthesized drugs, the safety of a drug is based on its pharmacodynamic and pharmacokinetic properties, *not* its source.

Aqueous and Lipid Solubility

An important property of a drug is its solubility in various components of the body. For simplicity, the body can be considered to have aqueous compartments (extracellular and intracellular environments) and lipid compartments (lipid bilayer of all cell membranes). The aqueous solubility of a drug often depends on the degree of ionization or polarity of the molecule. Water molecules behave as dipoles and are attracted to charged molecules, forming an aqueous shell around them. Conversely, the lipid solubility of a molecule is inversely proportional to its charge.

Many drugs are weak bases or weak acids. For such molecules, the pH of the medium determines the fraction of ionized versus nonionized molecules. If the pKa (acid dissociation constant) of the drug and the pH of the medium are known, the fraction of molecules in the ionized state can be predicted from the Henderson-Hasselbalch equation (Equation [1]):

$$\text{Log (Protonated form/Unprotonated form)} = pK_a - pH \quad (1)$$

In Equation (1), "protonated" means associated with a proton (H^+). This equation applies to both acids and bases. Weak bases are ionized and, therefore, more polar and more water soluble when they are protonated. In contrast, weak acids are not ionized when they are protonated, and so are less water soluble. Equations (2) and (3) summarize these points for weak bases and weak acids:

$$\text{Weak base} \quad RNH_3^+ \quad \Leftrightarrow \quad RNH_2 + H^+ \quad (2)$$
$$\text{(Protonated)} \qquad \text{(Unprotonated)}$$

$$\text{Weak acid} \quad RCOOH \quad \Leftrightarrow \quad RCOO^- + H^+ \quad (3)$$
$$\text{(Protonated)} \qquad \text{(Unprotonated)}$$

The Henderson-Hasselbalch relationship is clinically important when it is necessary to estimate or alter the partition of drugs between compartments of differing pH. For example, most drugs are freely filtered at the glomeruli, but lipid-soluble drugs can be rapidly reabsorbed from the tubular urine. If a person takes an overdose of a drug that is a weak acid (eg, aspirin), the excretion of this drug is faster in alkaline urine. This is because a drug that is a weak acid dissociates to its charged, polar form in alkaline solution, and this form cannot readily diffuse from the renal tubule back into the blood. Therefore, the drug stays trapped in the tubule and is excreted into the urine. Conversely, excretion of a weak base (eg, pyrimethamine) is faster in acidic urine (Figure 3-1).

ROUTES OF ADMINISTRATION AND ABSORPTION

When drugs enter the body at sites remote from the target tissue, they require transport by the circulation to the intended site of action. To enter the blood, a drug must be absorbed from its site of administration. Absorption, therefore, describes the entry of the drug into the body. Not all routes of administration result in similar amounts of drug reaching the systemic circulation and the target tissue. In fact, for some drugs and certain routes, the amount absorbed may be only a small fraction of the amount administered. Thus, the rate and efficiency of a drug's absorption differ depending on its route of administration. The two main routes of administration are enteral and parenteral. Enteral routes involve the gastrointestinal (GI) system whereas parenteral routes bypass the GI system. Parenteral routes of drug administration include the vasculature, musculoskeletal, pulmonary, and integumentary systems. Table 3-1 lists the common routes of drug administration and their general characteristics.

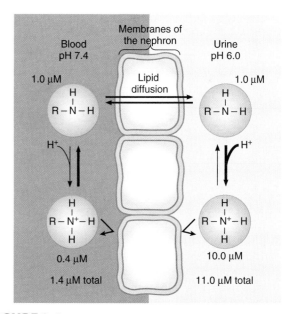

FIGURE 3-1 **Henderson-Hasselbalch principle applied to drug excretion in the urine.** Because the nonionized form diffuses readily across the lipid barriers of the nephron, this form may reach equal concentrations in the blood and urine; in contrast, the ionized form does not diffuse as readily. Protonation occurs within the blood and the urine according to the Henderson-Hasselbalch equation. Pyrimethamine, a weak base of pKa 7.0, is used in this example. In the blood at pH of 7.4, only 0.4 µmol of the protonated form is present for each 1.0 µmol of the unprotonated form. Thus, the total concentration in the blood is 1.4 µmol/L. In the urine at pH 6.0, 10 µmol of the nondiffusible ionized form will be present for each 1.0 µmol of the unprotonated, diffusible form. Therefore, the total urine concentration (11 µmol/L) may be almost 8 times higher than the blood concentration.

Enteral Administration

Enteral routes of administration include oral, sublingual or buccal, and rectal. Oral administration is defined as swallowing of the drug and absorption from the GI lumen. The majority of drugs currently prescribed are intended for oral delivery because this route offers maximum convenience and is preferred when chronic drug treatment is required. Oral absorption may be slower and less complete compared to some parenteral routes. When a drug is administered orally and absorbed from the stomach and intestine, the drug moves through the hepatic portal vein and through the liver. Enzymes within the liver may transform some percentage of the drug into an inactive form prior to entering the systemic circulation. This effect of the liver on oral administration of a drug is known as the first-pass effect (or, first-pass inactivation or metabolism), and is discussed later in the chapter. The extent of first-pass inactivation varies dramatically, depending on the drug. When first-pass effect is high, considerable fractions of these drugs are lost during absorption and the oral route is not clinically practical. All parenteral routes avoid the first-pass effect.

Sublingual administration involves placing the drug (eg, in form of a tablet, drop, or spray) under the tongue. Buccal

TABLE 3-1 Routes of administration, general characteristics, and bioavailability.

Route	Characteristics	Bioavailability (%)
Enteral		
Oral (PO)	Most convenient First-pass effect may be significant	5 to < 100
Sublingual/Buccal	Avoids first-pass effect	75 to < 100
Rectal (PR)	Less first-pass effect than oral	30 to < 100
Parenteral		
Intravenous (IV)	Most rapid onset	100 (by definition)
Intramuscular (IM)	Large volumes up to 5 mL often feasible May be painful	75 to ≤ 100
Subcutaneous (SC)	Smaller volumes than IM May be painful	75 to ≤ 100
Inhalation	Often very rapid onset	5 to < 100
Transdermal	Usually very slow absorption Prolonged duration of action	80 to ≤ 100

administration involves placing the drug into the pouch between the gums and cheek. These delivery routes are unusual in that they allow a drug to be placed in the mouth *without* a first-pass effect. These routes allow direct absorption of the drug into the systemic circulation because the veins that drain the oral mucosa go to the superior vena cava (avoiding the "first pass" through the liver). This process may be fast or slow depending on the physical formulation of the product. Several therapeutic drugs have been designed for sublingual administration, but the most familiar is nitroglycerin for relief of acute angina. In nicotine users, smokeless tobacco is placed in and absorbed directly from the buccal space.

The rectal route also offers partial avoidance of the first-pass effect, although not as completely as the sublingual or buccal routes. Rectal formulations are usually prescribed as suppositories and inserted into the lower rectum, but they tend to migrate upward into the upper rectum. Absorption from the upper rectum results in the drug undergoing the same bioavailability limitations as drugs administered orally. Larger amounts of drug and drugs with unpleasant tastes are better administered rectally than by the buccal or sublingual routes. However, some drugs administered rectally may cause significant local irritation.

Parenteral Administration

Vascular administration includes the intravenous and intra-arterial routes. The intravenous route offers instantaneous and complete absorption. This route is potentially more dangerous because of the high drug concentration reached if administration is too rapid. Intra-arterial routes are used much less frequently and are designed to administer a drug to a specific organ or tissue.

Drug absorption from an intramuscular injection site is often faster and has a higher bioavailability than oral administration. Sometimes, large volumes (eg, 5 mL into each buttock) may be administered. However, some drugs may not be administered via this route because of ADRs at the injection site. For example, parenteral anticoagulants, such as unfractionated heparin, may cause a hematoma when injected into the muscle.

Drug administration into the pulmonary system includes the intranasal and inhalation routes. This administration may be intended for either local or systemic effects. Intranasal administration of nasal decongestants is *intended* for localized effects to treat colds or rhinoconjunctivitis. Likewise, inhalation of bronchodilators and steroidal anti-inflammatory drugs is intended for localized effects in the airways of individuals with asthma or chronic obstructive pulmonary disease (COPD). However, some degree of systemic delivery may also be achieved with these routes of administration. For example, long-term use of inhaled glucocorticoids—especially when used in high doses—can result in systemic ADRs such as osteoporosis and thinning and bruising of the skin. Two intranasally administered drugs that are intended for systemic action include calcitonin and cocaine. Similarly, systemic delivery of nicotine occurs rapidly after inhaling tobacco smoke or nicotine vapor ("vaping").

The skin may also be used to administer drugs. If the intended target tissue is only the skin, then administration is described as cutaneous or topical. If the intended target tissue is deeper than the skin or the drug is applied to the skin with the intent of systemic effects, then administration is described as transdermal. In order for a drug applied to the skin to "go more than skin deep," the drug must be specifically designed for this application or a specialized delivery mode must be employed. For the former, many drugs (eg, opioids, scopolamine, sex hormones, nicotine) have been formulated to resist breakdown by enzymes within the skin and are packaged within "patches" that allows slow and prolonged drug concentration in the blood. Two transdermal delivery modes familiar to physical therapists include iontophoresis and phonophoresis. The former uses electrical current and the latter uses mechanical energy to theoretically enhance the delivery of anti-inflammatory and analgesic drugs to subcutaneous tissues. The last method of using the skin to administer drugs is subcutaneous injection. In this case, the drug is injected into the subcutaneous tissue (deepest skin layer) and is intended for systemic delivery. Insulin is the drug most commonly delivered via subcutaneous injection. For all routes of administration involving the skin, absorption is usually slow.

Intra-articular administration is utilized to achieve high concentration of a drug in the joint space to treat conditions such as arthritis or joint infection. Common drugs injected into joints include glucocorticoids, local anesthetics, opioids, and antibiotics. Viscosupplementation is an increasingly common procedure that involves injecting hyaluronic acid (artificial synovial fluid) into joints affected by osteoarthritis. Absorption of drugs from joints into the blood is usually slow and incomplete.

Other administration routes include localized delivery for the ocular or vaginal surfaces and injections into specific compartments such as the intrathecal space surrounding the spinal cord.

Several factors influence the time it takes for a drug to be absorbed from the delivery site to the drug's clinical effect. The first is blood flow to the site. High blood flow rapidly distributes the drug away from the application site and maintains a high drug depot to blood concentration gradient. The concentration of the drug at the site of administration is also important in determining the gradient between the depot and the blood (Box 3-1).

BOX 3-1 Fick's Law of Diffusion

Diffusion is a major determinant of the rate of absorption across a barrier such as the cell membrane, the epidermis, or vascular wall. Fick's law predicts that the rate of movement of molecules (diffusion rate) across a barrier is directly proportional to the concentration gradient ($C_1 - C_2$), the permeability coefficient for the molecule, and the area of diffusion; and inversely proportional to the thickness of the barrier (Equation [4]). This relationship quantifies the observation that drug absorption is faster from organs with large surface areas such as the small intestine compared to organs with smaller surface areas such as the stomach. Furthermore, drug absorption is faster from organs with thin membrane barriers such as the lung compared to those with thicker barriers such as the skin.

$$\text{Diffusion rate} = \frac{(C_1 - C_2) \times \text{Permeability coefficient} \times \text{Area}}{\text{Thickness}} \quad (4)$$

DISTRIBUTION

Most drugs must move from the site of administration to a *distant* target tissue. This movement of the drug within the body is called distribution. In order for a drug to be distributed, it must travel through barriers such as capillary walls and cell membranes. This movement within and between biologic compartments is called permeation.

Permeation

Permeation may involve several different processes including diffusion, specific transport carriers, and endocytosis along with exocytosis. Permeation of drugs by diffusion occurs in both aqueous and lipid environments. Some drugs require transport carriers or endocytosis and exocytosis to reach target tissues. In the latter case, these drugs may be too large or too lipid insoluble to otherwise reach their targets.

Diffusion

Diffusion involves the passive movement of molecules from an area of greater concentration to an area of lower concentration. The magnitude of diffusion is predicted by Fick's law (Box 3-1). Aqueous diffusion takes place through the watery extracellular and intracellular spaces. For example, the membranes of most capillaries have small water-filled pores that permit the aqueous diffusion of molecules up to the size of small proteins between the blood and the extravascular space. Lipid diffusion involves the movement of molecules through membranes and other lipid structures.

Transport Carriers

A large number of drugs are transported across barriers by carrier molecules that move similar endogenous substances. In general, these carriers are proteins that may be specific (eg, amino acid carriers in the blood-brain barrier) or they may transport a wide variety of compounds (eg, nonspecific acid and base transporters in renal tubules). Many neoplastic cells are capable of transporting out chemotherapeutic drugs via such carriers, thereby achieving considerable resistance to treatment. Fick's law does not govern carrier transport. Instead, transport is capacity limited by the number of carriers available.

Transport carriers may use several different transport mechanisms. Active transport requires the hydrolysis of adenosine triphosphate (ATP) to move a molecule *against* its diffusion gradient (from an area of lower concentration to one of higher concentration). The most common example of this mechanism is the sodium-potassium pump (Na^+/K^+ ATPase) in all animal cells used to transport sodium from the inside to the outside of a cell. In contrast, facilitated diffusion transports molecules *down* their diffusion gradient. This mechanism allows the permeation of polar molecules across lipid barriers that would otherwise occur at an extremely slow rate. Facilitated diffusion is the mechanism by which amino acids from the GI lumen are transported into epithelial cells lining the lumen.

Endocytosis and Exocytosis

Endocytosis is the process by which a molecule binds to a specialized receptor on the extracellular surface of the cell membrane and is then internalized by infolding of that area of the membrane. The contents of the resulting intracellular vesicle are subsequently released into the cytoplasm of the cell. Endocytosis permits very large molecules such as peptides or very lipid-insoluble chemicals to enter cells. A common physiological example of receptor-mediated endocytosis is that of vitamin B_{12}. Dietary vitamin B_{12} tightly binds to intrinsic factor (IF), a glycoprotein produced in the gastric epithelium. In the small intestine, a membrane protein that recognizes the IF-vitamin B_{12} complex participates in its endocytosis. Exocytosis is the reverse process; that is, the expulsion of membrane-encapsulated material from cells into the extracellular space.

Volume of Distribution

When determining the distribution of any drug, the body is assumed to represent one or more physical volumes in which the drug is sequestered, or separated by barriers. Specific variables may be used to predict these volumes of distribution.

Often, the distribution of a drug is not homogenous throughout the body, and the drug may concentrate in one or more tissues (eg, blood, fat, bone). These tissues are described as "physical compartments" and their volumes can be approximated based on an individual's weight and sex (Table 3-2). The calculated parameter for the volume of distribution (V_d) has no direct physical equivalent. Therefore, we say that drugs have an *apparent* V_d, which relates the amount of drug in the body to its plasma concentration (Equation [5]):

$$V_d = \text{Amount of drug in body/Plasma drug concentration}\quad(5)$$
$$(\text{Units} = \text{Liters or liters/kilogram})$$

Because the size of the compartments to which a drug may be distributed varies with body size, V_d is sometimes expressed as V_d per kilogram of body weight.

Determinants of V_d

Many drugs do not distribute equally in all compartments. Drug distribution to tissues varies and is dependent upon multiple variables including organ mass, blood flow, solubility of the drug, intravascular and extravascular binding, and comorbidities. The size of the organ determines the concentration gradient between blood and the organ. For example, skeletal muscle can take up a large amount of drug because the concentration in the muscle tissue remains low, and the blood to tissue gradient high. This gradient continues even after relatively large amounts of drug have been transferred because skeletal muscle is a very large organ. In contrast, because the brain is smaller, distribution of a smaller amount of drug into it will raise the tissue concentration and reduce the blood to tissue concentration gradient to zero.

Blood flow to the target tissue is an important determinant of the *rate* of uptake, although blood flow may not affect the steady-state amount of drug in the tissue. As a result, well-perfused tissues such as the brain, heart, kidneys, and splanchnic organs, will often achieve high tissue concentrations sooner than poorly perfused tissues such as fat, cartilage, and bone. If the drug is rapidly eliminated, the concentration in poorly perfused tissues may never rise significantly.

Figure 3-2 illustrates the relationship of drug solubility with respect to the vascular compartment and the extravascular compartment of the body. If the drug is highly soluble within the intracellular compartment (the largest compartment in the body), the drug will move down its concentration gradient from the extracellular compartment into the intracellular compartment. As a result, drug concentration in the perivascular extracellular compartment will be lower, facilitating diffusion from the blood vessel into the extravascular tissue compartment as the drug moves down its concentration gradient from the vascular, to the extravascular and into the intracellular compartment. Figure 3-2 also illustrates the relationship of drug binding on volume of distribution. If a drug binds to macromolecules in the blood or a tissue compartment, the drug's concentration tends to increase in that compartment. For example, warfarin is strongly bound to plasma albumin, which restricts the diffusion of warfarin out of the vascular compartment. Conversely, chloroquine is strongly bound to tissue proteins, which results in a marked reduction in the plasma concentration of chloroquine. As a result, warfarin has a low V_d, whereas chloroquine has a very high V_d (Table 3-3). Some organs, including the brain, have high lipid content and thus dissolve a high concentration of lipid-soluble drugs. As a result, some psychotropic drugs such as amitriptyline or fluoxetine will transfer out of the blood and into the brain tissue more rapidly and to a greater extent than a drug with low lipid solubility (Table 3-3).

Finally, the V_d of drugs may be altered by comorbidities. For instance, liver disease results in reduced plasma protein synthesis and kidney disease results in urinary loss of plasma proteins. Thus, the V_d of drugs that are normally bound to albumin may be increased by these comorbidities.

ELIMINATION

The duration of action for most drugs is determined by the dosage and the rate of elimination. Elimination is the disappearance of the biologically active compound from the body by metabolism (biotransformation) and/or excretion. Elimination may occur by several mechanisms. For drugs that are not metabolized, excretion is the mode of elimination. Various organs such as the kidney, skin, GI tract, or lungs may excrete the *active* compound out of the body. For most drugs, excretion is primarily by way of the kidneys. Major exceptions are anesthetic gases, which are excreted primarily by the lungs.

Metabolism (discussed later) of the drug may render it inactive. For drugs that have active metabolites, elimination of the parent molecule by biotransformation does not terminate

TABLE 3-2 **Physical volumes (in L/kg body weight) of some body compartments into which drugs may be distributed.**

Compartment and Physical Volume
Water
Total body water (0.6 L/kg[a])
Extracellular water (0.2 L/kg)
Blood (0.08 L/kg)
Plasma (0.04 L/kg)
Fat (0.2–0.35 L/kg)
Bone (0.07 L/kg)

kg, kilogram; L, liter.
[a]An average figure. Total body water in a young person might be 0.7 L/kg; in an obese person, 0.5 L/kg.

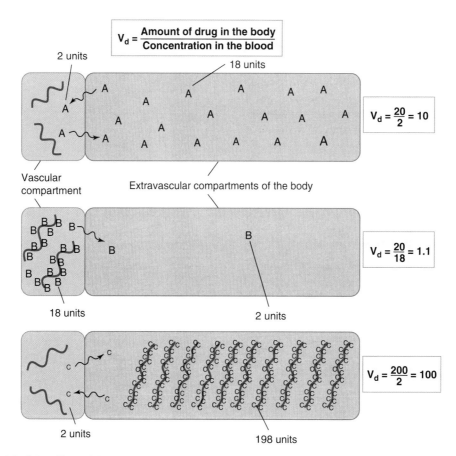

FIGURE 3-2 **Model of the effect of drug binding on the apparent volume of distribution (V_d).** Drug A diffuses freely between the two compartments and does not bind to macromolecules (heavy wavy lines) in the vascular or extravascular compartments. With 20 units of drug A in the body, the steady-state distribution leaves a blood concentration of 2 units. In contrast, drug B binds avidly to proteins in the blood. Drug B's diffusion is much more limited. At equilibrium, only 2 units of the total diffused into the extravascular volume, leaving 18 units still in the blood. In both cases, the total amount of drug in the body is the same (20 units), but the apparent V_d is very different. Drug C is avidly bound to molecules in peripheral tissues, so that a larger total dose (200 units) is required to achieve measurable plasma concentrations. At equilibrium, 198 units are found in peripheral tissues and only 2 units in the plasma, so that the apparent V_d is greater than the physical volume of the system.

TABLE 3-3 Apparent volumes of distributions (V_d) for several drugs.

Compartment and Volume[a]	Drug and V_d[a]
Plasma (0.04 L/kg)	Furosemide (0.11 L/kg), warfarin (0.14 L/kg)
Extracellular water (0.2 L/kg)	Gentamicin (0.29 L/kg), indomethacin (0.26 L/kg)
Total body water (0.6 L/kg)	Acyclovir (0.69 L/kg), lithium (0.79 L/kg)
Concentrated outside vasculature[b]	Fluoxetine (35 L/kg), chloroquine (186 L/kg)

L, liter; kg, kilogram.

[a]All volumes based on a 70-kg individual.

[b]Many drugs with high V_d are lipid-soluble and concentrate into both the central nervous system and adipose tissue. Chloroquine is the exception above, which concentrates in skeletal muscle. Although the V_d provides an indication of the concentration of the drug outside of the vasculature, it does not allow determination into which tissue the drug is being sequestered. Several drug V_d in the table represent averages from a published range.

its action because the metabolites have clinical effects. A small number of drugs combine irreversibly with their receptors, so that disappearance from the bloodstream is not equivalent to cessation of drug's action. For example, aspirin is an irreversible inhibitor of cyclooxygenase. Even after aspirin is eliminated from the blood, the receptors that were bound while the drug was circulating are still inactivated.

Clearance

Elimination of a drug is expressed as its clearance (CL). Clearance is the ratio of the rate of disappearance of the active molecule from the plasma to its plasma concentration (Equation [6]).

$$CL = \text{Rate of drug elimination/Plasma drug concentration} \quad (6)$$
$$(\text{Units} = \text{Liters per unit time})$$

Figure 3-3 graphically illustrates clearance, which is dependent upon the extraction ratio ($[C_i - C_o]/C_i$) and the blood flow (Q). The extraction ratio represents the ability of an organ to remove a drug from the perfusing blood during its passage through that organ, and is expressed as a percentage or fraction.

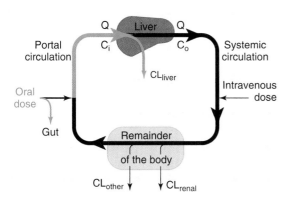

FIGURE 3-3 **The principles of organ extraction (clearance, CL) and first-pass effect.** Part of the administered oral dose (blue) is lost in the gut (in feces) and lost due to first-pass metabolism in the liver before it enters the systemic circulation. The volume of blood cleared of drug from the circulation by the liver (CL_{liver}) is proportionate to blood flow (Q) times the difference between drug concentration entering (C_i) and leaving (C_o) the liver.

As with V_d, CL is sometimes expressed as CL per kilogram body weight. There are multiple organs of clearance, and multiple mechanisms for clearing a drug from the blood. Although all tissues have some capacity to clear drugs, the major organs of clearance are the kidney, liver, lung, and GI tract. Mechanisms of clearance include extraction and binding by the tissue, metabolism of the drug to an inactive metabolite (as in the liver), or excretion of the active molecule or metabolite (as in the kidney). Following oral administration, the drug must pass through the GI mucosa and liver prior to entering the systemic circulation. A portion of the drug dose may be extracted and metabolized at these locations prior to reaching the systemic circulation (ie, first-pass effect). Drugs administered parenterally also undergo hepatic and renal clearance. After steady-state concentration in plasma has been achieved, the extraction ratio is one measure of the elimination of the drug by that organ.

The magnitudes of clearance for different drugs range from a small fraction of the blood flow to a maximum of the total blood flow to the organ of elimination. Clearance depends on the particular drug and the condition of the organs of elimination in the particular person. The clearance of a drug that is very effectively extracted by an organ is often flow limited; that is, the blood is completely cleared of the drug as it passes through the organ. For such a drug, the total clearance from the body is a function of, and is limited to, the blood flow through the eliminating organ.

Elimination Kinetics

Elimination of drugs is described as either first-order or zero-order kinetics. Most drugs in clinical use demonstrate first-order kinetics. In first-order kinetics, the rate of elimination of the drug is *proportional* to its concentration (ie, the clearance is constant). The higher the drug plasma concentration, the greater the amount of drug eliminated per unit time. The result is that the drug's concentration in the plasma decreases exponentially with time (Figure 3-4A). Drugs with first-order elimination have a characteristic half-life (discussed below) that is constant *regardless* of the amount of drug in the body. Thus, the concentration of such a drug in the blood will decrease by 50% for every half-life.

The term zero-order elimination implies that the rate of elimination is *constant* (ie, the clearance is not constant), regardless of the drug's concentration (Figure 3-4B). Zero-order elimination occurs with drugs that saturate their elimination mechanisms at clinically relevant concentrations. As a result, the concentrations of these drugs in plasma decrease in a linear (not exponential) fashion over time. Over most of its plasma concentration range, ethanol demonstrates zero-order elimination. This is why it can reasonably be predicted how long it will take for a person's blood alcohol content (BAC) to reach zero because only a fixed amount of alcohol is metabolized per hour. At high therapeutic or toxic concentrations, phenytoin and aspirin also demonstrate zero-order elimination.

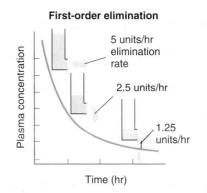

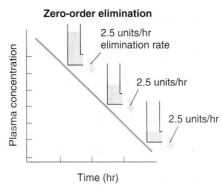

FIGURE 3-4 **Comparison of first-order and zero-order elimination.** For drugs with first-order kinetics (left), the rate of elimination is proportionate to the plasma concentration. First-order elimination is the more common process. In the case of zero-order elimination (right), the rate of elimination is constant and independent of concentration.

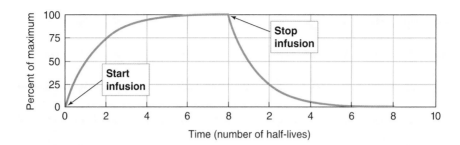

FIGURE 3-5 **Plasma concentration (plotted as percentage of maximum) of a drug given by constant intravenous infusion for 8 half-lives and then stopped.** The concentration rises smoothly with time and always reaches 50% of steady state after 1 half-life, 75% after 2 half-lives, 87.5% after 3 half-lives, and so on. The decline in plasma concentration after drug administration ceases follows the same type of curve: 50% is left after 1 half-life, 25% after 2 half-lives, and so on. The asymptotic approach to steady state on both increasing and decreasing limbs of the curve is characteristic of drugs following first-order kinetics.

Half-Life

Half-life ($t_{1/2}$) is a parameter determined by the drug's volume of distribution and clearance. Similar to clearance, half-life is a constant for drugs that follow first-order kinetics. Half-life can be determined graphically from a plot of the drug's plasma level versus time (Figure 3-5), or from the following relationship (Equation [7]):

$$t_{1/2} = 0.7 \times V_d/CL \qquad (7)$$

To predict changes in half-life, both primary variables (V_d and CL) must be known. Disease, age, and other variables usually alter the clearance of a drug much more than its volume of distribution. However, if the V_d decreases at the same time as the clearance, the half-life of a drug may not change. The half-life also determines the rate at which plasma concentration rises during a constant infusion and falls after administration is stopped (Figure 3-5). During an infusion, plasma levels of the drug generally reach a plateau and a steady-state equilibrium will be established after four to five half-lives. At steady state, the rate of administration and the rate of elimination are equal. Following the termination of the infusion, greater than 95% of the drug will be lost after five half-lives (for a drug with first-order elimination kinetics). The half-life for a drug is critical in developing pharmacokinetic models to estimate changes in drug plasma concentration over time (Box 3-2).

For clinicians, the concept of a drug's half-life is valuable for at least two reasons. First, consider a patient that discontinues a specific drug due to experiencing headaches and dizziness that were suspected ADRs. The physical therapist can use the knowledge of the drug's half-life to predict whether these symptoms are more or less likely to be attributed to the drug. For example, consider if the drug's half-life is 2 hours and the patient presented to the physical therapist 3 days after drug discontinuation. Within 10 hours (5 half-lives), 95% of the drug would have been eliminated from the body. If the patient presented to the clinic 72 hours after drug discontinuation with persistent and unchanged symptoms of headaches and dizziness, the therapist should consider other factors (eg,

BOX 3-2 Pharmacokinetic Models

The elimination of drugs from the body may be estimated based on a compartmental model. A model may be based on an assumption of equal distribution of the drug throughout all tissues with the body acting as a single compartment. Alternatively, the drug can be modeled as sequestered in two or more tissues with the body acting as multiple compartments. A few drugs may behave as if they are distributed to only one compartment, especially if they are restricted to the vascular compartment. Others have more complex distributions that require more than two compartments for construction of accurate mathematical models. After absorption into the circulation, many drugs undergo an early distribution phase followed by a slower elimination phase. Mathematically, this behavior can be modeled by means of a "two-compartment model" (Figure 3-6). Each phase is associated with a characteristic half-life: $t_{1/2\alpha}$ for the distribution phase and $t_{1/2\beta}$ for the elimination phase. When the concentration is plotted on a logarithmic axis, the elimination phase for a first-order drug is a straight line.

neuromusculoskeletal or vestibular impairments) likely contributing to the patient's symptomology in order to direct the physical examination. A second reason that the concept of a drug's half-life is advantageous to understand is to anticipate that for individuals with decreased clearance (eg, renal failure) and/or increased volume of distribution (eg, increased body fat for lipid-soluble drugs like anesthesia), drugs will have longer half-lives and thus these individuals will experience the effects of the drugs (whether beneficial or adverse) for longer.

BIOTRANSFORMATION

All organisms are exposed to foreign chemical compounds in the air, water, and food. Many tissues act as portals for entry of external molecules into the body. To ensure the elimination

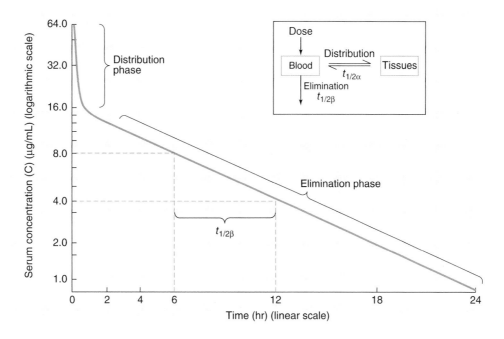

FIGURE 3-6 **Serum concentration-time curve after administration of a drug as an intravenous bolus.** This drug follows first-order kinetics and appears to occupy two compartments. Each phase is associated with a characteristic half-life ($t_{1/2}$). The initial curvilinear portion of the data represents the distribution phase and accompanying distribution half-life ($t_{1/2\alpha}$), with drug equilibrating between the blood compartment and the tissue compartment. The linear portion of the curve represents drug elimination. The elimination half-life ($t_{1/2\beta}$) can be extracted graphically as shown by measuring the time between any two plasma concentration points on the elimination phase that differ by twofold.

of pharmacologically active foreign chemicals (xenobiotics) as well as to terminate the action of many endogenous substances, metabolic pathways are available to alter their activity and increase their susceptibility to excretion. Biotransformation is the alteration of exogenous and endogenous chemical compounds by metabolic enzymes. The products of biotransformation are therefore called metabolites. Most drugs are relatively lipid soluble, a characteristic favorable to absorption and distribution across cellular plasma membranes. This same property would result in very slow removal from the body because the molecule would also be readily reabsorbed from the urine in the renal tubule. Enzymatic biotransformation hastens excretion by transforming many drugs to less lipid soluble and therefore more readily excreted forms.

Biotransformation Reactions

The liver is the primary organ for drug metabolism because it has the highest concentration of xenobiotic-metabolizing enzymes. The kidneys also play an important role in the metabolism of some drugs. A few drugs, such as esters, are metabolized in many tissues because of the broad distribution of esterases responsible for the metabolism of these molecules.

Biotransformation may be divided into phase I and phase II reactions. Phase I reactions include oxidation, reduction, deamination, and hydrolysis (Table 3-4). Many phase I reactions are mediated in part by the cytochrome P450 (abbreviated as CYP) group of enzymes, which are also called mixed-function

TABLE 3-4 **Examples of phase I drug-metabolizing reactions.**

Reaction Type	Typical Drug Substrates
Oxidations, P450 dependent	
Hydroxylation	Amphetamines, barbiturates, phenytoin, warfarin
N-dealkylation	Caffeine, morphine, theophylline
O-dealkylation	Codeine
N-oxidation	Acetaminophen, nicotine
S-oxidation	Chlorpromazine, cimetidine, thioridazine
Deamination	Amphetamine, diazepam
Oxidations, P450 independent	
Amine oxidation	Epinephrine
Dehydrogenation	Chloral hydrate, ethanol
Reductions	Chloramphenicol, clonazepam, dantrolene, naloxone
Hydrolyses	
Esters	Aspirin, clofibrate, procaine, succinylcholine
Amides	Indomethacin, lidocaine, procainamide

TABLE 3-5 Examples of phase II drug-metabolizing reactions.

Reaction Type	Typical Drug Substrates
Glucuronidation	Acetaminophen, diazepam, digoxin, morphine, sulfamethiazole
Acetylation	Clonazepam, dapsone, isoniazid, mescaline, sulfonamides
Glutathione conjugation	Ethacrynic acid, reactive phase I metabolite of acetaminophen
Glycine conjugation	Deoxycholic acid, nicotinic acid (niacin), salicylic acid
Sulfation	Acetaminophen, methyldopa
Methylation	Dopamine, epinephrine, histamine, norepinephrine, thiouracil

oxidases. There are many different families, or types, of CYP enzymes. However, approximately 75% of the drugs metabolized by phase I CYP pathways are metabolized by just two families: CYP3A4/5 or CYP2D6. Phase II reactions involve conjugation of hydrophilic subgroups to specific chemical structures (Table 3-5). These additions occur at hydroxyl (—OH), amine (—NH$_2$), and sulfhydryl (—SH) functions on the substrate molecule. The subgroups that are added include glucuronate, acetate, glutathione, glycine, sulfate, and methyl groups. Because most of these subgroups are relatively polar, their addition to the parent drug molecule increases the aqueous solubility of the metabolite, which enhances its ability to be excreted.

Determinants of Biotransformation Rate

The rate of biotransformation of a drug may vary markedly among different individuals. This variation is most often due to comorbidities, genetic differences, or drug-drug interactions. Hepatic metabolism often decreases with age and liver disease. For a few drugs, age or disease-related differences in drug metabolism are significant. Metabolism may also be decreased by pharmacodynamic factors. For example, propranolol reduces hepatic blood flow. Sex is important for only a few drugs. For instance, first-pass metabolism of ethanol is lower in women than in men. Because biotransformation rates are often the primary determinant of clearance, these rate variations in drug metabolism are a significant determinant of plasma drug levels in patients.

Genetic Factors

It has been well recognized that several drug-metabolizing systems differ among families or populations in genetically determined ways. The developing field of pharmacogenomics ties together pharmacology and genomics (the study of genes and their functions). Pharmacogenomics aims to understand how genes affect an individual's responses to drugs, with the ultimate goal of developing effective and

safe medications at doses that are specifically tailored to a person's genetic profile. Although a complete discussion of pharmacogenomics is beyond this chapter, Box 3-3 highlights key examples of the role of pharmacogenomics in clinical pharmacology.

Drug-Drug Interactions

A significant factor affecting drug metabolism is drug-drug interactions. Coadministration of certain agents may alter the disposition of many drugs. CYP enzymes can be *induced* or *inhibited* by drugs, some dietary supplements, and even some foods. Enzyme induction usually results from increased synthesis of CYP enzymes in the liver. Many isozymes (families) of the CYP family exist and inducers selectively increase subgroups of these isozymes. For example, cigarette smoking induces CYP1A2 isozymes in the liver and lung. If a smoker is concurrently taking another drug metabolized by the CYP1A2 family such as duloxetine (commonly taken for depression or neuropathic pain), the metabolism of duloxetine may be increased. Thus, the plasma concentration of duloxetine may be lower than the *intended* effective plasma concentration.

Table 3-6 is a partial list of common inducers of a few isozymes and the drugs whose metabolism is increased. Several days are usually required to reach maximum induction. Likewise, a similar amount of time is required to return the affected CYP enzymes to normal levels after withdrawal of the inducer. The most common CYP inducers involved in serious drug interactions are carbamazepine, phenobarbital, phenytoin, and rifampin. In patients comedicated with these CYP inducers, the half-life of other drugs metabolized by the same CYP isozyme may be decreased.

In contrast, some drugs inhibit their own metabolism and the metabolism of other agents. Table 3-7 lists some common enzyme inhibitors and the drugs whose metabolism is diminished. Classic CYP inhibitors involved in serious drug interactions are amiodarone, cimetidine, furanocoumarins (present in grapefruit juice), ketoconazole and related antifungal agents, and the human immunodeficiency virus (HIV) protease inhibitor ritonavir. For example, if an individual is consistently consuming grapefruit, the furanocoumarins within the fruit *inhibit* CYP3A4 isozymes in the liver. If the person is taking a statin (to lower blood cholesterol)—which is also metabolized by the CYP3A4 family of enzymes—the metabolism of the statin will be *decreased*. The plasma concentration of the statin may be higher than the *intended* effective plasma concentration and may result in an increased risk of ADRs such as statin-induced myopathy. Many medications carry the warning that consumption of grapefruit may turn a "safe dose of medicine to an overdose." This patient-friendly language is intended to translate the concern that CYP inhibition by grapefruit may effectively increase the plasma concentration of a medication by decreasing the drug's metabolism.

Last, *suicide inhibitors* are drugs that are metabolized to products that irreversibly inhibit the metabolizing enzyme.

Variations in specific genes, known as polymorphisms, may result in differences in the control or expression of molecules involved in drug pharmacokinetics. These changes may be due to single or multiple nucleotide polymorphisms.

Phase I Reactions

Of the 100 known polymorphisms for CYP2D6, currently at least 9 are clinically significant. One of these variations results in ultra-rapid conversion of codeine (a *moderate* agonist at μ-opioid receptors) to morphine (a *full* agonist at μ-opioid receptors), with subsequent deaths in children due to this enhanced conversion. The CYP2C19 gene is responsible for metabolism of a small number of significant drugs, including clopidogrel, an antiplatelet prodrug. One polymorphism for CYP2C19 results in decreased conversion of clopidogrel to the active drug, resulting in enhanced clotting risk. In contrast, another CYP2C19 polymorphism results in an increased risk of bleeding due to increased conversion of clopidogrel to the active form. The presence of multiple enzyme polymorphisms is also important. For example, individuals with a combination of reduced function polymorphisms in CYP2C9 and vitamin K epoxide reductase VKOR have an increased bleeding risk from the anticoagulant warfarin.

Phase 2 Reactions

Uridine 5'-diphospho-(UDP)-glucuronosyltransferase (UGT1A1) and thiopurine S-methyltransferase (TPMT) are enzymes involved in the clearance or inactivation of anticancer drugs. Reduced polymorphisms of UGT1A1 results in increased concentration of the metabolite of irinotecan (a drug indicated for treating metastatic colorectal cancer) and bone marrow depression. The reduced polymorphism of TPMT results in decreased activation of azathioprine (an immunosuppressant), which is a prodrug, and decreased metabolism of its active metabolites. These polymorphisms result in altered therapeutic efficacy and increased toxicity.

Transporters

The organic anion transporter (OATP) 1B1 is responsible for removing both endogenous compounds and drugs such as statins from the blood into hepatocytes. Reduced function polymorphisms in the SLCO1B1 gene that expresses OATP1B1 results in increased concentration of statins in the blood with subsequent risk for skeletal muscle myopathy.

Human Leukocyte Antigens

Finally, human leukocyte antigen (HLA) polymorphisms have been associated with increased risk for drug-associated liver injury, Stevens-Johnson syndrome, and epidermal necrolysis.

TABLE 3-6 A partial list of drugs that significantly induce CYP450-mediated drug metabolism in humans.

CYP Family Induced	Important Inducers	Drugs Whose Metabolism Is Induced
1A2	Benzo[a]pyrene (from tobacco smoke), carbamazepine, phenobarbital, rifampin, omeprazole	Acetaminophen, clozapine, haloperidol, theophylline, tricyclic antidepressants, (R)-warfarin
2C9	Barbiturates[a] (especially phenobarbital), phenytoin, primidone, rifampin	Barbiturates, celecoxib, chloramphenicol, chlorpromazine, doxorubicin, ibuprofen, phenytoin, steroids, tolbutamide, (S)-warfarin
2C19	Carbamazepine, phenobarbital, phenytoin, rifampin	Diazepam, phenytoin, topiramate, tricyclic antidepressants, (R)-warfarin
2E1	Ethanol[a], isoniazid	Acetaminophen, enflurane, ethanol (minor), halothane
3A4	Barbiturates, carbamazepine, glucocorticoids, efavirenz, phenytoin, rifampin, pioglitazone, St. John's wort	Antiarrhythmics, antidepressants, azole antifungals, benzodiazepines, calcium channel blockers, cyclosporine, delavirdine, doxorubicin, efavirenz, erythromycin, estrogens, HIV protease inhibitors, nefazodone, paclitaxel, proton pump inhibitors, rifabutin, rifampin, sildenafil, SSRIs, statins, tamoxifen, trazodone, vinca alkaloids

CYP, cytochrome P450; HIV, human immunodeficiency virus; SSRI, selective serotonin reuptake inhibitor.
[a]Some drugs, such as barbiturates and ethanol, may be both inducers and substrates for metabolism.

TABLE 3-7 **A partial list of drugs that significantly inhibit CYP450-mediated drug metabolism in humans.**

CYP Family Inhibited	Important Inhibitors	Drugs Whose Metabolism Is Inhibited
1A2	Cimetidine, fluoroquinolones, grapefruit juice, macrolides, isoniazid, zileuton	Acetaminophen, clozapine, haloperidol, theophylline, tricyclic antidepressants, (R)-warfarin
2C9	Amiodarone, chloramphenicol, cimetidine, isoniazid, metronidazole, SSRIs, zafirlukast	Barbiturates, celecoxib, chloramphenicol, chlorpromazine, doxorubicin, ibuprofen, phenytoin, steroids, tolbutamide, (S)-warfarin
2C19	Fluconazole, omeprazole, SSRIs	Diazepam, phenytoin, topiramate, (R)-warfarin
2D6	Amiodarone, cimetidine, quinidine, SSRIs	Antiarrhythmics, antidepressants, β-blockers, clozapine, flecainide, lidocaine, mexiletine, opioids
3A4	Amiodarone, azole antifungals, cimetidine, clarithromycin, cyclosporine[a], diltiazem, erythromycin, fluoroquinolones, grapefruit juice, HIV protease inhibitors[a], metronidazole, quinine, SSRIs, tacrolimus	Antiarrhythmics, antidepressants, azole antifungals, benzodiazepines, calcium channel blockers, cyclosporine, delavirdine, doxorubicin, efavirenz, erythromycin, estrogens, HIV protease inhibitors, nefazodone, paclitaxel, proton pump inhibitors, rifabutin, rifampin, sildenafil, SSRIs, statins, tamoxifen, trazodone, vinca alkaloids

CYP, cytochrome P450; HIV, human immunodeficiency virus; SSRI, selective serotonin reuptake inhibitor

[a]Some drugs, such as cyclosporine and HIV protease inhibitors, may be both inhibitors and substrates for metabolism.

Such agents include allopurinol, ethinyl estradiol, spironolactone, secobarbital, and propylthiouracil.

Drugs that Inhibit Intestinal P-Glycoprotein Transporters

The P-glycoprotein transporters comprise a family of ATP-dependent transporters that have been identified in the epithelium of the GI tract, in the blood-brain barrier, and in cancer cells. These transporter proteins decrease absorption of drugs from the GI system by transporting drugs from the intestinal mucosa back into the GI lumen (where they will be excreted in the feces).

Drugs such as verapamil and furanocoumarin inhibit intestinal P-glycoprotein transporters, resulting in increased absorption and decreased fecal excretion of several other drugs and thus increasing those drugs' plasma concentration. Important drugs normally expelled by these GI transporters include digoxin, cyclosporine, and saquinavir. Thus, P-glycoprotein inhibitors may result in toxic plasma concentrations of the latter drugs when given at normally nontoxic dosages.

Biotransformation Metabolites

Drug metabolism is not synonymous with drug inactivation. In fact, there are several biotransformation outcomes. Often, metabolism results in the production of an *inactive* metabolite. For example, the actions of many drugs such as the sympathomimetics and phenothiazines are terminated before they are excreted because they are metabolized to biologically inactive derivatives. Biotransformation can also result in metabolites that are biologically active. Several benzodiazepines have active metabolites. Thus, if individuals have renal disease that compromises the excretion of active metabolites, the duration of the drug's clinical effect will be increased. Some drugs are metabolized from an inactive form—known as a prodrug—into an active form. For instance, dexamethasone phosphate is inactive as administered; the drug must be metabolized in the body to become the active anti-inflammatory compound. Finally, certain drugs (eg, lithium) are not modified by the body and continue to act until they are excreted.

Biotransformation may produce toxic metabolites. A clinically relevant example is the metabolism of acetaminophen. At therapeutic dosages, acetaminophen is conjugated to harmless glucuronide and sulfate metabolites by phase II reactions. If a large overdose is taken, a CYP-dependent phase I reaction converts some of the acetaminophen to a reactive metabolite that combines with available intracellular glutathione in the liver to a harmless metabolite. However, when hepatic glutathione levels are depleted, the reactive metabolite may combine with essential hepatic cell proteins, resulting in death of those cells. In severe liver disease, stores of phase II conjugates may be depleted, making phase I metabolic reactions more prominent, and the patient more susceptible to hepatic toxicity with near-normal doses of acetaminophen. Also, enzyme inducers such as ethanol may increase acetaminophen toxicity because they increase phase I metabolism compared to phase II metabolism, resulting in increased production of the reactive acetaminophen metabolites.

BIOAVAILABILITY

The bioavailability of a drug is the fraction of the administered dose that reaches the systemic circulation, and is specific to both the drug and the route of administration

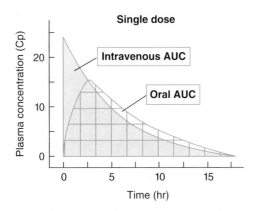 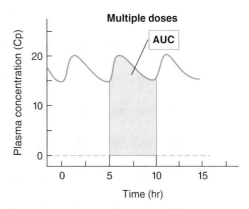

FIGURE 3-7 **The area under the curve (AUC) is used to calculate the bioavailability of a drug.** The AUC can be derived from either single-dose studies (left) or multiple-dose measurements (right). Bioavailability is calculated from $AUC_{(route)}/AUC_{(IV)}$.

(Table 3-1). In the case of intravenous administration, the bioavailability is 100%. Bioavailability by other routes may be much lower. Mechanisms that account for reduced bioavailability include incomplete absorption from the site of administration, P-glycoprotein-mediated transport back into the lumen of the GI tract, binding in tissues prior to reaching the systemic circulation, or biotransformation at the application site or prior to entering the systemic circulation. The first-pass effect following oral administration accounts for the fact that some drugs have low bioavailability when given orally. Even for drugs with equal bioavailabilities, entry into the systemic circulation occurs over varying periods of time depending on the drug formulation and other factors. To account for such factors, the plasma drug concentration is integrated over time to obtain an integrated total area under the curve (AUC) (Figure 3-7). The AUC assists in determining the bioequivalence of different formulations of the drug.

DOSAGE REGIMENS

A dosage regimen is a plan for drug administration over a period of time. The regimen may be divided into *loading* and *maintenance* doses. Ideally, the dosing regimen is based on knowledge of the therapeutic window (Chapter 2) and the drug's clearance and volume of distribution. An appropriate dosage regimen results in the achievement of therapeutic levels of the drug in the blood while staying within the therapeutic window.

If the therapeutic concentration must be achieved rapidly and the V_d is large, a large loading dose may be needed at the onset of therapy. The loading dose is a function of the V_d for the drug (Equation [8]):

$$\text{Loading Dose} = \frac{(V_d \times \text{Desired plasma concentration})}{\text{Bioavailability}} \quad (8)$$

Note that clearance does not enter into this calculation. If the V_d is much larger than blood volume and the loading dose

is very large, the dose should be given slowly to avoid plasma levels in the toxic dose range during the distribution phase.

During chronic therapy, maintenance dosing is required so that the rate of drug administration is equivalent to the rate of elimination (ie, steady state is maintained). Calculation of the maintenance dosage is a function of clearance (Equation [9]).

$$\text{Maintenance Dosage} = \frac{(CL \times \text{Desired plasma concentration})}{\text{Bioavailability}} \quad (9)$$

Note that V_d is not directly involved in the above calculation. The dosing rate calculated for maintenance dosage is the average dose per unit time. For chronic therapy, oral administration is desirable. The number of doses to be given per day is usually determined by the drug's half-life and the therapeutic window. To encourage adherence to the dosing regimen, doses should be given only once or a few times per day. If maintaining a concentration within the therapeutic window is important, either a larger dose may be given at long time intervals or smaller doses at more frequent intervals. If the therapeutic window is narrow, then smaller and more frequent doses must be administered to decrease the likelihood of ADRs.

Theoretical Dosing Regimen

Figure 3-8 illustrates a hypothetical scenario involving the development of a dosing regimen using pharmacodynamic and pharmacokinetic principles. Theophylline, a drug used in the treatment of asthma or COPD, is associated with ADRs including nausea, vomiting, headache, and irritability. Theophylline has a minimum therapeutic concentration range of 7-10 mg/L and a minimum toxic concentration range of 15-20 mg/L. Thus, for a given patient, the therapeutic window might be fixed in the range of 7.5-15.0 mg/L. In Figure 3-8A, a comparison of three dosing regimens is presented: continuous intravenous (IV) infusion, three 224-mg doses at 8-hour intervals, and a single 672-mg dose once per day. Notice that while all three dosing regimens achieve the same *mean* plasma

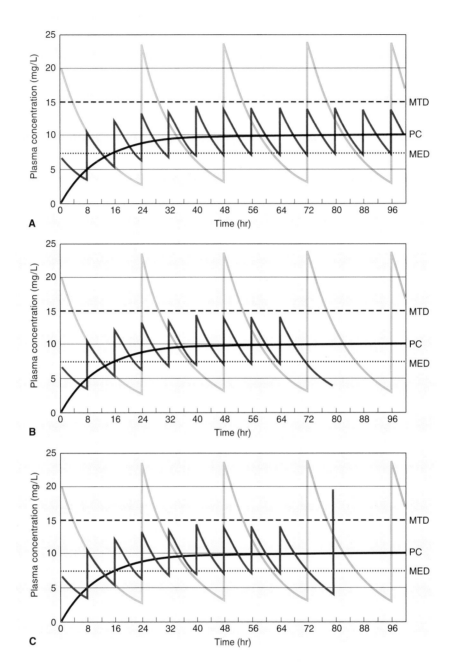

FIGURE 3-8 The therapeutic window for theophylline in a hypothetical patient, and the relationship between frequency of dosing, minimum effective dose (MED) (dotted black line), and minimum toxic dose (MTD; dashed black line). **Panel A** shows that the MED was 7.5 mg/L; the MTD was 15 mg/L. The half-life of theophylline is ~ 8 hours. The desired steady-state plasma concentration (PC) was 10 mg/L. The smoothly rising solid black line represents the PC achieved with an intravenous infusion at 28 mg/h. The doses at 8-hour intervals (red lines) are 224 mg, and for 24-hour intervals are 672 mg (blue lines). To maintain the PC within the therapeutic window, the theophylline must be given at least once every half-life because the MED is half the MTD and the PC will decay by 50% in each half-life. In each of the three dosing regimens, the average steady-state PC is 10 mg/L. **Panel B** shows the effects of missing a maintenance dose. **Panel C** shows the effect of subsequently taking a double 8-hour maintenance dose at the next dosing interval.

drug concentration, each presents unique clinical ramifications. The continuous infusion achieves the desired plasma concentration with minimal variation, but this administration format is impractical for chronic therapy. The once-a-day dosage achieves the desired plasma concentration part of the time, but plasma concentrations spike into the toxic levels and increase the risk of ADRs. In addition, the once-a-day regimen results in plasma concentrations decreasing *below* the therapeutic window prior to the next dose. Last, the 8-hour interval dosage regimen achieves the desired mean plasma concentration with minimal time spent in either toxic or subtherapeutic ranges. Figure 3-8 also illustrates that the time to reach a steady-state average plasma theophylline level is approximately 4-5 half-lives, *regardless* of the frequency of administration.

Patient compliance with regular dosing is a significant problem. Figure 3-8 examines the effects of noncompliance on systemic theophylline plasma concentrations. In Figure 3-8B, the patient missed the 224-mg dose at the 72-hour time point. At the 80-hour time point (one half-life later), plasma theophylline concentration was 50% below the therapeutic window (at 4 mg/L). At that time, the patient decided to correct the error by taking two 8-hour doses together, a total of 448 mg (Figure 3-8C). Now, the theophylline plasma concentration increased (to 19 mg/L)—above the therapeutic window and into the toxic range. These figures illustrate why maintaining regular dosing is required to both achieve a drug's therapeutic benefits and to minimize the risk of ADRs. Unfortunately, there are some medications for which the therapeutic and toxic concentrations vary significantly among individuals. In these cases, it is impossible to predict the therapeutic window in a given person and such medications must be titrated individually in each patient.

Medication Adherence

Medication adherence affects all healthcare professionals—not *just* prescribers. Skipping a dose or taking the wrong dose or at the wrong time are common examples of medication noncompliance. Other examples include: failing to fill prescriptions, failing to follow recommendations for consumption with food or avoidance of certain foods, using incorrect techniques with inhalers or nasal sprays, premature discontinuation (due to ADRs, fear of dependency, lack of funds, etc). Physical therapists have roles in monitoring and helping to improve medication adherence. For most therapists, reviewing or taking a patient's medication history is not a new practice. However, more specific questioning such as "Have you been taking your medicines *as prescribed*?" and "Are you taking *any other* over-the-counter medications or dietary supplements or herbal medications that you have not listed?" represents a fuller appreciation of the complexity of pharmacodynamics and pharmacokinetics and how medications influence patients' clinical presentation and/or the course of physical therapy.

CHAPTER 3 QUESTIONS

1. Which of the following requires the conversion of adenosine triphosphate (ATP) to adenosine diphosphate (ADP) as a protein moves a molecule against its concentration gradient?

   a. Active transport
   b. Facilitated transport
   c. Passive diffusion
   d. Endocytosis

2. At what pH must the urine be to optimally trap an acid with a pKa of 7.50?

   a. 7.75
   b. 8.50
   c. 7.25
   d. 5.50

3. Which of the following is *not* a parenteral route of administration?

   a. Intravenous
   b. Transdermal
   c. Rectal
   d. Inhalation

4. The drug has a volume of distribution of 0.20 L/kg. What is the distribution of the drug in the body?

   a. Limited to the plasma
   b. Concentrated outside of the plasma
   c. Total body distribution
   d. Limited to plasma and extracellular space

5. The plasma concentration of a drug is 100 mcg/L and its half-life is 3 hours. What is the concentration of the drug 12 hours later?

   a. 6.25 mcg/L
   b. 25.0 mcg/L
   c. 3.125 mcg/L
   d. 12.50 mcg/L

6. The half-life ($t_{1/2}$) is calculated by which of the following formulas?

   a. Clearance multiplied by the drug dose
   b. Volume of distribution divided by the clearance
   c. Volume of distribution multiplied by the clearance
   d. Volume of distribution multiplied by the drug dose

7. Which of the following is *not* involved in a maintenance dosage for a drug?

   a. Clearance
   b. Half-life
   c. Volume of distribution
   d. Bioavailability

8. Which of the following is the biotransformation reaction in which acetate or glutathione subgroups are added to a drug molecule to increase the rate of elimination?

   a. Phase 4 reactions
   b. Phase 1 reactions
   c. Phase 3 reactions
   d. Phase 2 reactions

9. Pharmacogenomics may be defined as which of the following?

    a. How genes affect an individual's responses to drugs
    b. The rate at which a drug is eliminated from the body
    c. The distribution of drugs through the body
    d. The mechanism by which drugs are absorbed by the body

10. Which of the following routes of delivery would *not* avoid the "first-pass effect"?

    a. Sublingual delivery
    b. Oral delivery
    c. Intravenous delivery
    d. Inhaled delivery

Introduction to Autonomic Pharmacology

The autonomic nervous system (ANS) provides bidirectional communication (afferent and efferent fibers) between the brain and smooth muscle, cardiac muscle, and exocrine and endocrine glands. Its name is derived from the fact that the activities of the ANS are largely independent (ie, autonomous) of direct conscious control. The ANS is concerned primarily with necessary visceral functions like modification of blood flow to organs, digestion, and regulation of cardiac output. Afferent (sensory) fibers provide information regarding the internal and external environment and modify motor output through reflex arcs of varying size and complexity.

The ANS shares several commonalities with the endocrine system, the other major system that regulates bodily functions. These properties include high-level integration in the brain, the ability to influence processes in distant regions of the body, and extensive use of negative feedback. In the nervous system, information is transmitted between neurons and their effector cells via chemical transmission. Chemical transmission takes place through the release of small amounts of transmitter substances from the nerve terminals into the synapse. The transmitter diffuses across the synaptic cleft and binds to its specific receptor, which either activates or inhibits the postsynaptic cell.

Drugs that either mimic or block the actions of chemical transmitters can be used to selectively modify many autonomic functions such as blood pressure, heart rate, smooth muscle contraction, vasodilation, glandular secretion, and release of neurotransmitter from presynaptic nerve terminals. Drugs affecting the ANS are useful in many clinical conditions. Unfortunately, many drugs used for other purposes also have unwanted effects on autonomic function.

ANATOMY OF THE AUTONOMIC NERVOUS SYSTEM

The ANS is anatomically divided into two major portions: the sympathetic (thoracolumbar) division and the parasympathetic (craniosacral) division (Figure 4-1). Both divisions originate in nuclei within the central nervous system (CNS) and give rise to preganglionic efferent fibers that exit from the brainstem or spinal cord and terminate in motor ganglia. The sympathetic preganglionic fibers leave the CNS through the thoracic and lumbar spinal nerves. The parasympathetic preganglionic fibers leave the CNS through several of the cranial nerves and the third and fourth sacral spinal nerve roots.

The majority of sympathetic preganglionic fibers terminate in ganglia located in the paravertebral chains that lie on either side of the spinal column. Some sympathetic preganglionic fibers terminate in the prevertebral ganglia on the ventral surface of the aorta. From these ganglia, postganglionic sympathetic fibers traverse to the innervated tissues. The majority of parasympathetic preganglionic fibers terminate on ganglion cells in the walls of the organs innervated; others terminate in parasympathetic ganglia located just outside the innervated organs.

In addition to these clearly defined peripheral motor portions of the ANS, large numbers of afferent fibers run from the periphery and ultimately terminate in the integrating centers within the hypothalamus and medulla and evoke motor activity that is carried to the effector cells by the efferent fibers described above.

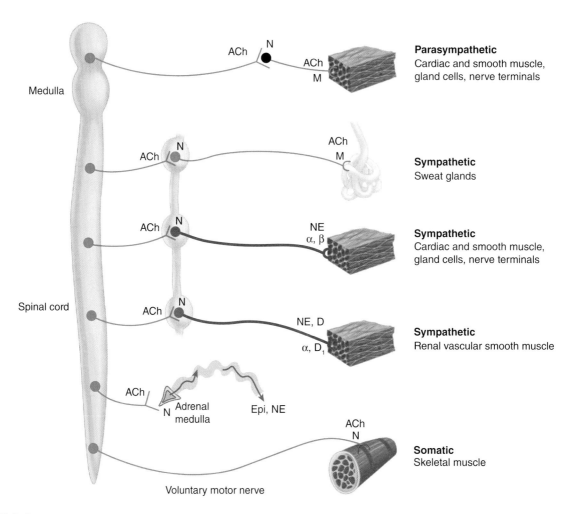

FIGURE 4-1 **Diagram comparing key anatomic and neurotransmitter features of autonomic and somatic motor nerves.** Only primary neurotransmitters are shown. Parasympathetic ganglia are not shown as discrete structures because most are in or near the wall of the innervated organ. Note that some sympathetic postganglionic fibers release acetylcholine or dopamine rather than norepinephrine. The adrenal medulla, a modified sympathetic ganglion, receives sympathetic preganglionic fibers and releases mainly epinephrine and some norepinephrine into the blood. ACh, acetylcholine; D, dopamine; Epi, epinephrine; M, muscarinic receptors; N, nicotinic receptors; NE, norepinephrine.

NEUROTRANSMITTER CHEMISTRY OF THE ANS

Traditionally, autonomic nerves are classified based on whether the primary neurotransmitter released from the postganglionic presynaptic terminals or varicosities is acetylcholine or norepinephrine (Figure 4-1). All preganglionic efferent autonomic fibers (regardless of whether they are sympathetic or parasympathetic) synthesize and release acetylcholine and are thus termed cholinergic. In addition, most parasympathetic postganglionic fibers are cholinergic. Some parasympathetic postganglionic neurons also utilize nitric oxide (eg, in the vascular endothelium) or peptides for transmission (Table 4-1). Most sympathetic postganglionic fibers release norepinephrine. These are referred to as noradrenergic, or simply, adrenergic fibers. A few sympathetic postganglionic fibers release acetylcholine (eg, innervation to the sweat glands). Dopamine, an important neurotransmitter in the CNS, is released by some peripheral sympathetic fibers in the cardiac, gastrointestinal, and renal systems. Adrenal medullary cells, which are embryologically analogous to postganglionic sympathetic neurons, release a mixture of epinephrine and norepinephrine, though higher quantities of epinephrine, into the blood.

There are five main potential targets for pharmacological manipulation of ANS function: neurotransmitter synthesis, neurotransmitter storage, neurotransmitter release, termination of neurotransmitter action, and receptor effects.

Cholinergic Transmission

Synaptic terminals and varicosities of cholinergic neurons contain large numbers of membrane-bound vesicles that contain most of the acetylcholine (Figure 4-2). Farther from the synaptic membrane, a smaller number of large dense-cored vesicles contain peptide cotransmitters with or without acetylcholine (Table 4-1). Vesicles are initially synthesized in the cell

TABLE 4-1 Some of the transmitter substances found in the ANS.

Acetylcholine (ACh)	Primary transmitter at ANS ganglia and at all postganglionic parasympathetic and limited sympathetic nerve endings
Norepinephrine (NE)	Primary transmitter at most postganglionic sympathetic nerve endings
Dopamine	Possible postganglionic sympathetic transmitter in renal blood vessels
Adenosine triphosphate (ATP)	Acts as a transmitter or cotransmitter at many ANS-effector synapses
Neuropeptide Y (NPY)	Cotransmitter in many parasympathetic postganglionic neurons and sympathetic postganglionic noradrenergic vascular neurons. Causes long-lasting vasoconstriction
Nitric oxide (NO)	Probable transmitter for parasympathetic-evoked vasodilation

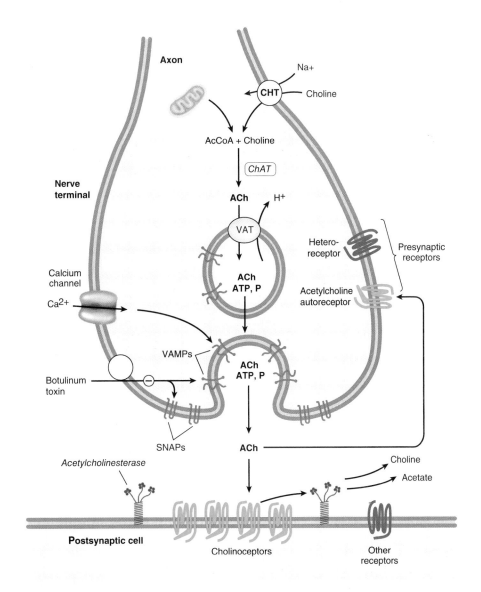

FIGURE 4-2 **Illustration of a generalized cholinergic junction with cholinergic receptors (cholinoceptors) in the postsynaptic membrane.** Choline is transported into the presynaptic nerve terminal by a sodium-dependent choline transporter (CHT). Acetylcholine (ACh) is synthesized from acetyl coenzyme A (AcCoA) and choline by the cytoplasmic enzyme choline acetyltransferase (ChAT). ACh is transported into the synaptic vesicle by a second carrier called a vesicle-associated transporter (VAT). Peptides (P) and adenosine triphosphate (ATP) are also stored in the vesicle. Transmitter release occurs when voltage-sensitive calcium channels in the terminal membrane open. The resulting increase in intracellular calcium causes fusion of vesicle-associated membrane proteins (VAMPs) with synaptosome-associated proteins (SNAPs) on the inner membrane surface and expulsion of ACh and cotransmitters into the synapse. Botulinum toxin blocks this last step. Stimulation of Ach autoreceptors and heteroreceptors on presynaptic terminals regulates additional release of ACh. Acetylcholine's action is terminated by acetylcholinesterase in the synaptic space.

body of the neuron and transported to the terminal. Vesicles may also be recycled several times within the terminal. Acetylcholine is synthesized from acetyl coenzyme A (acetyl CoA) and choline (Figure 4-2). Acetyl CoA is synthesized within the plentiful mitochondria in the synaptic terminal; choline is transported from the extracellular fluid into the terminal. Once synthesized, acetylcholine is transported from the cytoplasm into the vesicles. Acetylcholine synthesis occurs rapidly to enable a very high rate of transmitter release. Within each synaptic vesicle, roughly 1000-50,000 molecules of acetylcholine are stored; the acetylcholine within each vesicle is called a "quanta." Neurotransmitter release from the vesicles is dependent on extracellular calcium, and occurs when an action potential reaches the synaptic terminal and triggers a sufficient influx of calcium ions. Increased intracellular Ca^{2+} concentration initiates fusion of the vesicle membranes with the presynaptic terminal membrane. Fusion of the membranes results in release of the neurotransmitter contents of the vesicle into the synapse. Depolarization of an *autonomic* postganglionic nerve terminal or varicosity releases less quanta and over a much larger area than does depolarization of a *somatic* motor nerve. After release from the presynaptic terminal, acetylcholine molecules may bind to and activate an acetylcholine receptor. Rapidly, all of the acetylcholine diffuses within range of an acetylcholinesterase molecule, which enzymatically splits acetylcholine into choline and acetate, terminating its action (Figure 4-2). Most cholinergic synapses have a high concentration of acetylcholinesterase. Consequently, the half-life of acetylcholine in the synapse is less than a second.

Adrenergic Transmission

Adrenergic neurons transport tyrosine (the amino acid precursor) into the axon terminal where norepinephrine is synthesized and finally stored in membrane-bound vesicles (Figure 4-3). Figure 4-4 outlines the biosynthesis of the catecholamine neurotransmitters (dopamine, epinephrine, and norepinephrine). In most sympathetic postganglionic neurons, norepinephrine is the final product that is packaged and stored within synaptic vesicles. In the adrenal medulla and certain areas of the brain, norepinephrine is further converted to epinephrine. In dopaminergic neurons of the CNS, the synthetic process terminates with dopamine. Several processes that occur within sympathetic nerve terminals are potential sites of drug action.

Neurotransmitter release from noradrenergic nerve endings is similar to the calcium-dependent process previously described for cholinergic terminals. Termination of transmission results from diffusion of norepinephrine away from the receptor site with eventual metabolism in the plasma or liver or reuptake into presynaptic or postsynaptic locations (Figure 4-3). Metabolism of norepinephrine and epinephrine may occur by enzymes such as monoamine oxidase (MAO) in the presynaptic terminal or by catechol-O-methyltransferase (COMT) in other tissues (Figure 4-4). Certain chemicals in the diet (eg, tyramine, an amine highly concentrated in some aged cheeses) or drugs (eg, amphetamines) can be taken up

into presynaptic noradrenergic nerve endings by the norepinephrine transporter (NET; Figure 4-3). Once taken up, these compounds result in increased norepinephrine activity in the synapse either by displacing norepinephrine from storage vesicles or by inhibiting the enzyme responsible for metabolic inactivation of norepinephrine.

AUTONOMIC RECEPTORS

Unique autonomic receptor subtypes have been defined based on careful comparisons of the potency of a series of autonomic agonists and antagonists (Table 4-2). There are two primary cholinergic receptor subtypes—muscarinic and nicotinic—named after the alkaloids muscarine and nicotine originally used in their identification. The adrenergic receptors (adrenoceptors) are subdivided into three primary subtypes: alpha (α), beta (β), and dopamine (D) receptors. Whereas α and β receptor subtypes bind mainly norepinephrine, D receptors preferentially bind dopamine. The development of more selective antagonists led to the discovery of subclasses within these major subtypes. Within the α receptor subtype, α_1 and α_2 receptors have been characterized. Within the β receptor subtype, β_1, β_2, and β_3 receptors have been defined. Table 4-3 lists the peripheral tissue locations of the adrenoceptors as well the physiological actions resulting from receptor activation.

FUNCTIONAL ORGANIZATION OF AUTONOMIC ACTIVITY

Drugs that affect the ANS can often evoke significant reflex (ie, compensatory) effects. To appreciate or anticipate such actions, it is essential to understand how autonomic nerves interact with each other and with their effector organs. Autonomic reflexes are particularly important in understanding cardiovascular responses to drugs that affect the ANS. For example, the primary controlled variable in cardiovascular function is mean arterial pressure (MAP). A change in any variable, such as decreased heart rate due to the administration of a drug that blocks β_1 receptors, will decrease MAP. This drop in MAP may trigger powerful autonomic reflexes such as increased renin release from the kidneys, in an effort to compensate for the drug-induced drop in MAP. The reflexive response to restore homeostasis may even be sufficient enough to reverse the drug's effect on heart rate (Figure 4-5).

Central Integration

Autonomic function is integrated and regulated at many levels from the CNS to the effector cells. The two divisions of the ANS and the endocrine system are integrated with each other in the midbrain and medulla, with sensory input, and with information from higher CNS centers. Within each organ system of the body, the interactions between the sympathetic and parasympathetic divisions of the ANS are often in opposition to each other (Table 4-4). The parasympathetic nervous system (PNS) is a trophotropic system that promotes

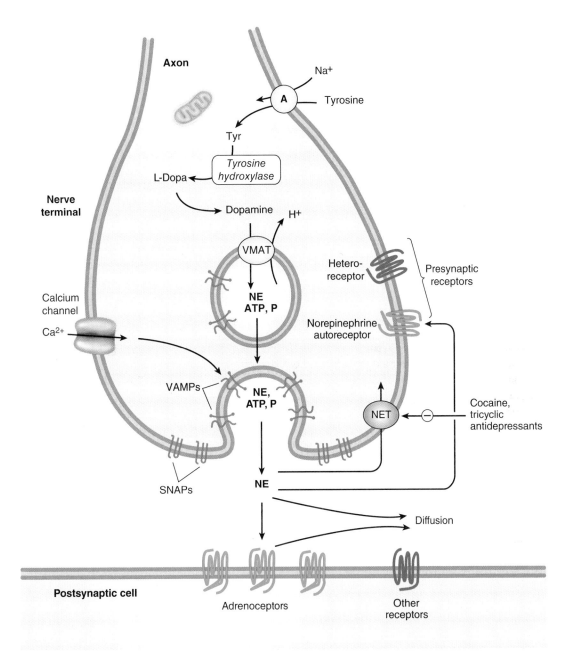

FIGURE 4-3 **Illustration of a generalized noradrenergic junction with adrenergic receptors (adrenoceptors) in the postsynaptic membrane.** Tyrosine is transported into the noradrenergic ending by a carrier (A). Tyrosine is converted to dopamine, which is then transported into the vesicle by the vesicular monoamine transporter (VMAT). VMAT also transports norepinephrine (NE) and several other amines into the vesicle. Within the vesicle, dopamine is converted to NE. Peptides (P) and adenosine triphosphate (ATP) are also stored in the vesicle. Release of transmitter occurs when an action potential opens voltage-sensitive calcium channels and increases intracellular calcium. Fusion of vesicles with the surface membrane results in expulsion of NE and cotransmitters into the synapse. After release, NE diffuses out of the synaptic cleft or is transported back into the cytoplasm of the presynaptic terminal by the norepinephrine transporter (NET), or into the postsynaptic cells. The NET may be inhibited by cocaine, which results in increased transmitter in the synaptic space. Stimulation of NE autoreceptors and heteroreceptors on presynaptic terminals regulates additional release of NE.

growth, while the sympathetic nervous system (SNS) is an ergotropic system that leads to energy expenditure. For example, activation of the PNS includes slowing of the heart rate and stimulation of digestive activity ("rest and digest"). In contrast, activation of the SNS results in cardiac stimulation (rate and force), increased blood glucose, and cutaneous vasoconstriction—all responses that are suited to fighting or surviving an attack ("fight or flight"). At a more subtle level of interactions in the brainstem and spinal cord, there are important cooperative interactions between the parasympathetic and sympathetic systems. For some organs, the sensory (afferent) fibers of the PNS exert reflex control over motor outflow in the

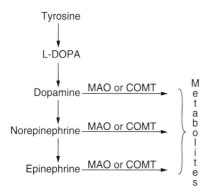

FIGURE 4-4 **Biosynthesis of catecholamines from tyrosine through epinephrine.** Metabolism of dopamine, norepinephrine, or epinephrine by either monoamine oxidase (MAO) or catechol-*O*-methyltransferase (COMT) results in the production of inactive metabolites.

sympathetic system. For example, when baroreceptors detect a drop in blood pressure, the firing rate of the carotid sinus nerve (traveling in cranial nerve IX) decreases. This input into the vasomotor center in the medulla leads to increased sympathetic outflow (increased heart rate, contractility and venous and arteriolar constriction) to increase blood pressure.

Peripheral Integration

In peripheral tissues, integration of autonomic function may occur at presynaptic or postsynaptic locations. Presynaptic regulation is the use of negative or positive feedback control to regulate neurotransmitter release from synaptic terminals. A well-documented mechanism involves α_2 receptors located on noradrenergic nerve terminals. When norepinephrine and similar molecules activate these receptors, further release of norepinephrine from that nerve ending diminishes. In contrast,

TABLE 4-2 Autonomic receptor types with documented or probable effects on effector tissues.

Receptor	Typical Location(s)	Result of Receptor Binding and Activation
Cholinergic		
M_1	CNS neurons, sympathetic postganglionic neurons, some presynaptic sites	Formation of second messengers and increases in intracellular calcium
M_2	Myocardium, smooth muscle, some presynaptic sites	Opening of potassium channels, inhibition of adenylate cyclase
M_3	Exocrine glands, vessels (smooth muscle and endothelium)	Formation of second messengers and increases in intracellular calcium
M_4	Possible vagal nerve endings	Opening of potassium channels, inhibition of adenylate cyclase
M_5	Vascular endothelium, especially in the CNS	Formation of second messengers and increases in intracellular calcium
N_N	Postganglionic neurons, some presynaptic cholinergic terminals	Opening Na^+/K^+ channels, depolarization
N_M	Skeletal muscle motor end plate	Opening Na^+/K^+ channels, depolarization
Adrenergic		
α_1	Postsynaptic effector cells, especially smooth muscle	Formation of second messengers and increases in intracellular calcium
α_2	Presynaptic adrenergic nerve terminals, platelets, adipocytes, vascular and visceral smooth muscle, postsynaptic neurons in brainstem and spinal cord	Inhibition of adenylate cyclase
β_1	Postsynaptic effector cells: heart, adipocytes, brain, presynaptic adrenergic and cholinergic nerve terminals	Stimulation of adenylate cyclase
β_2	Postsynaptic effector cells: smooth muscle and cardiac muscle, liver, pancreas, lungs	Stimulation of adenylate cyclase
β_3	Postsynaptic effector cells: adipocytes, urinary bladder	Stimulation of adenylate cyclase
Dopaminergic		
D_1, D_5	Brain, effector tissues: smooth muscle of renal vasculature	Stimulation of adenylate cyclase
D_2	Brain, effector tissues: smooth muscle, presynaptic nerve terminals	Inhibition of adenylate cyclase increased opening K^+ channels
D_3	Brain	Inhibition of adenylate cyclase
D_4	Brain, cardiovascular system	Inhibition of adenylate cyclase

CNS, central nervous system; α, alpha; β, beta; D, dopamine; M, muscarinic; N, nicotinic.

TABLE 4-3 Types of adrenoceptors,[a] some of the peripheral tissues in which they are found, and major effects of their activation.

Type[b]	Tissue	Action
α_1	Most vascular smooth muscle	Contracts (increases vascular resistance)
	Pupillary dilator muscle	Contracts (mydriasis)
	Pilomotor smooth muscle	Contracts (erects hair)
α_2	Adrenergic and cholinergic nerve terminals	Inhibits transmitter release
	Platelets	Stimulates aggregation
	Some vascular smooth muscle	Contracts
	Adipocytes	Inhibits lipolysis
	Pancreatic β cells	Inhibits insulin release
β_1	Heart	Stimulates rate and force
	Juxtaglomerular cells	Stimulates renin release
β_2	Respiratory, uterine, and vascular smooth muscle	Relaxes
	Liver (human)	Stimulates glycogenolysis
	Pancreatic β cells	Stimulates insulin release
	Somatic motor nerve terminals	Causes tremors
β_3 (β_1, β_2 may also contribute)	Adipocytes	Stimulates lipolysis
	Detrusor muscle	Relaxation
D_1	Renal and other splanchnic blood vessels	Dilates (decreases resistance)
D_2	Nerve terminals	Inhibits adenylate cyclase

[a]Adrenoceptor distribution in the CNS is discussed in Chapter 12.
[b]See Table 4-2 for abbreviations.

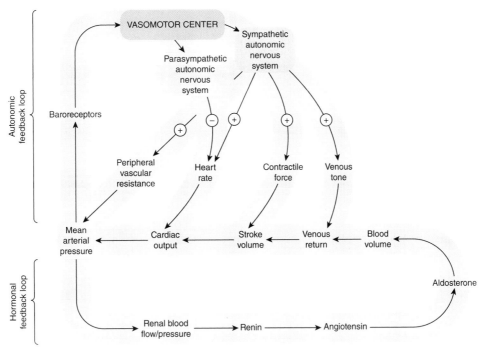

FIGURE 4-5 Autonomic and hormonal control of cardiovascular function. Note that two feedback loops are present: the autonomic loop and the hormonal loop. The sympathetic nervous system directly influences four major variables: peripheral vascular resistance, heart rate, contractile force, and venous tone. The sympathetic system also directly modulates renin production (not shown). The parasympathetic nervous system directly influences heart rate. In addition to its role in stimulating aldosterone secretion, angiotensin II directly increases peripheral vascular resistance and facilitates sympathetic effects (not shown). The net feedback effect of each loop is to compensate for changes in mean arterial pressure. Thus, decreased blood pressure due to blood loss would evoke increased sympathetic outflow and renin release. Conversely, elevated pressure due to the administration of a vasoconstrictor drug would cause reduced sympathetic outflow, reduced renin release, and increased parasympathetic (vagal) outflow.

TABLE 4-4 Direct effects of autonomic nerve activity on some organ systems.

| Organ | Effect of | | | |
| | Sympathetic Activity | | Parasympathetic Activity | |
	Action[a]	Receptor[b]	Action	Receptor
Eye				
Iris radial muscle	Contracts	α_1	—	—
Iris circular muscle			Contracts	M_3
Ciliary muscle	[Relaxes]	β	Contracts	M_3
Heart				
Sinoatrial node	Accelerates	β_1, β_2	Decelerates	M_2
Ectopic pacemakers	Accelerates	β_1, β_2	—	
Contractility	Increases	β_1, β_2	Decreases (atria)	M_2
Blood vessels				
Skin and splanchnic vessels	Contracts	α	—	
Skeletal muscle vessels	Relaxes	β_2	—	
	[Contracts]	α	—	
	Relaxes	M^c	—	
Endothelium			Releases EDRF[d]	$M_3, M_5{}^e$
Bronchiolar smooth muscle	Relaxes	β_2	Contracts	M_3
Gastrointestinal tract				
Smooth muscle				
Walls	Relaxes	$\alpha_2,{}^f \beta_2$	Contracts	M_3
Sphincters	Contracts	α_1	Relaxes	M_3
Secretion	Decreases	α_2	Increases	M_3
Genitourinary smooth muscle				
Bladder wall	Relaxes	β_3	Contracts	M_2 and M_3
Sphincter	Contracts	α_1	Relaxes	M_3
Uterus, pregnant	Relaxes	β_2	—	
	Contracts	α	Contracts	M_3
Penis, seminal vesicles	Ejaculation	α	Erection	M
Skin				
Pilomotor smooth muscle	Contracts	α	—	
Sweat glands				
Thermoregulatory	Increases	M	—	
Apocrine (stress)	Increases	α	—	
Metabolic functions				
Liver	Gluconeogenesis	β_2, α	—	
Liver	Glycogenolysis	β_2, α	—	
Adipocytes	Lipolysis	β_3	—	
Kidney	Renin release	β_1	—	
Autonomic nerve endings				
Sympathetic	—	—	Decrease NE release	M^g
Parasympathetic	Decreases ACh release	α	—	

NE, norepinephrine.

[a]Less important actions are shown in brackets.

[b]Specific receptor type: α = alpha, β = beta, M = muscarinic.

[c]Vascular smooth muscle in skeletal muscle has sympathetic cholinergic dilator fibers.

[d]The endothelium of most blood vessels releases EDRF (endothelium-derived relaxing factor), which causes marked vasodilation, in response to muscarinic stimuli. However, unlike the receptors innervated by sympathetic cholinergic fibers in skeletal muscle blood vessels, these muscarinic receptors are not innervated and respond only to circulating muscarinic agonists.

[e]Cerebral blood vessels dilate in response to M_5 receptor activation.

[f]Probably through presynaptic inhibition of parasympathetic activity.

[g]Probably through M_1, but M_2 may participate in some locations.

activation of presynaptic β receptors appears to facilitate the release of norepinephrine. Presynaptic receptors that respond to the primary transmitter substances released by the nerve ending are called autoreceptors (Figures 4-2 and 4-3). Autoreceptors are usually inhibitory, but many cholinergic fibers, especially somatic motor fibers, have excitatory nicotinic autoreceptors. Control of transmitter release is not limited to modulation by the neurotransmitter itself. Nerve terminals also carry regulatory receptors that respond to many other substances. Such heteroreceptors (Figures 4-2 and 4-3) may be activated by substances released from other nerve terminals that synapse with the nerve ending. For example, some efferent vagal fibers in the myocardium synapse on sympathetic noradrenergic nerve terminals and inhibit norepinephrine release. Alternatively, compounds may diffuse to these receptors from the blood or from nearby tissues. Presynaptic regulation by a variety of endogenous chemicals probably occurs in all nerve fibers.

Postsynaptic regulation can be considered from two perspectives. The first is modulation by the prior history of activity at the primary receptor, that is, receptor up-regulation or down-regulation, or receptor desensitization (Chapter 2). Up-regulation occurs in response to decreased activation of the receptors. In contrast, down-regulation and desensitization occurs in response to increased activation of the receptors. Alternatively, receptor modulation may occur by other temporally associated conditions such as electrolyte levels inside or outside of the effector cell, or circulating hormones.

PHARMACOLOGIC MODIFICATION OF AUTONOMIC FUNCTION

Figure 4-6 summarizes the major steps in impulse transmission. Modifying any step in this process may increase or decrease the amount of neurotransmitter released and available to bind to the appropriate receptors. Depending on which step (or steps) is targeted, drugs can produce generalized effects or have a highly specific effect. Drugs that block action potential propagation are very nonselective in their action, since these drugs act on a process that is common to all neurons. On the other hand, drugs that act on the biochemical processes involved in neurotransmitter release and turnover are more selective. Direct-acting antagonists bind to postsynaptic receptors, but have no efficacy (ie, they block the endogenous agonist from binding to the receptor). Indirect-acting antagonists inhibit neurotransmitter synthesis, storage, or release, which results in less neurotransmitter available to bind with postsynaptic receptors. Direct and indirect adrenergic antagonists are called sympatholytics; that is, these drugs inhibit the activity of the SNS. In contrast, sympathomimetics are drugs that increase the activity of (ie, mimic) the sympathetic system. They can also act directly or indirectly. Direct-acting agonists have both affinity and efficacy for their respective postsynaptic receptors. Examples of indirect-acting agonists include **cocaine**, which decreases the reuptake of neurotransmitter, and **selegiline**, which inhibits the enzyme responsible for neurotransmitter breakdown. Both of these indirect mechanisms result in increased neurotransmitter

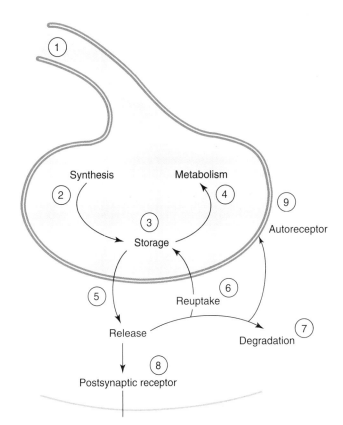

FIGURE 4-6 **Potential sites of pharmacologic modulation at synapses.** Electrical impulses propagate down the axon. At the presynaptic membrane, an influx of extracellular calcium results in fusion of the synaptic vesicle with the presynaptic membrane and release of neurotransmitter into the synapse. The neurotransmitter may interact with presynaptic autoreceptors and postsynaptic receptors. Eventually, the neurotransmitter may be taken back up into the presynaptic terminal or postsynaptic terminal or it may diffuse from the synaptic space. Neurotransmitter metabolism (ie, degradation) may occur at any of these locations. Pharmacologic manipulation can occur at many locations. Local anesthetics inhibit the action potential in the axon (1). An indirect-acting antagonist may inhibit synthesis, storage, or release of the neurotransmitter (2, 3, 5). Direct-acting antagonists inhibit postsynaptic receptors (8). Indirect-acting agonists may augment neurotransmitter action by inhibiting metabolism, reuptake, or degradation of the neurotransmitter (4, 6, 7). Finally, stimulation of presynaptic autoreceptors often leads to a decrease in further neurotransmitter release from the presynaptic nerve terminal (9).

in the synapse and increased postsynaptic receptor stimulation. Similar direct-acting and indirect-acting classifications exist for the agonists and antagonists that interact with cholinergic receptors in the PNS.

Because the biochemistry of adrenergic transmission is very different from that of cholinergic transmission, activation or blockade of either adrenergic or cholinergic receptors on effector cells offers maximum flexibility and selectivity of effect. Furthermore, individual subgroups of receptors (eg, within the larger subtype β-adrenergic receptors) can often be selectively activated or blocked. Subsequent chapters in this section (Chapters 5-10) provide examples of how selective receptor activation or blockade is critical in the clinical use of these drugs.

CHAPTER 4 QUESTIONS

1. Cholinergic nerve fibers release which of the following?

   a. Acetylcholine
   b. Dopamine
   c. Epinephrine
   d. Norepinephrine

2. Which of the following is the neurotransmitter found in the synapse between pre- and postganglionic nerve fibers in the autonomic nervous system?

   a. Norepinephrine
   b. Dopamine
   c. Epinephrine
   d. Acetylcholine

3. Which of the following is the enzyme in the presynaptic nerve terminal responsible for degrading norepinephrine?

   a. Acetylcholinesterase
   b. Dopa decarboxylase
   c. Monoamine oxidase
   d. Catechol-*O*-methyltransferase

4. Which of the following is a presynaptic autoreceptor that when stimulated diminishes additional norepinephrine release from the nerve terminal?

   a. Angiotensin-2
   b. Alpha-2
   c. Beta-2
   d. Nicotinic

5. The sympathetic nervous system is also known as which of the following?

   a. Craniosacral
   b. Craniolumbar
   c. Thoracosacral
   d. Thoracolumber

6. In the sympathetic nervous system, where is acetylcholine the neurotransmitter?

   a. Sweat glands
   b. Blood vessels
   c. Myocardium
   d. Urinary bladder

7. Which of the following receptor subtypes is located on the postsynaptic side of the synapse at the neuromuscular junction?

   a. Alpha
   b. Beta
   c. Nicotinic
   d. Muscarinic

8. Stimulation of which of the following receptors on blood vessels results in vasoconstriction?

   a. Alpha-1
   b. Beta-1
   c. Beta-3
   d. Beta-2

9. What is the final product in catecholamine neurotransmitter synthesis?

   a. Acetylcholine
   b. Dopamine
   c. Epinephrine
   d. Norepinephrine

10. A drug that inhibits neurotransmitter synthesis, storage, or release would be defined as which of the following?

    a. Indirect-acting antagonist
    b. Direct-acting antagonist
    c. Indirect-acting agonist
    d. Direct-acting agonist

Drugs Affecting the Cholinergic System

CASE STUDY

T.J. is a 25-year-old male who was involved in a motorcycle accident 4 weeks ago and transferred to an inpatient rehabilitation facility yesterday. He is scheduled for transfer training in the open gym immediately after breakfast today. As a result of the accident, T.J. has a stable spinal cord injury (SCI) at the T10 neurological level. The patient has no cardiovascular dysfunction. He is currently taking drugs to reduce spasticity, including tolterodine to reduce neurogenic detrusor overactivity (spastic bladder). The therapist and patient begin with a sliding board transfer from the wheelchair to the plinth. The patient urinates involuntarily during his initial attempt with the sliding board activities. The patient is embarrassed and states that this happened before when he attempted to sit up and reposition himself with his hands. The patient requests that this morning's rehabilitation session be terminated. In the afternoon, T.J. does not want to come to the gym because he is concerned that the same problem will occur.

REHABILITATION FOCUS

This chapter covers drugs that either enhance or inhibit the actions of cholinergic transmission. Cholinomimetics amplify cholinergic transmission and have the potential to improve or inhibit the rehabilitation process. Prescriptions for either direct-acting or indirect-acting cholinomimetics may be prescribed for glaucoma, hypotonic bladder function, myasthenia gravis, or Alzheimer's disease. In individuals with Alzheimer's dementia, scheduling rehabilitation when these drugs are at their maximal plasma level may enhance functional or cognitive activities and assist the therapist in providing a positive outcome. In contrast, many patients may also be self-medicating with nicotine (a direct-acting agonist at nicotinic receptors) via inhalation or buccal (ie, smoking or dipping) absorption. These patients may experience various adverse sympathetic or parasympathetic responses based on other comorbidities. The therapist should encourage these patients to abstain from these activities prior to rehabilitation interventions (or permanently, if possible).

The second half of the chapter covers muscarinic and nicotinic antagonists that inhibit cholinergic transmission. Muscarinic antagonists may be prescribed for patients with spastic bladder and incontinence, parkinsonism, or pulmonary dysfunction. For individuals with spastic bladder and incontinence due to SCI, inadvertent voiding may be reduced by scheduling rehabilitation interventions during peak plasma levels of the drug. During sustained periods of exertion, hyperthermia may occur due to the inhibition of eccrine sweat glands by antimuscarinic agents. The clinical application for antimuscarinics in the treatment of parkinsonism and pulmonary dysfunction are discussed in Chapters 17 and 35, respectively. Cholinergic antagonists that act at nicotinic acetylcholine receptors in skeletal muscle are commonly used in patients undergoing major surgery requiring mechanical ventilation. In these patients, normal musculoskeletal function returns following elimination of the drug. If possible, the therapist should establish and review treatment plans with patients prior to surgery when cognitive and musculoskeletal function is higher than immediately following surgery.

CHOLINOMIMETIC DRUGS

When synaptic transmission depends on acetylcholine as the primary neurotransmitter, it is called *cholinergic*. Acetylcholine's activity is terminated very quickly by the enzyme acetylcholinesterase (AChE), which is found in high concentration in cholinergic synapses. There are two major subtypes of cholinergic receptors: muscarinic (M) and nicotinic (N). Drugs that mimic the effects of acetylcholine are referred to as cholinomimetics; some are agonists at cholinergic receptors, whereas others *indirectly* increase acetylcholine's actions by inhibiting AChE (Figure 5-1).

The seven identified subtypes of cholinergic receptors (cholinoceptors) and their respective receptor signaling mechanisms are laid out in Table 5-1. Selective agonists for several muscarinic receptor subtypes are available. In contrast, agonist selectivity for nicotinic receptors is very limited. Instead, direct-acting nicotinic agonists are broadly classified

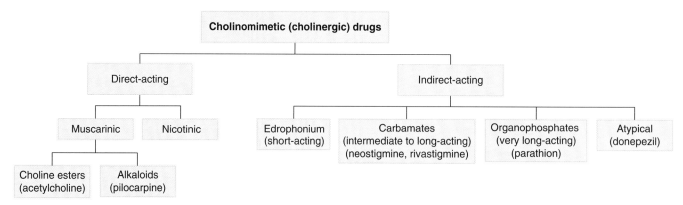

FIGURE 5-1 **Cholinomimetics.** These drugs include direct-acting agonists at muscarinic or nicotinic receptors and indirect-acting drugs that inhibit acetylcholinesterase, the enzyme that terminates the action of endogenous acetylcholine. Example drugs are in parentheses.

on the basis of whether ganglionic (N_N) or neuromuscular (N_M) stimulation predominates. Activation of both nicotinic receptor subtypes opens an ion channel selective for sodium and potassium, resulting in cellular depolarization. In general, activation of muscarinic receptors modulates the formation of second messengers or the activity of ion channels.

The physiologic responses of direct-acting agonists result from their selective interaction with either muscarinic or nicotinic receptors. In contrast, indirect-acting agonists are not specific in selective receptor stimulation because they inhibit the hydrolysis and inactivation of endogenous acetylcholine. These drugs increase endogenous acetylcholine concentration where acetylcholine is normally released and therefore amplify the effect of endogenous acetylcholine. Table 5-2 outlines the spectrum of action of typical direct- and indirect-acting cholinomimetics and a summary of their pharmacokinetics.

TABLE 5-1 Subtypes and characteristics of cholinoceptors.

Receptor Type	Location	Postreceptor Mechanism[a]
Muscarinic (M)		
M_1	Nerves	IP_3, DAG cascade
M_2	Heart, nerves, smooth muscle	Inhibition of cAMP production, activation of K^+ channels
M_3	Glands, smooth muscle, endothelium	IP_3, DAG cascade
M_4	CNS	Inhibition of cAMP production
M_5	CNS	IP_3, DAG cascade
Nicotinic (N)		
N_M	Skeletal muscle neuromuscular junction (end plate receptor)	Na^+, K^+ depolarizing ion channel
N_N	CNS, autonomic postganglionic cell bodies, dendrites	Na^+, K^+ depolarizing ion channel

[a]Mechanisms of receptor signaling include either formation of the second messengers diacylglycerol (DAG) and inositol-1, 4, 5-trisphosphate (IP_3) or inhibition of the formation of cyclic adenosine monophosphate (cAMP), or ion channel activation for sodium (Na^+) influx or potassium (K^+) efflux.

Source: Data from Millar NS, Gotti C: Diversity of vertebrate nicotinic receptors. *Neuropharmacology* 2009;56:237.

DIRECT-ACTING CHOLINERGIC AGONISTS

Direct-acting agonists are divided into two groups based on chemical structure (Figure 5-1). The first group consists of choline esters, typified by **acetylcholine**, **carbachol**, and **bethanechol**. The second group includes naturally occurring alkaloids such as **nicotine**, **muscarine**, and **pilocarpine**. Further classification is based on whether the agents primarily activate muscarinic or nicotinic receptors.

Physiologic Effects

Most of the physiologic effects of direct-acting muscarinic agonists are predictably parasympathomimetic based on the known distribution of muscarinic receptors (Table 5-3). There are two important exceptions to this generality. First, direct-acting muscarinic agonists stimulate muscarinic receptors located on eccrine sweat glands and cause sweating. This thermoregulation function is physiologically under sympathetic, not parasympathetic, nerve control. Second, muscarinic agonists cause vasodilation due to release of endothelial-derived relaxing factor (EDRF) from uninnervated muscarinic receptors on the endothelial cells lining vascular walls. The resulting vasodilation may produce a drop in blood pressure.

The physiologic response to nicotinic receptor stimulation depends on whether N_N or N_M receptors are activated. The effects of N_N receptor stimulation in the autonomic ganglia depends on the organ system involved. Since blood

TABLE 5-2 Cholinomimetics: spectrum of action and pharmacokinetics.

Drug	Spectrum of Action	Pharmacokinetic Features
Direct-acting		
Acetylcholine	B	Rapidly hydrolyzed by cholinesterase (ChE); duration of action 5-30 sec; poor lipid solubility
Bethanechol	M	Resistant to ChE, orally active, poor lipid solubility; duration of action 30 min to 2 hr
Carbachol	B	Like bethanechol
Pilocarpine	M	Not an ester; good lipid solubility; duration of action 30 min to 2 hr
Nicotine	N	Not an ester; duration of action 1-6 hr; high lipid solubility
Indirect-acting		
Edrophonium	B	Alcohol, quaternary amine, poor lipid solubility, not orally active; duration of action 5-15 min
Neostigmine	B	Carbamate, quaternary amine, poor lipid solubility, orally active; duration of action 30 min to 2 hr
Physostigmine	B	Carbamate, tertiary amine, lipid soluble; duration of action 30 min to 2 hr
Pyridostigmine	B	Carbamates like neostigmine, but longer duration of action (4-8 hr)
Echothiophate	B	Organophosphate, moderate lipid solubility; duration of action 2-7 days
Parathion	B	Organophosphate insecticide, high lipid solubility; duration of action 7-30 days

M, muscarinic; N, nicotinic; B, both.

TABLE 5-3 Effects of cholinoceptor stimulation.

Organ	Response[a]
Muscarinic Receptors	
CNS	Complex stimulatory effects: mild alerting reaction (nicotinic), tremor, emesis, excitation of respiratory centers, convulsions
PNS	Complex stimulatory effects: stimulation of autonomic ganglia results in either parasympathetic or sympathetic response depending on each organ system (nicotinic)
Eye	
Sphincter muscle of iris	Contraction (miosis)
Ciliary muscle	Contraction (accommodation for near vision, cyclospasm)
Heart	
Sinoatrial node	Decrease in rate (negative chronotropy)
Atria	Decrease in contractile strength (negative inotropy); decrease in refractory period
Atrioventricular node	Decrease in conduction velocity (negative dromotropy); increase in refractory period
Ventricles	Small decrease in contractile strength
Blood vessels	Dilation (via EDRF)
Bronchi	Contraction (bronchoconstriction)
Gastrointestinal tract	
Motility	Increase
Sphincters	Relaxation (via enteric nervous system)
Urinary bladder	
Detrusor	Contraction
Trigone and sphincter	Relaxation; voiding
Glands	Increased secretion: thermoregulatory sweat, lacrimal, salivary, bronchial, gastric, intestinal glands
Nicotinic Receptors	
N_M: skeletal muscle	Activation of neuromuscular end plates; contraction of muscle, followed by paralysis upon continued stimulation
N_N: autonomic ganglia	Variable. Depending on the organ system, sympathetic or parasympathetic activity may be augmented

EDRF, endothelial-derived relaxing factor. Evidence suggests EDRF is nitric oxide (NO).

[a]Only the direct effects are indicated; homeostatic responses to these direct actions may be important.

vessels are dominated by sympathetic innervation, activation of nicotinic receptors on postganglionic neurons results in vasoconstriction. In contrast, the gastrointestinal (GI) system is dominated by parasympathetic control. Here, stimulation of the postganglionic neurons results in increased motility and secretion. The physiologic response to activation of N_M receptors at the neuromuscular junction depends on the duration of agonist exposure. Acute activation of N_M by direct-acting nicotinic agonists results in fasciculations and muscle spasms. Prolonged stimulation of N_M receptors (eg, nicotine or AChE inhibitors) results in receptor desensitization and muscle paralysis.

Clinical Uses

Table 5-4 lists several clinical applications of direct-acting muscarinic and nicotinic agonists. Bethanechol, a muscarinic

TABLE 5-4 Clinical applications of some cholinomimetics.

Drug	Action	Clinical Applications
Direct-Acting Agonists		
Bethanechol (M)	Activates bowel and bladder smooth muscle	Postoperative and neurogenic ileus and urinary retention
Nicotine (N)	Replaces rapid-onset actions (cigarette) with slower action	Smoking deterrence (patch, chewing gum)
Indirect-Acting Agonists		
Neostigmine (carbamate)	Amplifies effects of endogenous ACh	Treatment of myasthenia gravis
Pyridostigmine (carbamate)		Reversal of neuromuscular blockade by nondepolarizing drugs
Edrophonium (alcohol)		
Physostigmine (carbamate)	Amplifies effects of endogenous ACh	Glaucoma
Echothiophate (organophosphate)		
Donepezil (atypical)	Amplifies effects of endogenous ACh in the CNS	Alzheimer's disease
Galantamine (atypical)		
Rivastigmine (carbamate)		

ACh, acetylcholine; CNS, central nervous system; M, muscarinic; N, nicotinic.

agonist, is used to assist in micturition (voiding) in individuals with hypotonic bladder after surgery or SCI. Nicotine's clinical application is as an adjunct in tobacco abstention. In the form of nicotine replacement therapy (patch, chewing gum), nicotine may produce sustained desensitization of central nicotinic receptors, which is thought to facilitate smoking cessation. **Succinylcholine** is an agonist at N_M receptors. However, its stimulation of the motor end plate receptors results in a depolarizing neuromuscular blockade. Thus, succinylcholine is used to provide skeletal muscle paralysis as an adjuvant to general anesthesia; it will be discussed with the nicotinic antagonists in the last section of this chapter.

Adverse Effects

For muscarinic agonists, adverse effects include both central nervous system (CNS) and peripheral tissue responses. The CNS effects may include generalized stimulation and even hallucinations or seizures. In the eye, miosis (pupillary constriction) and spasm of ocular accommodation may occur, resulting in blurriness when the individual attempts to view distant objects. At higher doses, the peripheral responses can be predicted based on excessive parasympathomimetic stimulation: bronchoconstriction, excessive mucus production, GI distress, bladder spasms with increased frequency of voiding, and hypotension. Bradycardia may occur, but the hypotension usually evokes a reflex tachycardia. Finally, stimulation of muscarinic receptors on eccrine sweat glands may result in sweating.

Centrally acting nicotinic agonists may initiate seizures, coma, and respiratory depression. In the peripheral tissues, stimulation of the autonomic N_N receptors results in either parasympathetic or sympathetic manifestations, depending upon the organ system, as previously discussed. Significant clinical manifestations may include hypertension and cardiac arrhythmias. Prolonged stimulation of N_M receptors at the neuromuscular junction with subsequent muscle paralysis leads to decreased respiratory muscle function and hypoventilation. Nicotine in small doses, as incurs with smoking, is strongly addictive. Chronic exposure to nicotine linked with tobacco use is associated with pathologies such as several cancers, GI ulcers, vascular disease, and sudden coronary death.

INDIRECT-ACTING CHOLINERGIC AGONISTS

Indirect-acting cholinergic agonists are acetylcholinesterase (AChE) inhibitors. These fall into four major classes based on their chemical structure and duration of effect (Figure 5-1). Three classes are alcohols (**edrophonium**), carbamates (eg, **neostigmine**), and organophosphates (eg, **echothiophate**). The fourth class falls into none of the above and is labeled "atypical" in Figure 5-1. Both the carbamate and organophosphate classes bind to AChE and undergo hydrolysis. Following this enzymatic activity, the metabolite is released slowly, which prevents the binding and inactivation of endogenous acetylcholine. Metabolites of carbamates unbind from AChE over a period of hours, whereas the organophosphates require days to weeks to be released by AChE. Thus, the duration of action for carbamates ranges from 2 to 8 hours whereas the duration of action for organophosphates is much longer and can extend up to 30 days in the case of **parathion**. The alcohol class (containing only edrophonium) binds to the active site of AChE by hydrogen bonds. The binding is short-lived, accounting for its short duration of action (5-15 minutes). **Donepezil** and **galantamine** are atypical AChE inhibitors. They are structurally dissimilar and do not fall into any of the other three chemical classes. Finally, some indirect-acting cholinergic agonists also have some direct-acting agonist activity. For example, neostigmine both inhibits AChE and directly activates the postsynaptic N_M receptor at the neuromuscular junction.

Physiologic Effects

By inhibiting AChE, these drugs amplify the actions of endogenous acetylcholine at both muscarinic and nicotinic synapses. Thus, these drugs may augment sympathetic or parasympathetic functions in peripheral tissues. The response varies

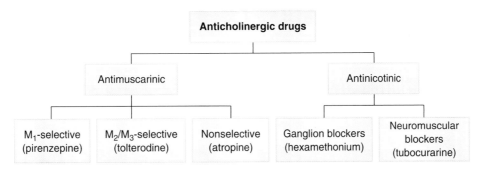

FIGURE 5-2 **Cholinoceptor antagonists based on their inhibition of either muscarinic (M) or nicotinic (N) receptors.** Example drugs are in parentheses.

based on the organ system. In the heart, GI tract, bladder, and lungs, parasympathetic activity predominates. At the neuromuscular junction, these drugs initially increase the force of muscle contractions, followed by fibrillations at higher concentrations, and ultimately ending with paralysis. In the CNS, cholinergic activity parallels what was previously described for the direct-acting cholinergic agonists (Table 5-3), except that the indirectly acting drugs do not typically cause vasodilation because endothelial cells are uninnervated, and do not release EDRF when these drugs are administered.

Clinical Uses

The clinical application of indirect-acting agonists (Table 5-4) differs somewhat from the direct-acting muscarinic and nicotinic agonists. The carbamates receive wider clinical use compared to the alcohol edrophonium or the organophosphates. Carbamates are used to treat myasthenia gravis, urinary retention, glaucoma, Alzheimer's disease, and to reverse neuromuscular blockade. For edrophonium, use is limited due to its short-acting nature; its primary use is in the diagnosis of myasthenia gravis and to treat a myasthenic crisis. Organophosphates are rarely used clinically. Echothiopate is one example of an organophosphate that is used in ophthalmic solution to treat glaucoma. Organophosphates have also been used as insecticides (eg, parathion) or as nerve gases in terrorist attacks (eg, **sarin**). The last group of AChE inhibitors is not placed in the traditional classification of indirect-acting cholinomimetics. These two drugs—donepezil and galantamine—are used exclusively in the treatment of Alzheimer's disease. Although these drugs do not stop, decelerate, or reverse the disease progression, they may promote small and temporary beneficial effects on cognition and functional improvements that may help patients remain independent for longer and assist their caregivers.

Adverse Effects

The adverse clinical manifestations of indirect-acting agonists parallel those of the direct-acting agonists with the following exceptions. First, vasodilation is late and uncommon, and bradycardia is more common than reflex tachycardia. The CNS manifestations are common following organophosphate

overdose, with convulsions followed by respiratory and cardiovascular depression. A mnemonic for remembering the spectrum of adverse effects is DUMBBELSS (diarrhea, urination, miosis, bronchoconstriction, bradycardia, excitation of skeletal muscle and the CNS, lacrimation, salivation, and sweating). As with nicotinic agonists, prolonged stimulation of the N_M receptors at the neuromuscular junction eventually results in muscle paralysis due to depolarizing nerve block, and is a hazard of pesticides containing these indirect-acting agonists.

ANTICHOLINERGIC DRUGS

Drugs that inhibit the effects of acetylcholine are antagonists at muscarinic or nicotinic receptors and are referred to as anticholinergics. Direct-acting cholinoceptor antagonists are classified based on their blockade of muscarinic or nicotinic receptors (Figure 5-2). There are nonspecific muscarinic receptor antagonists that block all subtypes (**atropine** is the prototype) and selective antagonists for certain muscarinic receptor subtypes. M_1 receptors are located on CNS neurons, autonomic postganglionic cell bodies, and many presynaptic sites. M_2 receptors are located in the heart, smooth muscle organs, and some neurons. M_3 receptors are mostly located on smooth muscle or glandular cells. Nicotinic antagonists are subdivided based on whether the drug inhibits postsynaptic N_M receptors at the neuromuscular junction or postsynaptic N_N receptors at the parasympathetic and sympathetic ganglia. The former are used as general anesthesia adjuvants to induce skeletal muscle paralysis. The latter drugs have limited clinical applications and will be discussed briefly.

MUSCARINIC ANTAGONISTS

Beyond receptor selectivity, muscarinic antagonists may be further subdivided based on their clinical application and target organ system. Drugs used for either CNS or ophthalmic applications must be sufficiently lipid soluble to cross specific hydrophobic barriers such as the blood-brain-barrier. A major determinant for the pharmacokinetics is the presence or absence of a permanently charged quaternary amine group

TABLE 5-5 Effects of muscarinic receptor antagonists.

Organ	Effect	Mechanism
CNS	Sedation, anti-motion sickness action, antiparkinson action, amnesia, delirium	Block of muscarinic receptors, unknown subtypes
Eye	Cycloplegia (inability to focus on nearby objects), mydriasis (pupil dilation)	Block of M_3 receptors
Bronchi	Bronchodilation, especially if constricted	Block of M_3 receptors
Gastrointestinal tract	Relaxation, slowed peristalsis	Block of M_1, M_3 receptors
Genitourinary tract	Relaxation of bladder wall, increased bladder capacity	Block of M_2 and M_3 receptors
Heart	Initial bradycardia, especially at low doses; then tachycardia	Tachycardia from block of M_2 receptors in sinoatrial node
Blood vessels	Block of muscarinic vasodilation; not manifest unless a muscarinic agonist is present	Block of M_3 receptors on endothelium of vessels
Glands	Marked reduction of salivation; moderate reduction of lacrimation, sweating; less reduction of gastric secretion	Block of M_1, M_3 receptors
Skeletal muscle	None	

TABLE 5-6 Clinical applications of some antimuscarinic drugs.

Organ System	Drugs	Clinical Applications
CNS	Benztropine Biperiden Trihexyphenidyl	Treat manifestations of Parkinson's disease
	Scopolamine	Prevent or reduce motion sickness
Eye	Cyclopentolate Homatropine Tropicamide	Produce mydriasis and cycloplegia
Bronchi	Aclidinium Ipratropium Tiotropium	Reverse bronchospasm in asthma and chronic obstructive pulmonary disease
Gastrointestinal tract	Dicyclomine Glycopyrrolate Methscopolamine	Reduce transient hypermotility
Genitourinary tract	Oxybutynin Tolterodine Trospium Solifenacin	Treat urinary urgency or incontinence

on these drugs. Presence of this charged group diminishes the penetration across hydrophobic barriers and, to some extent, the uptake by the GI system. Atropine, the prototypical nonselective muscarinic antagonist, is a plant alkaloid and is lipid soluble.

Physiologic Effects

The effects of muscarinic receptor inhibition are presented in Table 5-5. The peripheral actions of muscarinic blockers are mostly predicted by considering the removal of parasympathetic function on various organ systems. At therapeutic doses, cardiovascular effects include an initial bradycardia, possibly as a result of the blockade of postganglionic-presynaptic muscarinic receptors on vagal nerve endings. Bradycardia is followed by tachycardia and increased atrioventricular conduction rate that would be predicted from the blockade

of parasympathetic activity on the heart. In the respiratory system, bronchodilation and reduced secretion occurs. Inhibition of parasympathetic activity in the GI system results in decreased motility and reduction in gastric secretions. In the genitourinary system, decreased detrusor muscle tone results in increased bladder capacity. Lacrimation, salivation, and sweating are also reduced because these secretions are all mediated by cholinergic transmission. The reader should remember that lacrimation and salivation are under parasympathetic control, whereas the eccrine sweat glands are under sympathetic control. Antimuscarinic CNS effects are less predictable. Most common are sedation, decreased motion sickness, and improved motor function in individuals with parkinsonism.

Clinical Uses

Table 5-6 highlights clinical applications of muscarinic antagonists. Reversal of bronchospasm and treatment of parkinsonism are discussed in Chapters 17 and 35, respectively. Direct ocular application of muscarinic antagonists inhibits accommodation in the eye and causes dilation of the pupils. Centuries ago, extract of belladonna, the source of atropine, was used as a cosmetic to dilate the pupil. **Scopolamine**, typically applied as a transdermal patch, decreases motion sickness. **Oxybutynin** or **tolterodine** can be used to decrease urgency and relieve stress incontinence by decreasing hypertonicity of the bladder resulting from neural damage above the micturition reflex arc. Oxybutynin can be taken orally or applied as a transdermal patch; tolterodine is oral only. Newer drugs for incontinence are more selective for antagonism of M_2 and M_3 receptors. Though these drugs may be used in cardiovascular or GI dysfunction, other drug classes with fewer adverse effects have largely replaced them.

Adverse Effects

A traditional mnemonic for antimuscarinic toxicity is "Dry as a bone, hot as a pistol, blind as a bat, red as a beet, and mad as a hatter." This description reflects both the predictable antimuscarinic effects and some unpredictable actions. "Dry as a bone" refers to the inhibition of sweating, salivation, and lacrimation. Patients medicated with these drugs and involved in aerobic activities may also experience hyperthermia ("hot as a pistol") due to inhibited action of thermoregulatory eccrine sweat glands. Moderate tachycardia is also common; other arrhythmias are less common, but could be life-threatening. In the geriatric population, these drugs may exacerbate acute angle-closure glaucoma ("blind as a bat") and urinary retention, especially in men with benign prostate hyperplasia. However, blurred vision can occur in all age groups. With high doses, cutaneous blood vessels dilate, accounting for the "red as a beet" description. In the CNS, sedation, amnesia, and delirium with hallucinations contribute to the "mad as a hatter" description.

NICOTINIC ANTAGONISTS AT THE NEUROMUSCULAR JUNCTION (N_M)

Skeletal muscle contraction is evoked by activation of postsynaptic N_M receptors at the motor end plate. Activation of this nicotinic acetylcholine receptor results in channel opening, with subsequent influx of Na^+ and efflux of K^+ (ie, motor end plate potential). If depolarization is large enough, the motor end plate potential triggers action potential propagation along the entire muscle fiber. Drugs that block the N_M receptor at the neuromuscular junction are clinically useful in producing muscle relaxation as an adjunct to major surgery. Because these drugs are hydrophilic quaternary amines related to acetylcholine, they must be administered parenterally, and do not cross the blood-brain barrier. Neuromuscular blockers are divided based on their mechanism of action as nondepolarizing or depolarizing (Figure 5-3). All of these drugs produce a reversible blockade of the postsynaptic N_M receptor. In general, they are metabolized and eliminated by either the kidneys or the liver.

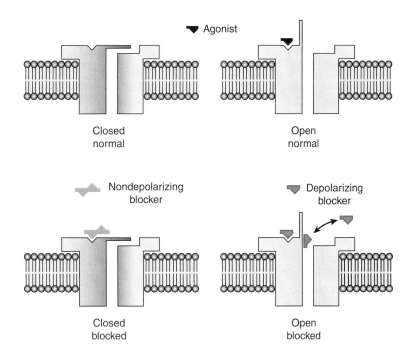

FIGURE 5-3 **Drug interactions with postsynaptic nicotinic cholinergic receptor at the skeletal muscle motor end plate. Top:** Binding of the agonist acetylcholine, resulting in opening of the ion channel (not shown: receptor has two binding sites for acetylcholine). **Bottom left:** Nondepolarizing blocker binds to receptor, preventing binding by endogenous acetylcholine. **Bottom right:** Depolarizing blocker (succinylcholine) both binds to the receptor and blocks the channel. Succinylcholine causes initial depolarization (muscle fasciculations) and then persistent depolarization of the channel (muscle paralysis). Normal closure of the channel gate is prevented and the blocker may move rapidly in and out of the pore. An additional effect on the motor end plate may occur through changes in the lipid environment surrounding the channel (not shown).

TABLE 5-7 Adverse effects of some neuromuscular blocking drugs.

Drug	Effect on Autonomic Ganglia	Effect on Cardiac Muscarinic Receptors	Ability to Release Histamine
Nondepolarizing			
Atracurium	None	None	Slight
Cisatracurium	None	None	None
Pancuronium	None	Moderate block	None
Rocuronium	None	Slight block	None
Tubocurarine	Weak block	None	Moderate
Vecuronium	None	None	None
Depolarizing			
Succinylcholine	Stimulation	Stimulation	Slight

Most neuromuscular blocking agents are N_M receptor antagonists of the nondepolarizing type. The prototype, **tubocurarine**, has a duration of action of approximately an hour, whereas **rocuronium** has a very rapid onset time (1-2 minutes) and a shorter duration of action of 10-20 minutes. Succinylcholine is the only clinically relevant depolarizing neuromuscular blocker drug. Succinylcholine is a direct-acting agonist that binds to the postsynaptic N_M receptor, resulting in depolarization of the motor end plate. This initial depolarization is like that produced by endogenous acetylcholine, but greatly prolonged. Initially, this presents as twitching and fasciculation. Because skeletal muscle is unable to maintain tension without the normal periodic depolarization and repolarization at the motor end plates, the depolarized muscle undergoes relaxation and a paralysis called "Phase I blockade." With continued exposure to the depolarizing neuromuscular blocker, the motor end plate depolarization ceases and repolarization occurs. Even so, the motor end plate cannot undergo depolarization because it is now desensitized (Phase II blockade). The mechanism for this desensitization is uncertain; however, blockade of the channel by succinylcholine may be important.

Physiologic Effects

Both nondepolarizing and depolarizing neuromuscular blockers produce flaccid muscle paralysis. The order of sensitivity of muscles to the nondepolarizing drugs proceeds from the smaller muscles (the first to undergo paralysis, and the last to recover) to the larger ones, with the diaphragm being the most resistant. For succinylcholine, paralysis appears initially in the legs and arms followed by paralysis of the axial musculature.

Clinical Uses

Nondepolarizing blockers are used frequently in major surgery to provide relaxation throughout the procedure. They are occasionally used in intensive care units to prevent respiratory complications when patients are on ventilators. The time of onset and duration of action varies with each drug. Due to its short half-life (minutes), succinylcholine is used almost exclusively to provide brief relaxation during intubation (ie, placing an endotracheal tube) when patients are being prepared for mechanical ventilation.

Adverse Effects

Several nondepolarizing blockers can have cardiovascular effects (Table 5-7) because of the action these drugs have on autonomic ganglia and cardiac muscarinic receptors, or interaction with the general anesthetic. Respiratory paralysis occurs as a direct result of the inhibition of the intercostal muscles and diaphragm, and thus mechanical ventilation is required. With older agents, hypotension occurs as a result of generalized histamine release.

Several adverse events are unique to succinylcholine. Some commonly used inhaled anesthetics, such as **isoflurane**, strongly enhance and prolong the effects of succinylcholine at the neuromuscular junction. Hyperkalemia may occur in patients with burns or SCI, peripheral nerve dysfunction, or muscular dysfunction. Emesis may occur as a result of increased intragastric pressure. Myalgia is a common postoperative complaint, and muscle damage may occur. Therapists should consider these muscular effects the day after succinylcholine is used, and adjust treatment goals accordingly. Finally, malignant hyperthermia is a rare autosomal dominant genetic disorder of skeletal muscle that occurs in certain individuals receiving general anesthetics with succinylcholine. The pathophysiologic mechanism appears to be an increase in intracellular free calcium from the sarcoplasmic reticulum. The syndrome has a rapid onset with tachycardia and hypertension and hallmark muscle rigidity and hyperthermia. Hyperkalemia and eventual acidosis may also occur. Treatment includes **dantrolene**, a drug that inhibits intracellular calcium release from the sarcoplasmic reticulum, as well as measures that decrease body temperature and blood pressure.

NICOTINIC ANTAGONISTS AT AUTONOMIC GANGLIA (N_N)

Postsynaptic N_N receptors are located in both parasympathetic and sympathetic ganglia. Similar to the N_M receptors, N_N receptors are susceptible to both nondepolarizing and depolarizing inhibition. The drugs used clinically are all nondepolarizing competitive antagonists (eg, **hexamethonium**, **mecamylamine**, **trimetaphan**). However, there is evidence that some of these drugs may also block the ion channel.

Physiologic Effects

Table 5-8 shows the physiologic effects of these drugs. Due to the inhibition of sympathetic control of venous tone, these drugs cause venous pooling and orthostatic hypotension. Moderate tachycardia and decreased cardiac output due to the reduction in venous return and decreased contractility may also occur.

TABLE 5-8 Physiologic effects of ganglion-blocking drugs (nicotinic N_N receptor antagonists).

Organ	Effects
CNS	Antinicotinic actions may include reduction of nicotine craving and amelioration of Tourette syndrome (mecamylamine only)
Eye	Moderate mydriasis and cycloplegia
Bronchi	Little effect; asthmatics may note bronchodilation
Gastrointestinal tract	Markedly reduced motility; constipation may be severe
Genitourinary tract	Reduced bladder contractility; impairment of erection and ejaculation
Heart	Moderate tachycardia in young adults; reduction in force of contraction and cardiac output at rest; block of exercise-induced changes
Blood vessels	Reduction in arteriolar tone; marked reduction in venous tone; decreased blood pressure; orthostatic hypotension may be severe
Glands	Reductions in salivation, lacrimation, sweating, and gastric secretion
Skeletal muscle	No significant effect

Clinical Uses

Due to the fact that the adverse effects of these drugs are severe, patients are only able to tolerate these drugs for a limited period. In addition, some drugs demonstrate short half-lives or are not orally active, reducing their clinical value. At present, two N_N antagonists may be used clinically. Mecamylamine, a lipophilic synthetic amine that crosses into the CNS, is being studied to decrease nicotine addiction and to treat Tourette syndrome. Trimetaphan may be used during a hypertensive crisis or to produce controlled hypotension in some surgical scenarios. Because these drugs inhibit the autonomic nervous system, they are rarely used and typically only for acute situations.

REHABILITATION RELEVANCE

The cholinergic or anticholinergic adverse effects most likely to affect rehabilitation activities are summarized below.

Cholinomimetic Drugs

- **Dyspnea** may occur with either direct- or indirect-acting muscarinic agonists. Bronchoconstriction may decrease the ability to participate in aerobic activities. To minimize dyspnea, aerobic activities should be designed to allow the patient more time to achieve aerobic goals. Consider patient education on "pursed lip breathing" and pacing techniques.
- **Decreased exercise performance** may occur when nonprescribed sources of nicotine (eg, cigarettes, dipping tobacco) are used prior to exercise. Decreased performance may result from unanticipated increases in blood pressure *beyond that* resulting from the exercise. Additionally, smoking may increase plasma carbon monoxide, which decreases oxygen-carrying capacity of blood. Angina pectoris is a potential outcome from these factors. Educate patients of the potential problems of consuming nonprescribed nicotine prior to aerobic activities. Therapists should also account for the potential for increased blood pressure prior to exercise when patients are *prescribed* nicotine in the form of patches, gum, or other formulations.
- **Increased urination frequency** may occur with muscarinic agonists. Provide patient education on the fact that abdominal contraction may *increase* the need to void.
- **Prevention of pupillary dilation** in response to decreased light may result from muscarinic agonists. Low light levels in the room, especially in conjunction with sedation, increase the chance of falls. Fall risk reduction strategies should be employed.

Anticholinergic Drugs

- **Hyperthermia** may result during aerobic activities due to perspiration inhibition caused by antimuscarinic drugs. Hyperthermia should be taken into account when developing a treatment plan. Aerobic activities should be conducted in cooler, well-ventilated areas.

- **Increased heart rate** and possibly arrhythmias may result from antimuscarinic drug effects.
- **Decreased pupillary constriction** in response to bright light may occur from antimuscarinic agents. Therapists should be aware that patients may be sensitive to bright lights and adjust light accordingly.
- **Sedation and decreased cognitive function** may occur with muscarinic receptor antagonists. High doses may also cause hallucinations, especially in older adults. If adverse effects decrease patients' understanding of instructions

and/or participation in rehabilitation programs, consider scheduling therapy sessions at the end of a dosage period when plasma drug level will be lowest.

- **Decreased muscle force, myalgia**, and potential muscle damage can occur with succinylcholine (depolarizing nicotinic receptor antagonist). Decreased muscle force may inhibit functional activities, especially in the early postoperative period. Alter functional training to allow for decreased maximal muscle force.

CASE CONCLUSION

During the initial sliding board transfer, contraction of abdominal musculature in conjunction with a Valsalva maneuver increased pressure on the patient's spastic bladder, which resulted in incontinence. When tolterodine is used to decrease bladder spasticity, it is frequently prescribed twice daily. The patient's first daily dosage was taken at breakfast just prior to rehabilitation activities. After an oral dose, plasma level peaks 1-2 hours later, and the elimination

half-life is approximately 2 hours. Insufficient time had elapsed for the initial tolterodine dose to reach peak plasma levels prior to rehabilitation activity. Thus, the dose may not have been sufficient to decrease contraction of the overactive bladder muscles. Rehabilitation activity should be rescheduled for approximately 1-2 hours after tolterodine is taken to maximize pharmacologic effect and minimize the patient's incontinence.

CHAPTER 5 QUESTIONS

1. Inhibition of muscarinic receptors may result in which of the following adverse effects?
   a. Muscle weakness
   b. Hyperactive bladder
   c. Hyperthermia
   d. Hypertension

2. Inhibition of which of the following receptors would result in skeletal muscle paralysis?
   a. Nicotinic type-N (N_N) receptors
   b. Nicotinic type-M (N_M) receptors
   c. Muscarinic-1 (M_1) receptors
   d. Muscarinic-2 (M_2) receptors

3. Malignant hyperthermia is a potential adverse effect associated with which of the following drugs?
   a. Succinylcholine
   b. Pancuronium
   c. Oxybutynin
   d. Neostigmine

4. Which of the following drug classes may be clinically used to improve muscle weakness in individuals with myasthenia gravis?
   a. Muscarinic agonists
   b. Nicotinic type-N (N_N) antagonists
   c. Muscarinic antagonists
   d. Indirect-acting cholinergic agonists

5. Which of the following drugs has addictive potential?
   a. Neostigmine
   b. Nicotine
   c. Tubocurarine
   d. Physostigmine

6. Which of the following drug classes may decrease hyperactivity of the bladder in a person with a spinal cord injury?
   a. Muscarinic agonists
   b. Nicotinic type-N (N_N) antagonists
   c. Muscarinic antagonists
   d. Nicotinic type-M (N_M) antagonists

7. Which of the following is an adverse effect associated with muscarinic agonists?
   a. Constipation
   b. Miosis
   c. Bronchodilation
   d. Hypertension

8. Which of the following drugs has clinical application for motion sickness?
   a. Edrophonium
   b. Nicotine
   c. Scopolamine
   d. Carbachol

9. Which of the following is the mechanism of action for all nicotinic receptors?

    a. Increasing diacylglycerol (DAG) as a second messenger
    b. Increasing cyclic adenosine monophosphate (cAMP) as a second messenger
    c. Increasing inositol-1, 4, 5-triphosphate (IP_3) as a second messenger
    d. Depolarization as a result of opening a Na^+/K^+ channel

10. Which of the following drugs increases cholinergic activity by inhibiting acetylcholinesterase?

    a. Bethanechol
    b. Vecuronium
    c. Rivastigmine
    d. Nicotine

Sympathomimetics and Sympatholytics

CASE STUDY

A physical therapy clinic is associated with a wellness center where the practice provides consulting advice on aerobic and resistance exercise training. D.J. is a 47-year-old man who works as an accountant for a local business. Recently, his physician told him that he had hypertension and that his "good" cholesterol was low. The physician suggested that D.J. begin a regular exercise program to lower his blood pressure and to help improve his cholesterol profile. At his last medical evaluation, measurements of resting blood pressure and heart rate were 135/84 mm Hg and 84 beats per minute (bpm), respectively. His body mass index was 29 kg/m^2. D.J. is currently taking no prescription drugs. The physical therapist developed an aerobic and upper extremity strength training program that D.J. has been performing three times per week during the past month, without incident. D.J. arrived today (Monday) to participate in his program. He stated that he missed Friday due to a cold. Over the weekend, he began taking over-the-counter cold medications to relieve his symptoms. These preparations included the topical decongestant Afrin (oxymetazoline) to relieve nasal congestion and oral Advil Cold and Sinus (ibuprofen and pseudoephedrine). During the conversation, the therapist notices that D.J. is moving his left arm in a circular motion and rubbing his left shoulder. He states that his left shoulder has been hurting intermittently for the past couple days just as it is now.

REHABILITATION FOCUS

Drugs with sympathomimetic and sympatholytic properties are used in a broad spectrum of pathophysiologic conditions to either mirror or inhibit the role of the sympathetic nervous system (SNS) and catecholamine neurotransmitters in the central nervous system (CNS). Drugs with sympathomimetic or sympatholytic properties are found in many other drug groups and are discussed in several chapters. Sympathomimetic drugs are prescribed to treat upper and lower respiratory dysfunctions (Chapter 35). Sympatholytic drugs are used in the treatment of various cardiovascular pathophysiologies (Chapters 7-10). Less obvious drugs that have either sympathomimetic clinical uses or adverse effects include tricyclic antidepressants and MAO$_A$ inhibitors used to treat depression (Chapter 19) and MAO$_B$ and COMT inhibitors used to treat parkinsonism (Chapter 17).

BACKGROUND

Receptors found in the SNS may be divided into alpha (α) or beta (β) adrenergic receptors (adrenoceptors) or dopamine (D) receptors. Drugs that bind to these receptors and augment the system are called sympathomimetics, while those that bind to these receptors and inhibit or prevent the binding of *endogenous* ligands are called sympatholytics. The sympathomimetics constitute an important group of agonists used for cardiovascular, respiratory, and other conditions. Sympathomimetics are readily divided into subgroups based on their spectrum of affinity for α, β, or D receptors. Alternatively, these agents may be divided into subgroups based on whether their mode of action is direct or indirect. Sympatholytics are antagonists frequently used in cardiovascular conditions, but are also used in diverse conditions such as urinary hesitancy and open-angle glaucoma. Sympatholytics are divided into primary subgroups on the basis of their adrenoceptor (α and β) selectivity.

SYMPATHOMIMETIC DRUGS

Mode of Action

Sympathomimetics may be divided into those that *directly* activate adrenoceptors and those that *indirectly* increase the concentration of catecholamine transmitter in the synapse (Figure 6-1). Indirect-acting agonists can release stored catecholamines (eg, amphetamine derivatives and tyramine) or inhibit the reuptake of catecholamines by the presynaptic

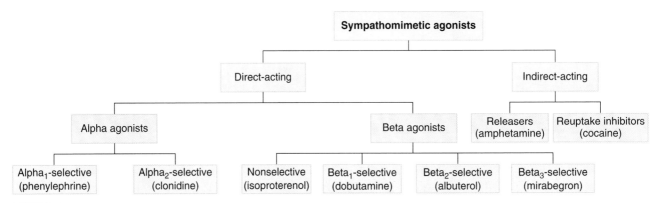

FIGURE 6-1 **Sympathomimetic agonists can be classified into subgroups on the basis of which receptors they activate: alpha (α) or beta (β) adrenergic receptors (adrenoceptors) or dopamine (D) receptors (not shown).** Sympathomimetics are also divided into subgroups based on whether their mode of action is direct (at postsynaptic receptors) or indirect (other than at postsynaptic receptors). Prototype drugs are in listed in parentheses.

nerve terminals that release them (eg, **cocaine** and tricyclic antidepressants; Figure 4-3). Although inhibition of enzymes involved in catecholamine metabolism (ie, blockade of catechol-*O*-methyltransferase [COMT] and monoamine oxidase [MAO]) has little direct effect on autonomic activity, MAO inhibition increases catecholamine stores within adrenergic synaptic vesicles and thus may potentiate the action of other indirect-acting sympathomimetics.

Spectrum of Action

Both α and β adrenoceptors are further subdivided into subtypes. The distribution of these receptors is set forth in Table 4-3. **Epinephrine** may be considered a single prototype with agonist effects at all adrenoceptor subtypes (α_1, α_2, β_1, β_2, and β_3). Separate prototypes—**phenylephrine** for α receptors and **isoproterenol** for β receptors—have also been characterized. Dopamine receptors constitute a third class of adrenoceptors. The just-mentioned drugs have relatively little effect on dopamine receptors. In contrast, when dopamine is given as a drug, it can activate β receptors at intermediate doses and α receptors at large doses. The relative affinities of representative drugs are presented in Table 6-1.

Chemistry and Pharmacokinetics

The endogenous adrenoceptor agonists (epinephrine, **norepinephrine**, and **dopamine**) are catecholamines that are rapidly metabolized by the endogenous enzymes COMT and MAO. As a result, these adrenoceptor agonists are inactive when given orally. When norepinephrine, epinephrine, and dopamine are released from presynaptic nerve terminals, they are subsequently taken up into these same presynaptic nerve terminals as well as into perisynaptic cells; this uptake may also occur when they are given as drugs. Isoproterenol is a synthetic catecholamine that is not readily taken up into presynaptic nerve terminals. When given parenterally, these agonists have a short duration of action and do not enter the CNS in significant amounts.

Indirect-acting sympathomimetics that can release stored transmitter from noradrenergic nerve terminals include amphetamines, **ephedrine**, and tyramine. Phenylisopropylamine derivatives are modified from phenylethylamine, which is the parent compound from which sympathomimetic drugs are derived. These drugs are resistant to breakdown by MAO; most of them are not catecholamines and are therefore also resistant to COMT. These agents are orally active, enter the CNS, and have effects that last much longer than those of catecholamines. Amphetamines and ephedrine are examples of phenylisopropylamine derivatives. Tyramine, a by-product of tyrosine metabolism in the body and an amine found in certain foods, is rapidly metabolized by MAO except in patients who are taking an MAO inhibitor drug. MAO inhibitors are sometimes used in the treatment of depression (Chapter 19).

TABLE 6-1 **Relative selectivity of adrenoceptor agonists.**

	Relative Receptor Affinities
Alpha agonists	
Phenylephrine	$\alpha_1 > \alpha_2 >>>>> \beta$
Clonidine	$\alpha_2 > \alpha_1 >>>>> \beta$
Mixed α and β agonists	
Norepinephrine	$\alpha_1 = \alpha_2; \beta_1 >> \beta_2$
Epinephrine	$\alpha_1 = \alpha_2; \beta_1 = \beta_2$
Beta agonists	
Dobutamine[a]	$\beta_1 > \beta_2 >>>> \alpha$
Isoproterenol	$\beta_1 = \beta_2 >>>> \alpha$
Terbutaline, metaproterenol, albuterol	$\beta_2 >> \beta_1 >>>> \alpha$
Dopamine agonists	
Dopamine	$D_1 = D_2 >> \beta >> \alpha$
Fenoldopam	$D_1 >> D_2$

α, alpha; β, beta; D, dopamine.
[a]Dobutamine is a relatively β_1-selective synthetic catecholamine.

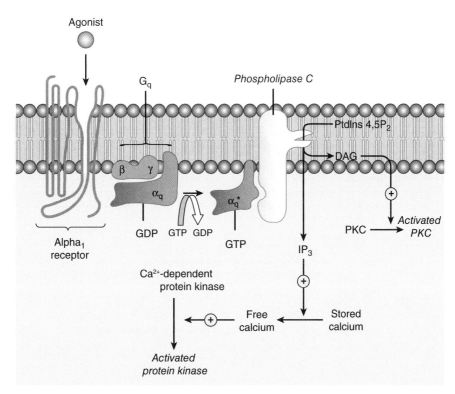

FIGURE 6-2 **Activation of α_1 responses.** Stimulation of α_1 receptors by an agonist leads to activation of a G_q coupling protein. The activated α subunit (α_q*) of this G protein activates the membrane-bound effector, phospholipase C, which leads to the release of IP_3 (inositol 1,4,5-trisphosphate) and DAG (diacylglycerol) from phosphatidylinositol 4,5-bisphosphate (PtdIns 4,5-P_2). IP_3 stimulates release of intracellular calcium stores, leading to increased concentration of cytoplasmic Ca^{2+}. The Ca^{2+} may then activate Ca^{2+}-dependent protein kinases, which in turn phosphorylate their substrates. DAG activates protein kinase C (PKC).

Mechanisms of Action

When catecholamines bind to and activate α_1 receptors, the effects are mediated by the coupling protein G_q. When G_q is activated, the protein activates the phosphoinositide cascade and causes the release of inositol-1,4,5-trisphosphate (IP_3) and diacylglycerol (DAG) from membrane lipids (Figure 6-2). Calcium is subsequently released from intracellular stores. Opening of calcium channels may also play a role in increasing intracellular calcium concentration. In smooth muscle cells, this elevated intracellular calcium results in contraction. In contrast, binding and activation of α_2 receptors results in inhibition of adenylate cyclase via the coupling protein G_i, and subsequent decrease of the second messenger cyclic adenosine monophosphate (cAMP) (Figure 6-3).

Activation of β receptors (β_1, β_2, and β_3) stimulates adenylate cyclase via the coupling protein G_s, which leads to an increase in intracellular cAMP. Cyclic AMP acts as a second messenger mediating the cellular response to β-receptor stimulation (Figure 6-3).

Agonist binding of D_1 receptors activates adenylate cyclase in neurons and vascular smooth muscle cells. D_2 receptors are more important in the brain, but probably also play a significant role as presynaptic receptors on peripheral nerves. These receptors inhibit adenylate cyclase activity, open potassium channels, and decrease calcium influx.

Physiologic Effects

CNS

Catecholamines do not enter the CNS effectively. Sympathomimetics such as amphetamines that do enter the CNS have a spectrum of stimulant effects, beginning with mild alerting or reduction of fatigue, and progressing to anorexia, euphoria, and insomnia. Some central effects probably result from the release of dopamine in certain dopaminergic tracts. Very high doses of amphetamines lead to marked anxiety or aggressiveness, paranoia, and, rarely, convulsions. Direct-acting α_2 agonists such as clonidine act quite differently in that they *decrease* sympathetic neuronal outflow and have sedative effects.

Eye

Topical phenylephrine and similar α_1 adrenergic agonists activate the pupillary dilator muscle. Accommodation is not significantly affected. Alpha$_2$ agonists increase the outflow of aqueous humor from the eye and can clinically be used to reduce intraocular pressure.

Gastrointestinal Tract

The gastrointestinal tract has an abundance of α and β receptors, located on both smooth muscle cells and neurons of the enteric nervous system. Activation of either α or β receptors

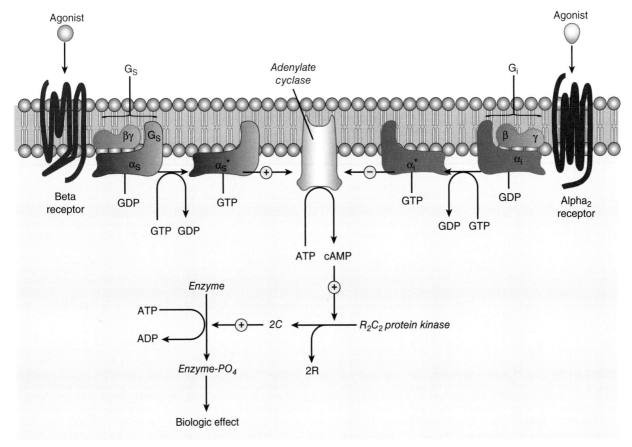

FIGURE 6-3 **Activation and inhibition of adenylate cyclase by agonists that bind to catecholamine receptors.** Binding to β adrenoceptors stimulates adenylate cyclase by activating the stimulatory G protein (G_s), which leads to dissociation of its α subunit charged with GTP. This α_s subunit directly activates adenylate cyclase, resulting in an increased rate of synthesis of cyclic adenosine monophosphate (cAMP). α_2-adrenoceptor ligands inhibit adenylate cyclase by causing dissociation of the inhibitory G protein (G_i) into its subunits: an α_i subunit charged with GTP and a β-γ unit. The mechanism by which these subunits inhibit adenylate cyclase is uncertain. cAMP binds to the regulatory subunit (R) of cAMP-dependent protein kinase, leading to the liberation of active catalytic subunits (C) that phosphorylate specific protein substrates and modify their activity. These catalytic units also phosphorylate the cAMP response element binding protein that which modifies gene expression (not shown).

leads to relaxation of the smooth muscle. Alpha$_2$ agonists may decrease salt and water secretion into the intestine.

Genitourinary Tract

Alpha adrenergic receptors in the bladder trigone and sphincter area mediate contraction of the sphincter. Thus, some sympathomimetics can be used to increase sphincter tone and promote urinary continence. In contrast, the selective β$_3$-agonist **mirabegron** relaxes bladder smooth muscle, so it is used in the treatment of overactive bladder. Beta$_2$ agonists may cause significant uterine relaxation in pregnant women near term, but the doses required also cause significant tachycardia.

Vascular Smooth Muscle

The response of blood vessels to catecholamine binding depends on the dominant receptor type within that particular vascular bed. Selective α$_1$ agonists (eg, phenylephrine) constrict skin and splanchnic blood vessels. Because these drugs increase blood pressure, they often evoke a compensatory reflex bradycardia. Selective α$_2$ agonists (eg, **clonidine**) cause vasoconstriction when administered intravenously or topically (as a nasal spray). However, when given orally they accumulate in the CNS and *reduce* sympathetic outflow and blood pressure as described in Chapter 7. Selective β$_1$ agonists have relatively little effect on blood vessels. Beta$_2$ agonists (eg, **terbutaline**) significantly reduce arteriolar tone in the skeletal muscle vascular bed and can therefore reduce peripheral vascular resistance and blood pressure. Dopamine, via activation of D$_1$ receptors, causes vasodilation in the splanchnic and renal vascular beds. This effect has been used in the treatment of renal failure associated with shock. D$_1$ receptors may also mediate natriuresis, with subsequent excretion of sodium and water and a potential lowering of blood pressure. At higher doses, dopamine also activates β receptors in the heart and elsewhere; at still higher doses, α receptors are activated.

Heart

The heart is well supplied with β$_1$ and β$_2$ receptors, though β$_1$ receptors predominate in some parts of the heart. Activation of both receptor subtypes results in increased normal and

TABLE 6-2 Effects of prototypical sympathomimetics on vascular resistance, blood pressure, and heart rate.

Drug	Effect on				
	Skin and splanchnic vasculature resistance	Skeletal muscle vasculature resistance	Renal vasculature resistance	Mean blood pressure	Heart rate
Phenylephrine	↑↑↑	↑	↑	↑↑	↓[a]
Isoproterenol	—	↓↓	—	↓↓	↑↑
Norepinephrine	↑↑↑↑	↑	↑	↑↑↑	↓[a]

[a]Compensatory reflex response.

abnormal pacemaker activity (chronotropic), contractility (inotropic), and conduction (dromotropic) responses.

Summary of Cardiovascular Actions

Table 6-2 summarizes the effects of prototypical sympathomimetics on vascular resistance, blood pressure, and heart rate. Sympathomimetics with both α and β_1 effects (eg, norepinephrine) increase blood pressure and activate the baroreceptor reflex. The increased afferent baroreceptor activity ultimately results in increased efferent vagal activity. This reflex vagal effect often dominates over any direct β-induced effects on heart rate, so that a slow infusion of norepinephrine typically causes increased blood pressure and bradycardia. The feedback regulation of blood pressure is further discussed in Chapter 4 (Figure 4-5). Note that a pure α agonist (phenylephrine) routinely slows heart rate via the baroreceptor reflex, in response to increased MAP. In contrast, a pure β agonist (isoproterenol) almost always increases heart rate, in response to a decreased MAP. Diastolic blood pressure is primarily affected by peripheral vascular resistance and heart rate. The adrenoceptors with the greatest effects on vascular resistance are α receptors and β_2 receptors. Systolic pressure is the sum of the diastolic and the pulse pressures. The pulse pressure is determined mainly by the stroke volume (a function of contractility), which is influenced by β_1 receptors.

Bronchi

Bronchial smooth muscle relaxes markedly in response to β_2 agonists. These agents are the most efficacious and reliable drugs available for reversing bronchospasm in asthma (Chapter 35).

Metabolic and Hormonal Effects

Beta$_1$ agonists increase renal renin secretion, which can result in increased blood pressure. Beta$_2$ agonists increase insulin secretion by the pancreas. Activation of β_1 and β_2 receptors increases glycogenolysis in the liver. The resulting hyperglycemia is countered by the increased insulin levels. Transport of glucose out of the liver is associated initially with hyperkalemia; transport into peripheral organs (especially skeletal muscle) is accompanied by movement of potassium into these cells, resulting in a later hypokalemia. Activation of β adrenoceptors in fat cells increases lipolysis.

Clinical Uses

Table 6-3 lists clinical applications for select sympathomimetics.

Anaphylaxis

Epinephrine is the drug of choice for the immediate treatment of anaphylactic shock. Sometimes, it may be supplemented with antihistamines and glucocorticoids, but neither of these drug classes is as efficacious or rapidly acting as epinephrine.

CNS

Phenylisopropylamines such as amphetamines are widely abused for their ability to defer sleep and elevate mood (Chapter 21). Clinical indications include narcolepsy, attention deficit disorder, and, with appropriate controls, weight reduction. The anorexiant effect may be helpful in initiating weight loss, but is insufficient to maintain weight loss unless individuals also receive intensive dietary and psychological counseling and support.

Eye

Alpha agonists, especially phenylephrine, are often used topically to cause pupil dilation (mydriasis) and to reduce the conjunctival itching and congestion caused by irritation or allergy. These drugs do not cause cycloplegia (loss of accommodation). Epinephrine has been used topically in the treatment of glaucoma. Phenylephrine has also been used for glaucoma, mainly outside the United States. **Apraclonidine** and **brimonidine** are α_2-selective agonists commonly used as topical therapies to reduce increased intraocular pressure associated with glaucoma.

Cardiovascular Applications

The cardiovascular applications of sympathomimetics may be broadly divided into clinical conditions in which the goal is to increase blood flow, decrease blood flow, or increase blood pressure. Increased blood flow is desired in acute heart failure

TABLE 6-3 Pharmacokinetics and clinical applications of some sympathomimetics.

Drug	Oral Activity	Duration of Action	Clinical Applications
Catecholamines			
Epinephrine	No	Minutes	Anaphylaxis (to cause vasoconstriction and bronchodilation)
			Glaucoma
			To cause vasoconstriction
Norepinephrine	No	Minutes	To cause vasoconstriction in hypotension
Isoproterenol	Poor	Minutes	Asthma
			Atrioventricular block (rare)
Dopamine	No	Minutes	Shock
Dobutamine			Heart failure
Other Sympathomimetics			
Albuterol	Moderate	Hours	Asthma
Amphetamines	Yes	Hours	Attention deficit disorder
Mirabegron	Yes	Hours	Urinary incontinence
Oxymetazoline	Yes	Hours	Nasal congestion
Xylometazoline			
Phenylephrine	Poor	Hours	Nasal congestion
			To cause mydriasis or vasoconstriction

and some types of shock. In these clinical situations, an increase in cardiac output and blood flow to the tissues is needed. Beta$_1$ agonists may be useful because they increase cardiac contractility and reduce afterload (to some degree) by decreasing the impedance to ventricular ejection through a small β$_2$ effect. This latter effect is because these drugs have a lesser capacity to stimulate β$_2$ receptors as well as β$_1$ receptors (Table 6-1). In contrast, certain clinical conditions require vasoconstriction to either decrease blood flow (in the case of hemorrhage) or to increase blood pressure (in the case of spinal shock). Alpha$_1$ agonists are useful vasoconstrictors in these situations. When used to decrease blood flow, α agonists are often mixed with local anesthetics to reduce the loss of the anaesthetic from the area of injection into the circulation. In spinal shock, α agonists may temporarily maintain blood pressure and perfusion of the brain, heart, and kidneys. On the other hand, shock due to septicemia or myocardial infarction is often made worse by vasoconstrictors because sympathetic discharge is usually already increased. Chronic orthostatic hypotension due to inadequate sympathetic tone can also be treated with an orally active α$_1$ agonist such as **midodrine**. Alternatively, orally active **droxidopa** is a prodrug that is converted to norepinephrine and has also been approved for neurogenic orthostatic hypotension.

Upper and Lower Respiratory System

Alpha$_1$ agonists are used to vasoconstrict the nasal vasculature and thus decrease sinus congestion. Both short- and long-acting β$_2$-selective agonists are used to relieve bronchoconstriction in asthma and chronic obstructive pulmonary disease. The short-acting β$_2$-selective agonists are not recommended for prophylaxis of bronchoconstriction (except for exercise-induced asthma), but they are effective and may be lifesaving during an acute asthma attack. The long-acting β$_2$-selective agonists

are recommended for bronchoconstriction prophylaxis, when combined with controller medications (Chapter 35).

Genitourinary Tract

Beta$_2$ agonists (**ritodrine**, terbutaline) are used to suppress premature labor, but the cardiac stimulant effect may be hazardous to both mother and fetus. Nonsteroidal anti-inflammatory drugs, calcium channel blockers, and magnesium are also used for this indication. The β$_3$-selective agonist mirabegron is used in the treatment of overactive bladder because of its ability to relax the detrusor muscle and allow bladder filling, which reduces the frequency of micturition. Long-acting oral sympathomimetics such as ephedrine are sometimes used to improve urinary continence in children with enuresis and in older adults. This action is mediated by α receptors in the trigone of the bladder and, in men, the smooth muscle of the prostate.

Adverse Effects

Because of their limited penetration into the brain, catecholamines have little CNS toxicity when given systemically. In the periphery, adverse effects result from activation of α and β receptors: excessive vasoconstriction, cardiac arrhythmias, myocardial infarction, and pulmonary edema or hemorrhage.

The phenylisopropylamines cross the blood-brain barrier and produce mild to severe CNS toxicity, depending on dosage. In small doses, they induce nervousness, anorexia, and insomnia; in higher doses, they may cause anxiety, aggressiveness, or paranoid behavior. Convulsions may occur.

Peripherally acting agents have toxicities that are predictable on the basis of the receptors they activate. Thus, α$_1$ agonists cause hypertension and β$_1$ agonists cause sinus tachycardia and serious arrhythmias. Beta$_2$ agonists cause tremors,

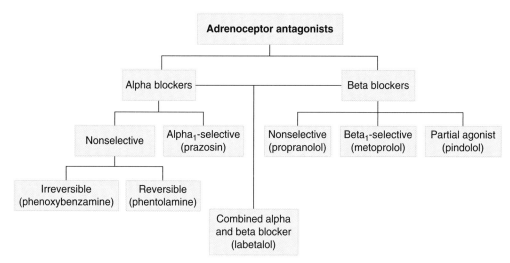

FIGURE 6-4 **Antagonists at α and β receptors are divided into subgroups on the basis of their receptor selectivity.** Prototype drugs are listed in parentheses.

and at higher doses, cardiac arrhythmias. Both β_1- and β_2-receptor stimulation may increase blood glucose levels. Note that none of the β agonists is purely selective; thus, at high doses, β_1-selective agents have β_2 actions and vice versa. The major adverse effect of β_3-selective agents is increased blood pressure. Other adverse effects occur at less than 5% incidence. Cocaine is of special importance as a drug of abuse (Chapter 21). The major toxicities of this drug include cardiac arrhythmias or myocardial infarction and convulsions. A fatal outcome is more common with acute cocaine overdose than with any other sympathomimetic.

SYMPATHOLYTIC DRUGS

Drugs that inhibit SNS activity are divided into subgroups based on their α and β adrenoceptor selectivity and then further divided based on their respective receptor *subtype* selectivity (Figure 6-4). Table 6-4 shows the relative receptor selectivity for certain adrenoceptor antagonists.

α-BLOCKING DRUGS

Subdivisions of the α-receptor antagonists are based on the selective affinity for α_1 versus α_2 receptors. Other features of classification are their reversibility and duration of action. **Phentolamine** is a competitive, reversible, nonselective α-blocker. **Phenoxybenzamine** is an irreversible, long-acting antagonist that is only slightly α_1 selective. Because there are clinical advantages to α_1-selective blockade, several drugs have been developed for this characteristic: **prazosin**, **doxazosin**, **terazosin**, and **tamsulosin**. Except for phenoxybenzamine, other α-adrenoceptor antagonists are competitive, meaning that their effects may be surmounted by increased concentrations of an agonist for the α receptor.

Alpha adrenergic receptor antagonists are active by oral and parenteral routes, though phentolamine is rarely given orally. Phentolamine has a duration of action of about

2-4 hours when used orally, and 20-40 minutes when given parenterally. Phenoxybenzamine has a short elimination half-life but a long duration of action (~ 48 hours) because it binds covalently to its receptor. Prazosin has a short duration of action (2-4 hours), while the other α_1-selective receptor antagonists act for 8-24 hours.

Physiologic Effects

Nonselective α-receptor antagonists (eg, phenoxybenzamine) cause a predictable blockade of the α-mediated responses to sympathetic discharge (Table 4-3) and to exogenous sympathomimetics. The most important effects of nonselective α-receptor antagonists are those on the cardiovascular system. Although there are no significant *direct* cardiac effects, the resulting reduction in vascular tone decreases arterial and venous pressures. This drop in mean arterial pressure activates baroreceptor reflex-mediated tachycardia (Figure 4-5), which may be exaggerated due to blockade of α_2 autoreceptors on

TABLE 6-4 **Relative selectivity of antagonists for adrenoceptors.**

Drug	Receptor Affinity
α Antagonists	
Prazosin, terazosin, doxazosin	$\alpha_1 \ggg\gg \alpha_2$
Phenoxybenzamine	$\alpha_1 > \alpha_2$
Phentolamine	$\alpha_1 = \alpha_2$
Mixed Antagonists	
Labetalol, carvedilol	$\beta_1 = \beta_2 \geq \alpha_1 > \alpha_2$
β Antagonists	
Metoprolol, acebutolol, alprenolol, atenolol, betaxolol, celiprolol, esmolol	$\beta_1 \ggg \beta_2$
Propranolol, carteolol, penbutolol, pindolol, timolol	$\beta_1 = \beta_2$

the presynaptic side of cardiac sympathetic nerve terminals. Normally, activation of α_2 autoreceptors reduces norepinephrine release; with blockade, net release of norepinephrine is increased (Figure 4-3). Phentolamine also has some non-α-mediated vasodilating effects. Because prazosin and other α_1-selective receptor antagonists block vascular α_1 receptors much more effectively than the presynaptic α_2 autoreceptors on SNS fibers innervating the heart, these drugs cause much less tachycardia than the nonselective α-blockers when reducing blood pressure.

Clinical Uses

Nonselective α-blockers have limited clinical applications. The main application is in presurgical management of pheochromocytoma (tumors that secrete catecholamines). Individuals with this condition may have severe hypertension and reduced blood volume, which should be corrected before subjecting the patient to the stress of surgery. Phenoxybenzamine is usually used during this preparatory phase; phentolamine is sometimes used during surgery. Phenoxybenzamine also has a serotonin receptor-blocking effect, which justifies its occasional use in carcinoid tumor. The drug also has an H_1 antihistamine effect, which leads to its use in mastocytosis. If potent α *agonists* such as norepinephrine are accidentally infiltrated into the body, tissue ischemia and necrosis may occur if not promptly reversed. In this case, phentolamine is sometimes infiltrated into the affected ischemic area to prevent tissue damage. Overdose with drugs of abuse such as amphetamine, cocaine, or **phenylpropanolamine** (a sympathomimetic previously found in cold-remedy and weight-control products that have since been withdrawn from the United States market) may lead to severe hypertension because of their indirect sympathomimetic actions. This hypertension usually responds well to α-receptor antagonists. Sudden cessation of clonidine therapy leads to rebound hypertension; this phenomenon can be treated with phentolamine.

Generic names for the selective α_1-blockers often end in "-osin." Prazosin, doxazosin, and terazosin are used in the management of hypertension (Chapter 7) and in urinary hesitancy and prevention of urinary retention in men with benign prostate hyperplasia (BPH). Tamsulosin is replacing many of the previously used α_1-blocking agents in the treatment of BPH because this drug has more specificity for the α_{1A} receptor–mediated contraction in prostate smooth muscle than for the other α_1-receptor subtypes present in vascular smooth muscle. Thus, tamsulosin relaxes prostate smooth muscle, but with minimal orthostatic hypotension effects.

Adverse Effects

The most important toxicities of the α-blockers are simple extensions of their α-blocking effects. The main manifestations are orthostatic hypotension and, in the case of the nonselective agents, marked reflex tachycardia. Tachycardia is less common and less severe with α_1-selective receptor antagonists. In patients with coronary disease, angina may be precipitated by

the tachycardia. Oral administration of any of these drugs may cause nausea and vomiting. The α_1-selective agents are associated with an exaggerated orthostatic hypotensive response shortly after initiation of treatment. Therefore, the first dose is usually small and taken just before going to bed.

β-BLOCKING DRUGS

All of the clinically used β-receptor antagonists (β-blockers) are competitive inhibitors. **Propranolol** is the prototype. Beta blockers are usually classified into subgroups on the basis of β_1 selectivity, partial agonist activity, local anesthetic action, and lipid solubility (Tables 6-4 and 6-5). General nomenclature for β-blockers is that generic drug names end in "-lol."

Labetalol and **carvedilol** have combined β- and α-blocking actions. Nadolol, propranolol, and timolol are typical nonselective β-receptor antagonists. These full antagonists may cause severe bronchospasm in people with obstructive lung disease due to their action at β_2 receptors. Drugs such as **acebutolol**, **atenolol**, **esmolol**, and **metoprolol** demonstrate a greater selectivity for β_1 receptors compared to β_2 receptors. This property may be advantageous when treating individuals with asthma because inhibition of β_2 receptor–mediated bronchodilation is minimized. **Pindolol** is a partial agonist at β receptors that has some intrinsic sympathomimetic activity. The use of partial agonists may also benefit individuals with asthma, as incomplete activation of the receptors may provide some bronchodilation. **Betaxolol** and metoprolol are β_1-selective agents that may be classified as inverse agonists. That is, they may reduce the constitutive β-receptor activity in some tissues. Physiologically, this results in a decreased baseline activity mediated by these receptors. The clinical value of these inverse agonists is undefined at present.

Beta blockers have been developed for chronic oral use. Table 6-5 slows that the duration of action for these drugs varies widely. Nadolol is the longest acting β-receptor antagonist. Acebutolol, atenolol, and nadolol are less lipid-soluble than other β-receptor antagonists and probably enter the CNS to a lesser extent. Several of these drugs demonstrate a local anaesthetic action, also known as "membrane-stabilizing" action. The clinical value of this membrane stabilizing effect is minimal since plasma concentrations do not achieve sufficient concentrations for this effect in tissues. However, beta blockers with local anesthetic actions (eg, pindolol) should not be used as eye drops because of the potential to inadvertently cause damage resulting from lack of sensation.

Physiologic Effects

Most of the organ-level effects of β-blockers are predictable from blockade of the β receptor–mediated effects. Mechanisms of blood pressure reduction include an initial reduction in cardiac output, but after a few days, their action may include a decrease in vascular resistance as a contributing effect. The latter physiologic response may be accounted for by reduced angiotensin II levels resulting from decreased

TABLE 6-5 Properties of several β-receptor antagonists.

Drug	Selectivity	Partial Agonist Activity	Local Anesthetic Action	Lipid Solubility	Elimination Half-Life
Acebutolol	β_1	Yes	Yes	Low	3-4 hr
Atenolol	β_1	No	No	Low	6-9 hr
Carvedilol[a]	None	No	No	Moderate	7-10 hr
Esmolol	β_1	No	No	Low	10 min
Labetalol[a]	None	Yes	Yes	Low	5 hr
Metoprolol	β_1	No	Yes	Moderate	3-4 hr
Nadolol	None	No	No	Low	14-24 hr
Pindolol	None	Yes	Yes	Moderate	3-4 hr
Propranolol	None	No	Yes	High	3.5-6 hr
Timolol	None	No	No	Moderate	4-5 hr

[a]Also cause α_1-receptor blockade.

β receptor–mediated renin release from the kidney. Individual drugs may have additional relevant cardiovascular effects that reduce blood pressure. For example, **nebivolol** releases endothelial nitric oxide, **celiprolol** also acts as a β_2-partial agonist, and carvedilol inhibits atherosclerotic plaque progression and smooth muscle proliferation.

Clinical Uses

The clinical applications of β-blockade are remarkably broad (Table 6-6). Cardiovascular clinical applications are discussed in Chapters 7–10. The treatment of open-angle glaucoma involves the use of β-blocking drugs as well as other agents.

Adverse Effects

Cardiovascular adverse effects are extensions of the β-blockade induced by these agents and include bradycardia, atrioventricular blockade, and acute heart failure. People with obstructive lung disease may suffer severe bronchospasm. Cold hands and feet during the winter months is an effect possibly mediated by inhibition of β_2 receptors on the skeletal muscle arteries, which leads to vasoconstriction. Experimentally, β-receptor antagonists

TABLE 6-6 Clinical applications of β-receptor antagonists.

Application	Drugs	Effect
Hypertension	Nadolol, propranolol, timolol	Reduced cardiac output, reduced renin secretion
Angina pectoris	Propranolol, metoprolol, others	Reduced heart rate and contractility
Arrhythmia prophylaxis after myocardial infarction	Atenolol, metoprolol, others	Reduced automaticity of all cardiac pacemakers
Heart failure	Bisoprolol, carvedilol, metoprolol	Decreased mortality; mechanism not understood
Hypertrophic cardiomyopathy	Propranolol	Improved stroke volume
Migraine	Propranolol and others	Prophylactic; mechanism uncertain
Tremor, "stage fright"	Propranolol	Reduced β_2 effects on neuromuscular transmission; possible CNS effects
Hyperthyroidism "thyroid storm"	Propranolol	Reduced heart rate and arrhythmogenesis; other mechanisms may be involved
Open angle glaucoma	Timolol and others	Reduced secretion of aqueous humor

have been shown to reduce insulin secretion, but this does not appear to be a clinically important effect. However, β-receptor antagonists may mask some initial symptoms of hypoglycemia such as tremor, tachycardia, and anxiety due to overdosage with insulin or oral hypoglycemics. Beta blockers may also decrease mobilization of glucose from the liver. The combined adverse effects of decreased heart rate, limitation of bronchodilation and vasodilation within the musculature, and hepatic glucose mobilization decreases exercise tolerance.

CNS adverse effects of β-receptor antagonists include mild sedation, sleep alterations, and occasionally depression. Atenolol, nadolol, and several other less lipid-soluble β-receptor antagonists are claimed to have less marked CNS action because they do not enter the CNS as readily as other β-blockers. Beta blocker therapy is also associated with slightly elevated low-density lipoprotein and triglyceride plasma concentrations and decreased high-density lipoprotein levels. Chronic use of these drugs may result in upregulation of β receptors on the myocardium. Abrupt discontinuation of these drugs following chronic use may result in increased risk of adverse cardiovascular events, such as rebound tachycardia. This is especially true of shorter-acting drugs such as propranolol and metoprolol. Prudence dictates that care should be used if the therapist is aware that a patient has abruptly terminated these medications.

REHABILITATION RELEVANCE

Both sympatholytic and sympathomimetic drugs can influence rehabilitation outcomes. Many sympatholytic drugs allow patients to safely participate in aerobic activities while minimizing increases in blood pressure, angina, or cardiac dysrhythmias. People with asthma, especially exercise-induced asthma, or other respiratory dysfunction may benefit from the bronchodilating effect of β_2 agonists before or during exercise. At the same time, several adverse effects of these drugs can occur:

- **Restlessness and insomnia** may result from CNS stimulation with sympathomimetics.
- **Increased blood pressure** may result from the use of α_1 agonists. This may precipitate angina pectoris, especially during aerobic activities. **Increased heart rate** or blood pressure may result from the use of β_2 agonists that may stimulate β_1 receptors in the heart and precipitate angina pectoris or cardiac dysrhythmias. Monitor blood pressure and heart rate prior to exercise and during the postrecovery period.
- **Orthostatic hypotension** is a problem that varies among drug classes. Alpha receptor antagonists precipitate orthostatic hypotension with greater frequency than β-receptor antagonists. Orthostatic hypotension may cause patients to faint when transferring from seated or supine positions to standing, exiting from warm aquatherapy area, or if aerobic exercise is terminated without an appropriate cool-down period. To prevent fainting associated with orthostatic hypotension, assist patients with positional changes (eg, slowing the speed of transitions, using other techniques to increase venous return such as deep breathing and ankle pumps). Always provide a cool-down period following exercise.
- **Bronchoconstriction** is an adverse effect whose incidence varies within the class of β-receptor antagonists. Nonselective receptor antagonists have the greatest potential, with partial agonists and β_1-selective antagonists demonstrating a lower incidence. Dyspnea may decrease aerobic capacity.
- **Depressed heart rate** may occur at rest and during exercise as a result of β-receptor antagonists. Therefore, heart rate should not be used as a marker of exercise intensity or exertion for individuals taking these drugs. Allow increased time to complete aerobic tasks to prevent dyspnea and account for depressed cardiac activity.

CASE CONCLUSION

The therapist recognized that the patient had just ascended one flight of stairs from the men's locker room to the main workout area and is now complaining of left shoulder pain. The therapist asked the patient to sit quietly and immediately measured his blood pressure and heart rate, which were 145/92 mm Hg and 102 bpm, respectively. The therapist realized that the patient might be presenting with manifestations of exertional angina, which may have been precipitated by cold medications that contain the α_1 agonists oxymetazoline and pseudoephedrine. The resulting elevated blood pressure increased cardiac workload. The drug-induced cardiac changes combined with the exertion of climbing the flight of stairs resulted in insufficient blood flow to the heart—manifested as angina. The therapist recommended that the patient terminate his exercise program and contact his physician immediately for further evaluation. For additional information on angina pectoris, see Chapter 8; for nasal decongestants, see Chapter 35.

CHAPTER 6 QUESTIONS

1. Stimulation of which of the following receptors results in bronchodilation?

   a. β_2
   b. β_1
   c. α_1
   d. α_2

2. Which of the following drugs would delay the clinical manifestations of hypoglycemia?

   a. Mirabegron
   b. Doxazosin
   c. Propranolol
   d. Clonidine

3. Which of the following receptors is coupled to a G_q coupling protein?

    a. β_1
    b. α_1
    c. α_2
    d. Dopamine

4. Stimulation of which of the following receptors would result in a reflex bradycardia?

    a. β_1
    b. α_1
    c. β_2
    d. Dopamine

5. Which of the following drugs would result in a reflex tachycardia?

    a. Albuterol
    b. Metoprolol
    c. Phenylephrine
    d. Doxazosin

6. Which of the following drugs inhibit both alpha and beta receptors?

    a. Labetalol
    b. Doxazosin
    c. Metoprolol
    d. Phenylephrine

7. Which of the following is *not* a positive effect resulting from stimulation of β_1 receptors in the heart?

    a. Phenotropic
    b. Chronotropic
    c. Dromotropic
    d. Inotropic

8. Which of the following drugs would most likely exacerbate dyspnea in an individual with chronic obstructive lung disease?

    a. Atenolol
    b. Metoprolol
    c. Pindolol
    d. Timolol

9. Which of the following drugs would be used in the treatment of overactive bladder?

    a. Mirabegron
    b. Tamsulosin
    c. Cocaine
    d. Dopamine

10. Which of the following drugs would most likely precipitate orthostatic hypotension?

    a. Nadolol
    b. Phenylephrine
    c. Terazosin
    d. Mirabegron

Antihypertensive Drugs

R.T. is a 46-year-old right-handed man who had attended college on a 4-year baseball pitching scholarship. He pitched for 3 years and was sidelined as a result of overuse injury toward the end of the fourth season. R.T. is currently employed in a manufacturing facility. His job requires constant standing and lifting heavy boxes (often overhead). His right shoulder has been persistently painful for the last 2 years, but the pain has increased over the last few weeks such that he is unable to lift anything over his head. Outside of work, he has a sedentary lifestyle, except for walking 10 minutes per day to the train station. He has occasionally sought medical care for complaints of right shoulder pain. He has a 5-year history of essential hypertension that is stable on current drugs. He has no other co-morbidities. One week ago, R.T. had elective arthroscopic right shoulder girdle repair. He was referred to an outpatient physical therapy clinic. His body mass index is 27 kg/m². Resting vitals are as follows: blood pressure 130/82 mm Hg; heart rate 66 bpm. R.T.'s current medication includes hydrochlorothiazide and labetalol and an opiate analgesic to reduce postsurgical pain. During initial evaluation, the therapist assessed

right upper extremity pain-free passive range of motion. Active range of motion was significantly limited by pain and postsurgical guidelines. R.T. expressed extreme urgency in regaining right arm function in order to return to work. The therapist has worked closely with the referring surgeon. The established treatment protocol involves immersion in a pool to allow buoyancy to facilitate pain-free movement of the upper extremity. The 35°C temperature promotes muscle relaxation and decreases guarding. R.T. entered the pool up to his neck and under the guidance of the therapist, began right upper extremity movements. After 15 minutes in the water, R.T. complained of shortness of breath and started up the pool stairs with the assistance of the therapist. At the top of the stairs, the patient felt lightheaded and was assisted to a chair; he fainted, losing consciousness for several seconds. Once the patient was stable, his vitals were taken in a seated position as quickly as possible: blood pressure 90/50 mm Hg and heart rate 74 bpm. The patient was coherent and returned to standing after several minutes.

REHABILITATION FOCUS

Hypertension is the most common cardiovascular disease as well as a precursor to other cardiovascular dysfunctions. The prevalence of hypertension increases with age, and varies based on race/ethnicity, education, and coexisting morbidities. Sustained arterial hypertension damages blood vessels; such changes in the kidney, heart, and brain lead to an increased incidence of renal failure, coronary disease, cardiac failure, and stroke.

Clinical research has consistently documented that aerobic activity is an effective nonpharmacologic approach for controlling hypertension and its sequelae. Other nonpharmacologic therapies include a diet low in sodium and fat (eg, Dietary Approaches to Stop Hypertension, DASH diet), weight reduction, smoking cessation, and moderate alcohol intake.

Antihypertensive drugs are used by individuals in all rehabilitation settings. While aerobic capacity may improve as a result of taking antihypertensive drugs, adverse drug reactions

while performing aerobic activities are not uncommon. Hypotension, especially *orthostatic hypotension*, is a common effect of antihypertensive drugs. The physical therapist should be aware of this possibility, especially in situations that result in peripheral vasodilation such as aquatic therapy in a warm pool, whirlpool of an entire lower extremity, and in the absence of a cool-down period following aerobic activity. Patients should be encouraged to exit the pool or whirlpool slowly and be provided with physical support, as needed. After aerobic activities, a cool-down period of less intense activity may be required to avoid syncope. The therapist should also recognize that heart rate responses to exercise might be blunted by certain classes of antihypertensives such as β-receptor antagonists and some calcium channel blockers. In contrast, direct-acting vasodilators and α_1-receptor antagonists may cause reflex tachycardia that may be exacerbated by exercise. Beta-receptor antagonists may also blunt exercise-induced bronchodilation and decrease respiratory capacity. Several classes of diuretics may cause significant plasma electrolyte imbalances. These electrolyte changes may predispose some individuals to arrhythmias, either directly or as a result of other drug interactions, and exercise may precipitate arrhythmias.

Hypertension is known as the "silent killer" because clinical consequences such as heart attack or stroke often do not occur until years later. Individuals taking antihypertensive medication may experience adverse effects that compromise regular medication use. Such nonadherence not only increases the risk of cardiovascular events, but may also predispose the person to adverse events during rehabilitation because of the increased sympathetic activity that occurs with exercise, functional return-to-work programs, and any procedure that causes discomfort or pain (eg, wound healing interventions). If individuals abruptly discontinue taking certain long-term medications, adverse effects like arrhythmias (in the case of β-receptor antagonists) or rebound hypertension (in the case of α_2-receptor agonists) may occur.

BACKGROUND

The autonomic nervous system, especially the sympathetic branch, plays a significant role in the regulation of blood pressure. A general discussion of autonomic responses was presented in Chapter 4, specifically Table 4-3 and Figure 4-5. According to the hydraulic equation, arterial blood pressure (BP) is directly proportional to the product of the blood flow and the resistance to passage of blood through the vessels. The estimate for blood flow is cardiac output (CO) and the determinant for resistance is peripheral vascular resistance (PVR). Thus, the equation is

$$BP = CO \times PVR$$

In both normotensive and hypertensive individuals, blood pressure is maintained by moment-to-moment regulation of cardiac output and peripheral vascular resistance (Figure 7-1). Vascular locations that regulate blood pressure are the arterioles, the venules, and the heart. The kidneys contribute slower, longer-lasting maintenance of blood pressure by regulating intravascular fluid volume.

The baroreceptor reflex is responsible for rapid *moment-to-moment* adjustments in blood pressure (eg, transitioning from a recumbent to an upright posture) that prevent orthostatic hypotension and syncope. The baroreceptor reflexes act in combination with the renin-angiotensin-aldosterone system, to coordinate function at these four control sites and to maintain normal blood pressure. Local release of hormones is also involved in the regulation of vascular resistance. For example, nitric oxide (NO) and some prostaglandins dilate blood vessels, whereas other local hormones such as endothelins constrict vessels.

Figure 7-2 outlines the baroreceptor reflex arc. Carotid baroreceptors are stimulated when the vessel walls are stretched, which occurs with an increase in blood pressure (**item 1** in Figure 7-2). Baroreceptor activation *inhibits* central sympathetic discharge (**item 2**) because neurons arising from the vasomotor area of the medulla are tonically active (**item 3**). Conversely, reduction in vessel wall stretch results in reduced baroreceptor activity. Thus, when a person transitions from a recumbent to an upright posture, baroreceptors sense reduced arterial pressure that results from pooling of blood in the veins below the level of the heart as reduced vessel wall stretch in the carotid sinus, and efferent sympathetic activity is increased (**items 4 and 5**). The postganglionic neuron usually releases norepinephrine,

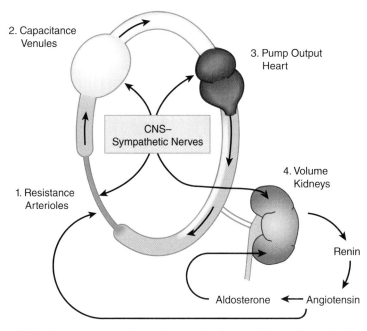

FIGURE 7-1 Anatomic sites of blood pressure control: vascular tone in the arterioles and venules (1 and 2), pump output by the heart (3), and regulation of intravascular fluid volume by the kidneys (4).

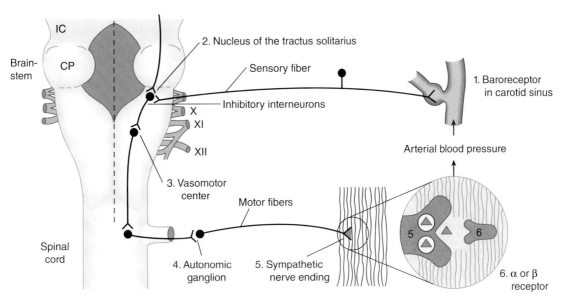

FIGURE 7-2 **Baroreceptor reflex arc.** See text for discussion of items 1 through 6.

activating α or β receptors (**item 6**). Vasoconstriction of the arterioles increases peripheral vascular resistance, vasoconstriction of the veins increases venous return to the heart, and increased heart rate and contractility increase cardiac output. Together, these sympathetic responses restore normal blood pressure. Recognize that the baroreceptor reflex acts in response to *any* event that lowers blood pressure, including a primary reduction in peripheral vascular resistance (which occurs with vasodilators) or a reduction in intravascular volume (which occurs with diuretics). Conversely, the baroreceptor reflex arc responds to an increase in blood pressure with *activation* of the vagus nerve thus slowing down the heart rate.

The kidneys—by controlling blood volume—are primarily responsible for *long-term* blood pressure control. If perfusion pressure to the kidney is reduced, blood flow within the kidney is redistributed and salt and water reabsorption is increased. In addition, sympathetic neural activity (via β-adrenoceptors) and decreased pressure in renal arterioles stimulate production of the hormone renin. Renin mediates conversion of the plasma protein angiotensinogen to angiotensin I. Angiotensin I is converted to angiotensin II by angiotensin-converting enzyme (ACE). Angiotensin II directly and indirectly increases blood pressure. First, angiotensin II potently constricts resistance vessels by acting on angiotensin II receptor type 1 (AT$_1$) receptors. Second, angiotensin II stimulates aldosterone synthesis in the adrenal cortex. Aldosterone is the hormonal regulator for the sodium/potassium/proton exchange process in the distal convoluted tubules and collecting ducts of the kidney. Aldosterone stimulates renal sodium reabsorption with a resulting increase in intravascular blood volume (which increases blood pressure). The last important hormone involved in blood pressure regulation is vasopressin (or, antidiuretic hormone, ADH). Vasopressin is released from the posterior pituitary gland in response to decreased blood volume or increased plasma osmolality. It plays

a role in maintenance of blood pressure through its ability to regulate water reabsorption in the collecting duct cells.

HIGH BLOOD PRESSURE

A specific cause of hypertension (HTN) can be established in only 10-15% of patients. In patients with no identified cause, high blood pressure is said to be "essential hypertension." In most cases, cardiac output is normal but there is an overall increase in resistance to blood flow through arterioles. No primary single abnormality has been identified as the cause of this increased peripheral vascular resistance. Rather, hypertension is usually a multifactorial condition. Epidemiologic evidence points to factors such as genetic inheritance, environmental, and dietary factors such as increased salt and decreased potassium or calcium intake. The heritability of essential hypertension is estimated to be about 30%. Functional variations of the genes for angiotensinogen, ACE, and the β$_2$ adrenoceptor appear to contribute to some cases of essential hypertension. Mutations in several genes have been linked to various rare causes of hypertension. Aging-associated increases in blood pressure are not as significant in populations that have low daily sodium intake. In contrast, a positive association exists between increased salt intake and increasing blood pressure.

ANTIHYPERTENSIVE DRUGS

Blood pressure in a hypertensive individual is controlled by the same mechanisms that operate in a normotensive individual. What *differs* is that the baroreceptors and the renal blood volume-pressure control systems appear to be "set" at a higher level of blood pressure in the hypertensive person. All antihypertensive drugs act by interfering with the normal blood

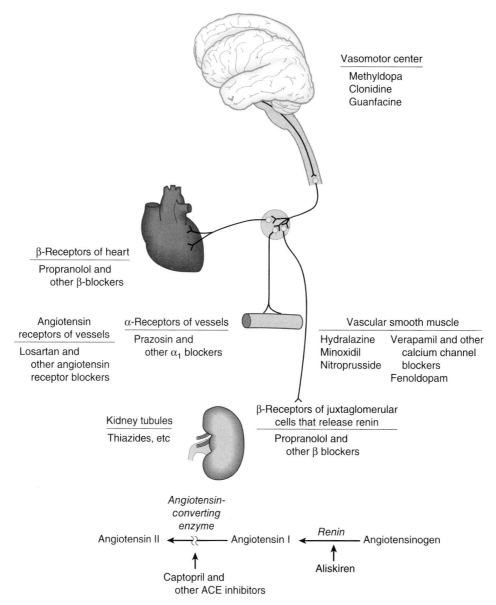

FIGURE 7-3 **Sites of actions of major classes of antihypertensive drugs.**

pressure regulation mechanisms. Figure 7-3 illustrates sites of action at which antihypertensive drugs interfere with blood pressure regulation. These sites include inhibition of sympathetic tone (sympatholytics), inhibition of vascular smooth muscle contraction (vasodilators), inhibition of angiotensin II formation (renin inhibitors and ACE inhibitors) and receptor activation (AT_1 receptor antagonists), and reduction of blood volume (diuretics).

Figure 7-4 outlines the various classes of antihypertensive drugs. Effective lowering of blood pressure prevents damage to blood vessels and substantially reduces morbidity and mortality rates. A "stepped" approach is used in the pharmacologic treatment of hypertension. This means that if a single drug does not adequately reduce blood pressure, another drug/s with different sites of action can be added to reduce

blood pressure while minimizing toxicity. In addition, several drug classes used in the treatment of hypertension result in compensatory responses (discussed at the end of the chapter). These compensatory responses can be minimized by treatment with lower dosages and/or with additional drugs with different mechanisms of action.

SYMPATHOLYTIC DRUGS

Clinically relevant drugs that decrease blood pressure by inhibiting the SNS include antagonists at adrenoceptors and drugs that decrease sympathetic outflow from the CNS (Figure 7-3). Older drugs that act at autonomic ganglia or postganglionic nerve terminals are rarely used clinically for control of blood pressure, so they are not discussed in this chapter.

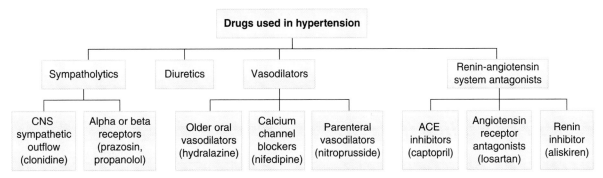

FIGURE 7-4 **Various classes of drugs used in the treatment of hypertension.** The general pharmacologic mechanisms include decreasing sympathetic tone (sympatholytics), decreasing blood volume (diuretics), relaxation of vascular smooth muscle (vasodilators), and inhibition of the effects of renin-angiotensin-aldosterone system (renin-angiotensin system antagonists). Prototype drugs are listed in parentheses.

Adrenoceptor Antagonists

The α_1, α_2, and β_1 receptors all play a modulatory role in controlling blood pressure. Mechanisms of action and the physiologic effects of inhibiting these receptors were discussed in Chapter 6.

The α_1-selective receptor antagonists such as **prazosin**, **doxazosin**, and **terazosin** (generic drug names often end in "-osin") are used for chronic treatment of hypertension as well as benign prostatic hyperplasia. These drugs decrease blood pressure by vasodilation of the *arterial* vasculature and, to a lesser extent, the venous vasculature. Adverse effects include orthostatic hypotension (especially with initial doses) and, less commonly, reflex tachycardia. Alpha blockers should not be used as monotherapy for this reason.

The β-receptor antagonists (β-blockers) such as **propranolol** and **metoprolol** are used not only for hypertension, but also for angina, cardiac arrhythmias, and chronic heart failure. Adverse effects of β-blockers include bradycardia, atrioventricular blockade, and acute heart failure. If individuals abruptly terminate use of β-blockers, additional care should be taken to monitor for tachycardia or other rhythm disturbances.

CNS-Acting Drugs

α_2-selective agonists such as **methyldopa**, **clonidine**, and **guanfacine** decrease sympathetic outflow via activation of α_2 receptors in the CNS (Figure 7-3). Given orally, these drugs readily enter the CNS and reduce blood pressure by reducing cardiac output, vascular resistance, or both. One advantage of these drugs is that they cause minimal orthostatic hypotension, a trait not shared by many of the other antihypertensive drug classes. Methyldopa is a prodrug that is converted in the brain to methylnorepinephrine; its clinical use is primarily restricted to hypertension during pregnancy. Guanfacine does not appear to have clinical advantages over clonidine and is rarely used.

The major compensatory response to the α_2-receptor agonists is salt retention. Sudden discontinuation of clonidine may cause rebound hypertension, which may be quite severe. This rebound increase in blood pressure can be controlled by reinstitution of clonidine therapy. Clonidine also increases the risk of depression and should be used with caution in patients at risk. Methyldopa occasionally causes hematologic immunotoxicity, and in some patients progresses to hemolytic anemia. All drugs in this class may cause sedation and dry mouth, methyldopa more so.

VASODILATORS

For some hypertensive patients, vasodilating drugs that act directly on smooth muscle cells via mechanisms that are *not* mediated by the SNS are useful. Vasodilators work by four major mechanisms: release of nitric oxide, opening of potassium channels (which leads to hyperpolarization), blockade of L-type calcium channels, and activation of D_1 dopamine receptors (Table 7-1). Compensatory responses such as salt retention and reflex tachycardia are prominent for some vasodilators, especially hydralazine and minoxidil.

TABLE 7-1 **Mechanism of action of vasodilators.**

Mechanism of Smooth Muscle Relaxation	Examples
Release of nitric oxide from drug or endothelium	Nitroprusside Hydralazine
Hyperpolarization of vascular smooth muscle through opening of potassium channels	Minoxidil sulfate Diazoxide
Reduction of calcium influx through L-type calcium channels	Nifedipine (dihydropyridines): vessels > heart Verapamil, diltiazem: heart ≥ vessels
Activation of dopamine$_1$ receptors	Fenoldopam

Release of Nitric Oxide

Hydralazine is an older vasodilator that has more effect on arterioles than on veins. The drug is orally active and suitable for chronic therapy. Hydralazine apparently acts through the release of nitric oxide (NO) from endothelial cells. However, the drug is rarely used at high dosages because of its toxicity. Toxicities include tachycardia, salt and water retention, and drug-induced lupus erythematosus. The latter effect is uncommon at dosages below 200 mg/d and is reversible upon stopping the drug. **Nitroprusside** is a short-acting agent (duration of action is a few minutes) that must be infused continuously and is used in hypertensive emergencies. The drug's mechanism of action involves the release of NO from the drug molecule itself. The released NO stimulates guanylate cyclase and increases cGMP concentration in smooth muscle, resulting in smooth muscle relaxation and vasodilation. The toxicity of nitroprusside includes excessive hypotension, tachycardia, and, if infusion is continued over several days, plasma accumulation of cyanide or thiocyanate.

Smooth Muscle Cell Hyperpolarization

Minoxidil is also an older vasodilator that has more effect on arterioles than on veins and is orally active. Minoxidil is a prodrug; its metabolite, minoxidil sulfate, hyperpolarizes and relaxes vascular smooth muscle by opening potassium channels. Minoxidil is reserved for severe hypertension because of multiple adverse effects including edema and tachycardia. Clinical use of minoxidil generally requires coadministration of a diuretic and a β-blocker to minimize these responses. Additional toxicities of minoxidil include hirsutism and pericardial abnormalities. **Diazoxide** is a parenteral vasodilator previously used in hypertensive emergencies. Given as intravenous bolus or as an infusion, its duration of action is several hours. Like minoxidil sulfate, diazoxide opens potassium channels, which hyperpolarizes and relaxes smooth muscle cells. Diazoxide also reduces insulin release and can be used to treat hypoglycemia caused by insulin-producing tumors. Adverse effects of diazoxide include hypotension, hyperglycemia, and salt and water retention.

Calcium Channel Blockade

L-type voltage-gated calcium channels are highly distributed in the cardiovascular system—both in cardiac muscle cells and in smooth muscle cells in the vasculature. Prototypical L-type calcium channel blockers (CCBs) include **nifedipine**, **verapamil**, and **diltiazem**. Select CCBs have been designed to have more or less affinity for calcium channels in the heart versus those in the blood vessels. Because they are orally active, these drugs are suitable for chronic use in hypertension. Many dihydropyridine analogs of nifedipine are also available. Because they produce fewer compensatory responses, CCBs are usually preferred to hydralazine and minoxidil. Their mechanism of action and toxicities are discussed in detail in Chapter 8.

Dopamine (D$_1$) Receptor Activation

Fenoldopam is a dopamine D$_1$ receptor agonist that causes prompt and marked arteriolar vasodilation, making it an effective drug for hypertensive emergencies. It is intravenously infused and its duration of action is approximately 10 minutes.

DRUGS THAT INHIBIT THE RENIN-ANGIOTENSIN-ALDOSTERONE SYSTEM

Figure 7-5 summarizes the sequence of events leading to the formation of angiotensin II. When the renin-angiotensin-aldosterone system is activated, blood pressure is increased. Drugs that inhibit this system not only reduce blood pressure, but may also decrease pathologic myocardial and vascular remodeling mediated by this system.

Three drug classes alter the actions of this system at different stages: renin inhibitors, angiotensin-converting enzyme inhibitors (ACE inhibitors), and angiotensin II receptor antagonists, which are also called angiotensin receptor blockers (ARBs) or AT$_1$ receptor blockers. The more extensively used classes are the ACE inhibitors and the ARBs. These drug classes have a low incidence of serious adverse effects, *except* in

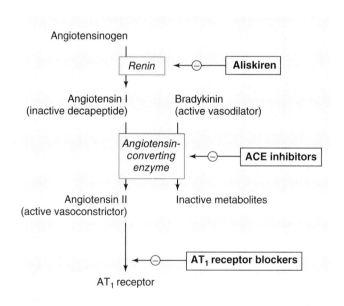

FIGURE 7-5 **Sites of action of renin inhibitors (aliskiren), angiotensin-converting enzyme inhibitors (ACE inhibitors), and angiotensin-II receptor (AT$_1$) antagonists in inhibiting the formation or action of angiotensin II.** Renin converts angiotensinogen to angiotensin I. ACE converts angiotensin I into angiotensin II and inactivates bradykinin, a vasodilator normally present in very low concentrations. ACE inhibitors decrease production of the vasoconstrictor angiotensin II and increase levels of the vasodilator bradykinin. Renin inhibitors and AT$_1$ receptor antagonists do not affect bradykinin levels, which may contribute to the lower incidence of cough observed with these drug classes.

pregnancy. ACE inhibitors and ARBs cause fetal renal toxicity. Though this effect has not been demonstrated with renin inhibitors, the use of all three classes is contraindicated in pregnancy.

In addition to being a potent vasoconstrictor, angiotensin II is a major stimulant of aldosterone release. Renin inhibitors, ACE inhibitors, and ARBs all reduce aldosterone levels. In addition, there are direct aldosterone receptor inhibitors (eg, spironolactone, eplerenone) that are discussed with the diuretics. Blockade of aldosterone release and its effects may lead to hyperkalemia. This potassium accumulation may be marked, especially if the patient has renal impairment, is consuming a high-potassium diet, or is taking potassium-sparing diuretics. Under these circumstances, potassium concentrations may reach toxic levels.

Renin Inhibitors

Inhibition of renin production prevents initiation of the renin-angiotensin-aldosterone cascade (Figure 7-5). **Aliskiren** is an orally active renin inhibitor that produces a dose-dependent decrease in angiotensin I and II, and aldosterone. Clinically, aliskiren produces a dose-dependent reduction in blood pressure in patients with essential hypertension. The most important adverse effect is decreased glomerular filtration rate. When used alone, hyperkalemia is minimal in individuals with normal renal function. Concomitant use of aliskiren with another drug that inhibits the renin-angiotensin-aldosterone system or with a potassium-sparing diuretic increases the risk of hyperkalemia. Hyperuricemia, gastrointestinal distress, and skin rash are also associated with use.

Angiotensin-Converting Enzyme Inhibitors (ACE Inhibitors)

ACE inhibitors—whose generic drug names end in "- pril" (eg, **captopril**, **lisinopril**)—*reduce* blood levels of angiotensin II and aldosterone and probably *increase* endogenous vasodilators of the kinin family such as bradykinin (Figure 7-5). Thus, both actions reduce blood pressure primarily by decreasing peripheral vascular resistance without significant changes in cardiac output or heart rate. ACE inhibitors have a low incidence of serious adverse effects. In contrast to the vasodilators, ACE inhibitors do not cause reflex tachycardia so their use is safer in individuals with ischemic cardiac disease. In up to 30% of patients, ACE inhibitors produce a chronic cough, which may be due to increased bradykinin and other substances that increase airway irritation. Decreases in glomerular filtration rate may occur in patients with preexisting renal vascular disease, although these drugs are protective in diabetic nephropathy. In fact, ACE inhibitors have been recommended for individuals with diabetes and significant albuminuria even in the absence of hypertension because they decrease albuminuria and stabilize renal function. Hyperkalemia may occur in up to 11% of patients taking these drugs; this effect is exacerbated when combined with potassium-sparing diuretics, renin and ACE inhibitors, or ARBs.

Angiotensin Receptor Blockers (ARBs) or AT₁ Receptor Blockers

The orally active ARBs—whose generic drug names end in "- artan" (eg, **losartan**, **valsartan**)—selectively block the actions of angiotensin II at AT_1 receptors (Figure 7-5). ARBs appear to be as effective in lowering blood pressure as the ACE inhibitors and have a similar adverse effect profile. However, there is a minimal incidence of chronic cough because ARBs do not have any effect on bradykinin metabolism. ARBs are most often used in individuals who have had adverse reactions to ACE inhibitors.

DIURETICS

Diuretics are drugs that increase urine volume (promote diuresis). Drug-mediated diuresis occurs by directly increasing the loss of water (aquaresis) or indirectly by increasing the loss of sodium (natriuresis). In natriuresis, sodium remaining in the renal tubules prevents the reabsorption of water, ultimately resulting in the loss of water into the urine. Diuretics are divided into several subgroups based on their inhibition of different transporters that regulate solute, electrolyte, and water loss from the renal tubules (Figure 7-6). Because the mechanisms for these various diuretic subgroups differ, their adverse effects differ.

To understand how diuretics increase urine volume, a review of the physiology of tubular transport systems in each segment of the nephron is helpful. Figure 7-7 provides an overview of the passage of fluid through the nephron, the tubular transport systems unique to each segment, and the sites of action of diuretic classes.

At the glomerulus, plasma is filtered through the glomerular membrane into Bowman's space. Because the total plasma volume (~ 4 L) is filtered many times (~ 180 L/day), the major function of the remainder of the nephron is to *reabsorb* essential substances so that they are not lost into the urine. The proximal convoluted tubule carries out isosmotic reabsorption of amino acids, glucose, and numerous ions. The proximal tubule is responsible for 60-70% of the total reabsorption of sodium chloride (NaCl) and water and is also the major site for reabsorption of sodium bicarbonate ($NaHCO_3$). Bicarbonate itself (HCO_3^-) is poorly reabsorbed through the luminal membrane (urinary side of the epithelium), but conversion of HCO_3^- to carbon dioxide (CO_2) via carbonic acid permits rapid reabsorption of the CO_2. Bicarbonate can then be regenerated from CO_2 within the tubular cell and transported into the interstitium and back into the blood. Carbonic anhydrase is required for the HCO_3^- reabsorption process. This enzyme, which resides on the brush border and in the cytoplasm of proximal convoluted tubule cells, is the target of carbonic anhydrase inhibitors (Figure 7-7: 1). Sodium is separately reabsorbed in exchange for hydrogen ions at the luminal surface of the cells and then transported into the interstitial space by the sodium pump at the basolateral surface. Active secretion and reabsorption of weak acids and bases also occurs in

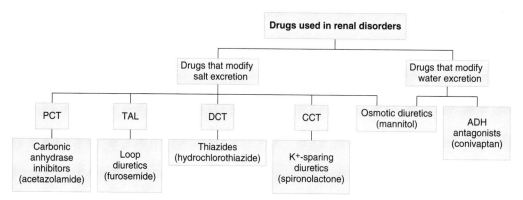

FIGURE 7-6 **Diuretic subclasses are based on sites of action within the nephron.** Effects of diuretics are predictable based on knowledge of the function of the segment of the nephron in which they act. Each nephron segment has a different mechanism for reabsorption of sodium and other ions. Prototype drugs are listed in parentheses. CCT, cortical collecting tubule; DCT, distal convoluted tubule; PCT, proximal convoluted tubule; TAL, thick ascending limb of the loop of Henle.

the proximal tubule. Uric acid transport is especially important and is targeted by some of the drugs used in treating gout (Chapter 34).

The thick ascending limb actively reabsorbs sodium, potassium, and two chloride molecules out of the lumen into the interstitium of the kidney via the action of a single $Na^+/K^+/2Cl^-$ (NKCC2) cotransporter (Figure 7-8). The NKCC2 cotransporter is the target of loop diuretics (Figure 7-7: 3). This cotransporter provides the concentration gradient for the countercurrent-concentrating mechanism in the kidney and is

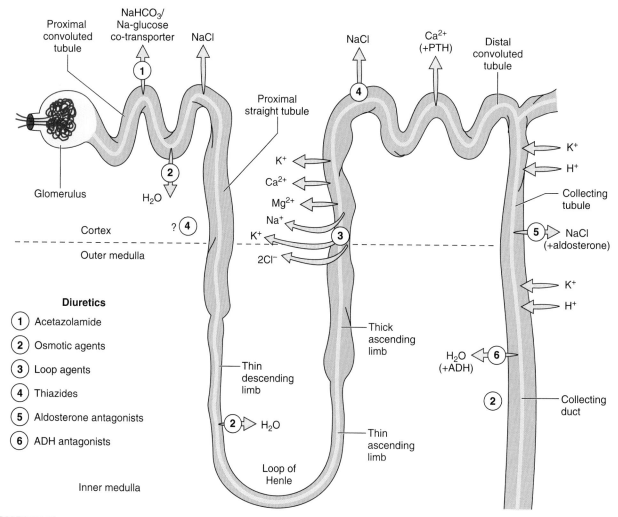

FIGURE 7-7 **Overview of renal tubule transport systems.** Numbers represent location of sites of action of classes of diuretics or prototypical examples.

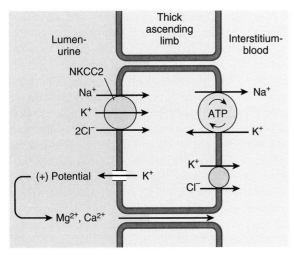

FIGURE 7-8 **Thick ascending limb cell: ion transport pathways across luminal and basolateral membranes.** As in all tubular cells, Na$^+$/K$^+$ ATPase in the basolateral membrane creates an electrochemical gradient. The major cotransporter is a Na$^+$/K$^+$/2Cl$^-$ (NKCC2) located in the luminal membrane. The positive electrical potential in the lumen is created by the back diffusion of K$^+$. This potential drives the reabsorption of divalent (Mg^{2+} and Ca^{2+}) and monovalent cations via the paracellular pathway.

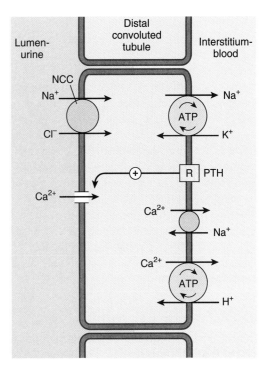

FIGURE 7-9 **Distal convoluted tubule cell: ion transport pathways across luminal and basolateral membranes.** The major Na$^+$ and Cl$^-$ cotransporter (NCC) in the luminal membrane is electrically neutral. "R" represents the parathyroid hormone (PTH) receptor.

responsible for the reabsorption of 20-30% of the sodium filtered at the glomerulus. Because potassium is pumped into the cell from both the luminal and basal sides, an escape route must be provided; this occurs via a potassium-selective channel on the luminal surface of the cells. Because the potassium diffusing through these channels is not accompanied by an anion, a net positive charge is set up in the lumen. This positive potential drives the intercellular reabsorption of calcium and magnesium.

The distal convoluted tubule actively pumps NaCl out of the lumen of the nephron via the electrically neutral (NCC) cotransporter (Figure 7-9). This cotransporter is the target of thiazide diuretics (Figure 7-7: 4). The distal convoluted tubule is responsible for approximately 5-8% of sodium reabsorption. Calcium is also reabsorbed in this segment under the control of parathyroid hormone (PTH); its role in osteoporosis is discussed in Chapter 25. Reabsorption of calcium from the tubule requires the Na$^+$-Ca^{2+} exchanger. Inhibition of the NCC cotransporter by thiazide diuretics increases Na$^+$-Ca^{2+} exchanger activity and thus facilitates Ca^{2+} reabsorption from the tubule.

The collecting tubule is the final segment of the nephron and the last site for modification of the filtrate. Here, sodium reabsorption is controlled by aldosterone (Figure 7-10). This segment is responsible for reabsorbing 2-5% of total filtered sodium. Sodium reabsorption occurs via channels and is accompanied by an equivalent loss of potassium or hydrogen ions. The collecting tubule is thus the primary site of potassium *excretion* and of urine acidification. The aldosterone receptor and the sodium channels are the sites of action for potassium-sparing diuretics (Figure 7-7: 5). Reabsorption of water occurs in the medullary portion of the collecting tubule

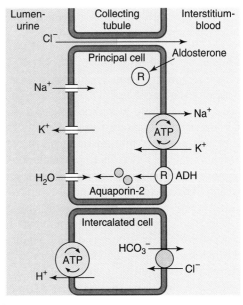

FIGURE 7-10 **Collecting tubule and collecting duct cells: ion transport pathways across luminal and basolateral membranes.** Diffusion of Na$^+$ from the lumen leaves a lumen-negative potential, which drives reabsorption of Cl$^-$ and efflux of K$^+$. The Na$^+$-K$^+$ exchange function is regulated by aldosterone, which binds to an intracellular receptor (R). Antidiuretic hormone (ADH) acts on its receptor (R) to facilitate insertion of aquaporin-2 channels (water channels) into the luminal surface, allowing reabsorption of water from the tubule. Hydrogen ion (H$^+$) secretion into the tubule with bicarbonate (HCO$_3^-$) reabsorption is also regulated here.

(Figure 7-10) and is under the control of antidiuretic hormone (ADH). ADH antagonists inhibit the effects of ADH in the collecting tubules (Figure 7-7: 6).

There are six subgroups of diuretics classified by their mechanisms or sites of action: carbonic anhydrase inhibitors, ADH antagonists, osmotic, loop, thiazide, and potassium-sparing (Figure 7-6). These drugs reduce vascular volume by either modifying salt excretion, water excretion, or both. Most diuretics act from the luminal side of the membrane, so they must be present in the urine. These drugs are filtered at the glomerulus and the weak acid-secretory carrier in the proximal tubule also secretes some diuretics. An exception is the aldosterone receptor antagonists that enter the collecting tubule cell from the basolateral side because they must bind to the cytoplasmic aldosterone receptor. Only the loop, thiazide, and potassium-sparing diuretics are commonly used in the treatment of hypertension.

Carbonic Anhydrase Inhibitors

The carbonic anhydrase inhibitors (eg, **acetazolamide**) significantly decrease HCO_3^- reabsorption. These diuretics are used to reduce intraocular pressure in glaucoma, to treat acute high-altitude sickness, and for edematous conditions associated with metabolic alkalosis. Because HCO_3^- is lost from the filtrate at more proximal regions of the nephron, increased NaCl reabsorption occurs in the rest of the nephron. Thus, the diuretic efficacy of acetazolamide decreases greatly over several days. Due to the loss of HCO_3^-, metabolic acidosis is a significant adverse effect, but this is a benefit in treating metabolic alkalosis.

Osmotic Diuretics

Mannitol, the prototypical osmotic diuretic, is given intravenously. Because it is freely filtered at the glomerulus but poorly reabsorbed from the tubule, mannitol remains in the lumen and "holds" water by virtue of its osmotic effect. The major location for this action is the proximal convoluted tubule. Reabsorption of water is also reduced in the descending limb of the loop of Henle and the collecting tubule. Most filtered solutes will also be excreted in larger amounts unless they are actively reabsorbed. Sodium excretion is usually increased because the rate of urine flow through the tubule is greatly accelerated and sodium transporters cannot handle the volume rapidly enough. Osmotic diuretics are useful in reducing intraocular pressure in acute glaucoma and intracranial pressure in neurologic conditions. Because water is removed from the intracellular compartment, hyponatremia and pulmonary edema may occur. As water is excreted into the urine, hypernatremia, hyperkalemia, and dehydration may follow. Headache, nausea, and vomiting are common, due to these shifts.

Loop Diuretics

Furosemide is the prototypical loop diuretic. Furosemide, **bumetanide**, and **torsemide** are chemically related sulfonamide derivatives. **Ethacrynic acid** is a phenoxyacetic acid derivative but acts by the same mechanism. Loop diuretics inhibit the cotransport of sodium, potassium, and chloride at the ascending loop of Henle (Figure 7-8). The loop of Henle is responsible for a significant fraction of total renal NaCl reabsorption; therefore, a full dose of a loop diuretic produces massive NaCl diuresis. If tissue perfusion is adequate, edema fluid is rapidly excreted and blood volume may be significantly reduced. The diluting ability of the nephron is reduced because the loop of Henle is the site of significant dilution of urine. Inhibition of the $Na^+/K^+/2Cl^-$ cotransporter also results in loss of the lumen-positive potential, which reduces reabsorption of divalent cations. As a result, calcium and magnesium excretion are significantly increased. The presentation of large amounts of sodium to the collecting tubule may result in significant potassium and proton excretion that may result in hypokalemic alkalosis.

Another mechanism by which loop diuretics increase urine volume is by increasing the formation of renal-generated prostaglandin E2 (PGE_2). Prostaglandin E2 inhibits sodium transport in the loop of Henle; thus, this additional action further limits sodium reabsorption. Inhibition of renal prostaglandin production by nonsteroidal anti-inflammatory drugs (Chapter 34) may blunt the diuretic effect of these drugs.

The major clinical application of loop diuretics is in the treatment of edematous states including heart failure and ascites. They are relatively short-acting in that diuresis usually occurs over a 4-hour period following a dose. Loop diuretics are particularly valuable in acute pulmonary edema, in which the pulmonary vasodilating action of renal PGE_2 plays a useful role. They are used in hypertension if response to thiazides is inadequate, but their short duration of action is a disadvantage for this indication. A less common but important application is in the treatment of severe hypercalcemia, which may occur in malignancy.

A major adverse effect of loop diuretics is potassium wasting (ie, significant loss of potassium into the urine), which can ultimately result in hypokalemia (Table 7-2). Due to the large amount of sodium presented to the collecting tubules, potassium is excreted by the collecting tubules in an effort to conserve sodium. If hypokalemia is severe, metabolic alkalosis may also occur. Because loop diuretics are so efficacious, they can cause hypovolemia and associated orthostatic hypotension and reflex tachycardia. At high doses, ototoxicity is an important adverse effect of the loop agents. The sulfonamides in this group may cause sulfonamide allergy.

Thiazide Diuretics

Hydrochlorothiazide (HCT) is the prototypical drug in this class. Thiazides are active by the oral route and have a duration of action of 6-12 hours, considerably longer than the loop diuretics. The major action of thiazides is to inhibit NaCl transport in the early segment of the distal convoluted tubule (Figure 7-9). In full doses, thiazides produce moderate but sustained sodium and chloride diuresis. Hypokalemic

TABLE 7-2 Electrolyte and systemic pH changes produced by diuretic subgroups.

Group	Amount in Urine			Body pH
	NaCl	NaHCO₃	K⁺	
Carbonic anhydrase inhibitors	↑[a]	↑↑↑[a]	↑[a]	Acidosis[b]
Loop diuretics	↑↑↑↑	—	↑	Alkalosis
Thiazides	↑↑	↑, —	↑	Alkalosis
K⁺-sparing diuretics	↑	—	↓	Acidosis

[a]Self-limited (2-3 days).
[b]Not self-limited.

metabolic alkalosis may occur (Table 7-2). Reduction in the transport of sodium into the tubular cell reduces intracellular sodium and promotes sodium-calcium exchange. As a result, *reabsorption* of calcium from the urine is increased and urine calcium content is decreased—the opposite of the effect of loop diuretics. Because they act in a diluting segment of the nephron, thiazides may interfere with excretion of water and cause dilutional hyponatremia.

The major application of thiazides is in hypertension, for which their long duration and moderate intensity of action are particularly useful. The maximal blood pressure-lowering effect occurs at doses lower than the maximal diuretic doses. When a thiazide is used with a loop diuretic, a synergistic effect occurs with marked diuresis. Chronic therapy of edematous conditions such as mild heart failure is another important application, although loop diuretics are preferred. Chronic calcium kidney stone formation can sometimes be controlled with thiazides because of their ability to reduce urine calcium concentration.

As with loop diuretics, chronic thiazide therapy is often associated with potassium wasting potentially resulting in hypokalemia. Diabetic patients may experience significant hyperglycemia. Serum uric acid and lipid levels are increased in some individuals. While uncommon, massive sodium diuresis with hyponatremia is a dangerous early effect of thiazides. Last, thiazides are sulfonamides; thus all diuretics in this class have sulfonamide allergenic potential.

Potassium-Sparing Diuretics

Spironolactone and **eplerenone** are steroid derivatives that act as antagonists of aldosterone in the collecting tubules (Figure 7-10). By binding to the intracellular aldosterone receptor and blocking the binding of aldosterone, these drugs reduce the expression of genes controlling the *synthesis* of epithelial sodium ion channels and Na⁺/K⁺ ATPase. Due to this mechanism of action, their onset of action is slow and duration of action is long-lasting (48-72 hours). In contrast, **amiloride** and **triamterene** act by directly *inhibiting* these sodium channels. Thus, these drugs have a faster onset of action (2-4 hours) and a shorter duration of action (7-9 hours). Regardless of the

precise mechanism of action, all potassium-sparing diuretics increase sodium excretion and decrease potassium and hydrogen ion excretion.

Individuals may be prescribed potassium-sparing diuretics if chronic therapy with loop or thiazide diuretics causes hypokalemia that cannot be controlled by dietary potassium supplements. The most common use is in the form of products that combine a thiazide with a potassium-sparing agent in a single tablet or capsule. The aldosterone receptor antagonists of this group are also used to treat elevated serum aldosterone levels (aldosteronism). Secondary aldosteronism occurs in hepatic cirrhosis and heart failure. In heart failure, spironolactone and eplerenone have been shown to have significant long-term benefits (Chapter 9). Some of this effect may be due to the drugs' inhibition of the pathologic remodeling of the ventricular walls that is mediated by aldosterone.

The most important adverse effect is hyperkalemia, which may be accompanied by metabolic acidosis (Table 7-2). These drugs should never be taken with potassium supplements or potassium-containing salt substitutes. Other drug that interfere with aldosterone release such as renin inhibitors, ACE inhibitors, and ARBs, if used at all, should be used with great caution. In men, gynecomastia may result from spironolactone binding to the androgen receptor. This occurs with lower incidence with eplerenone because eplerenone has a higher specificity for the mineralocorticoid receptor than the androgen receptor.

Antidiuretic Hormone (ADH) Antagonists

Figure 7-10 illustrates the site of action of the newer ADH antagonists such as **conivaptan** or **tolvaptan** (generic drug names end in "- vaptan"). These drugs are used to decrease the water retention that results from excessive ADH secretion, especially in congestive heart failure (CHF) and the syndrome of inappropriate ADH secretion (SIADH). Individuals with CHF who are on diuretics often develop hyponatremia secondary to excessive ADH secretion. SIADH is associated with some neoplasms, neurologic and pulmonary pathophysiologies, and as an adverse effect of some drugs.

REHABILITATION RELEVANCE

When an individual takes an antihypertensive medication, the body frequently produces compensatory responses. Drug-mediated decreases in blood pressure result in activation of both the baroreceptor reflex and the renin-angiotensin-aldosterone system in an attempt to return to the premedicated (hypertensive) pressure. Two common examples of compensatory responses to decreased blood pressure are tachycardia and salt and water retention. Thus, it is not uncommon for an individual to be prescribed an additional antihypertensive drug to minimize the body's compensatory response to decreased pressure that was caused by the *initial* antihypertensive drug. Figure 7-11 shows how reflexive tachycardia may be counteracted with β-receptor antagonists, and salt and water retention may be minimized with diuretics or drug classes that interfere with the renin-angiotensin-aldosterone system.

Table 7-3 summarizes the physiologic compensatory responses and adverse effects to different antihypertensive drug classes, some of which may influence various facets of rehabilitation.

In general, antihypertensive drugs allow individuals to safely participate in aerobic activities while minimizing increases in blood pressure. Summarized below are adverse effects of drugs or drug classes mostly likely to affect rehabilitation.

- **Orthostatic hypotension** is one of the most common problems associated with many classes of antihypertensive drugs, especially vasodilators, diuretics, and the dihydropyridine subclass of the CCBs. Orthostatic hypotension may cause patients to faint when transferring from sitting or supine positions to standing, exiting from a warm aquatherapy area, or if aerobic exercise is terminated without an appropriate cool-down period. To prevent syncope, assist patients with positional changes and when exiting a warm pool. Always provide a cool-down period following exercise.
- **Dyspnea** may occur with β-receptor antagonists (β-blockers), even if they are β_1-selective antagonists. Bronchoconstriction may decrease aerobic capacity. To minimize dyspnea, aerobic activities should be designed to allow the patient increased time to achieve aerobic goals. Consider patient education on "pursed lip breathing" and pacing techniques.
- Beta blockers may blunt several early manifestations of **hypoglycemia**, but dizziness and sweating may still occur. For diabetic individuals medicated with hypoglycemic drugs, glucose levels should be checked prior to aerobic activities.
- **Negative chronotropic effect**. Both β-blockers and, to lesser extent, verapamil and diltiazem (CCBs) depress resting and maximal heart rate. Allow increased time to perform aerobic activity to account for depressed heart rate. Heart rate should not be used as a marker of exertion for patients taking β-blockers. Instead, use perceived exertion scales (eg, Borg rating of perceived exertion) when prescribing or determining the intensity of aerobic activity.
- **Negative inotropic effect**. β-blockers and, to lesser extent, verapamil and diltiazem, depress cardiac contractility. Cardiac output, and thus, aerobic capacity may be decreased. Allow patients more time during aerobic activities to achieve aerobic goals.
- **Altered plasma potassium levels**. Loop and thiazide diuretics may cause hypokalemia, whereas potassium-sparing diuretics may cause hyperkalemia. Disruptions in plasma

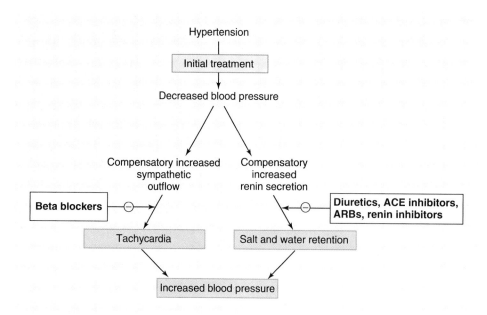

FIGURE 7-11 **Compensatory responses to decreased blood pressure when treating hypertension.** Arrows with minus signs indicate drug classes used to minimize the compensatory response. ACE, angiotensin-converting enzyme inhibitor; ARB, angiotensin receptor blocker.

TABLE 7-3 Compensatory responses and adverse effects of antihypertensive drugs.

Class and Drug	Compensatory Responses	Adverse Effects
Diuretics		
Potassium-wasting		
Furosemide	Minimal	Hypokalemia, hyperuricemia, allergic reactions, metabolic alkalosis, ototoxicity, hypomagnesemia, orthostatic hypotension
Hydrochlorothiazide	Minimal	Hypokalemia, hyperlipidemia, hyperuricemia, hyperglycemia, orthostatic hypotension, metabolic alkalosis, allergic reactions
Potassium-sparing		
Spironolactone	Minimal	Hyperkalemia, metabolic acidosis
Others		
Mannitol	Minimal	Pulmonary edema (acutely)
ADH receptor antagonist		Dehydration (chronically)
Conivaptan	Minimal	Hypernatremia, nephrogenic diabetes insipidus
CNS-mediated sympatholytics		
Clonidine	Salt and water retention	Dry mouth; severe rebound hypertension if drug is suddenly stopped
α₁-selective antagonists		
Doxazosin	Salt and water retention Slight tachycardia	Orthostatic hypotension (limited to first few doses)
β-selective antagonists		
Metoprolol	Minimal	Sleep disturbances, sedation, impotence, cardiac disturbances, decreased bronchodilation
Vasodilators		
Hydralazine	Salt and water retention; marked tachycardia	Lupus-like syndrome and vasculitis
Minoxidil	Marked salt and water retention, very marked tachycardia	Hirsutism, pericardial effusion, orthostatic hypotension
Nitroprusside	Salt and water retention	Excessive hypotension, cyanide toxicity (CN- released)
Calcium channel blockers		
Nifedipine	Minor salt and water retention	Constipation
ACE inhibitors		
Captopril	Minimal	Cough, decreased glomerular filtration rate, exacerbation of preexisting renal disease, fetal nephrotoxicity
Angiotensin II receptor antagonists		
Losartan	Minimal	Decreased glomerular filtration rate, exacerbation of preexisting renal disease, fetal nephrotoxicity
Renin inhibitor		
Aliskiren	Minimal	Decreased glomerular filtration rate, hyperuricemia, fetal nephrotoxicity

ACE, angiotensin-converting enzyme; ADH, antidiuretic hormone; CNS, central nervous system.

potassium levels affect *all* excitable cells. Thus, paresthesias, decreased skeletal muscle function, and cardiac arrhythmias (often perceived by the patient as heart palpitations) can occur. Manifestations of hypokalemia include increased excitability of ectopic pacemakers and corresponding arrhythmias, muscle cramps, and weakness. Hyperkalemia may be caused by potassium-sparing diuretics, β-blockers, and drugs that inhibit the renin-angiotensin-aldosterone system. Hyperkalemia depresses cardiac output. As with hypokalemia, the risk of cardiac arrhythmias increases and muscle weakness is possible (although the underlying mechanism is different). If a patient reports symptoms of altered (low or high) potassium levels, his/her physician should be notified because the most significant adverse effect is cardiac arrhythmias.

CASE CONCLUSION

The therapist contacted the referring physician to report the incident and to discuss whether referral back would be required prior to additional rehabilitation activities. R.T.'s initial difficulty in breathing was likely due to a combination of the effect of the nonselective β-receptor antagonist labetalol (which diminished bronchodilation during exertional activities) and the hydrostatic pressure on the chest (from submersion up to the neck in the pool). The subsequent hypotension was likely multifactorial. The warm pool caused systemic vasodilation. Then, upon leaving the pool, gravity exacerbated peripheral pooling of the blood. In addition, the β-receptor antagonist and thiazide diuretic partially inhibited homeostatic baroreflexes when R.T. started standing in order to exit the pool. Normally, the baroreceptor reflex should have increased heart rate and venous return to the heart to increase cardiac output (and thus blood flow to the brain), preventing the dizziness. The lack of reflexive tachycardia with the further decrease in blood pressure due to standing was due to effects of labetalol. Finally, the opiate analgesic may also have diminished respiratory drive by its effects on respiratory centers in the brainstem (see Chapter 20 for opiates).

CHAPTER 7 QUESTIONS

1. For which of the following drugs would heart rate *not* be an appropriate marker of exertion?

    a. Captopril
    b. Furosemide
    c. Propranolol
    d. Minoxidil

2. Which of the following drugs decreases sympathetic outflow from the central nervous system?

    a. Clonidine
    b. Hydralazine
    c. Losartan
    d. Doxazosin

3. Combination of losartan with which of the following drugs would increase the risk of hyperkalemia?

    a. Guanfacine
    b. Diazoxide
    c. Prazosin
    d. Metoprolol

4. Which of the following drugs produces a vasodilatory effect mediated by nitric oxide?

    a. Hydralazine
    b. Minoxidil
    c. Diazoxide
    d. Fenoldopam

5. The antihypertensive effect for which of the following drugs is mediated by inhibiting α_1 receptors?

    a. Clonidine
    b. Propranolol
    c. Prazosin
    d. Nifedipine

6. Which of the following drugs does *not* have reflex tachycardia as an adverse effect?

    a. Doxazosin
    b. Hydralazine
    c. Lisinopril
    d. Hydrochlorothiazide

7. A chronic cough is an adverse effect for which of the following drugs?

    a. Captopril
    b. Valsartan
    c. Aliskiren
    d. Propranolol

8. Dyspnea during exercise may be an adverse effect of which of the following drugs?

    a. Bumetanide
    b. Conivaptan
    c. Propranolol
    d. Lisinopril

9. Hyperkalemic metabolic acidosis is an adverse effect of which of the following drugs?

    a. Mannitol
    b. Bumetanide
    c. Hydrochlorothiazide
    d. Spironolactone

10. Hypokalemic metabolic alkalosis is an adverse effect of which of the following drugs?

    a. Mannitol
    b. Bumetanide
    c. Hydrochlorothiazide
    d. Spironolactone

Drugs Used in the Treatment of Angina Pectoris

J.M. is a 52-year-old man with a 14-year history of hypertension and coronary artery disease. He works as a union pipe fitter employed at a shipyard. A major component of his work includes climbing on scaffolding for activities performed in the process of ship construction. Three days ago, he fell 8 ft to the ground off a platform, resulting in a compound fracture of the right femur. Relevant history includes moderate alcohol intake, 25-year history of smoking one-half pack of cigarettes per day (12.5 pack-year), and a body mass index of 32. Current daily drugs include metoprolol, hydrochlorothiazide, and quinapril for chronic treatment of hypertension, and additional medications for pain control. The patient is also prescribed sublingual nitroglycerin, as needed. Two days ago, the compound femur fracture was reduced via internal fixation with a medullary rod; surgeon-prescribed weight-bearing status is weight-bearing as tolerated. On postoperative day one (POD 1), the physical therapist observed that the patient had normal upper body strength and trunk control and that he was independent in squat pivot transfers from bed to chair. In the morning of POD 2, the therapist brings the patient to the inpatient gym in a wheelchair for initial assessment of standing and ambulation in the parallel bars. Seated, resting vitals signs are 135/88 mm Hg, 60 bpm. The patient expresses considerable apprehension about today's therapy goals due to fear of excessive pain. The physical therapist convinces the patient to attempt to stand in the parallel bars with the use of a gait belt plus another assistant. The patient comes to a complete standing position with both hands on the parallel bars for assistance. Prior to taking his first step, the patient complains of left-sided chest pain that begins to radiate down the left arm. The patient is quickly assisted to a seated position, and the therapist records the following vitals: 145/92 mm Hg, 78 bpm. The therapist notes that the patient is pale and diaphoretic and asks the assistant to notify the nurse of the patient's current status and position. The patient declined an afternoon physical therapy session.

REHABILITATION FOCUS

A structured, individualized, and supervised exercise program is a key component of cardiac rehabilitation following a myocardial infarction, and has been shown to yield physical, psychological, and financial benefits to the patient. In addition, regular moderate exercise appears to reduce the potential for subsequent myocardial infarction, and may do so at a reduced financial cost to the patient and the healthcare system. Aerobic components of these programs are not limited to use of a treadmill, but may also utilize upper body activities or functional activities related to returning to work. Physical therapists, nurses, or exercise physiologists can safely supervise exercise programs. Healthcare professionals working with this patient population require an understanding of the potential benefits and liabilities of antianginal drug effects during periods of increased functional activity or exercise.

Patients may experience angina either as the sole manifestation or as a component of a larger cardiovascular pathophysiologic presentation. Antianginal drugs are prescribed to reduce the frequency of anginal attacks as well as to relieve an anginal episode. In the case of prevention, the therapist must confirm that the patient has taken the drug as prescribed prior to participating in the rehabilitation activity. In case of anginal relief, the therapist must confirm that the patient has the (unexpired) drug at hand during the assessment or treatment because the drug may be needed. Many activities in rehabilitation increase sympathetic stimulation of the heart, which can precipitate an anginal attack. Aerobic exercise or functional/strength conditioning can also increase the incidence of anginal attacks. In addition, the physical therapist must remember that pain, fear, and apprehension all stimulate the sympathetic nervous system. Pain occurring during wound debridement or postoperative mobilization or apprehension preceding or during functional activities following a stroke or surgery can also induce an anginal attack.

Finally, the physical therapist must recognize that some antianginal drugs may affect exercise tolerance due to effects on other organs in the body. For example, transdermal nitroglycerin may benefit the patient during functional activity.

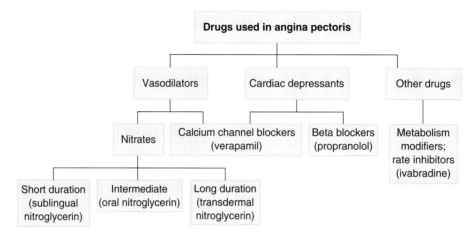

FIGURE 8-1 **Drug classes used in the treatment of angina pectoris.** Prototype drugs are listed in parentheses.

In contrast, β-receptor antagonists may reduce bronchodilation or cause bronchospasm and adversely affect physiologic responses to exercise.

BACKGROUND

Angina pectoris (or simply angina) refers to paroxysmal strangling or pressure-like chest pain caused by cardiac ischemia. Classically, angina is described as substernal pain that often radiates to the neck and left upper extremity. Occasionally, anginal pain may present in the right upper extremity or in the epigastrium. However, not all cardiac ischemia presents as pain. Women are less likely to present with classic anginal symptoms, but may present with anginal equivalents such as nausea, abdominal pain, and shortness of breath.

This chapter reviews the pathophysiology and therapeutic strategies for angina. Pharmacologic treatments are divided into vasodilators and cardiac depressants (Figure 8-1). In addition to medications, individuals with angina are often treated with lipid-lowering drugs to minimize additional plaque formation, as well as antithrombotics or anticoagulants to limit thrombosis formation and expansion at the site of these plaques. These drugs are discussed in Chapters 11 and 26.

DETERMINANTS OF CARDIAC OXYGEN DEMAND

The pharmacologic treatment of insufficient blood flow to the heart is based on physiologic factors that control how much oxygen the heart requires. The major determinant of the heart's oxygen requirement is myocardial fiber tension: the higher the tension, the greater the oxygen requirement. Figure 8-2 outlines the diastolic and systolic variables that contribute to fiber tension.

Among the diastolic factors, venous tone determines the amount of blood sequestered in the veins versus the amount that is returned to the heart. Venous tone is maintained by sympathetic activity and increases when sympathetic activity increases. Total blood volume and venous tone together determine preload, which is the major diastolic determinant of myocardial oxygen requirement.

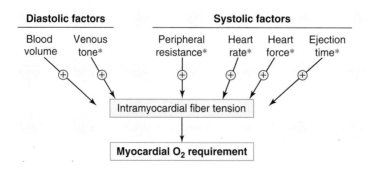

FIGURE 8-2 **Determinants of the volume of oxygen required by the heart.** Both diastolic and systolic factors contribute to the oxygen requirement; most of these factors are directly influenced by sympathetic discharge (venous tone, peripheral resistance, heart rate, and heart force) as noted by the asterisks.

Systolic factors that determine how much oxygen the heart needs include afterload, heart rate, contractility, and ejection time. Afterload is the pressure that the ventricle must overcome to eject blood into the arterial system. Afterload is determined by arterial blood pressure and the stiffness of large arteries. Heart rate contributes to the heart's oxygen demand because at fast heart rates, myocardial fibers spend more time in the contracted state. However, since faster heart rates abbreviate the time spent in diastole (when coronary perfusion is maximal), this leads to decreased myocardial perfusion. Heart rate and systolic blood pressure may be multiplied to yield the rate pressure product (RPP), a measure of cardiac work and therefore of oxygen requirement. In patients with atherosclerotic angina, effective drugs reduce the RPP. Contractility, or the force of cardiac contraction, is another systolic factor controlled mainly by sympathetic activity to the heart. Finally, ejection time for ventricular contraction is inversely related to force of contraction but is also influenced by impedance to outflow. Increased ejection time increases myocardial oxygen requirement.

ANGINA PECTORIS

Atherosclerotic angina is also known as exertional, stable, or classic angina. This form of angina is associated with atherosclerotic plaques that partially occlude one or more coronary arteries. When cardiac work increases (eg, during exercise), insufficient blood flow to the heart results in the accumulation of acidic metabolites and ischemic changes that stimulate myocardial visceral afferent fibers. This "referred" pain results from the convergence of visceral and somatic afferent fibers onto spinothalamic tract cells in thoracic spinal segments. Rest usually leads to relief of myocardial ischemic pain within 5-15 minutes. Atherosclerotic angina constitutes about 90% of angina cases.

Vasospastic angina is also known as rest angina, variant angina, or Prinzmetal angina and accounts for less than 10% of cases. Vasospastic angina involves reversible spasm of large coronary arteries, usually at the site of a plaque. Spasm may occur at any time, even during sleep. Vasospastic angina superimposed on atherosclerotic angina may deteriorate into unstable angina, also known as crescendo angina or acute coronary syndrome. Unstable angina is characterized by increased frequency and severity of anginal attacks that result from a combination of atherosclerotic plaques, platelet aggregation at fractured plaques, and vasospasm. Unstable angina is thought to be the immediate precursor of a myocardial infarction and is treated as a medical emergency. Finally, painless myocardial ischemia can proceed to necrosis, which is referred to as a silent myocardial infarction.

DRUGS TO TREAT ANGINA

The defect that causes angina is inadequate coronary oxygen delivery relative to the myocardial oxygen requirement. Strategies to correct this defect include reducing the oxygen requirement and/or increasing oxygen delivery (Figure 8-3). Currently popular pharmacologic therapies include nitrates,

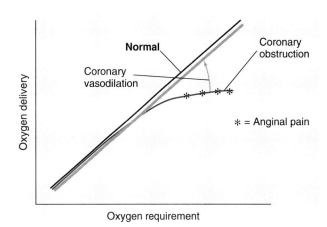

FIGURE 8-3 **Strategies for the treatment of exertional angina.** When coronary flow is adequate, O_2 delivery increases as O_2 requirement increases with exercise (black line). Angina is characterized by reduced coronary oxygen delivery versus oxygen requirement (red line), and anginal pain occurs as the oxygen debt increases. In some cases, this debt may be corrected by increasing oxygen delivery (revascularization or, in the case of reversible vasospasm, nitrates, and calcium channel blockers, brown line). More often, drugs are used to reduce oxygen requirement (nitrates, β-blockers, and calcium channel blockers) and slow progress along the red line.

calcium channel blockers, and β-receptor antagonists. These three drug classes reduce the heart's oxygen requirement in atherosclerotic angina. Nitrates and calcium channel blockers (but not β-receptor antagonists) can also increase oxygen delivery by reducing vasospasm, a useful effect only in vasospastic angina. Newer strategies help balance myocardial oxygen delivery and requirement by reducing sinoatrial discharge (eg, ivabradine) or decreasing myocardial fiber tension during diastole (eg, ranolazine). Another pharmaceutical strategy is to decrease oxidative stress during myocardial ischemia (eg, allopurinol). Many individuals with persistent angina also undergo myocardial revascularization to correct coronary artery obstructions. Therapy for unstable angina differs from that for exertional or vasospastic angina. Urgent revascularization is the treatment of choice in most cases. Antithrombotic drugs such as clopidogrel, prasugrel, ticagrelor, and/or aspirin are used to prevent platelet aggregation (Chapter 11). Intravenous nitroglycerin is sometimes of value.

NITRATES

The drugs comprising this pharmacologic class are sometimes referred to as "organic nitrates." **Nitroglycerin** (glyceryl trinitrate) is the prototypical agent of this class and the most important of the therapeutic nitrates. Sublingual nitroglycerin, used for the treatment of acute anginal attacks, has an onset of action of 1-3 minutes and duration of action of at least 25 minutes. Because the transdermal formulation has a longer

TABLE 8-1 Pharmacokinetically distinct forms of nitrate drugs used in angina.

Category	Example	Timeframe of Action
Short acting	Sublingual nitroglycerin	Rapid onset (1 min) Short duration of action (at least 25 min)
Intermediate acting	Oral regular or sustained-release nitroglycerin or isosorbide dinitrate or mononitrate	Slow onset Duration of action: 2-4 hr to 6-10 hr (in some formulations, effect is due to active metabolites)
Long acting	Transdermal nitroglycerin patch	Slow onset Long duration of action: 24 hr

duration of action (10-12 hours), it is used to prevent anginal attacks (Table 8-1).

Glyceryl trinitrate is rapidly denitrated in the liver and in smooth muscle to glyceryl dinitrate and then more slowly to glyceryl mononitrate. While glyceryl dinitrate retains a significant vasodilating effect, the mononitrate is much less active. Because of rapid enzymatic breakdown in the liver, there is a large first-pass effect for nitroglycerin (~90%). Sublingual nitroglycerin avoids the first-pass effect and its effect is primarily the result of the unchanged drug. The lower efficacy of swallowed nitroglycerin probably results from high levels of circulating glyceryl dinitrate (Chapter 3). Parenteral passive transdermal delivery is also available. Patches or ointment containing nitroglycerin provide maintenance therapy by providing therapeutic blood levels for up to 24 hours.

Isosorbide dinitrate, another commonly used nitrate, is available in sublingual and oral forms. Although isosorbide dinitrate is also rapidly denitrated in the liver and smooth muscle, the resulting isosorbide mononitrate is an active vasodilating agent, which is available as a separate drug for oral use. Several other nitrates are available for oral use and, like the oral nitroglycerin preparation, have an intermediate duration of action of 4-6 hours.

At the cellular level, nitrates cause smooth muscle relaxation. Denitration of the nitrates within smooth muscle cells releases nitric oxide (NO), which stimulates guanylate cyclase. Increased guanylate cyclase activity increases the second messenger cGMP, ultimately leading to smooth muscle relaxation by dephosphorylation of myosin light chain phosphate (Figure 8-4). This mechanism is identical to that of the direct-acting vasodilator, nitroprusside (Chapter 7).

At the level of the cardiovascular system, nitrates cause many effects (Table 8-2). Veins are the most sensitive to the action of nitrates, arteries less so, and arterioles are least sensitive. Venodilation leads to decreased venous return to the

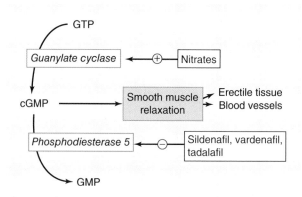

FIGURE 8-4 Mechanism of vasodilation by nitrates and drugs used in erectile dysfunction. Nitrate-stimulated guanylate cyclase activity increases cyclic guanosine monophosphate (cGMP) resulting in smooth muscle relaxation and vasodilation. Sildenafil and similar drugs used in erectile dysfunction inhibit a phosphodiesterase isoform (PDE-5) that metabolizes cGMP in smooth muscle of the corpora cavernosa. Increased cGMP relaxes erectile smooth muscle, allowing for greater inflow of blood and more effective and prolonged erection. This effect occurs to a lesser extent in the smooth muscle of other tissues. Because nitrates and PDE-5 inhibitors both increase cGMP by complementary mechanisms, they can have a synergistic effect on decreasing blood pressure.

heart (decreased preload) and subsequent reduction of intra-cardiac volume during diastole. The decreased end diastolic volume reduces myocardial fiber tension, which reduces myocardial oxygen demand. Vasodilation of the arterioles reduces

TABLE 8-2 Beneficial and deleterious cardiovascular effects of nitrates in the treatment of angina.

Effect	Mechanism of Action and Result
Potential Beneficial Effects	
Decreased ventricular volume	Decreased myocardial oxygen requirement
Decreased arterial pressure	
Decreased ejection time	
Vasodilation of epicardial coronary arteries	Relief of coronary artery spasm
Increased collateral flow	Improved perfusion to ischemic myocardium
Decreased left ventricular diastolic pressure	Improved subendocardial perfusion
Potential Deleterious Effects	
Reflex tachycardia	Increased myocardial oxygen requirement; decreased diastolic perfusion time and coronary perfusion
Reflex increase in contractility	Increased myocardial oxygen requirement

afterload, which can contribute to an increased ejection volume and further decrease in cardiac size (amount of filling). Arteriolar dilation reduces total peripheral resistance and blood pressure. These changes result in an overall reduction in myocardial fiber tension, oxygen consumption, and the RPP. Thus, the primary mechanism for nitrates' therapeutic benefit in atherosclerotic angina is reduction of the heart's oxygen requirement. An increase in coronary flow via collateral vessels in ischemic areas has also been proposed. In vasospastic angina, a reversal of coronary spasm and increased flow has been demonstrated. Intravenous nitroglycerin is sometimes used in unstable angina and has been demonstrated to reduce platelet aggregation. When nitroglycerin reduces blood pressure, a significant reflex tachycardia and increased force of contraction are predictable. The effects of nitrates are not isolated to the smooth muscle in the cardiovascular system. However, their effects on smooth muscle of the bronchi, gastrointestinal tract, and genitourinary tract are too small to be clinically useful.

Vasodilators such as nitroprusside used in hypertension and nitrates used in angina both act by releasing nitric oxide. However, nitroprusside and other drugs in this class are strong arteriolar vasodilators, whereas nitrates are relatively less effective on arterioles. The more limited arteriolar vasodilation caused by nitrates ensures that excessive dilation will not occur in normal vessels to the detriment of flow through partially obstructed ones. Drugs such as nitroprusside would vasodilate both partially obstructed and normal coronary arterioles, and more so in the latter. Blood flow in the unobstructed arteriole then would increase disproportionately compared to the partially obstructed coronary arteriole, ultimately decreasing blood flow through the partially obstructed coronary arteriole and potentially exacerbating the tissue hypoxia (termed "coronary steal"). For this reason, drugs such as nitrates that act primarily on veins are very useful in angina because they demonstrate minimal coronary steal.

Nitroglycerin is available in several formulations (Table 8-1). Standard treatment of acute exertional angina is sublingual tablet, which has a duration of action of at least 25 minutes. Isosorbide dinitrate is similar or slightly longer in duration of action. Swallowed normal-release nitroglycerin has a duration of action of 4-6 hours. Sustained-release oral forms have a somewhat longer duration of action. Transdermal formulations, in ointment or patch, can maintain therapeutic blood levels for up to 24 hours. Tolerance develops after 8-10 hours, with rapidly diminishing effectiveness thereafter. Therefore, conventional medical practice is to recommend that nitroglycerin patches be removed after 10-12 hours to allow recovery of sensitivity to the drug. A new patch may be applied after a 12-hour patch-free period.

The most common adverse effects of nitrates are the responses evoked by vasodilation (Table 8-2). These include tachycardia (due to the baroreceptor reflex), orthostatic hypotension (due to venodilation), and throbbing headache (due to meningeal artery vasodilation). Nitrates interact with

sildenafil and similar drugs promoted for erectile dysfunction. Both classes of drugs increase cGMP in vascular smooth muscle, causing a synergistic relaxation of vascular smooth muscle that could result in potentially dangerous hypotension and hypoperfusion of critical organs, as well as priapism, an erection lasting longer than 4 hours which can cause damage to the surrounding tissues. (Figure 8-4).

β-RECEPTOR ANTAGONISTS

β-adrenergic receptor antagonists (β-blockers; BBs) are described in detail in Chapter 6. Generic drug names for these drugs end in "-lol". All β-receptor antagonists are effective in the prophylaxis of atherosclerotic angina attacks. Beneficial effects include decreases in heart rate, cardiac contractility, and blood pressure. Like the nitrates and calcium channel blockers, the β-receptor antagonists reduce the RPP.

These drugs are used for prophylactic therapy of angina, but are of no value in an acute anginal attack. They are extremely effective in preventing exertional angina, but are ineffective against the vasospastic form. The combination of β-receptor antagonists with nitrates is useful in the treatment of angina because the adverse compensatory effects (increased end diastolic pressure and increased ejection time) are minimized. For additional adverse effects, see Chapter 6.

CALCIUM CHANNEL BLOCKERS

Calcium channel blockers (CCBs) were discussed in the treatment of hypertension (Chapter 7). Several of these drugs are approved for use in angina (Table 8-3), and may be divided into two main classes: dihydropyridines and miscellaneous agents. **Nifedipine** is the prototypical dihydropyridine, while **diltiazem** and **verapamil** are familiar examples of the miscellaneous class. Although CCBs differ markedly in structure, all are orally active and most have half-lives of 3-6 hours. These drugs inhibit the movement of calcium ions through voltage-gated L-type calcium channels, the calcium channels most important in cardiac and smooth muscle. These drugs decrease calcium influx during action potentials in a frequency- and voltage-dependent manner. As a result of the reduced intracellular calcium, cardiac and vascular smooth muscle contractility is decreased. None of the CCBs interfere with calcium-dependent neurotransmission or hormone release because these processes do not utilize L-type calcium channels.

CCBs decrease cardiac contractility, relax blood vessels and, to a lesser extent, relax the uterus, bronchi, and gut. The physiologic response to these drugs varies with the specific agent. Diltiazem and verapamil have a greater inhibitory effect on heart rate and contractility than on vasodilation. Because they inhibit calcium-dependent conduction in the atrioventricular (AV) node, verapamil and diltiazem may be used to treat AV nodal arrhythmias (Chapter 10). In contrast,

TABLE 8-3 Clinical indications and toxicities of some calcium channel blockers (CCBs).

Drug	Indications	Adverse Effects
Dihydropyridines		
Amlodipine	Angina, hypertension	Headache, peripheral edema
Felodipine	Hypertension, Raynaud's phenomenon	Dizziness, headache
Isradipine	Hypertension	Headache, fatigue
Nicardipine	Angina, hypertension	Peripheral edema, dizziness, headache, flushing
Nifedipine	Angina, hypertension, migraine, Raynaud's phenomenon	Hypotension, dizziness, flushing, nausea, constipation, dependent edema
Nimodipine	Subarachnoid hemorrhage, migraine	Headache
Nisoldipine	Hypertension	Probably similar to nifedipine
Nitrendipine	Investigational for angina, hypertension	Probably similar to nifedipine
Miscellaneous		
Diltiazem	Angina, hypertension, Raynaud's phenomenon	Hypotension, dizziness, flushing, bradycardia
Verapamil	Angina, hypertension, arrhythmias, migraine	Hypotension, myocardial depression, constipation, dependent edema

nifedipine and other dihydropyridines evoke greater vasodilation, and the resulting sympathetic reflex prevents bradycardia and may actually increase heart rate. All CCBs reduce blood pressure and reduce the RPP in individuals with angina.

CCBs are effective prophylactic therapy in both exertional and vasospastic angina. Nifedipine has also been used to abort acute anginal attacks. In atherosclerotic angina, these drugs are particularly valuable when combined with nitrates. In addition to well-established uses in angina, hypertension, and supraventricular tachycardia, some CCBs are used in the treatment of migraines, preterm labor, and Raynaud's syndrome (Table 8-3). Finally, **nimodipine**, another dihydropyridine, is approved only for the management of stroke associated with subarachnoid hemorrhage.

Adverse effects of these drugs include constipation, pretibial edema, nausea, flushing, and dizziness. More serious adverse effects include acute heart failure, AV blockade, and sinoatrial node depression; these are more common with verapamil than with the dihydropyridines. Table 8-3 presents a summary of the adverse events when CCBs are used alone.

ALTERNATIVE ANTIANGINAL PHARMACOLOGIC STRATEGIES

Several new drugs or older drugs that have been used for other indications are used to treat angina. **Allopurinol**, a common anti-inflammatory agent used to treat gout, inhibits xanthine oxidase (Chapter 34), an enzyme that contributes to oxidative stress and endothelial dysfunction. High-dose allopurinol has been shown to prolong exercise time in patients with atherosclerotic angina. Most common adverse effects include skin rash, increased liver enzymes, and GI dysfunction.

Ivabradine is a so-called bradycardic drug because of its relative selective inhibition of hyperpolarization-activated sodium channels that control the rate of sinoatrial nodal depolarization and subsequent heart rate. This inhibition reduces cardiac rate and workload. No other significant hemodynamic

effects have been reported. Ivabradine appears to reduce anginal attacks with an efficacy similar to that of CCBs and β-blockers. Due to the negative chronotropic effects, bradycardia is a potential adverse effect. Other limited adverse effects include visual disturbances, vertigo, and syncope. Ivabradine is approved for use in angina and heart failure outside the United States.

Nicorandil is a drug that has properties of an organic nitrate and is also an agonist at K_{ATP} cardiac channels, which means that it increases potassium conductance. While the drug has vasodilating properties in normal coronary arteries, its effects are more complex in individuals with angina. Clinical studies suggest that nicorandil reduces both preload and afterload and also provides some myocardial protection via preconditioning by activation of K_{ATP} cardiac channels. One large trial showed a significant reduction in the relative risk of fatal and nonfatal coronary events in patients receiving the drug. Adverse effects include weakness, myalgia, and reflex tachycardia. Currently, nicorandil is approved for use in the treatment of angina in many European and Asian countries, but not in the United States.

Ranolazine appears to act by reducing a late sodium current in cardiac muscle, with subsequent decrease in intracellular calcium levels (Chapter 9) and reduced diastolic tension, cardiac contractility, and work. Ranolazine is approved for use in angina in the United States. Relatively infrequent (< 10%) adverse effects include bradycardia, dizziness, orthostatic hypotension, and weakness. Finally, ranolazine prolongs the QT interval in patients with coronary artery disease, but shortens it in patients with long QT syndrome. The drug has not been associated with torsade de pointes, a polymorphic ventricular tachycardia.

COMBINING ANTIANGINAL AGENTS

Table 8-4 summarizes the beneficial effects compared to the adverse effects of organic nitrates, CCBs, or β-blockers used

TABLE 8-4 **Effects of nitrates alone and with beta blockers or calcium channel blockers (CCBs) in angina pectoris.**

	Nitrates Alone	β-Blockers or CCBs Alone	Combined Nitrate and β-Blockers or CCBs
Heart rate	*Reflex increase*	**Decrease**	**Decrease**
Arterial pressure	**Decrease**	**Decrease**	**Decrease**
End-diastolic pressure	**Decrease**	*Increase*	**Decrease**
Contractility	*Reflex increase*	**Decrease**	No effect or decrease
Ejection time	**Reflex decrease**	*Increase*	No effect
Net myocardial oxygen requirement	**Decrease**	**Decrease**	**Decrease**

Undesirable effects that increase myocardial oxygen requirement are shown in *italics*; major therapeutic effects are shown in **bold and underlined**.

alone, or in combination with each other. Notably, when each drug class is used alone, it has undesirable clinical effects that can often be mitigated when used in combination with other agents.

NONPHARMACOLOGIC THERAPY

Myocardial revascularization can be achieved by coronary artery bypass grafting (CABG) or percutaneous coronary intervention (PCI). The latter procedure includes both percutaneous transluminal coronary angioplasty (PTCA; or simply, angioplasty) to dilate the vessel, followed by placement of an intraluminal stent to maintain vessel patency. These procedures are extremely important in the treatment of severe angina. They are the only methods capable of consistently increasing coronary flow in atherosclerotic angina and increasing the RPP.

REHABILITATION RELEVANCE

Administration of drugs such as nitrates prior to aerobic activities or painful treatments such as wound debridement can help prevent exertional angina. Anti-anginal drugs also have an ergogenic (*ie*, performance-enhancing) effect, allowing extended exercise duration when compared to their absence (Figure 8-5). For individuals with exertional angina exercising on a treadmill, the RPP when taking no drug (control) was similar to the RPP obtained during three dosages of diltiazem, a CCB. This suggests that an ergogenic effect - *not* an analgesic effect - allowed patients to exercise for a longer period of time. Although Figure 8-5 shows the effect of diltiazem, other anti-anginal drug classes have demonstrated similar results.

Many of the drugs clinically used for angina are also used in the treatment of hypertension, so the adverse effects are similar to those discussed in Chapter 7.

- **Orthostatic hypotension** is a problem that varies among drug classes and sometimes among drugs within the same

class. Organic nitrates and the dihydropyridines (CCBs) demonstrate a higher risk, while β-blockers carry a lower risk. Orthostatic hypotension may cause patients to faint when transferring from sitting or supine positions to standing, exiting from a warm aquatherapy area, or if aerobic exercise is terminated without an appropriate cool-down period. To prevent symptomatic orthostatic hypotension, assist patients with slow positional changes and when exiting a warm pool. Always provide a cool-down period following exercise.

- **Bronchoconstriction** is a problem with β-blockers. Resulting dyspnea may limit aerobic capacity. The incidence of this adverse effect is lower with β_1-selective receptor antagonists and partial β-receptor antagonists compared to nonselective β-receptor antagonists. Allow patients increased time to complete aerobic tasks to prevent dyspnea.

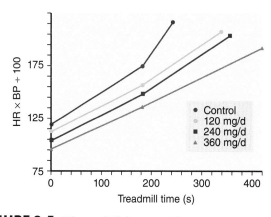

FIGURE 8-5 **Effects of diltiazem on the rate pressure product (heart rate × systolic blood pressure) in a group of 20 patients with exertional angina.** In a double-blind study using a standard protocol, patients were tested on a treadmill during treatment with placebo and three doses of the drug. Heart rate (HR) and systolic blood pressure (BP) were recorded at 180 seconds of exercise (midpoints of lines) and at the time of onset of anginal symptoms (rightmost points). Note that the drug treatment decreased the rate pressure product at all times during exercise and prolonged the time to appearance of symptoms.

- β-blockers **blunt early manifestations of hypoglycemia** occurring during aerobic activities. For diabetics taking hypoglycemia drugs, have patients check glucose levels prior to aerobic activities.
- Several antianginal drugs **depress heart rate**. Heart rate should not be used as a marker of exertion for patients taking β-blockers. Instead, perceived exertion scales (eg, Borg rating of perceived exertion scale) should be utilized to measure and prescribe exercise intensity.
- Several antianginal drugs **depress cardiac contractility**, which depresses cardiac output and further limits aerobic capacity.
- Nitrates and dihydropyridines cause **reflex tachycardia**.

CASE CONCLUSION

The patient was apprehensive prior to standing because he feared increased pain with weight-bearing on his right lower extremity. Upon rising, the patient likely experienced increased pain due to the femur injury and surgical repair. The combination of anticipatory pain prior to standing and increased pain during standing resulted in increased sympathetic discharge to the heart (increased heart rate and contractility). The combination of pain-associated sympathetic discharge with the pain due to the exertional activity of rising from the chair resulted in increased cardiac oxygen demand. The increased oxygen demand clinically manifested as exertional angina. To minimize a recurrence of this exertional angina, the physical therapist should request that the nursing staff provide his prescribed sublingual nitroglycerin for the patient to carry with him to the next therapy session. The patient could then take the drug 5-10 minutes prior to the expected exertion during physical therapy sessions. If angina occurs, the patient should take the medication as prescribed to relieve the exertional angina.

CHAPTER 8 QUESTIONS

1. The three forms of angina are exertional angina, unstable angina, and variant angina.

   a. True
   b. False

2. Which of the following cardiovascular drug classes is *not* utilized to treat the various forms of angina pectoris?

   a. Calcium channel blockers
   b. Nitroglycerin and other organic nitrates
   c. β-receptor antagonists
   d. α_1-receptor agonists

3. Pharmacologic mechanism(s) for the various classes of antianginal agents does *not* include which of the following?

   a. Decreasing cardiac preload by vasodilation
   b. Decreasing cardiac afterload by vasodilation
   c. Decreasing coronary blood flow
   d. Negative chronotropic and inotropic effects on the heart

4. Sublingual or buccal administration of nitroglycerin achieves a faster therapeutic systemic blood level of the drug compared to oral administration.

   a. True
   b. False

5. Which of the following is *not* an adverse effect associated with organic nitrates?

   a. Orthostatic hypotension
   b. Tachycardia
   c. Bronchoconstriction
   d. Headache

6. Which of the following drugs is thought to decrease anginal manifestation by inhibiting oxidative stress?

   a. Allopurinol
   b. Propranolol
   c. Diltiazem
   d. Nicorandil

7. Which of the following drugs decreases anginal effects by depressing myocardial function?

   a. Isosorbide dinitrate
   b. Labetalol
   c. Amlodipine
   d. Allopurinol

8. Which of the following drugs decreases anginal effects by depressing myocardial function?

   a. Isosorbide dinitrate
   b. Verapamil
   c. Amlodipine
   d. Allopurinol

9. Reflex tachycardia would most likely be an adverse effect of which of the following drugs?

    a. Isosorbide dinitrate
    b. Labetalol
    c. Diltiazem
    d. Allopurinol

10. Which dual combination of drugs directly increases the risk of acute heart failure?

    a. Nitroglycerin and diltiazem
    b. Metoprolol and verapamil
    c. Isosorbide dinitrate and amlodipine
    d. Metoprolol and amlodipine

Drugs Used in Heart Failure

T.S. is a 75-year-old man with heart failure resulting from long-standing cardiomyopathy. The patient has a history of coronary artery disease including a triple coronary artery bypass graft 5 years ago. He has a body mass index (BMI) of 30 kg/m² and a 45-pack-year history of smoking, though he quit smoking 8 years ago. Ten days ago, T.S. had a right total knee arthroplasty and spent 3 days in the hospital and 5 days in a rehabilitation facility. He was discharged from the rehabilitation facility with minimal assistance for sit to stand transfers and household distance ambulation with a front-wheeled walker. He was referred to outpatient physical therapy to continue transfer and gait training and to increase his aerobic endurance. On initial evaluation, the physical therapist measured his blood pressure at 135/75 mm Hg and pulse at 68 bpm. His current drug list includes daily carvedilol, benazepril, furosemide, and spironolactone. In addition, he takes an opiate analgesic as needed for pain relief. The patient arrives this morning for his second therapy appointment. As T.S. walked with his front-wheeled walker approximately 15 ft from his car to the clinic, the therapist noted that he appeared pale. Before initiating the session, the therapist stated her observation and concern. T.S. said that he has consistently been taking all his drugs as prescribed on the preceding days. The therapist measured his blood pressure as 145/90 mm Hg for and pulse at 70 bpm. Prior to beginning gait training with a cane, the physical therapist notices that the patient's legs appear significantly swollen. She assesses bilateral 3+/5 pitting edema at his ankles. T.S. shares that he had dinner last night at the new barbecue restaurant where he had a delicious barbecue platter with French fries and "bottomless" iced tea. Cautiously, the therapist assists T.S. to standing and begins gait training with the cane. After approximately 35 ft, T.S. becomes extremely dyspneic with audible wheezing and is diaphoretic around his head, neck, and hands. A chair is immediately brought up behind the patient and the therapist assists him to a seated position. His vital signs are 160/94 mm Hg and 86 bpm.

REHABILITATION FOCUS

Heart failure (HF) occurs when cardiac output is inadequate to provide the oxygen needed by the body. HF does not have a single cause. Preexisting heart conditions such as hypertension, coronary artery disease, and myocardial infarction increase the risk of HF because over time these conditions gradually sap the heart of its strength—leaving it too weak or too stiff to pump efficiently. In the United States, the most common cause of HF is coronary artery disease.

Epidemiologically, about one third of HF is due to systolic dysfunction in which ejection fraction is reduced because of decreased contractility (systolic failure). Another third of HF results from decreased myocardial wall relaxation during diastole that limits ventricular filling (diastolic failure). The remaining cases are a combination of systolic and diastolic dysfunction. Heart failure is a highly lethal condition, with a 5-year mortality rate of approximately 50%. The prevalence of HF is increasing because cardiovascular conditions such as myocardial infarction are being treated more effectively and more individuals are surviving long enough to develop the condition. Although research suggests that the primary defect in early HF resides in the excitation-contraction coupling machinery of the heart, the clinical condition involves many other processes and organs, including the baroreceptor reflex, the sympathetic nervous system (SNS), the kidneys, angiotensin II and other peptides, and death of cardiac cells.

This chapter reviews normal cardiac contractility and the pathophysiology and major clinical manifestations of HF. Drugs used to treat HF include positive inotropic agents to increase cardiac contractility as well as vasodilators and several miscellaneous drug classes that act at both cardiac and noncardiac sites to decrease the workload on the heart (Figure 9-1). Several drugs acting at noncardiac sites, such as the vasculature, kidneys and central nervous system, have been discussed in Chapters 6 through 8.

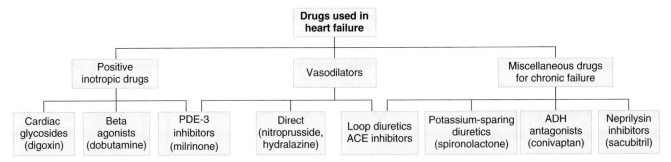

FIGURE 9-1 **Drugs used in the treatment of heart failure.** Several drug classes have many physiologic effects and do not fall into a single category. Prototype drugs are listed in parentheses. ACE, angiotensin-converting enzyme; ADH, antidiuretic hormone; PDE-3, phosphodiesterase type 3.

CONTROL OF NORMAL CARDIAC CONTRACTILITY

The force of contraction of heart muscle (contractility) is determined by several processes that ultimately lead to the movement of actin and myosin filaments in the cardiac sarcomere (Figure 9-2). During systole, calcium interacts with the actin-troponin-tropomyosin system to make the binding site on actin available for myosin to bind and the sarcomeres to shorten. The calcium required for this interaction is that which is released from the sarcoplasmic reticulum (SR), a cytoplasmic organelle that stores calcium. The amount of calcium released depends on the amount previously stored in the SR and on the amount of "trigger" calcium that initially enters the cell during the action potential.

Several factors related to intracellular calcium physiology regulate cardiac contractility. The first factor is sensitivity of the contractile proteins to calcium (Figure 9-2, **site 6**). Increased sensitivity of these proteins to calcium improves cardiac contractility; however, the determinants of calcium sensitivity (ie, the curve relating shortening of cardiac sarcomeres to cytoplasmic calcium concentration) are incompletely understood. Next, increasing the amount of calcium stored and released from the SR improves cardiac contractility. The SR membrane contains a very efficient calcium transporter (**site 4**), which maintains free cytoplasmic calcium at very low levels during diastole by pumping calcium into the SR. The amount of calcium *sequestered* in the SR is determined in part by the amount available for transport into the SR. This in turn is dependent on the balance of calcium influx (primarily through voltage-gated L-type calcium channels; **site 3**) and calcium efflux (calcium removed from the cell primarily via the Na^+/Ca^{2+} exchanger; **site 2**). The amount of calcium *released* from the SR (**site 5**) is regulated in part by the calcium influx through opening of L-type calcium channels (**site 3**) that occurs during the action potential. The amount of calcium that enters the cell depends on the number of L-type calcium channels and the duration of their opening. (As described in Chapter 4, sympathetic stimulation of the heart increases calcium influx through L-type calcium channels.) Ultimately, this small rise in free cytoplasmic calcium during

the action potential triggers the opening of calcium channels in the membrane of the SR, which produces a rapid release of a large amount of calcium into the cytoplasm in the vicinity of the actin-troponin-tropomyosin complex.

The Na^+/Ca^{2+} exchanger uses the influx of sodium during the action potential to move calcium against its concentration gradient from the cytoplasm to the extracellular space (**site 2**). Under physiologic conditions, extracellular concentrations of these ions are much less labile than intracellular concentrations. The ability of the Na^+/Ca^{2+} exchanger to carry out this transport is thus strongly dependent on the intracellular concentrations of both calcium and sodium, especially sodium. By removing intracellular sodium, the Na^+/K^+ ATPase (**site 1**) is the major determinant of sodium concentration in the cell. The sodium influx through voltage-gated channels, which occurs as a normal part of almost all cardiac action potentials, is another determinant. As described below, the Na^+/K^+ ATPase appears to be the primary target of cardiac glycosides.

PATHOPHYSIOLOGY

The fundamental physiologic defect in HF is a decrease in cardiac contractility or a decrease in filling. Decreased contractility results in cardiac output that is inadequate to maintain homeostasis. This is best shown by the ventricular function curve, also known as the Frank-Starling curve (Figure 9-3). The ventricular function curve can be used to illustrate the body's compensatory responses to HF as well as the response to drugs. As ventricular ejection decreases, the end-diastolic fiber length increases as shown by the shift from point A to point B in Figure 9-3. Contraction at point B is intrinsically less efficient than operation at shorter fiber lengths because of the increase in myocardial oxygen requirement associated with increased fiber stretch (Figure 8-2).

Figure 9-4 summarizes some of the body's compensatory responses to depressed cardiac output. These are mediated primarily by the SNS and the renin-angiotensin-aldosterone system. The baroreceptor reflex appears to be reset in HF such that sympathetic outflow is increased and parasympathetic outflow is decreased. Increased sympathetic outflow results

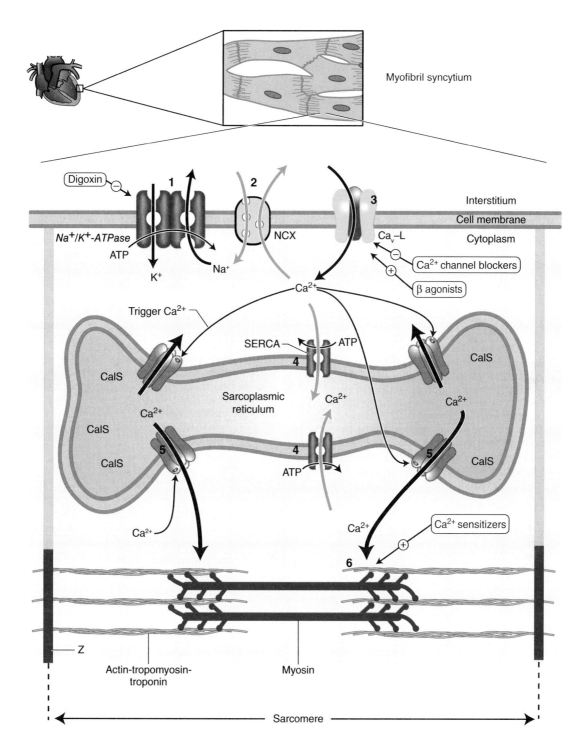

FIGURE 9-2 **Schematic diagram of a cardiac muscle sarcomere with key sites numbered (see text).** Site 1: Na⁺/K⁺ ATPase (sodium/potassium pump), which is the site of action of cardiac glycosides. Site 2: Na⁺/Ca²⁺ exchanger (NCX). Site 3: voltage-gated L-type calcium channel (Ca$_v$-L). Calcium entering through this channel is referred in the text as "trigger" calcium. Site 4: SR Ca²⁺-ATPase (SERCA) that pumps calcium into the SR. CalS inside the SR is calcium bound to calsequestrin, a high-capacity Ca²⁺-binding protein. Site 5: calcium channel in SR membrane that is activated to release calcium stored in the SR. Release of this stored Ca²⁺ is initiated by an influx of "trigger" calcium (site 3). Site 6: actin-troponin-tropomyosin complex at which calcium released from the SR brings about interaction of actin and myosin. Black arrows represent processes that initiate contraction or support basal tone. Green arrows represent processes that promote relaxation. SR, sarcoplasmic reticulum; Z, Z-line.

in tachycardia, increased contractility, and increased vascular tone (afterload). The decrease in renal blood flow due to HF activates the renin-angiotensin-aldosterone system and release

of antidiuretic hormone (ADH), resulting in further increases in vascular tone and increased blood volume. Later in HF, the heart enlarges and contractile tissue undergoes remodeling,

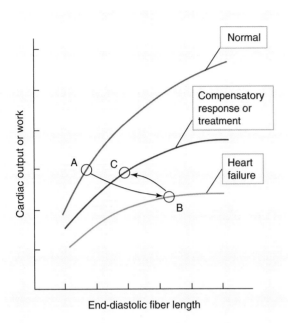

FIGURE 9-3 **Ventricular function (Frank-Starling) curves.** The *x*-axis can be any measure of preload-fiber length (eg, filling pressure, pulmonary capillary wedge pressure, etc). The *y*-axis is a measure of external cardiac work (eg, stroke volume, cardiac output, etc). In heart failure, cardiac output is reduced at all fiber lengths and the heart dilates because ejection fraction is decreased. As a result, the heart moves from point A to point B. Due to compensatory sympathetic discharge or effective clinical treatment the heart ejects more blood (moving from point B to point C).

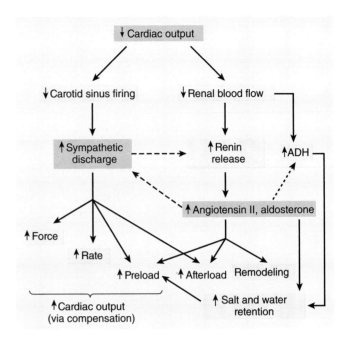

FIGURE 9-4 **Compensatory responses that play an important role in the progression of heart failure.** These include increased sympathetic discharge, increased activation of the renin-angiotensin-aldosterone system, and increased release of antidiuretic hormone (ADH).

with loss of functional myocardial cells and further reduction of contractile function. These cardiomegalic changes are mediated by increased sympathetic tone, angiotensin II, and possibly aldosterone. Although these compensatory responses *temporarily* improve cardiac output, they also increase cardiac workload. Eventually, the increased load contributes to further long-term decline in cardiac function.

Key clinical signs and symptoms of HF include tachycardia, decreased exercise tolerance, dyspnea, and cardiomegaly. Patients manifest varying degrees of impaired cardiac reserve and exercise intolerance. Additional cardiac arrhythmias (besides tachycardia) may be present. Increased salt and water retention results in weight gain, peripheral edema, and pulmonary edema. Edema in dependent lower extremities often manifests as pitting edema and patients' complaints of "heavy feet or legs." Pulmonary edema results in exertional dyspnea, orthopnea, and paroxysmal nocturnal dyspnea. When these clinical signs of congestion are present, the condition has been described as congestive heart failure.

Clinically, HF may be divided into chronic *compensated* heart failure and acute *decompensated* heart failure. The New York Heart Association subdivides chronic HF into four classes. Class I is associated with no limitations on ordinary activities and symptoms that occur only with greater than

ordinary exercise. Class II is characterized by some limitation of ordinary activities that results in fatigue and palpitations. Class III results in no symptoms at rest, but fatigue and other clinical manifestations appear with *less than* ordinary physical activity. Class IV is associated with symptoms even when the patient is at rest. In contrast, acute HF manifests as fairly rapid (hours to days) development of worsening peripheral edema, respiratory distress with exertion and later at rest, and diaphoresis and cyanosis. Acute HF requires increased medical intervention.

PHARMACOLOGICAL STRATEGIES

Figure 9-1 presents all drug classes used in the treatment of HF, while Table 9-1 outlines drug class preferences for *acute* versus *chronic* HF. Traditionally, diuretics and cardiac glycosides (digoxin) have been considered first-line therapy for HF. While diuretics are still a fundamental component of medical management for both systolic and diastolic HF, studies indicate that digoxin has been greatly overused.

Pharmacologic therapies for HF include the removal of retained salt and water with diuretics, direct treatment of the depressed heart with positive inotropic drugs (cardiac glycosides, β-receptor agonists, and phosphodiesterase inhibitors), reduction of preload and afterload with vasodilators, and reduction of afterload and retained salt and water with angiotensin inhibitors. In addition, considerable evidence suggests that angiotensin inhibitors diminish pathologic structural

TABLE 9-1 Drug classes used in heart failure.

Chronic Heart Failure	Acute Heart Failure
Diuretics	Diuretics
Aldosterone receptor antagonists	Vasodilators
Angiotensin-converting enzyme inhibitors	Beta receptor agonists
Angiotensin receptor antagonists	Phosphodiesterase inhibitors-3
Beta receptor blockers	Natriuretic peptide
Cardiac glycosides	
Vasodilators	
Neprilysin Inhibitors	

cardiac changes that often follow myocardial infarction and lead to HF. Current clinical evidence suggests that *acute* HF should be treated with a loop diuretic, a prompt-acting positive inotropic agent such as a β-receptor agonist or a phosphodiesterase type-3 (PDE-3) inhibitor, and vasodilators as required to optimize filling pressures and blood pressure. In contrast, in *chronic* HF, therapy directed at noncardiac targets may be more valuable than traditional drugs such as digoxin that focus on improving cardiac contractility. Thus, chronic HF is best treated with diuretics, plus angiotensin-converting enzyme (ACE) inhibitors or angiotensin receptor antagonists (ARBs), neprilysin inhibitors and ARBs, or if tolerated, a β-receptor antagonist for rate control, improved diastolic filling and cardiac output, and to reduce progression of chronic HF. Positive inotropic drugs such as cardiac glycosides reduce symptoms in chronic failure, if systolic dysfunction is prominent.

POSITIVE INOTROPIC AGENTS

Cardiac Glycosides

The cardiac glycosides are often called *digitalis* because several are derived from *Digitalis purpurea*, or foxglove. **Digoxin** is the prototype agent and the only one commonly used in the United States. A very similar molecule, digitoxin, which also comes from foxglove, is no longer available in the United States. The primary mechanism of action of digoxin is inhibition of Na$^+$/K$^+$ ATPase (the "sodium/potassium pump") within the myocardial cell membrane (Figure 9-2, **site 1**). This results in a small increase in *intracellular* sodium, which alters the driving force for the Na$^+$/Ca^{2+} exchanger so that less calcium is removed from the cell (**site 2**). The increased intracellular calcium is pumped into and stored within the sarcoplasmic reticulum (**site 4**) and, upon release (**site 5**), increases contractile force (**site 6**). Although other mechanisms of action for digoxin have been proposed, these are probably not as important as inhibition of the myocardial Na$^+$/K$^+$ ATPase. Digoxin also has a cardioselective parasympathomimetic effect. This action involves sensitization and increased firing of the baroreceptors resulting in decreased efferent sympathetic activity and increased vagal stimulation. Muscarinic transmission in atrial and atrioventricular nodal cells is also facilitated.

Physiologic Response

Digoxin causes mechanical and electrical effects that result from direct actions on cardiac membranes and indirect actions mediated through enhanced parasympathetic activity on the heart (Table 9-2). Mechanical effects include increased contractility (resulting in increased ventricular ejection), decreased end-systolic and end-diastolic dilation, increased cardiac output, and increased renal perfusion. These beneficial effects permit a decrease in the compensatory sympathetic

TABLE 9-2 Major effects of digoxin on electrical activity in the heart. Digoxin-induced arrhythmias are listed in the last row of the table.

| Variable | Tissue | | |
	Atrial Muscle	AV Node	Purkinje System Ventricles
Effective refractory period	↓[a]	↑[a]	↓[b]
Conduction velocity	↑[a]	↓[a]	Negligible
Automaticity	↑[b]	↑[b]	↑[b]
Electrocardiogram (before arrhythmias)	Negligible	↑ PR interval	↓ QT interval; T wave inversion; ST segment depression
Arrhythmias[c]	Tachycardia fibrillation	Tachycardia blockade	Premature ventricular contractions, bigeminy, tachycardia, fibrillation

AV, atrioventricular.

[a]Parasympathomimetic action.

[b]Direct membrane action.

[c]Digoxin-induced arrhythmias are more likely in the presence of hypokalemia, hypomagnesemia, or hypercalcemia.

and renal responses previously described. The decrease in sympathetic tone is especially beneficial; reduced heart rate, preload, and afterload allow the heart to function more efficiently (Figure 9-3, point C).

The electrical effects of digoxin include early cardiac parasympathomimetic responses and later detrimental arrhythmogenic responses. The overall effect of digoxin is to slow ventricular rate. Digoxin decreases atrioventricular (AV) conduction velocity, which can be seen on the electrocardiogram (ECG) as an increased PR interval. Flattening of the T wave is also often seen. The increase in AV nodal refractory period is particularly important when atrial flutter or fibrillation is present because the refractoriness of the AV node determines the ventricular rate in these arrhythmias. The effects on the atria and AV node are largely parasympathetic in origin. Later, shortened QT, inversion of the T wave, and ST segment depression may occur.

Clinical Uses

Digoxin has been and still is the traditional positive inotropic agent used in the treatment of chronic HF. However, careful clinical studies indicate that while digoxin improves functional status by reducing symptoms, it does not prolong life. As discussed later, other agents such as diuretics, ACE inhibitors or ARBs, and vasodilators may be equally effective, less toxic in some individuals, and some of these alternative drug therapies *do* prolong life. In individuals with atrial flutter and fibrillation, reduction of conduction velocity, or increasing the refractory period of the AV node, is *desirable* so that ventricular rate is controlled at a level compatible with efficient ventricular filling and ejection. The parasympathomimetic action of digoxin often accomplishes this therapeutic objective, although high doses may be required. Alternative drugs for rate control include β-blockers and calcium channel blockers. However, these drugs have negative inotropic effects that would not be beneficial in this population. Because the half-life of digoxin ranges from 36 to 48 hours in adults without renal failure, significant amounts of the drug may accumulate in the body, and dosing regimens must be carefully designed and monitored.

Adverse Effects

The therapeutic effect of increased contractility is a direct result of the increase in myocardial intracellular calcium. However, this accumulation of intracellular calcium is also the most important manifestation of its toxicity and contributes to its narrow therapeutic window. Increased intracellular calcium results in delayed after-depolarizations (depolarizations that appear after normal evoked action potentials), which may evoke extrasystoles (ectopic beats), tachycardia, or fibrillation in any part of the heart. In the ventricles, extrasystoles are recognized as premature ventricular contractions (PVCs). When PVCs are coupled to normal beats in a 1:1 fashion, the rhythm is called bigeminy.

The toxicity of digoxin is increased by hypokalemia, hypomagnesemia, and hypercalcemia. These electrolyte imbalances could result from *other* medications. For example, loop diuretics and thiazides, which are also key medications used in treating HF, may induce hypokalemia and hypomagnesemia, and thus precipitate digoxin toxicity. Digoxin-induced vomiting may induce hypomagnesemia and similarly facilitate toxicity.

The major signs of digoxin toxicity ("dig toxicity") are arrhythmias, nausea, vomiting, and diarrhea. Rarely, confusion or hallucinations and visual aberrations occur. Treatment of digoxin-induced arrhythmias is imperative because this manifestation of digoxin toxicity is common and dangerous. Table 9-2 lists common arrhythmias noted with chronic digoxin intoxication. Acute severe intoxication is caused by suicidal or accidental extreme overdose and results in cardiac depression leading to cardiac arrest rather than tachycardia or fibrillation.

β-receptor Agonists

Dobutamine and **dopamine** are useful in many cases of acute HF in which systolic function is markedly depressed. These agents activate cardiac β_1 adrenoceptors and enhance calcium influx (Figure 9-2, site 3). The increased calcium influx increases cardiac contractility and—in individuals in HF—does so with *minimal* increase in heart rate. However, β_1-adrenoceptor agonists are not appropriate for chronic HF because of tolerance and lack of oral efficacy. Manifestations of toxicity include significant arrhythmias, angina, and gastrointestinal distress.

Phosphodiesterase Type-3 Inhibitor

Milrinone is the major representative of this infrequently used group. This drug increases cyclic adenosine monophosphate (cAMP) by inhibiting its breakdown by PDE-3, which results in increased myocardial intracellular calcium. Similar to the effect produced by β_1-adrenoceptor agonists, the increase in contractility occurs with a minimal increase in heart rate in those with HF. PDE-3 inhibitors also cause vasodilation, which may be responsible for a major part of their beneficial effect. At sufficiently high concentrations, these agents may also increase the sensitivity of the contractile protein system to calcium (Figure 9-2, site 6). PDE-3 inhibitors are used in the treatment of *acute* HF. They should not be used in chronic HF because they have been shown to increase morbidity and mortality. Adverse effects include nausea, vomiting, thrombocytopenia, hepatic and bone marrow toxicities, and arrhythmias.

VASODILATORS

Direct-acting vasodilators and nitrates were previously discussed in Chapters 7 and 8. Vasodilator therapy with nitroprusside or nitroglycerin is often used for acute severe HF with congestion. Vasodilators are used because they decrease preload (which reduces cardiac size and improves mechanical efficiency) and also decrease afterload (which decreases resistance to ventricular ejection). Vasodilator therapy can be dramatically effective, especially when increased afterload is a major factor in causing the failure, such as in continuing hypertension in an individual who has just had an infarct. Chronic HF sometimes responds favorably to oral combination of an arteriolar and venous dilator such as hydralazine and isosorbide dinitrate, especially in African Americans.

NATRIURETIC PEPTIDES

The atria and other tissues release a family of natriuretic peptides that promote excretion of sodium into the urine (natriuresis), which results in decreased blood volume. Natriuretic peptides include atrial natriuretic peptide (ANP), brain natriuretic peptide (BNP), and C-type natriuretic peptide (CNP). The kidney also produces urodilatin, a peptide found in low concentration in the general circulation that has similar biologic properties. Natriuretic peptides participate in the homeostatic regulation of sodium excretion and blood pressure. Release of natriuretic peptides appears to be triggered by blood volume expansion. ANP and BNP exhibit similar natriuretic, diuretic, and hypotensive effects. The physiologic role of CNP is unclear; it has less natriuretic and diuretic activity than ANP and BNP, but is a potent vasodilator.

Several factors increase the release of ANP from the heart. These include atrial stretch, volume expansion, changing from the standing to the supine position, and exercise. In each case, the increase in ANP release is probably due to increased atrial stretch. Increased sympathetic stimulation (specifically, activation of α_{1A} adrenoceptors) and release of glucocorticoids and vasopressin also stimulate ANP release. Physiologically, ANP decreases blood pressure not only by decreasing blood volume, but also by promoting vasodilation. ANP inhibits the renin-angiotensin-aldosterone system and the secretion of antidiuretic hormone (also known as vasopressin). Both of these changes increase sodium and water excretion. ANP's vasodilation effects result from relaxation of vascular smooth muscle via increased guanylate cyclase activity. ANP also reduces sympathetic tone to the peripheral vasculature and antagonizes the action of angiotensin II and other vasoconstrictors.

In various pathologic states including HF, primary aldosteronism, chronic renal failure, and the syndrome of inappropriate antidiuretic hormone (SIADH) secretion, plasma ANP concentration increases. In fact, high plasma levels of ANP and BNP have emerged as diagnostic and prognostic markers for HF. Plasma ANP concentration is closely correlated with the New York Heart Association functional class of symptomatic HF.

The recombinant forms of BNP and ANP are called **nesiritide** and **carperitide**, respectively. These drugs are only used in *acute* HF. Their clinical effects appear to be due mainly to vasodilation, although natriuretic effects may also contribute. The most common adverse effect is excessive hypotension; significant renal damage is also of serious concern. A newer approach to therapeutically utilizing natriuretic peptides is by increasing the concentration of endogenous natriuretic peptides via inhibition of the enzymes that break them down (see below).

NEPRILYSIN INHIBITORS

One of the enzymes responsible for degradation and inactivation of natriuretic peptides is neprilysin. Neprilysin is also responsible for the degradation of angiotensin II and bradykinin (among other vasoactive peptides). **Sacubitril** is a prodrug that is metabolized to a neprilysin inhibitor. The use of sacubitril alone has the beneficial effect of increasing circulating levels of natriuretic peptides, but it also increases levels of angiotensin II and bradykinin. The increase in angiotensin II and bradykinin minimizes the clinical benefit of increased natriuretic peptides and increases the risk of angioedema. Therefore, sacubitril is combined with an angiotensin II type 1 receptor antagonist such as **valsartan** (Chapter 7). Thus, valsartan is listed as an angiotensin receptor neprilysin inhibitor (ARNI). The sacubitril-valsartan combination (available as a single oral formulation) increases clinical efficacy while minimizing adverse effects. Specifically, this drug combination inhibits two pathophysiologic mechanisms associated with HF: the renin-angiotensin-aldosterone-ADH system and decreased physiologic sensitivity to natriuretic peptides. Sacubitril increases circulating levels of natriuretic peptide by inhibiting neprilysin and valsartan inhibits the elevation of circulating levels of angiotensin II that occurs as a result of neprilysin inhibition. Elevated circulating levels of bradykinin (resulting from sacubitril) are prevented by degradation of bradykinin by both ACE and aminopeptidase P. Treatment with the sacubitril-valsartan combination reduces morbidity and mortality for individuals with systolic HF. Hypotension is the most common significant adverse effect due to the ARNI. For individuals taking the sacubitril-valsartan combination, ACE inhibitors are contraindicated due to potential increases in bradykinin and associated angioedema.

ANTIDIURETIC HORMONE ANTAGONISTS

There are three recognized receptors for vasopressin or ADH: V_{1a}, V_{1b}, and V_2. The V_1 receptors are expressed in vascular smooth muscle and the central nervous system. V_2 receptors are expressed in the kidney tubules, particularly in the distal convoluted tubule and collecting duct cells. As discussed in Chapter 7, ADH is responsible for vasoconstriction and increased water reabsorption in the kidney (Figure 7-10). When ADH binds to V_2 receptors on collecting tubule cells, adenylate cyclase is activated and cAMP production is increased. The increased cAMP results in increased insertion of aquaporin proteins (water channels) into the collecting tubule membrane, which allows water to move out of the tubules and into the vasculature.

Vasopressin receptor antagonists have generic drug names that end in "vaptan." **Tolvaptan** is the prototypical orally active drug that is selective for V_2 receptors. **Conivaptan** is an intravenous ADH antagonist that binds to both V_{1a} and V_2 receptors. Thus, conivaptan not only inhibits water reabsorption (by binding to V_2 receptors), but also promotes vasodilation (by binding to V_1 receptors). These drugs are clinically used in the treatment of HF and in SIADH. However, the vaptans do not appear to reduce mortality in HF. The most serious adverse effect is nerve demyelination resulting from the rapid correction of hyponatremia caused by these drugs.

MISCELLANEOUS MEDICATIONS

Diuretics (loop, thiazide, and aldosterone antagonists), ACE inhibitors and ARBs, and β-receptor antagonists have been discussed in Chapters 6 and 7, especially in relation to their use as antihypertensives. This discussion will focus on the clinical benefit of these medications in the treatment of HF.

Diuretics are usually first-line medications in HF because of their ability to reduce high filling pressure, which subsequently decreases myocardial oxygen demand. **Furosemide**, a loop diuretic, is a very useful agent for immediate reduction of the pulmonary congestion and severe edema associated with acute or severe chronic failure. Thiazides, such as **hydrochlorothiazide**, are sometimes sufficient for mild chronic failure. **Spironolactone** and **eplerenone**, potassium-sparing diuretics that are aldosterone antagonists, have significant long-term benefits in chronic failure.

Angiotensin-converting enzyme inhibitors, such as **captopril**, have been shown to reduce morbidity and mortality in chronic HF. Although they have no direct positive inotropic action, these agents reduce aldosterone secretion, salt and water retention, and vascular resistance. They are now considered, along with diuretics, among the first-line drugs for chronic HF. Although the angiotensin receptor antagonists (the ARBs) such as **losartan** appear to have the same benefits as ACE inhibitors, there is less clinical experience with these drugs compared to the ACE inhibitors. However, for patients with asthma or chronic obstructive airway disease, ARBs may be an alternative as they have a reduced incidence of chronic coughs compared to ACE inhibitors.

Finally, long-term studies have shown that certain β-receptor antagonists (**carvedilol**, **labetalol**, **metoprolol**, and **nebivolol**) reduce progression of chronic HF. The benefit of these agents had long been recognized in individuals with hypertrophic cardiomyopathy, but benefits have also been demonstrated in those without cardiomyopathy. In acute HF, β-receptor antagonists are not of value and they may be detrimental if systolic dysfunction is marked.

REHABILITATION RELEVANCE

For individuals with HF, exercise programs including aerobic and resistance components result in improved exercise tolerance, endurance, and quality of life. Safe and effective cardiac rehabilitation programs occur in both inpatient and outpatient settings. The physical therapist must be cognizant of the interactions among the patient, the medications, and the exercise intervention. While drugs used to improve cardiac performance or decrease cardiac workload improve patient participation in cardiac rehabilitation programs, changes in dosage or introduction of additional medications are common and may result in adverse events previously discussed.

Therapists should monitor fluid overload (eg, increased lung congestion or edema in dependent extremities) in this population because this can be an indication of either a progression or acute exacerbation of HF. If fluid overload is present, exercise intensity must be decreased, or the exercise program terminated until the patient is medically reevaluated and medication changes are made, if necessary. For any patient taking medications that affect the heart and vascular system, therapists must anticipate orthostatic hypotension and provide appropriate assistance and guarding to prevent syncope. Appropriate cool-down periods are necessary following aerobic activities due to the increased peripheral vasodilation resulting from exercise *in conjunction with* the vasodilation induced by vasodilators and possibly decreased blood volume (in the case of diuretics).

The adverse effects relevant to rehabilitation depend on the specific drug or drug class. Many of these have been discussed in Chapters 6 through 8. Below is a select summary of adverse events, with emphasis on those caused by drugs or combination of drugs typically involved in the treatment of HF.

- **Arrhythmias** may be induced by cardiac glycosides such as digoxin. Aerobic activities may increase the potential for glycoside-induced arrhythmias. When possible, the therapist should monitor heart rate during sessions, especially when aerobic activities are a part of the therapy. Because of the narrow therapeutic window for digoxin and the potential for many drug-drug interactions, therapists should monitor for signs and symptoms of "dig toxicity" and relay any suspicion to the medical team.

- **Hypokalemia** may result from thiazide and loop diuretic use. These diuretics may *exacerbate* the effects of cardiac glycosides, increasing the risk of glycoside toxicity. In addition to arrhythmias, musculoskeletal manifestations of decreased plasma potassium levels include paresthesias, muscle weakness, and cramps. If the therapist recognizes any of these clinical manifestations, prompt review of the patient's drug list is indicated. If lab values are current and available, the therapist should confirm that plasma potassium level is within the normal range.

- **Hyperkalemia** may result from use of drug classes that inhibit the renin-angiotensin-aldosterone system (ie, ACE inhibitors, ARBs, aldosterone receptor antagonists). Hyperkalemia may *decrease* the effect of cardiac glycosides. The clinical manifestations of hyperkalemia are similar to those of hypokalemia. The therapist should follow the guidelines presented above for hypokalemia.

CASE CONCLUSION

The physical therapist should immediately contact the referring physician's office to determine whether the patient should be transferred to emergency facilities or to the referring physician's office. This patient's medical history and current medical problems are extensive. His slow postsurgical rehabilitation progress was likely multifactorial, including significant smoking history, high BMI, older age, and HF. The adverse event that occurred during this therapy session could have been precipitated by the previous evening's dinner that included a significant amount of sodium and water, which may have exceeded the action of the diuretic (furosemide), resulting in both systemic and pulmonary edema. Systemic edema was evident as bilateral pitting edema in the dependent extremities; pulmonary edema may have provoked or contributed to the patient's exertional dyspnea. In addition, carvedilol, a nonselective β-receptor antagonist, may have exacerbated the dyspnea by limiting bronchodilation that typically occurs with exercise. Although not documented as a comorbidity, T.S. may have chronic obstructive pulmonary disease, given his significant smoking history. Last, the opiate for pain may have decreased respiratory drive (see Chapter 20 for Opiates). The physical therapist can play a large role in the treatment of HF by encouraging patients to weigh themselves every morning—after urination and before breakfast. Typically, a weight gain of 2-3 lb or more in a day indicates fluid retention, which requires lowering the intensity of exercise, or even holding exercise interventions because fluid overload places a greater workload on the heart.

CHAPTER 9 QUESTIONS

1. A decrease in ejection fraction due to decreased myocardial fiber contraction characterizes which of the following?

   a. Systolic heart failure
   b. Diastolic heart failure
   c. Combined systolic/diastolic heart failure
   d. High output heart failure

2. Which of the following drugs increases cardiac contractility by inhibiting the $Na^+/K^+/ATPase$?

   a. Dopamine
   b. Dobutamine
   c. Digoxin
   d. Sacubitril

3. Which of the following drugs may exacerbate the pharmacologic effects of digoxin and increase the risk of an adverse effect?

   a. Captopril
   b. Furosemide
   c. Metoprolol
   d. Spironolactone

4. Which of the following drugs increases cardiac contractility by acting as an agonist at cardiac β receptors?

   a. Captopril
   b. Digoxin
   c. Dobutamine
   d. Hydrochlorothiazide

5. Which of the following drugs increases cardiac contractility by increasing intracellular cyclic adenosine monophosphate (cAMP) by inhibiting phosphodiesterase?

   a. Labetalol
   b. Digoxin
   c. Dobutamine
   d. Milrinone

6. Which of the following drugs is combined with sacubitril to minimize the adverse effects of inhibiting neprilysin?

   a. Furosemide
   b. Propranolol
   c. Captopril
   d. Valsartan

7. Which of the following drugs acts only by inhibiting vasopressin 2 (V_2) receptors in the kidney?

   a. Vasopressin
   b. Conivaptan
   c. Tolvaptan
   d. Antidiuretic hormone

8. With respect to its use in heart failure, dopamine would be considered which of the following?

   a. ADH antagonist
   b. Neurotransmitter
   c. Positive inotropic drug
   d. Vasodilator

9. Which of the following drug classes is used in acute heart failure?

   a. Beta-receptor agonists
   b. Beta-receptor antagonists
   c. Cardiac glycosides
   d. Angiotensin-converting enzyme inhibitors

10. Which of the following drugs acts in part as a natriuretic?

    a. Carvedilol
    b. Nesiritide
    c. Digoxin
    d. Dopamine

Antiarrhythmic Drugs

S.M. is a 42-year-old woman with a history of paroxysmal atrial fibrillation and mitral valve prolapse since childhood. The patient is under the care of a cardiologist for these conditions. She has a body mass index of 25 kg/m^2 and no other documented comorbidities. Her job requires her to examine carbon fiber aerospace components at the end of the manufacturing process. The required physical motions include stacking objects weighing 8-15 lb and bending over repetitively during an 8-hour shift. Three weeks ago, S.M. felt a sudden and extreme pain in the right lumbar area while bending over to retrieve a component that had fallen on the floor. She was transported to the emergency department and discharged with a prescription for meloxicam, a nonsteroidal anti-inflammatory drug. The patient was seen by the corporate physician 2 days later and referred to an outpatient physical therapy clinic for pain relief and a return-to-work program. At the first appointment, the therapist noted that S.M. needed assistance getting out of the vehicle passenger seat. Beyond activities of daily living and clinic visits, S.M. states that she has done almost no physical activity. She has remained in bed or on the couch. Her current medications include diltiazem and naproxen, an over-the-counter nonsteroidal anti-inflammatory drug that she started taking after she completed her prescription of meloxicam. The first three sessions of therapy were aimed at minimizing pain and improving functional mobility. Today, S.M. arrives to begin the functional return-to-work program. At rest, her heart rate is 78 bpm, regular rhythm and her blood pressure is 132/89 mm Hg. Fifteen minutes into the return-to-work exercises, the patient complains of chest palpitations that she recognizes as an arrhythmia. Determination of vital signs indicates her heart rate is 120 bpm, irregular rhythm and blood pressure is 159/98 mm Hg. After several minutes, her palpitations recede and heart rate becomes regular though still tachycardic at 102 bpm.

REHABILITATION FOCUS

Cardiac arrhythmias, or abnormal heart rhythms, can be brief or long lasting. They can be completely benign or life threatening. Arrhythmias often occur in the presence of preexisting heart disease. Arrhythmias occur in over 80% of individuals with an acute myocardial infarction and are the most common cause of death in those who have had a myocardial infarction. Electrolyte imbalances can also cause arrhythmias. Diuretics are significant sources of such imbalances. Treatment is required when cardiac rhythms are too rapid, too slow, asynchronous, or significantly reduce cardiac output. Certain arrhythmias may precipitate more serious or even lethal rhythm disturbances. For example, multiple premature ventricular contractions can precipitate ventricular fibrillation, which is fatal unless corrected promptly. In such cases, antiarrhythmic drugs may be lifesaving. In contrast, pharmacologic treatment of arrhythmias that are asymptomatic or minimally symptomatic is avoided because of the ability of many of these drugs to *induce* lethal arrhythmias. In this chapter, we review the conduction sequence and electrophysiology of the normal cardiac rhythm, highlight the mechanisms of arrhythmias, and discuss antiarrhythmic drugs used in their treatment.

Four classes of antiarrhythmic drugs are most widely recognized (Figure 10-1). Classification is based on mechanism of action: blockade of sodium channels (class 1); blockade of cardiac β_1 adrenergic receptors (class 2); blockade of potassium channels (class 3); and, blockade of calcium channels (class 4). A fifth miscellaneous class includes those antiarrhythmic drugs with different mechanisms of action.

ELECTROPHYSIOLOGY OF NORMAL CARDIAC RHYTHM

Cardiac Electrical Conduction Pathway

Figure 10-2 shows the intrinsic cardiac electrical activity with the simultaneous electrocardiogram (ECG) waveforms. The electrical impulse that triggers a normal cardiac contraction originates at regular intervals in the sinoatrial (SA) node, usually at a frequency of 60-100 bpm. This pacemaker impulse

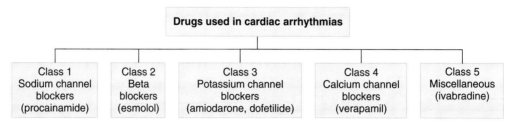

FIGURE 10-1 Drugs used in the treatment of cardiac arrhythmias. There are four major classes of antiarrhythmic drugs and an additional miscellaneous class. Prototype drugs are in parentheses.

spreads rapidly through the atria and enters the atrioventricular (AV) node, which is normally the only conduction pathway between the atria and ventricles. Conduction through the AV node is slow, requiring about 0.15 second. This delay is critical because it provides enough time for atrial contraction to propel blood into the ventricles. The impulse then propagates over the His-Purkinje system and invades all parts of the ventricles. Ventricular activation is complete in less than 0.1 second; therefore, contraction of all the ventricular muscle is synchronous and hemodynamically effective. *Arrhythmias*

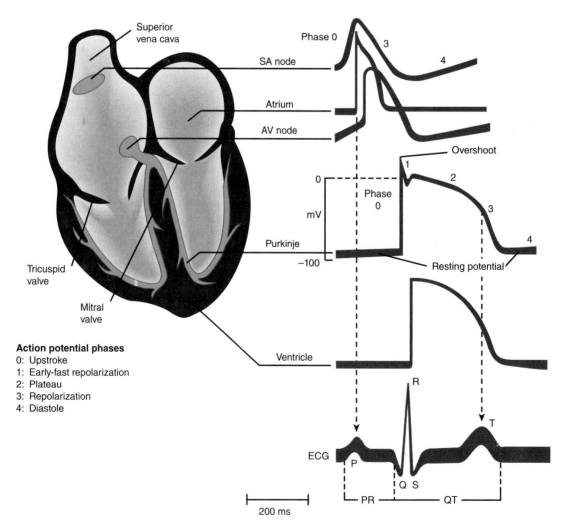

FIGURE 10-2   Diagram of the heart with normal electrical activity (intracellular recordings from areas indicated and corresponding electrocardiogram [ECG]). Sinoatrial (SA) node, atrioventricular (AV) node, and Purkinje cells display pacemaker activity (phase 4 depolarization). The ECG is the body surface manifestation of depolarization and repolarization waves of the heart. The P wave is generated by atrial depolarization, the QRS by ventricular muscle depolarization, and the T wave by ventricular repolarization. The PR interval is a measure of conduction time from atrium to ventricle, and the QRS duration indicates the time required for all of the ventricular cells to be activated (ie, the intraventricular conduction time). The QT interval reflects the duration of the ventricular action potential.

consist of cardiac depolarizations that deviate from the above description in one or more aspects (ie, abnormalities in pacemaker origin of the impulse, the rate or regularity, or the conduction pathway).

Action Potentials in the Cardiac Cell

The transmembrane potential of cardiac cells is determined by two factors: the concentrations of sodium (Na$^+$), potassium (K$^+$), calcium (Ca^{2+}), and chloride (Cl$^-$) on either side of the membrane and the permeability of the membrane to each ion. These water-soluble ions are unable to freely diffuse across the lipid plasma membrane. Ions can only move down their electrochemical gradients at specific times during the cardiac cycle when ion channels open. Individual channels are relatively ion-selective and a "gate" composed of a flexible peptide chain controls ion flux through each channel. Each type of ion channel has its own type of gate, and each type of gate is modulated by specific transmembrane voltage, ionic, and/or metabolic conditions. Once an ion channel opens, the movement of ions produces currents that form the basis of the cardiac action potential (AP).

In most parts of the heart, sodium channels are the most important determinant of AP conduction. The molecular and functional structure of sodium channels has been extensively characterized. Figure 10-3 illustrates a convenient way to describe the behavior of the sodium channel in terms of three functional states. The channel contains an activation

gate (m) and an inactivation gate (h). At rest, the activation gate is closed, and the inactivation gate is open (**panel 1**). Depolarization to the threshold voltage results in opening of the activation gate (**panel 2**). The sodium ion influx is brief because the inactivation gate closes soon after the opening of the activation gate (**panel 3**). Upon repolarization, recovery from inactivation (panel 3) takes place, making the sodium channels again available for excitation (panel 1). This reactivation requires energy in the form of conversion from ATP to ADP.

Most cardiac L-type calcium channels are activated and inactivated in a similar way as sodium channels. However, the transitions occur more slowly and at more positive potentials in cardiac L-type calcium channels than in sodium channels.

At rest, most cardiac cells are not significantly permeable to sodium, but at the start of each AP, they become permeable due to ion fluxes through voltage-gated channels and carrier mechanisms. Figure 10-4 describes the ion fluxes that comprise each phase of the cardiac AP. In normal atrial, Purkinje, and ventricular cells, the AP upstroke (phase 0) is dependent on sodium current (I_{Na}). After a very brief activation of the m gate, the sodium channel enters a more prolonged period of inactivation due to closing of the h gate. At the SA and AV nodes, calcium current (I_{Ca}) dominates the phase 0 upstroke. The characteristic plateau of the cardiac AP (phases 1 and 2) results from calcium *depolarizing* current (I_{Ca}) occurring simultaneously with potassium *repolarizing* current (I_K). At the end of the plateau (when calcium channels close), I_K causes

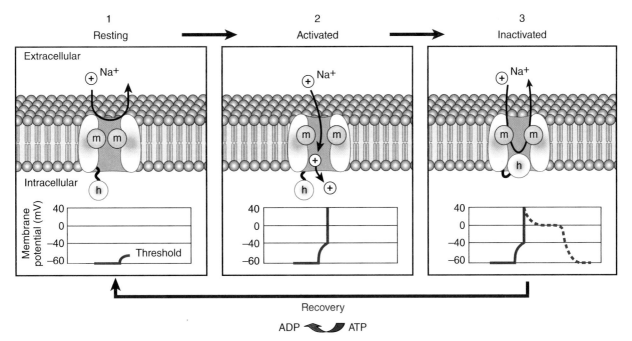

FIGURE 10-3 **Schematic representation of a Na$^+$ channel cycling through different conformational states during the cardiac action potential.** Transitions between resting, activated, and inactivated states are dependent on membrane potential and time. The activation gate is shown as *m* and the inactivation gate as *h*. Potentials typical for each state are shown under each channel schematic as a function of time. The dashed line indicates that part of the action potential during which most Na$^+$ channels are completely or partially inactivated and unavailable for reactivation. Reactivation of the channel (movement from panel 3 back to panel 1) requires energy via conversion of ATP to ADP. ADP, adenosine diphosphate; ATP, adenosine triphosphate.

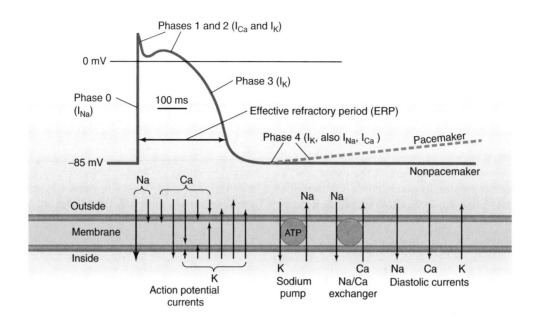

FIGURE 10-4 Ion permeability changes and transport processes that occur during an action potential in a typical Purkinje or ventricular cardiac cell. Each phase (0-4) is generated by specific ionic currents. The sodium pump and sodium-calcium exchanger are mainly involved in maintaining ionic steady state during repetitive activity. In nonpacemaker cells (solid line), the outward potassium current during phase 4 is sufficient to maintain a stable negative resting potential. In pacemaker cells (dashed line at right end of tracing), the potassium current is smaller and the depolarizing currents (sodium, calcium, or both) during phase 4 are large enough to gradually depolarize the cell during diastole. ATP, adenosine triphosphate.

rapid repolarization (phase 3). During the plateau of the AP, most sodium channels are inactivated. There is a relatively long time between phase 0 and sufficient recovery of sodium channels (in phase 3) before a new AP can be propagated in response to an external stimulus. This duration is termed the refractory period. Thus, the effective refractory period (ERP) of a cardiac cell is a function of how rapidly sodium channels recover from inactivation. Any prolongation of this recovery time results in an increase in the ERP and is dependent upon the membrane potential, which varies with repolarization time and extracellular potassium concentration. A more positive resting membrane potential results in fewer sodium channels opening and a depressed sodium current. The carrier processes, such as the Na^+/K^+-ATPase pump and the sodium-calcium exchanger, contribute little to the *shape* of the AP; however, they are critical for maintaining the electrochemical gradients on which the sodium, calcium, and potassium currents depend. Antiarrhythmic medications act on I_{Na}, I_{Ca}, or I_K, individually or in combination, or on the second messenger systems that modulate these currents.

ARRHYTHMOGENIC MECHANISMS

Factors precipitating arrhythmias include ischemia, hypoxia, acidosis or alkalosis, electrolyte abnormalities, excessive catecholamine exposure, autonomic influences, toxicity due to **digitalis** or antiarrhythmic drugs, overstretching of cardiac fibers, and the presence of scarred or otherwise diseased cardiac tissue. All arrhythmias result from disturbances in impulse *formation* and/or disturbances in impulse *conduction*.

The rate of impulse formation from the SA node can be accelerated or decelerated. Increased SA nodal rates result from stimulation of cardiac β_1 receptors, positive chronotropic drugs, fiber stretch, acidosis, and partial depolarization by injury currents. In contrast, decreased SA nodal rates result from vagal discharge and β_1-receptor antagonists. In some pathophysiologic conditions such as ischemia, hypoxia, hyperkalemia or hypokalemia, latent pacemaker cells and normally quiescent atrial and ventricular cells can also demonstrate abnormal pacemaker activity.

Disturbances in impulse conduction are a major cause of cardiac arrhythmias. Severely depressed conduction may result in a simple block such as at the AV node. AV blockade (often termed "nodal block") is particularly significant because the AV node is normally the only conduction pathway between the atria and ventricles.

Another common conduction abnormality is called re-entry or "circus movement" (Figure 10-5). In re-entry rhythms, a single impulse re-enters in a retrograde direction and excites areas of the heart more than once. The path of the re-entering impulse may be confined to a very small area such as within or near the AV node. Alternatively, multiple re-entry circuits, determined by the properties of the cardiac tissue, may meander through the heart in apparently random paths.

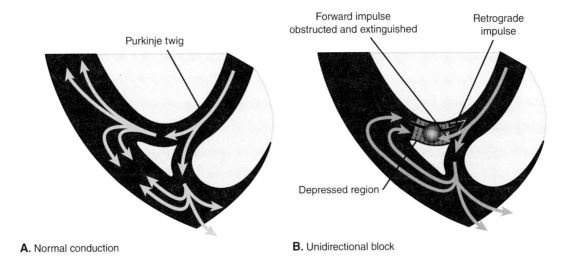

Purkinje twig

Forward impulse
obstructed and extinguished

Retrograde
impulse

Depressed region

A. Normal conduction

B. Unidirectional block

FIGURE 10-5 **Diagram of a re-entry circuit that might occur in small bifurcating branches of the Purkinje system where they enter the ventricular wall.** (**A**) Normally, electrical excitation branches around the circuit, is transmitted to the ventricular branches, and becomes extinguished at the other end of the circuit due to collision of impulses from opposite directions. (**B**) An area of unidirectional block develops in one of the branches, preventing anterograde impulse transmission, but allowing retrograde impulse transmission through the block if the impulse finds excitable tissue that is not in its refractory period. This impulse then re-excites tissue it had previously passed through, and a re-entry arrhythmia is established.

Furthermore, the circulating impulse gives off "daughter impulses" that can spread to the rest of the heart. Depending on how many round trips through the pathway the impulse makes before dying out, the arrhythmia may manifest as one or a few extra beats or as a sustained tachycardia. In order for re-entry to occur, three conditions must coexist. First, there must be an anatomic or physiologic obstacle to typical (forward) conduction in order to establish a circuit around which the re-entrant wavefront can propagate. Second, there must be unidirectional block at some point in the circuit (ie, conduction must die out in one direction but continue in the opposite direction). Third, the conduction time around the circuit must be long enough so that the retrograde impulse does not enter the refractory tissue as it travels around the obstacle (ie, the conduction time must exceed the ERP for the tissue). Under such conditions, as shown in Figure 10-5B, the normal impulse gradually decreases as it invades progressively more depolarized tissue and finally stops. Several classes of antiarrhythmic drugs suppress arrhythmias by altering the refractory period in cardiac tissue where the re-entry occurs. If the refractory period in tissue near the site of the block is lengthened, it is more likely that the tissues will *still* be refractory when re-entry is attempted (thus inhibiting propagation of the re-entry impulse). Alternatively, if the refractory period in the depressed region is shortened, it is less likely that unidirectional block will occur.

Clinically important arrhythmias include atrial flutter, atrial fibrillation (AF), atrioventricular nodal re-entry (a common type of supraventricular tachycardia [SVT]), premature ventricular contractions (PVCs), ventricular tachycardia (VT), and ventricular fibrillation (VF). Figure 10-6 shows example

ECG recordings of normal sinus rhythm and several common arrhythmias. Torsade de pointes is a ventricular arrhythmia characterized by polymorphic ventricular tachycardia, often displaying waxing and waning QRS amplitude on the ECG. Torsade de pointes has great pharmacologic importance because this rhythm is often *induced* by antiarrhythmic drugs and other drugs that prolong the QT interval. This arrhythmia is also associated with long QT syndrome, a heritable abnormal prolongation of the QT interval caused by mutations in the I_K or I_{Na} channel molecules.

ANTIARRHYTHMIC DRUGS

Arrhythmias are caused by abnormal pacemaker activity and/or abnormal impulse propagation. Thus, the goals of pharmacologic therapy are to reduce the activity of ectopic pacemakers (ie, sites outside of the SA node that are acting as pacemakers) and to modify conduction or refractoriness in re-entry circuits to disable circus movement. The major mechanisms of antiarrhythmic drugs include blockade of sodium channels (class 1), cardiac β_1 receptors (class 2), potassium channels (class 3), and calcium channels (class 4).

Antiarrhythmic drugs decrease the automaticity of ectopic pacemakers more than that of the SA node. They also reduce conduction and excitability and increase the refractory period to a greater extent in depolarized tissue than in normally polarized tissue. This is accomplished chiefly by using sodium or calcium channel-blocking agents that have a high affinity for activated channels during phase 0, or inactivated channels during phases 2 and 3, but very low affinity

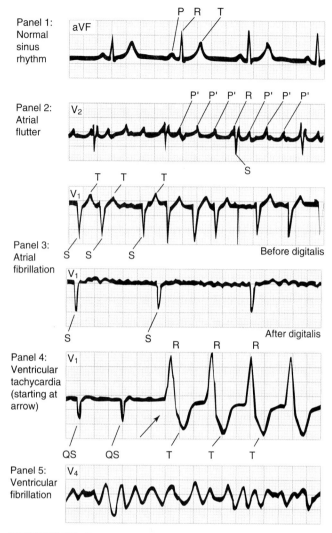

FIGURE 10-6 **Typical ECGs of normal sinus rhythm and some common arrhythmias.** Major waves (P, Q, R, S, and T) are labeled in each ECG except in panel 5, in which electrical activity is completely disorganized and none of the deflections are recognizable.

for resting channels during phase 4 (Figure 10-4). As a result, these drugs preferentially block electrical activity when there is a tachycardia during which many channel activations and inactivations occur per unit time. These drugs also block electrical activity in cells that are resting at *less negative* potentials (such as occurs in hypoxic tissue) when many channels are inactivated. In summary, antiarrhythmic drugs are more likely to block channels that are being used frequently (as would occur in a tachycardia) or are in an inactivated state (as would occur in hypoxic cells).

In ectopic pacemaker cells, most antiarrhythmic agents reduce the slope of phase 4 of the AP by blocking either sodium or calcium channels. By reducing the ratio of influx to efflux of positive ions, the result is a *slower* depolarization. In addition, some agents may increase the activation threshold for the AP in susceptible cells.

In re-entry arrhythmias, which depend on critically depressed anterograde conduction, most antiarrhythmic agents slow conduction by one or both of two mechanisms. First, agents may decrease the steady-state number of available unblocked channels, which reduces the excitatory currents to a level below that required for AP propagation. Second, these drugs may increase the ERP by prolonging the recovery time of the channels still able to reach the rested and available state. As a result, early extrasystoles (ectopic beats) are unable to propagate at all; later impulses propagate more slowly and are subject to bidirectional conduction block.

The mechanisms described above enable antiarrhythmic drugs to suppress the electrical activity of ectopic pacemakers and abnormal conduction occurring in depolarized cells. Table 10-1 shows the effect of common agents on key waveforms of the ECG. Antiarrhythmic drugs minimally affect electrical activity in normal repolarized myocardial cells. However, as dosage is increased, most agents also depress conduction in normal tissue, eventually resulting in drug-induced arrhythmias. Furthermore, a drug concentration that inhibits arrhythmias under the initial circumstances of treatment may promote arrhythmias during tachycardia, acidosis, hyperkalemia, or ischemia.

Class 1 Antiarrhythmics (Sodium Channel Blockers)

Class 1 agents are the oldest group of antiarrhythmic drugs and are still widely used. They are local anesthetics that slow or block conduction (especially in depolarized cells) and slow or abolish abnormal pacemakers wherever these processes depend on sodium channels. Useful sodium channel-blocking drugs bind to their receptors much more readily when the channel is open or inactivated than when it is fully repolarized and recovered from its previous activity. Ion channels in arrhythmic tissue spend more time in the open or inactivated states than do channels in normal tissue. Therefore, these antiarrhythmic drugs block channels in abnormal tissue more effectively than channels in normal tissue. As a result, antiarrhythmic sodium channel blockers selectively depress tissue that is frequently depolarizing (eg, during a tachycardia) or is relatively depolarized during rest (eg, hypoxic tissue).

By blocking sodium channels, all class 1 drugs slow the phase 0 depolarization. Class 1A drugs (eg, **procainamide**) prolong the AP, whereas class 1B drugs (eg, **lidocaine**) shorten the AP in some cardiac tissues. Class 1C drugs (eg, **flecainide**) have no effect on AP duration. Figure 10-7 illustrates the effects of class 1 agents on the cardiac AP.

Class 1A

Procainamide is the class 1A prototype. Other drugs with class 1A actions include **quinidine** and **disopyramide**. These three drugs can be used in all types of atrial and ventricular arrhythmias. Procainamide is also commonly used in arrhythmias

TABLE 10-1 Properties of the prototype antiarrhythmic drugs.

Drug	Class	Half-Life	PR Interval	QRS Duration	QT Interval
Disopyramide	1A	7-8 hr	↓ or ↑^{a}	↑↑	↑↑
Procainamide	1A	3-4 hr	↓ or ↑^{a}	↑↑	↑↑
Quinidine	1A	6 hr	↓ or ↑^{a}	↑↑	↑↑
Lidocaine	1B	1-2 hr	—	—^{b}	—
Mexiletine	1B	8-20 hr	—	—^{b}	↓^{c}
Flecainide	1C	20 hr	↑ (slight)	↑↑	—
Propafenone	1C	5-7 hr	↑	↑↑↑	—
Esmolol	2	10 min	↑↑	—	—
Propranolol	2	5 hr	↑↑	—	—
Amiodarone	1A, 2, 3, 4	weeks	↑	↑↑	↑↑↑↑
Ibutilide	3	6 hr	—	—	↑↑↑
Dofetilide	3	7 hr	—	—	↑↑
Sotalol	2, 3	7-12 hr	↑↑	—	↑↑↑
Diltiazem	4	4-8 hr	↑↑	—	—
Verapamil	4	7 hr	↑↑	—	—
Adenosine	Misc	< 10 sec	↑↑↑	—	—

^{a}PR may decrease through antimuscarinic action or increase through channel blocking action.
^{b}Lidocaine and mexiletine slow conduction velocity in ischemic, depolarized ventricular cells but not in normal tissue.
^{c}Decreased QT in Purkinje cells.

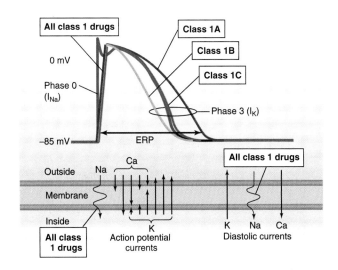

FIGURE 10-7 Diagram of the effects of class 1 agents. The top outline shows the cardiac action potential (AP); the bottom schematic shows the currents that cross the plasma membrane that contribute to the shape of the cardiac AP. All class 1 drugs reduce phase 0 and phase 4 sodium currents (wavy lines) in susceptible cells. Class 1A drugs also reduce phase 3 potassium currents (I_K) and prolong AP duration, resulting in significant prolongation of the effective refractory period. Class 1B and 1C drugs have different (or no) effects on I_K and shorten or have no effect on AP duration.

during the acute phase of myocardial infarction. **Amiodarone**, often categorized as a class 3 agent, also has typical class 1A actions. By blocking I_{Na}, class 1A antiarrhythmic drugs slow conduction velocity in the atria, Purkinje fibers, and ventricular cells. At high doses, some class 1 drugs also slow AV conduction. The drug-induced reduction in ventricular conduction velocity results in increased QRS duration in the ECG (Table 10-1). In addition, class 1A drugs block I_K. Therefore, they increase AP duration and the ERP, in addition to slowing conduction velocity and ectopic pacemakers. The increase in AP duration generates an increase in QT interval. Amiodarone has similar effects on sodium current and has the greatest AP-prolonging effect.

The most common adverse effect of class 1A drugs is precipitation of new arrhythmias. Hyperkalemia can exacerbate the cardiac toxicity of all class 1 drugs.

Torsade de pointes is particularly associated with quinidine and other drugs (except amiodarone) that prolong AP duration. Procainamide also causes hypotension (especially when used parenterally) and a reversible syndrome similar to lupus erythematosus. Quinidine causes cinchonism, which may manifest as headache, vertigo, tinnitus, cardiac depression, gastrointestinal upset, and autoimmune reactions such as thrombocytopenic purpura. Quinidine reduces the clearance of digoxin and thus may significantly increase the serum concentration of digoxin. Disopyramide has marked antimuscarinic effects and may precipitate heart failure.

Class 1B

Lidocaine is the class 1B prototype. Lidocaine selectively affects ischemic or depolarized Purkinje and ventricular tissue and has little effect on atrial tissue. Thus, lidocaine is useful in treating acute ventricular arrhythmias, especially those occurring in ischemic tissue, such as following myocardial infarction. Atrial arrhythmias are not responsive unless caused by digitalis. Lidocaine reduces AP duration, but because it slows recovery of sodium channels from inactivation, it does not shorten and may even prolong the ERP. Lidocaine is never given orally because it has a very high first-pass effect and its metabolites are potentially cardiotoxic. Instead, lidocaine is usually given intravenously, but intramuscular administration is possible. **Mexiletine** is another commonly used 1B agent. Mexiletine has similar effects to lidocaine, but is administered orally. Because these agents have little effect on normal cardiac cells, they have little effect on the ECG (Table 10-1). **Phenytoin**, an anticonvulsant and not a true local anesthetic, is sometimes classified with the class 1B antiarrhythmic agents because it can be used to reverse digitalis-induced arrhythmias. Phenytoin resembles lidocaine in lacking significant effect on the normal ECG.

Although class 1B drugs may precipitate arrhythmias, this is less common than with class 1A and 1C drugs. Lidocaine and mexiletine may cause typical local anesthetic toxicity. Such toxicity may result in CNS stimulation, possibly including convulsions and cardiovascular depression. Allergies such as rashes are also a potential effect and may extend to anaphylaxis.

Class 1C

Flecainide is the class 1C prototype. Class 1C drugs increase QRS duration on the ECG, but have no effect on ventricular AP duration or QT interval. They are *powerful* depressants of sodium current and can markedly slow conduction velocity in atrial and ventricular cells. As such, flecainide is approved only for certain intractable supraventricular arrhythmias and refractory ventricular tachycardias that tend to progress to VF at unpredictable times resulting in "sudden death." Flecainide is more likely than other antiarrhythmic agents to exacerbate or precipitate arrhythmias; for this reason, its use is now restricted for arrhythmias that fail to respond to other drugs. **Propafenone** is a class 1C agent that also possesses weak β-receptor antagonist activity (class 2). This drug is used for supraventricular arrhythmias, but also has the adverse effect of precipitating arrhythmias. In addition, propafenone may cause constipation and a metallic taste.

Class 2 Antiarrhythmics (β-Receptor Antagonists)

β-blockers are discussed in detail in Chapter 6. **Propranolol** and **esmolol** are the prototype antiarrhythmic β-receptor antagonists. Their mechanism in decreasing arrhythmogenesis is primarily cardiac β_1-receptor blockade with subsequent decreased production of cyclic adenosine monophosphate (cAMP). This results in reduced sodium and calcium currents

and the suppression of abnormal pacemakers. The AV node is particularly sensitive to β-receptor antagonists, which is reflected in prolongation of the PR interval (Table 10-1). Under some conditions, these drugs may have some direct local anesthetic effect in the heart (ie, sodium channel blockade), but this is probably rare at clinically relevant concentrations.

Propranolol, **metoprolol**, and **timolol** are commonly used to prevent recurrent infarction and sudden death in patients who have had a myocardial infarction. Because esmolol is very short-acting, it is used intravenously exclusively in acute arrhythmias.

The toxicities of β-receptor antagonists have been discussed in Chapter 6. Individuals with arrhythmias are often more prone to β-receptor antagonist-induced depression of cardiac output than are those with normal hearts. However, judicious use of these drugs reduces progression of chronic heart failure (Chapter 9) and the incidence of potentially fatal arrhythmias that occur in heart failure.

Class 3 Antiarrhythmics (Potassium Channel Blockers)

Sotalol, **dofetilide**, and **ibutilide** are the class 3 prototypes. Amiodarone is also typically considered a class 3 antiarrhythmic because of its action as a potassium channel blocker; however, amiodarone has several other actions. The hallmark of class 3 drugs is prolongation of the AP duration due to blockade of potassium channels (I_K) that are responsible for the repolarization phase of the AP (Figure 10-8). Prolongation of the AP results in an increase in the ERP and reduces the ability of the heart to respond to tachycardias. Sotalol, dofetilide,

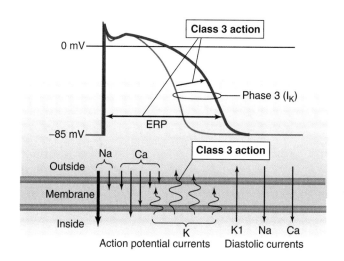

FIGURE 10-8 Diagram of the effects of class 3 drugs. The top outline shows the cardiac action potential (AP); the bottom schematic shows the currents that cross the plasma membrane that contribute to the shape of the cardiac AP. All class 3 drugs prolong the AP duration in susceptible cardiac cells by reducing the outward (repolarizing) phase 3 potassium current (I_K, wavy lines). The main effect is to prolong the effective refractory period (ERP). Note that the phase 4 diastolic potassium current (I_K) is not affected by these drugs.

ibutilide, and amiodarone produce this effect on most cardiac cells. The action of these drugs is therefore apparent in the ECG as an increase in QT interval. *N*-**acetylprocainamide** (acecainide), which is a metabolite of procainamide (class 1A), also significantly prolongs the AP and the QT interval.

Sotalol is commonly used and is available by the oral route (Table 10-1). Because of its action as a β-receptor antagonist, sotalol may cause sinus bradycardia or bronchoconstriction. Dofetilide and ibutilide are recommended for atrial flutter and fibrillation. All three of these drugs may induce torsade de pointes.

Amiodarone is effective in most types of arrhythmias and is considered the most efficacious of all antiarrhythmic drugs. This may be because it has a broad spectrum of activity—blocking β₁ receptors as well as sodium, calcium, and potassium channels. However, because of its toxicities, use of amiodarone is approved mainly for arrhythmias that are resistant to other drugs. Nevertheless, amiodarone is used extensively in a wide variety of arrhythmias. Amiodarone can cause microcrystalline deposits in the cornea and skin, hyper- or hypothyroidism, paresthesias, tremor, and pulmonary fibrosis. Amiodarone rarely causes new arrhythmias, perhaps because of its broad spectrum of action. **Dronedarone** is a deiodinated analog of amiodarone that has a similar mechanism of action. Unlike amiodarone, dronedarone does not affect thyroid function, though hepatotoxicity is a potential adverse effect.

Class 4 Antiarrhythmics (Calcium Channel Blockers)

Calcium channel blockers (CCBs) are discussed in detail in Chapters 7 and 8. **Verapamil** is the class 4 prototype. **Diltiazem** is also an effective antiarrhythmic drug, although it is not FDA-approved for this purpose. Nifedipine and the other dihydropyridines are not useful as antiarrhythmics probably because they decrease arterial pressure sufficiently to evoke a compensatory sympathetic discharge to the heart that facilitates rather than suppresses arrhythmias. Verapamil and diltiazem are most effective in arrhythmias that must traverse the AV node, a calcium-dependent tissue. These agents selectively depress calcium current moving through L-type calcium channels (Figure 10-9). The CCBs decrease conduction velocity and increase the ERP and PR interval (Table 10-1).

Calcium channel blockers are effective for converting AV nodal re-entry (also known as nodal tachycardia) to normal sinus rhythm. Their major use is in the prevention of nodal arrhythmias in individuals prone to recurrence. Diltiazem is also used for treatment of atrial flutter and fibrillation. CCBs are orally active, but are also available for parenteral use (Table 10-1). The most important toxicity of verapamil is excessive pharmacologic effect, including significant depression of contractility, AV conduction, and blood pressure. Diltiazem has less depressant effect on blood pressure.

Miscellaneous Antiarrhythmic Drugs

Several drugs used to treat arrhythmias do not fit within the typical 1-4 classification. Common agents include **ivabradine**, **ranolazine**, **adenosine**, and digitalis. Ivabradine inhibits pacemaker channels highly expressed in the SA node that act as nonselective voltage-gated cation channels. When ivabradine binds to the channel in the open position, the current—known as the "funny current" (I_f)—is inhibited. The resulting physiologic effect is a decrease in SA nodal pacemaker activity, and a negative chronotropic effect (decreased heart rate). Unlike β-blockers,

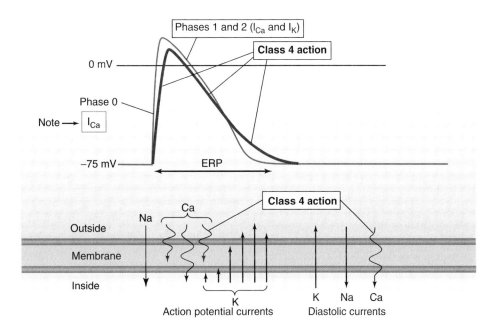

FIGURE 10-9 **Diagram of the effects of class 4 drugs in a calcium-dependent cardiac cell in the AV node (note that the AP upstroke in these cells is due mainly to calcium current).** Class 4 drugs reduce inward calcium current during the AP and during phase 4 (wavy lines). As a result, AV nodal conduction velocity is slowed and refractoriness is prolonged. Pacemaker depolarization during phase 4 is also slowed if caused by excessive calcium current. ERP, effective refractory period.

ivabradine does not prolong the PR interval or depress stroke volume; thus, the drug does not decrease intracardiac conduction or contractility. Adverse effects include bradycardia, visual disturbance, vertigo, and syncope. Although ivabradine is used as an antiarrhythmic drug elsewhere, this drug is currently approved in the United States only for use in heart failure to prevent tachycardia often present in this condition.

Ranolazine binds to and inhibits many types of voltage-gated sodium channels as well as a type of voltage-gated potassium channel. The *net* effect on the electrical properties of myocardial cells (eg, effect on AP duration) and on the ECG (eg, effect on QT interval) is dependent on the clinical presentation. Although ranolazine has been used in atrial fibrillation and ventricular arrhythmias such as ventricular tachycardia, the drug is only FDA-approved for chronic stable angina. Ivabradine and ranolazine are also briefly discussed in Chapter 8.

Adenosine is a normal compound found within every cell of the body. When given in high doses (6-12 mg) as an intravenous bolus, adenosine is extremely effective in abolishing AV nodal arrhythmias by markedly slowing or completely blocking conduction in the AV node (Table 10-1), probably by hyperpolarizing this tissue via increased I_K and reduced I_{Ca}. Because of its high efficacy, very low toxicity, and short duration of action (15 seconds), adenosine has become the drug of choice for rapid conversion of acute episodes of paroxysmal supraventricular tachycardia. Toxicity includes flushing, hypotension, chest pain, and dyspnea.

The use of digitalis as a positive inotrope in the treatment of heart failure is discussed in Chapter 9. Digoxin's parasympathomimetic action is sometimes exploited in the treatment of rapid atrial or AV nodal arrhythmias. In atrial flutter or fibrillation, digitalis slows AV conduction sufficiently to protect the ventricles from excessively high rates (Figure 10-6, panel 3). In AV nodal re-entrant arrhythmias, digitalis may exert enough depressant effect to abolish the arrhythmia. The latter use of digitalis has become less common since the introduction of CCBs and adenosine as antiarrhythmic drugs.

NONPHARMACOLOGIC THERAPY OF CARDIAC ARRHYTHMIAS

One of the most common adverse effects of antiarrhythmic drugs is precipitation of *another* arrhythmia that can, in some individuals, be lethal. Recognition of the long-term dangers of antiarrhythmic agents and the development of technological advances have led to effective nonpharmacologic therapy for several arrhythmias. At the start of the 20th century, experimental research suggested that transecting the re-entry circuit could permanently interrupt re-entry rhythms. This concept has now been applied to treat clinical arrhythmias that occur due to re-entry in anatomically delineated pathways. For example, individuals with Wolff-Parkinson-White syndrome have an accessory pathway or AV bypass tract that leads to early activation of the ventricles because action potentials can bypass the AV node via this defined accessory pathway. Interruption of the accessory AV bypass tract can permanently correct this

arrhythmia. Such interruption was originally performed via open-heart surgery. Now, accessory pathways can be precisely mapped and transected via cardiac catheter-based procedures using radiofrequency energy (radiofrequency ablation) or extreme cold (cryoablation). Since these cardiac catheter-based procedures cause minimal morbidity, they are being increasingly applied to other re-entry arrhythmias with defined pathways, such as AV nodal re-entry, atrial flutter, some forms of atrial fibrillation, and ventricular tachycardia. Other nonpharmacologic forms of therapy such as external cardiac defibrillation, implanted cardiac defibrillators (ICDs), and implanted pacemakers, have also become extremely important.

REHABILITATION RELEVANCE

Arrhythmias can be manifestations of several cardiovascular pathophysiologies and/or the effects of various drugs and electrolyte imbalances. In patients with a reported history of arrhythmias, both decreases and increases in arrhythmia incidence during rehabilitation have been reported. The prevention of arrhythmias with antiarrhythmic drugs in patients during rehabilitation has demonstrated mixed results. However, quality of life, as defined by emotional stability, satisfaction with work and social life, and return to work, are higher in these rehabilitated patients.

The cardiovascular stress of graded exercise in cardiac rehabilitation programs may increase the risk of an arrhythmic incident. The physical therapist should also remember that the potential for increased arrhythmias in patients with a documented history of arrhythmias is not restricted to cardiac rehabilitation. *Any* activity that increases sympathetic tone may increase the incidence of arrhythmias. The patient participating in a work-hardening program may be just as likely to have an arrhythmia as a patient in cardiac rehabilitation. Careful monitoring of patients with a known history of arrhythmias is strongly encouraged. Monitored ECG during ambulation and exercise training is the preferred method. When ECG monitoring is unavailable, the therapist can assess for the presence of dizziness or nausea during activities, monitor heart rate (with a portable pulse oximeter), and palpate for an abnormal heart rhythm. These subjective and objective findings may allow the therapist to detect arrhythmias during rehabilitation. If arrhythmias are suspected with physical activities, consultation with the primary care provider should include a request for the patient to participate in exercise in an environment with real-time ECG monitoring.

Control of arrhythmias with antiarrhythmic agents allows individuals to improve aerobic tolerance during cardiac rehabilitation, return-to-work conditioning, and other rehabilitation programs. Summarized below are adverse effects most likely to influence therapy sessions or goals and possible therapy solutions.

- **Arrhythmias** are the most common adverse effect of *almost all* antiarrhythmic drugs. The incidence of arrhythmias increases with tachycardia, acidosis, hypokalemia, or ischemia. Thus, monitoring of heart rate and rhythm whenever possible during exercise—when these precipitating conditions are more likely—is particularly important.

- **Bronchoconstriction** and associated dyspnea is a problem with class 2 antiarrhythmic drugs. Dyspnea may decrease aerobic capacity. Allow increased time to complete aerobic tasks to limit dyspnea and to account for depressed cardiac output.
- **Cardiac output** may be depressed during aerobic activities with any of the antiarrhythmic drug classes, but especially with class 2 agents and several drugs in class 4. Prescribed exercise intensity should be decreased and patients should be allowed more time to complete rehabilitation tasks.
- **Heart rate** may be decreased both at rest and during exercise. Thus, heart rate is not accurate as a marker of exertion for patients taking class 2 and some class 4 antiarrhythmic drugs. Use perceived exertion scales (eg, Borg rating of perceived exertion scale) to determine aerobic intensity.

- **Hypoglycemia** unawareness or delayed awareness may occur in diabetics taking class 2 antiarrhythmic drugs. If hypoglycemia is suspected, have patients check blood glucose level prior to and following exercise. Have simple carbohydrates readily available in clinic gym.
- **Orthostatic hypotension** is a potential adverse effect with class 2, class 4, and some class 3 antiarrhythmic drugs. Orthostatic hypotension may cause syncope when transferring from recumbent to upright positions, exiting from warm pools, or if aerobic exercise is terminated without appropriate cool-down period. To prevent fainting, assist patients with positional changes and when exiting a warm pool. Finally, always provide a cool-down period following aerobic activity.
- **Thyroid dysfunction** may occur with amiodarone. If either hyper- or hypothyroid dysfunction is suspected, the therapist should refer the patient for additional evaluation.

CASE CONCLUSION

The patient's elevated blood pressure and tachycardia during the functional return-to-work exercises may indicate that the activity induced the arrhythmia. This situation may have been precipitated by the patient's 3-week period of deconditioning since the accident. In addition, the corporate referring physician may not have been aware of the patient's preexisting cardiac disease. The therapist should alert both the referring physician and the patient's cardiologist of her hemodynamic response to initial aerobic training to determine if she should receive additional medical care prior to continuing the aerobic conditioning program.

CHAPTER 10 QUESTIONS

1. The arrhythmic mechanism of action for re-entry is due to which of the following?
   a. Unidirectional blockade of anterograde electrical conduction in the heart
   b. Bidirectional blockade of anterograde electrical conduction in the heart
   c. Increased excitability of ectopic pacemaker activity
   d. Decreased excitability of ectopic pacemaker activity

2. Which of the following electrolyte disturbances would increase the pharmacologic effect of class 3 antiarrhythmic drugs?
   a. Hyponatremia
   b. Hypocalcemia
   c. Hypokalemia
   d. Hypomagnesemia

3. Which of the following electrolyte disturbances would increase the pharmacologic effect of class 4 antiarrhythmic drugs?
   a. Hypokalemia
   b. Hyponatremia
   c. Hyperkalemia
   d. Hypocalcemia

4. Which of the following antiarrhythmic drugs has negative chronotropic, inotropic, and dromotropic effects?
   a. Dofetilide
   b. Adenosine
   c. Propranolol
   d. Lidocaine

5. Which of the following antiarrhythmic drugs has negative chronotropic, inotropic, and dromotropic effects?
   a. Lidocaine
   b. Verapamil
   c. Dofetilide
   d. Adenosine

6. Which of the following drugs inhibits both sodium channels and potassium channels?
   a. Procainamide
   b. Flecainide
   c. Propranolol
   d. Verapamil

7. Which of the following drug classes only increases QRS duration on the ECG?

   a. Class 1B
   b. Class 1C
   c. Class 2
   d. Class 4

8. Which of the following drugs is most associated with thyroid dysfunction?

   a. Amiodarone
   b. Dofetilide
   c. Quinidine
   d. Verapamil

9. Which of the following antiarrhythmic drugs only inhibits sodium channels?

   a. Propafenone
   b. Propranolol
   c. Disopyramide
   d. Verapamil

10. Which of the following drugs has a mechanism of action that makes it both a class 2 and class 3 antiarrhythmic?

    a. Procainamide
    b. Propranolol
    c. Sotalol
    d. Verapamil

Drugs Affecting the Blood

S.R. is a 66-year-old retired man who has been participating in a conditioning program at a wellness center for 2 months without incident. The program includes walking on a treadmill, upper extremity resistance exercises, and abdominal exercises. During the summer, the wellness center provides an area for clients to exchange produce from their gardens. S.R. has atrial fibrillation and stable angina pectoris and is currently taking warfarin in addition to antianginal drugs. S.R. participates in the conditioning program 4 days per week. A physical therapist reviews his status and modifies the exercise prescription every other week. Last week, S.R. was absent. This week, he participated on Monday and Tuesday, and the therapist reviewed his status on Wednesday. During the initial discussion, S.R. stated he was out of town visiting his grandchildren and he kept up with his medications but not his conditioning program. He also mentioned that he missed the fresh vegetables last week while away. Today, he complains of pain in his shoulders and knees. He figures it was the result of not keeping up with his exercise program last week and getting started again. The therapist notices a circumferential bruise around the right wrist that appears several days old. When questioned, S.R. states that the bruise must have been due to his grandchildren leading him by the wrist last week. The therapist asks the client whether he knows his current INR level. When S.R. responds that he has not had his INR level checked for the past few weeks, the therapist advises him to discontinue the conditioning program until he is certain that his anticoagulation level is within a safe therapeutic range.

REHABILITATION FOCUS

A considerable number of patients undergoing rehabilitation are treated with drugs that affect the blood and these medications have significant impacts on rehabilitation outcomes. Anemia is a problem experienced by many patients, especially those receiving cancer chemotherapy and those with renal or heart failure. Exercise programs combined with drug therapy improve quality of life in these patients and reduce morbidity and mortality. However, when patients are being treated with hematopoietic factors, aerobic capacity and immune responses may be depressed. Consistent review of hematocrit, hemoglobin, and blood cell counts prior to therapy interventions is warranted to determine the appropriateness and intensity of mobilization and exercise.

Anticlotting drugs are used to treat individuals with a variety of conditions including neurologic, cardiac, and postsurgical. Anticlotting medications may include anticoagulants and/or antiplatelet drugs. When available, clinicians should carefully monitor coagulation lab test results prior to beginning a treatment session, especially if interventions involve wound care, intense aerobic or resistance exercises, or significant joint mobilizations. This will ensure that the treatment session is appropriately scaled to the patient's level of medication. If patients are over-medicated, myalgia or arthralgia associated with bleeding into tissues may occur 1 or 2 days following a rehabilitation session involving impact-related physical activities.

Patients with bleeding disorders resulting from insufficient platelet activation or those who have been overmedicated with antiplatelet agents bleed from surfaces such as the gingiva and skin or demonstrate heavy menses. Patients with insufficient clotting activity tend to bleed into deep tissues such as joints or muscles for no apparent reason. Individuals with hemophilia-type bleeding disorders who are undermedicated may also present with myalgia and arthralgia following physical activity.

BACKGROUND

The first half of this chapter presents the hematopoietic factors (micronutrients and growth factors) that affect the formation of blood cells and platelets. The second half of the chapter includes the drugs used to treat disorders of coagulation.

Hematopoiesis is the production of circulating erythrocytes (red blood cells, RBCs), platelets, and leukocytes (white blood cells, WBCs) from undifferentiated stem cells. This remarkable

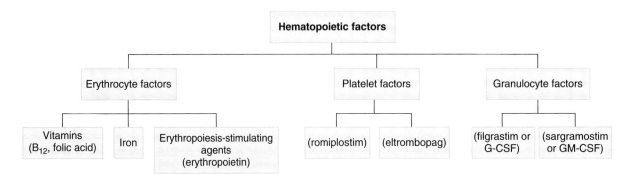

FIGURE 11-1 **Drugs used in the treatment of cytopenias.** Hematopoietic factors are initially classified based on the blood component stimulated. Erythrocyte factors include micronutrients and injectable erythropoiesis-stimulating agents. Platelet-stimulating drugs include injectable (romiplostim) and oral (eltrombopag). Granulocyte factors include G-CSF (granulocyte colony-stimulating factor) that specifically stimulates formation of granulocytes (eg, neutrophils) and GM-CSF (granulocyte-macrophage colony-stimulating factor) that stimulates both macrophage and granulocyte formation. Prototype drugs are in parentheses.

process produces over 200 billion new blood cells per day in the normal person and even greater numbers of cells in people with conditions that cause loss or destruction of blood cells. The hematopoietic machinery resides primarily in the bone marrow in adults and requires a constant supply of essential micronutrients such as iron, vitamin B_{12}, and folic acid. Hematopoietic growth factors—proteins that regulate the proliferation and differentiation of hematopoietic cells—are also required. Circulating blood cells play essential roles in oxygenation of tissues, coagulation, protection against infectious agents, and tissue repair. Blood cell deficiency is a relatively common occurrence that can have profound effects on health. Inadequate supply of either the growth factors or, more commonly, the essential micronutrients, results in a lack of functional blood cells.

Anemia is a deficiency of oxygen-carrying erythrocytes. Regardless of the cause, anemia presents clinically with pallor, fatigue, dizziness, exertional dyspnea, reduced exercise tolerance, and tachycardia. The most common causes are insufficient supply of iron, vitamin B_{12}, or folic acid. Treatment involves replacement of the missing nutrients. In certain types of anemia or other cytopenias (deficiencies in the number of mature blood cells), treatment requires administration of recombinant hematopoietic growth factors. These growth factors stimulate the production of various lineages of blood cells and regulate blood cell function. Almost a dozen glycoprotein hormones regulate the differentiation and maturation of stem cells within the bone marrow. Several growth factors produced by recombinant DNA technology have FDA approval for treatment of people with blood cell deficiencies. Figure 11-1 outlines the agents used to treat cytopenias.

MICRONUTRIENTS USED TO PREVENT OR CORRECT ANEMIAS

Iron

Iron is the essential metallic nonprotein component of heme, the molecule responsible for the bulk of oxygen transport in the blood. Iron is available in a variety of foods but is especially

abundant in meat. Heme iron, found only in animal proteins in the diet, is efficiently absorbed without having to be broken down into elemental iron. Nonheme iron from nonanimal dietary sources (eg, grains, beans) is absorbed less efficiently than heme iron (ie, its bioavailability is lower). Iron in the body is present in myoglobin, hemoglobin, transferrin, and ferritin. Both myoglobin and hemoglobin are heme-based proteins, the former found in muscle and the latter in red blood cells. Transferrin is an iron-binding transport protein and ferritin is an iron storage protein. Iron deficiency occurs most often in women (because of menstrual blood loss) and in vegetarians or malnourished individuals (because of inadequate dietary iron intake). Children and pregnant women have increased requirements for iron.

The body has a complex system for regulating the uptake and storage of iron. An adequate supply of iron is required for normal hematopoiesis, yet excess free iron is extremely toxic. Regulation of body iron content occurs through modulation of intestinal absorption. There is no mechanism for efficient excretion of iron. Thus, if gastrointestinal iron absorption is abnormally increased, iron overload (hemochromatosis) occurs, which can cause significant organ damage. Free iron from iron supplements and iron stripped from complexes in food is absorbed as the ferrous ion (Fe^{2+}) and oxidized in the intestinal mucosal cell to the ferric (Fe^{3+}) form. Heme iron is absorbed as a complex and the heme component is degraded to release free iron. Iron is stored as Fe^{3+} in the intestinal mucosa (in ferritin, a complex of iron and the protein apoferritin) or carried elsewhere in the body (bound to transferrin). Excess iron is stored as ferritin in the reticuloendothelial system and, in cases of gross overload, in parenchymal cells of the skin, liver, heart, and other organs. An accumulation of stored iron occurs in hemolytic anemias (due to excessive destruction of red blood cells) and in hemochromatosis (an inherited abnormality of iron absorption). Minimal amounts of iron are eliminated from the body with sweat and saliva and in exfoliated skin and intestinal mucosal cells.

The only indication for iron administration is to prevent or treat iron deficiency anemia (IDA). Iron deficiency can be diagnosed from red blood cell morphology (pale, microcytic cell size, diminished hemoglobin content) and from measurements of serum and bone marrow iron stores. IDA is treated by oral **ferrous iron** supplementation in a salt form (**iron sulfate**, **iron gluconate**, or **iron fumarate**). In special cases, parenteral administration of iron preparations (**iron dextran or sucrose, ferric gluconate complex**) is provided. Iron should not be given to patients with hemolytic anemia because their iron stores are elevated, not depressed.

Several adverse effects can result from iron supplementation. Acute iron toxicity is most common in children and usually occurs as a result of accidental ingestion of iron supplement tablets. Depending on the dose, necrotizing gastroenteritis, shock, metabolic acidosis, coma, and death may result. Chronic toxicity occurs most often in individuals who receive frequent transfusions (eg, individuals with sickle cell anemia) and in those with hemochromatosis. Immediate treatment of acute iron intoxication is necessary and usually consists of removal of unabsorbed tablets from the gut, correction of acid-base and electrolyte abnormalities, and administration of chelators for iron that has already been absorbed. **Deferoxamine** is a parenteral chelator that promotes urinary and fecal iron excretion. **Deferasirox** is an oral chelator that promotes fecal iron excretion. Chronic iron toxicity, such as in hemochromatosis, is usually treated by phlebotomy (therapeutic withdrawal of blood).

Vitamin B_{12} (Cobalamin)

Vitamin B_{12} is a cobalt-containing molecule that is produced by bacteria. Dietary sources high in vitamin B_{12} include meat (especially liver), eggs, dairy products, as well as many fortified cereals and other processed foods.

Vitamin B_{12}—sometimes referred to as extrinsic factor—is absorbed from the gastrointestinal tract only in the presence of intrinsic factor, a protein product of the parietal cells of the stomach. Defective secretion of intrinsic factor results in vitamin B_{12} deficiency and pernicious anemia, which is particularly common in older adults. Vitamin B_{12} is stored in the liver in large amounts; a normal individual has enough to last 5 years. *Nutritional* deficiency is rare, except in strict vegetarians after many years without meat, eggs, or dairy products. Vitamin B_{12} is transported in the blood bound to transcobalamin II. When parenteral vitamin B_{12} is given, any vitamin B_{12} that exceeds this transport protein's binding capacity is excreted.

Vitamin B_{12} is essential in two reactions: conversion of methylmalonyl-coenzyme A (CoA) to succinyl-CoA and conversion of homocysteine to methionine. The latter reaction is linked to folic acid metabolism and is required for the transfer of one-carbon units in DNA synthesis. Impairment of DNA synthesis affects all cells, but because red blood cells must be produced continuously, deficiency of either vitamin B_{12} or folic acid usually manifests first as anemia. In addition, an important manifestation of vitamin B_{12} deficiency is the development of neurologic defects, which may become irreversible if not treated promptly. The two forms of vitamin B_{12} available for therapeutic use are **cyanocobalamin** and **hydroxocobalamin**. In typical multivitamin supplements, vitamin B_{12} is present as cyanocobalamin, which the body converts to active forms of the vitamin. Although cyanocobalamin and hydroxocobalamin have equivalent effects, hydroxocobalamin has a longer circulating half-life because it is more firmly bound to plasma proteins.

The major clinical use of vitamin B_{12} is in the treatment of pernicious anemia and anemia that results from a lack of intrinsic factor following gastric resection. Because vitamin B_{12} deficiency anemia is almost always caused by inadequate gastrointestinal absorption of the vitamin, supplementation should be given by parenteral administration. Neither form of vitamin B_{12} (cyanocobalamin and hydroxocobalamin) has significant toxicity.

Folic Acid

Folate is the broad term for both the naturally occurring (primarily polyglutamated) folate found in food and folic acid (the monoglutamate form) that is contained in dietary supplements and fortified foods. In naturally occurring dietary folate, all but one of the glutamates is removed prior to absorption. The richest dietary sources of folate are yeast, liver, kidney, and green vegetables. Since 1998, all products made from enriched grains in the United States and Canada have been supplemented with folic acid in an effort to reduce the incidence of congenital neural tube defects.

Folic acid is readily absorbed from the gastrointestinal tract. Only modest amounts are stored in the body, so a decrease in dietary intake is followed by anemia within a few months. Like vitamin B_{12}, folic acid is required for normal synthesis of DNA, purines, and amino acids. Thus, rapidly dividing cells that require DNA synthesis are highly sensitive to folic acid deficiency. A deficiency in folic acid usually presents as megaloblastic anemia in which there are many immature and dysfunctional red blood cells that continue growing in size, but do not divide. During pregnancy, deficiency of folic acid increases the risk of fetal neural tube defects such as spina bifida.

Folic acid deficiency is most often caused by inadequate dietary consumption of folates or malabsorption. In addition, patients undergoing renal dialysis require folic acid supplementation because folates are removed from the plasma by the dialysis process. Anemia resulting from folic acid deficiency is readily treated by oral folic acid supplementation. Folic acid supplementation can correct the anemia, but not the neurologic deficits of vitamin B_{12} deficiency. Therefore, vitamin B_{12} deficiency must be ruled out before folic acid is used as the sole therapeutic agent in the treatment of a patient with megaloblastic anemia. Folic acid has no recognized toxicity.

HEMATOPOIETIC GROWTH FACTORS

Erythropoiesis-Stimulating Agents

Erythropoietin (EPO) is an important protein hormone produced by the kidney that activates specific receptors on erythroid progenitor cells contained in the bone marrow to stimulate the production of mature red blood cells and increase their release from the bone marrow. There are several engineered forms of EPO available for therapeutic use. **Epoetin alfa** is a recombinant human erythropoietin (rhEPO). **Darbepoetin alfa**, a glycosylated form of EPO with a much longer half-life, is often used to treat patients with anemia due to decreased EPO production as a result of chronic renal failure. **Methoxy polyethylene glycol-epoetin beta** is an even longer-lasting form of EPO that can be administered once or twice a month.

Erythropoiesis-stimulating agents (ESA) are routinely used for anemia associated with renal failure and are sometimes effective for individuals with other forms of anemia (eg, primary bone marrow disorders or anemia secondary to cancer or cancer chemotherapy, bone marrow transplantation, or acquired immune deficiency syndrome). These drugs are banned by most athletic organizations due to the ergogenic advantage they provide.

Patients receiving ESA therapy have their hemoglobin kept within the range of 10-12 g/dL even though normal hemoglobin ranges from 14 to 18 g/dL for adult men and 12-16 g/dL for adult women (see below). Current clinical lab testing calculates hemoglobin blood levels; hematocrit is then calculated based on the ratio that the hematocrit is approximately three times the hemoglobin (g/dL). Thus, except in the presence of specific comorbidities, hemoglobin and hematocrit parallel each other at the approximate 1:3 ratio.

The most serious adverse effects of ESA therapy are increased rate of all-cause mortality and cardiovascular events in renal dialysis patients and in cancer patients. These adverse effects are minimized by avoiding a rapid rise in hematocrit and keeping serum hemoglobin within the 10-12 g/dL range. Thus, individuals with hemoglobin levels less than 12 g/dL who are on these drugs may still have minimal exercise tolerance due to low oxygen-carrying capacity. When compared to other ESAs, methoxy polyethylene glycol-epoetin beta has been found to increase mortality when used for treatment of anemia caused by cancer chemotherapy.

Myeloid Growth Factors

Myeloid growth factors are agents that interact with specific receptors on myeloid progenitor cells in the bone marrow to enhance the production and maturation of megakaryocytes, erythrocytes, granulocytes (basophils, neutrophils, eosinophils), and monocytes. The two clinically available myeloid growth factors are **filgrastim** (granulocyte colony-stimulating factor; G-CSF) and **sargramostim** (granulocyte-macrophage colony-stimulating factor; GM-CSF). Both are made by recombinant DNA technology and stimulate the production and function of neutrophils. Sargramostim also stimulates the production of other myeloid and megakaryocyte progenitors. Filgrastim and, to a lesser degree, sargramostim also mobilize hematopoietic stem cells (ie, increase their concentration in peripheral blood). **Pegfilgrastim** is a covalent conjugation product of filgrastim and a form of polyethylene glycol that has a much longer serum half-life than filgrastim.

Both filgrastim and sargramostim are used to accelerate the recovery of neutrophils after cancer chemotherapy and to treat other forms of secondary and primary neutropenia (eg, aplastic anemia, congenital neutropenia). When given to patients soon after autologous stem cell transplantation, filgrastim reduces the time to engraftment (the process by which newly transplanted stem cells start to produce new blood cells) and the duration of neutropenia. Filgrastim is also used to mobilize peripheral blood stem cells in preparation for autologous stem cell transplantation. The toxicity of filgrastim is minimal, although the drug sometimes causes bone pain (ostealgia). Sargramostim can cause more severe reactions, including fever, arthralgias, and capillary damage with edema. Allergic reactions are rare.

Megakaryocyte Growth Factors

Megakaryocytes are large bone marrow progenitor cells responsible for the production of platelets that are necessary for blood clotting. **Oprelvekin** is the recombinant form of **interleukin-11** (**IL-11**), which is a key endogenous cytokine that regulates platelet production. Oprelvekin stimulates the growth of primitive megakaryocytic progenitors and increases the number of peripheral platelets by binding to the thrombopoietin receptor (Mpl). The drug is used to treat patients who have had a prior episode of thrombocytopenia after a cycle of cancer chemotherapy. In such patients, oprelvekin reduces the need for platelet transfusions. The most common adverse effects are fatigue, headache, dizziness, and fluid retention. The fluid retention may also result in anemia, dyspnea, and transient atrial arrhythmias. **Romiplostim** is a thrombopoietin receptor agonist that has no sequence homology with human thrombopoietin, thus minimizing antibody development. Romiplostim is injected subcutaneously in patients with chronic idiopathic thrombocytopenia who have failed to respond to conventional treatment. **Eltrombopag** is an orally active agonist for the thrombopoietin receptor. Eltrombopag is also used for patients with chronic idiopathic thrombocytopenia that is refractory to other agents. However, the risk of hepatotoxicity and hemorrhage has restricted the use of eltrombopag and liver function must be monitored. Rebound thrombocytopenia has been observed following termination of these drugs.

DRUGS USED IN COAGULATION DISORDERS

Hemostasis is the process by which bleeding from a damaged blood vessel stops. Hemostasis requires appropriate functioning of both the coagulation (clotting) cascade and platelets. The clotting cascade is a series of proteolytic reactions that produces active proteases that ultimately result in the production of thrombin (clotting factor IIa). Thrombin converts the soluble plasma protein fibrinogen into insoluble fibrin, a key structural component of a fibrous clot. In healthy vasculature, circulating blood platelets and clotting factors do not adhere

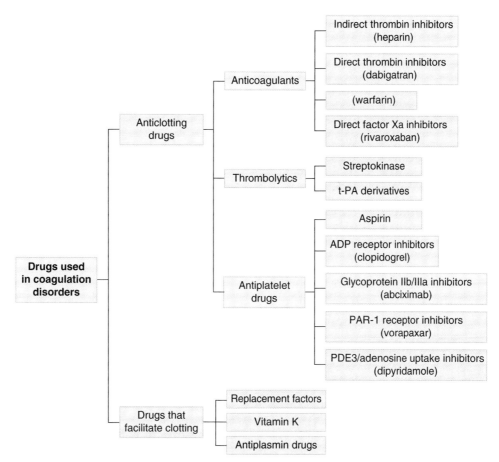

FIGURE 11-2 **Drugs used in the treatment of coagulation disorders are broadly divided into those that prevent or dissolve clots (anticlotting drugs) and those that facilitate clotting.** Anticlotting drugs are divided into 3 classes based on their mechanisms of action: anticoagulants, antiplatelet drugs, and thrombolytics. Drugs that facilitate clotting are divided into three classes: replacement clotting factors, vitamin K supplementation (required for the synthesis of clotting factors), and drugs that inhibit plasmin (an enzyme that degrades blood clots). Prototype drugs within drug classes are in parentheses. ADP, adenosine diphosphate; PAR-1, protease activated receptor type 1; PDE3, phosphodiesterase-3; t-PA, tissue plasminogen activator.

to the endothelial cells that line the blood vessels. However, when endothelial damage exposes the underlying tissue, platelets in the vicinity immediately undergo a reaction that cause them to stick to the exposed collagen (platelet adhesion) and to each other (platelet aggregation), and the coagulation cascade is activated. The platelet plug quickly arrests bleeding but must be reinforced by fibrin for long-term effectiveness. Disorders of hemostasis can be divided into excessive clotting (thrombosis) and excessive bleeding (bleeding diathesis).

Figure 11-2 outlines the drugs used to treat disorders of hemostasis. These can be broadly divided into two primary groups: (1) anticlotting drugs (anticoagulants, antiplatelet drugs, and thrombolytics) used to decrease clotting in individuals who either have evidence of a pathologic thrombus or are at risk for thrombotic vascular occlusion; and (2) drugs used to restore clotting in patients with clotting deficiencies. The first group includes some of the most commonly used drugs in the United States. Anticlotting drugs are used in the prevention and treatment of myocardial infarction and other acute coronary syndromes, atrial fibrillation, ischemic stroke, and deep vein thrombosis (DVT). The anticoagulant and thrombolytic drugs

are effective in treatment of *both* venous and arterial thrombosis, whereas antiplatelet drugs are used primarily for treatment or prevention of arterial thrombosis. Drugs used to facilitate clotting are critical for patients with excessive bleeding due to over-anticoagulation or other causes (eg, hemophilia).

ANTICLOTTING DRUGS

Anticoagulants

All anticoagulants have their effect by ultimately inhibiting the formation of fibrin clots. Four major types of anticoagulants are available. Indirect thrombin inhibitors such as heparin and its related low-molecular-weight products (enoxaparin and fondaparinux) must be administered parenterally. Direct thrombin inhibitors include the parenterally administered argatroban and orally active dabigatran. Warfarin, a coumarin derivative, is the oldest orally active anticoagulant. Last, the direct Xa inhibitors with suffixes ending in "-aban" represent the newest class of orally effective anticoagulants. The anticoagulant drug classes differ in their chemistry,

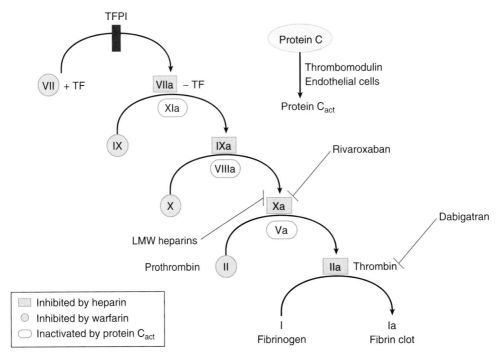

FIGURE 11-3 **A model of the coagulation cascade showing the series of enzymatic reactions that leads to activation (indicated by lowercase "a") of each clotting factor (indicated by Roman numerals).** Tissue factor (TF) is important in initiating the clotting cascade. Tissue factor pathway inhibitor (TFPI) inhibits the action of the VIIa–TF complex. High-molecular-weight heparin acts in the blood to directly activate antithrombin, which inactivates the clotting factors enclosed in green rectangles. The activated form of protein C (protein C$_{act}$), another anticlotting factor, inactivates the activated clotting factors shown in blue ovals. Warfarin acts in the liver to inhibit the synthesis of clotting factors enclosed in orange circles. Low-molecular-weight (LMW) heparins, rivaroxaban, and fondaparinux mainly inhibit factor Xa. Direct thrombin inhibitors (eg, dabigatran) inhibit thrombin (clotting factor IIa).

pharmacokinetics, and pharmacodynamics. Figure 11-3 illustrates the sites where different types of anticoagulants inhibit the coagulation cascade. Table 11-1 summarizes the mechanisms of action, pharmacokinetics, major clinical applications, and adverse effects of anticoagulants.

Indirect Thrombin Inhibitors

Indirect thrombin inhibitors produce their effect by binding to antithrombin and enhancing the *inactivation* of clotting factor Xa. **Heparin** is a large highly acidic sulfated polysaccharide polymer obtained from animal sources. Heparin is also referred to as unfractionated heparin or high-molecular-weight (HMW) heparin because each batch contains molecules of varying size, with an average molecular weight of 15,000-20,000. Heparin must be given parenterally (intravenously or subcutaneously). Intramuscular injection is avoided because of the risk of hematoma formation.

Figure 11-4 illustrates how heparin acts as an anticoagulant. HMW heparin binds to antithrombin III (ATIII), a powerful endogenous anticlotting protease. The heparin–ATIII complex then combines with and irreversibly breaks down thrombin (activated factor II) and several other factors, particularly factor Xa (Figure 11-3). In the presence of heparin, antithrombin III destroys thrombin and factor Xa approximately 1000-fold faster than in its absence. Because it acts on existing blood components,

heparin provides anticoagulation immediately after administration. The action of heparin is monitored with the activated partial thromboplastin time (aPTT) or partial thromboplastin time (PTT) laboratory tests. However, use of the factor Xa assay may have fewer confounding variables than the aPTT assay.

To provide greater and more consistent bioavailability and longer durations of action than HMW heparin, low-molecular-weight (LMW) fractions (2000-6000) of heparin have been developed (**enoxaparin**, **dalteparin**, and **tinzaparin**). Doses can be given subcutaneously less frequently (eg, once or twice per day) than heparin. **Fondaparinux** is a small synthetic drug that contains a key pentasaccharide present in pharmacologically active molecules of unfractionated and LMW heparins. Fondaparinux is administered subcutaneously once daily.

Like HMW heparin, LMW heparins and fondaparinux bind ATIII and form complexes that have the same inhibitory effect on factor Xa (Figure 11-4). However, LMW heparin–ATIII and fondaparinux–ATIII complexes provide a more selective action because they inhibit thrombin formation, but do not proteolytically degrade thrombin like the HMW heparin–ATIII complex. The aPTT test does not reliably measure the anticoagulant effect of the LMW heparins and fondaparinux. Because the LMW heparins and fondaparinux have fairly reliable pharmacokinetic properties, their use usually precludes the need for

TABLE 11-1 Properties of major classes of anticoagulants.

Subclass	Mechanism of Action	Pharmacokinetics	Clinical Applications	Adverse Effects
Heparins				
Unfractionated heparin[a]	Complexes with antithrombin III. Irreversibly inactivates clotting factors thrombin and factor Xa	Parenteral administration	Venous thrombosis, PE, MI, unstable angina, adjuvant to percutaneous coronary intervention (PCI) and thrombolytics	Bleeding (monitor with aPTT; protamine is reversal agent). Osteoporosis and thrombocytopenia with chronic use
Factor Xa inhibitors				
Rivaroxaban[b]	Binds to active site of factor Xa and inhibits its enzymatic action	Oral administration. Fixed dose. No routine monitoring (factor Xa test)	Venous thrombosis, PE, prevention of stroke in patients with nonvalvular atrial fibrillation	Bleeding. Andexanet alfa (recombinant modified factor Xa protein) is a reversal agent
Direct thrombin inhibitors				
Dabigatran[c]	Binds to thrombin's active site and inhibits its enzymatic action	Oral administration	Anticoagulation in patients with heparin-induced thrombocytopenia (HIT)	Bleeding (monitor with aPTT). Idarucizumab is a reversal agent
Coumadin anticoagulant				
Warfarin	Inhibits vitamin K epoxide reductase and thereby interferes with production of functional vitamin K–dependent clotting and anticlotting factors	Oral administration. Delayed onset and offset of anticoagulant activity. Many drug-drug and drug-CAMS interactions. Anticoagulant activity affected by dietary vitamin K	Venous thrombosis, PE, prevention of stroke in patients with nonvalvular atrial fibrillation	Bleeding (monitor with PT/INR). Thrombosis early in therapy due to protein C deficiency. Teratogen. Vitamin K₁ is a reversal agent

aPTT, activated partial thromboplastin time; CAMS: complementary and alternative medicine supplements; INR, international normalized ratio; MI, myocardial infarction; PE, pulmonary embolism; PT, prothrombin time.

[a]Low-molecular-weight heparins (LMW) heparins (enoxaparin, dalteparin, tinzaparin) have more selective anti-factor Xa activity. These drugs also have more reliable pharmacokinetics with renal elimination, and protamine reversal is only partially effective. There is less risk of thrombocytopenia. Fondaparinux effects are similar to those of LMW heparins.

[b]Apixaban and edoxaban are similar to rivaroxaban.

[c]Bivalirudin and argatroban are parenterally administered, all other parameters are similar to dabigatran.

laboratory monitoring of their anticoagulation effect. However, the lack of a readily available test for monitoring drug effect is a potential problem in special circumstances such as in patients with impaired renal function who may exhibit reduced drug clearance.

Because of its rapid effect, HMW heparin is used when anticoagulation is needed immediately (eg, initiation of anticoagulation therapy). Common uses include treatment of DVT, pulmonary embolism, and acute myocardial infarction. Heparin is used in combination with thrombolytics for revascularization procedures and in combination with glycoprotein IIb/IIIa inhibitors (antiplatelet agents) during angioplasty and placement of coronary stents. Because heparin does not cross the placenta, it is the drug of choice when an anticoagulant must be used in pregnancy. LMW heparins and fondaparinux have similar clinical applications.

Increased bleeding is the most serious hazard of heparin and the related molecules; the bleeding may result in

hemorrhagic stroke. HMW heparin causes moderate transient thrombocytopenia in many patients and severe thrombocytopenia and paradoxical thrombosis in a small percentage of patients. The latter individuals produce an antibody that binds to a complex of heparin and platelet factor 4. LMW heparins and fondaparinux are less likely to cause this immune-mediated thrombocytopenia. Prolonged use of full doses of HMW heparin for 3-6 months is associated with osteoporosis. In rare instances of dangerously elevated anticoagulation with excessive HMW heparin, heparin can be rapidly neutralized by intravenous administration of the highly basic protein **protamine**. Protamine only partially reverses the effects of LMW heparins and does not affect the action of fondaparinux.

Direct Thrombin Inhibitors

As their name implies, direct thrombin inhibitors inhibit coagulation by directly binding to the active site of thrombin

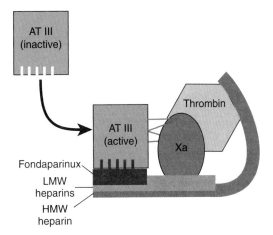

FIGURE 11-4 **Illustration of mechanism by which low-molecular-weight (LMW) heparins, fondaparinux (a small fragment of heparin), and high-molecular-weight (HMW, unfractionated) heparin act as anticoagulants.** Activated antithrombin III (AT III active) degrades thrombin, factor Xa, and several other factors. When HMW heparin combines with AT III active, the drug increases degradation of both factor Xa and thrombin. Combination of AT III active with fondaparinux or LMW heparins more selectively increases degradation of Xa.

(and inhibiting the downstream production of fibrin) without the presence of ATIII. Several direct thrombin inhibitors are derived from the protein hirudin made by *Hirudo medicinalis*, the medicinal leech. **Desirudin** and **bivalirudin** are modified forms of hirudin. **Argatroban** is a small, nonprotein molecule that may accumulate in patients with liver disease. All the direct thrombin inhibitors, except for **dabigatran etexilate**, are administered parenterally.

Direct thrombin inhibitors are used as alternatives to heparin primarily in patients with heparin-induced thrombocytopenia. Bivalirudin, which also inhibits platelet activation, is used in combination with aspirin during percutaneous coronary angioplasty. Like HMW heparin, the action of direct thrombin inhibitors is monitored with the aPTT laboratory test. In addition, these agents do not interact with cytochrome P450 (CYP)-interacting drugs.

Dabigatran is the only orally active direct thrombin inhibitor. The drug is approved for prevention of stroke and systemic embolism in nonvalvular atrial fibrillation. Advantages of dabigatran include predictable pharmacokinetics that allow for fixed dosing as well as a predictable immediate anticoagulant response that makes routine monitoring or overlap with other anticoagulants unnecessary. As with all anticoagulants, bleeding is the primary toxicity. If this occurs with dabigatran, its anticoagulant effect can be reversed by **idarucizumab**, which is a humanized monoclonal Fab fragment that binds to and reduces free dabigatran blood levels.

Coumarin Anticoagulants

Warfarin is the only member of the coumarin anticoagulants used in the United States. Warfarin is a small, lipid-soluble molecule that is readily absorbed after oral administration.

Because the drug crosses the placenta and has teratogenic effects, it is not used in pregnancy. Warfarin is highly bound to plasma proteins (> 99%), and its elimination depends on metabolism by CYP enzymes.

Warfarin interferes with posttranslational modification of clotting factors in the liver, a process that requires vitamin K. During the formation of factors II (thrombin), VII, IX, and X, vitamin K is oxidized to vitamin K epoxide. Vitamin K epoxide reductase then reduces the epoxide back to vitamin K. Warfarin competes with vitamin K epoxide for the reductase, decreasing the reduction of the epoxide and thus decreasing the *formation* of the above clotting factors in the liver (Figure 11-3). Because these clotting factors have half-lives of 8-60 hours in the plasma, the anticoagulant effect of warfarin is observed only after an 8-12 hour delay, which allows sufficient time for some existing clotting factors to begin to be consumed. The effect of warfarin is monitored by the prothrombin time (PT) corrected by means of the International Normalized Ratio (INR).

Warfarin has been used for chronic anticoagulation in all of the clinical situations described previously for heparin except those that occur in pregnant women. In addition, it is used for prophylaxis of venous thromboembolism in valvular disease and atrial fibrillation or flutter. Warfarin is contraindicated in pregnancy because the drug can cause bone defects and hemorrhaging in the developing fetus. Early in therapy, a period of hypercoagulability with subsequent dermal vascular necrosis can occur. This is most commonly due to reduced synthesis of protein C, an endogenous vitamin K–dependent anticoagulant with a relatively short half-life. If pharmacotherapy is being changed from indirect thrombin inhibitors to warfarin, a 5-7 day overlap between these drugs is required to minimize this hypercoagulable state that may initially occur with warfarin.

Bleeding is the most important adverse effect of warfarin. Because warfarin has a narrow therapeutic window, its involvement in drug and many supplement interactions is of major concern. CYP-inducing drugs (eg, barbiturates, carbamazepine, phenytoin) increase clearance of warfarin and reduce the anticoagulant effect of a given dose. CYP inhibitors (eg, amiodarone, selective serotonin reuptake inhibitors, cimetidine) reduce metabolism of warfarin and increase its anticoagulant effects. Many dietary supplements (eg, St. John's wort, ginkgo, arnica) also interact with warfarin and can alter the INR/PT. Because vitamin K is necessary for the production of functioning clotting factors, variations in dietary vitamin K (found in high concentrations in leafy green vegetables) can also alter the anticoagulant effects of warfarin. Increases in dietary vitamin K decrease the anticoagulant effect of warfarin, and decreases in dietary vitamin K have the opposite effect.

In the case of excessive anticoagulation effect, warfarin's action can be reversed with vitamin K_1 (**phytonadione**). However, recovery requires synthesis of new functional clotting factors and is therefore slow, requiring 6-24 hours. More rapid reversal can be achieved by transfusion with fresh or frozen plasma that contains normal clotting factors.

Direct Oral Factor Xa Inhibitors

The new class of orally active Xa inhibitors includes **rivaroxaban**, **apixaban**, and **edoxaban**. These small molecules directly bind to and inhibit both free factor Xa and factor Xa bound in the clotting complex (Figure 11-3). Given as fixed doses, they have a rapid onset of action, shorter half-lives than warfarin, and do not require monitoring. They undergo elimination by both CYP-dependent and CYP-independent processes.

All three drugs are approved for prevention of stroke in patients with atrial fibrillation, without valvular heart disease. Rivaroxaban and apixaban are approved for prevention and treatment of venous thromboembolism after hip or knee surgery. Adverse effects are similar to other anticoagulants in that they may cause bleeding. **Andexanet alfa** is the first potential antidote for the oral factor Xa inhibitors. The drug does not have procoagulant activity, but rather competes with factor Xa for binding to factor Xa inhibitors. Thus, by acting as a factor Xa "decoy" molecule, andexanet alfa binds these drugs and decreases their anticoagulant effect. Although andexanet alfa was developed to inhibit direct factor Xa inhibitors, the drug should theoretically also inhibit the actions of the LMW heparins and fondaparinux because they interact with antithrombin III to inactivate factor Xa. Andexanet alfa will have less of an inhibitory effect on the anticoagulant effect of HMW heparin because its interaction with antithrombin III inactivates thrombin in addition to factor Xa.

Antiplatelet Drugs

Platelet aggregation plays a central role in the clotting process and is especially important in clots that form in the arterial circulation, including those responsible for coronary and cerebral artery occlusion. Several endogenous substances *facilitate* platelet aggregation, including thromboxane A2, adenosine diphosphate (ADP), fibrin, and serotonin. There are also several endogenous substances that *inhibit* platelet aggregation including those that increase cyclic adenosine monophosphate (cAMP) formation in platelets (eg, prostacyclin).

Figure 11-2 outlines five main groups of antiplatelet agents. Figure 11-5 illustrates their mechanisms of interrupting platelet aggregation. All antiplatelet drugs significantly enhance the effects of other anticlotting agents. However, their inhibitory effects on hemostasis cannot be monitored with the aPTT or PT anticoagulation tests. Table 11-2 summarizes mechanisms of action and clinical parameters of the antiplatelet drugs.

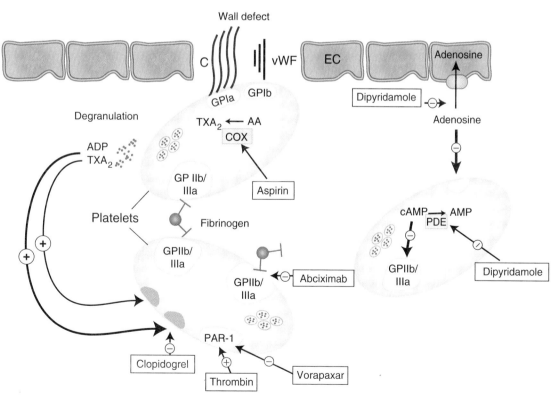

FIGURE 11-5 **Thrombus formation at the site of the damaged vascular wall (EC, endothelial cell) and the role of platelets and clotting factors.** Platelet membrane receptors include the glycoprotein Ia receptor (GPIa) binding to collagen (C), the GPIb receptor binding to von Willebrand factor (vWF), the GP IIb/IIIa receptor binding to fibrinogen and other macromolecules, and PAR-1 activated by thrombin. Aggregating substances released from the degranulating platelet include adenosine diphosphate (ADP) and thromboxane A2 (TXA₂). Mechanisms of action for prototypical antiplatelet drugs (aspirin, clopidogrel, abciximab, vorapaxar, and dipyridamole) are also shown. PAR-1, protease activated receptor type 1; PDE, phosphodiesterase.

TABLE 11-2 Major classes of antiplatelet drugs, their mechanisms of action, significant pharmacokinetics, and major clinical applications along with adverse effects.

Subclass	Mechanism of Action	Pharmacokinetics	Clinical Application	Adverse Effects
COX inhibitor				
Aspirin	Nonselective, irreversible COX inhibitor, reduces platelet production of thromboxane A2, potent stimulator of platelet aggregation	Duration of activity is longer than pharmacokinetic half-life due to irreversible action	Prevention and treatment of arterial thrombosis	Gastrointestinal toxicity, nephrotoxicity, hypersensitivity reaction due to increased leukotrienes; tinnitus, hyperventilation metabolic acidosis, hyperthermia, coma in overdose
Glycoprotein IIb/IIIa inhibitor (GP IIb/IIIa)				
Abciximab[a]	Inhibits platelet aggregation by interfering with GPIIb/IIIa binding to fibrinogen and other ligands	Parenteral administration	Used during PCI to prevent restenosis, acute coronary syndrome	Bleeding, thrombocytopenia with prolonged use
ADP receptor antagonists				
Clopidogrel[b,c]	Irreversibly inhibits platelet ADP receptor	Oral administration	Acute coronary syndrome, prevention of restenosis after PCI, prevention and treatment of arterial thrombosis	Bleeding, gastrointestinal disturbances, hematologic abnormalities
PAR-1 receptor antagonists				
Vorapaxar	Competitive inhibitor of PAR-1 (thrombin) receptor	Oral administration	Prophylaxis in individuals at risk of thrombotic cardiovascular events	Bleeding, rarely major hemorrhage, potentially intracranial bleeding
Additional antiplatelet drugs				
Dipyridamole[d]	Inhibits adenosine uptake and inhibits phosphodiesterase enzymes that degrade cyclic nucleotides (cAMP, cGMP)	Oral administration	Prevention of thromboembolic complications of cardiac valve replacement; combined with aspirin for secondary prevention of ischemic stroke	Headache, palpitations, contraindicated in congestive heart failure

[a]Eptifibatide and tirofiban are reversible GP IIb/IIIa inhibitors of smaller size than abciximab.

[b]Ticlopidine is an older ADP receptor antagonist with more toxicity, particularly leukopenia and thrombotic thrombocytopenic purpura.

[c]Prasugrel is newer drug, similar to clopidogrel with less variable kinetics, activation primarily by CYP3A4. Ticagrelor is a reversible ADP receptor antagonist that does not require activation.

[d]Cilostazol is similar to dipyridamole.

ADP, adenosine diphosphate; COX, cyclooxygenase; PAR-1, protease-activated receptor type 1; PCI, percutaneous coronary intervention.

Aspirin

Aspirin and the nonsteroidal anti-inflammatory drugs (NSAIDs) are discussed in Chapter 34. These drugs inhibit the formation of all prostaglandins, including thromboxane, by inhibiting the enzyme cyclooxygenase (COX). Although *all* NSAIDs impart an increased risk of bleeding, only aspirin is used therapeutically as an antiplatelet drug. Aspirin is particularly effective because of its irreversible inhibition of COX. In blood vessels, there is a delicate balance between the platelet-*inhibiting* effect of prostacyclin (produced by endothelial cells) and the platelet-*activating* effect of thromboxane (released by previously activated platelets). Platelets lack the ability to make new proteins, so they are unable to escape aspirin's inhibitory effect on thromboxane formation. In contrast, endothelial cells,

which contain a nucleus and the capacity to synthesize new proteins, continue to produce some COX and prostacyclin. Aspirin therapy therefore tips the prostacyclin/thromboxane balance toward prostacyclin and thus inhibition of platelet function (Figure 11-5). Since all of the other NSAIDs inhibit COX reversibly, they have a less selective antiplatelet effect. In fact, if other NSAIDs are administered concomitantly, they may decrease the antiplatelet effect of aspirin.

Aspirin is used to prevent future infarcts in individuals who have had one or more myocardial infarcts. Aspirin may also reduce the incidence of first infarcts. The drug is used extensively to prevent transient ischemic attacks (TIAs), ischemic stroke, and other thrombotic events. The dose of aspirin required for antithrombotic effect is lower than the anti-inflammatory dose. Aspirin causes adverse gastrointestinal, renal, and CNS effects (Chapter 34).

ADP Receptor Inhibitors

Clopidogrel, **prasugrel**, and **ticlopidine** irreversibly inhibit the ADP receptor, resulting in inhibition of ADP-mediated platelet aggregation (Figure 11-5). Because these drugs irreversibly modify the platelet ADP receptor, platelets are affected for the remainder of their approximately 10-day lifespan (as is the case with aspirin). Clopidogrel and prasugrel are prodrugs that require biotransformation; their metabolites inhibit the ADP receptors. Prasugrel has a faster antiplatelet onset due to a higher rate of biotransformation. Reversible ADP receptor antagonists are also available with oral (**ticagrelor**) or intravenous (**cangrelor**) administration.

Clopidogrel, prasugrel, and ticlopidine are useful in preventing TIAs and ischemic stroke, especially in individuals who cannot tolerate aspirin. Clopidogrel is also used to reduce thrombosis in patients who have recently received a coronary artery stent. Ticlopidine causes bleeding in up to 5% of patients and severe neutropenia in about 1%. Very rarely, thrombotic thrombocytopenic purpura, a serious condition characterized by hemolysis and end-organ damage, can occur. Clopidogrel is less hematotoxic. Ticagrelor has similar clinical uses and adverse effects. Due to its short half-life (3-6 minutes), the use of cangrelor is limited to percutaneous coronary interventions.

Glycoprotein IIb/IIIa Inhibitors

Glycoprotein IIb/IIIa is the most abundant receptor on the surface of activated platelets. Binding of fibrinogen (the primary ligand) and other ligands (eg, von Willebrand factor) to the glycoprotein IIb/IIIa receptor crosslinks platelets, resulting in platelet aggregation and formation of the platelet plug. Activation of the GP IIb/IIIa receptor is the final step in platelet aggregation. **Abciximab**, **eptifibatide**, and **tirofiban** reversibly block the glycoprotein IIb/IIIa receptor, inhibiting the binding of fibrinogen and other ligands to this receptor (Figure 11-5). The glycoprotein IIb/IIIa receptor antagonists have short half-lives and must be given by continuous infusion. These agents are used to prevent restenosis after coronary angioplasty and are used in acute coronary syndromes (eg, unstable angina and non-Q-wave acute myocardial infarction). Major toxicities are bleeding and, with chronic use, thrombocytopenia.

Protease Activated Receptor-1 (PAR-1) Inhibitors

Protease activated receptors (PAR) are a subfamily of G protein–mediated transmembrane receptors that are activated by enzymatic cleavage of the N-terminus region on the external surface of the cell membrane. This cleavage results in refolding of the protein and activation of the receptor. There are four major PAR receptors found in multiple tissue types; PAR-1 and PAR-4 receptors are found on platelets. Thrombin is a potent stimulus for platelet activation and aggregation.

Thrombin mediates this effect through enzymatic cleavage of the PAR receptor on platelets, with a higher affinity for PAR-1. **Vorapaxar** is an orally active PAR-1 competitive receptor antagonist (Figure 11-5). The drug does not interfere with the role of thrombin in the clotting cascade (ie, conversion of fibrinogen to fibrin). As such, vorapaxar does not alter clotting cascade activity, but works by inhibiting thrombin-related platelet aggregation. Vorapaxar does not alter platelet aggregation that occurs due to other activators such as ADP.

Vorapaxar is used to reduce the risk of thrombotic cardiovascular events in individuals who are at risk of subsequent myocardial infarction or have established peripheral cardiovascular disease. Bleeding is an associated risk and intracranial bleeding is a life-threatening risk, especially in people with previous hemorrhagic strokes.

Additional Antiplatelet-Directed Drugs

Dipyridamole and the newer **cilostazol** appear to have dual mechanisms of action to inhibit platelet function. First, these drugs inhibit phosphodiesterase-3 (PDE3), the enzyme that degrades cyclic adenosine monophosphate (cAMP) and cyclic guanosine monophosphate (cGMP). Cyclic AMP is a second messenger and an inhibitor of platelet aggregation. Cyclic GMP is a vasodilator. Thus, by inhibiting PDE3, increased cAMP is available to inhibit platelet aggregation. Second, these drugs inhibit the uptake of adenosine by endothelial cells and erythrocytes, thereby increasing the plasma concentration of adenosine (Figure 11-5). Adenosine acts through platelet adenosine A2 receptors to increase platelet cAMP and thus inhibit aggregation.

Dipyridamole has minimal clinical benefit when used alone. The drug is used in conjunction with drugs such as warfarin or aspirin to prevent thrombosis due to different cardiovascular pathophysiologies or for secondary prophylaxis of cerebrovascular ischemia. Cilostazol is used to treat intermittent claudication (muscle pain on exercise), a manifestation of peripheral arterial disease. The most common adverse effects of dipyridamole and cilostazol are headaches and palpitations.

Thrombolytic Drugs

All clots must eventually be broken down by the body. Thrombolytic enzymes catalyze the conversion of the inactive circulating precursor plasminogen to the active form of the enzyme called plasmin. Plasmin splits fibrin into fragments, thus promoting the breakdown and dissolution of clots (Figure 11-6). Thrombolytic drugs increase the formation of plasmin. All of these agents are given intravenously and rapidly break down thrombi. The thrombolytic drugs include **streptokinase**, **tissue plasminogen activator (t-PA)** and its recombinant human derivatives **alteplase**, **tenecteplase**, and **reteplase** (Figure 11-2).

Streptokinase

Streptokinase is a protein obtained from bacterial cultures. Streptokinase forms a complex with plasminogen, the inactive precursor of plasmin. The streptokinase-plasminogen

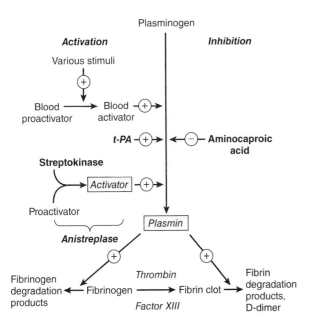

FIGURE 11-6 **Diagram of the fibrinolytic system.** The useful thrombolytic drugs are shown on the left in bold type. These drugs increase the formation of plasmin, the major fibrinolytic enzyme. The "activator" shown in the shaded box is a complex of streptokinase and plasminogen. Aminocaproic acid, a useful inhibitor of fibrinolysis, is shown on the right.

complex catalyzes rapid conversion of plasminogen to plasmin. The duration of action for streptokinase is 20-25 minutes. Streptokinase has clinical indications similar to t-PA and its derivatives discussed below. However, streptokinase is a bacterial protein and often evokes the production of antibodies. These antibodies can cause the bacterial protein to lose its effectiveness or induce severe allergic reactions on subsequent therapy. Patients who have had streptococcal infections may have preformed antibodies to the drug. Alteplase and other t-PA variants are not subject to this problem, but they are much more expensive than streptokinase and not much more effective.

Tissue Plasminogen Activator (t-PA)

t-PA is a large human protein that directly converts fibrin-bound plasminogen to plasmin (Figure 11-6). The drug has little activity unless it is bound to fibrin. In theory, this should make t-PA selective for the plasminogen that has already bound to fibrin (ie, in a clot), and should result in less danger of widespread production of plasmin and spontaneous bleeding. In fact, t-PA's selectivity appears to be quite limited. Alteplase is normal human plasminogen activator produced by recombinant DNA technology. Reteplase is a mutated form of human t-PA with similar effects, but slightly faster onset of action and longer duration of action. Tenecteplase is another mutated form of t-PA with a longer half-life. The duration of action for these drugs varies between 2 and 10 minutes.

The major application of the thrombolytic agents is as an alternative to percutaneous coronary angioplasty in the emergency treatment of coronary artery thrombosis. Under ideal conditions (ie, intravenous treatment within 6 hours), these agents can promptly restore blood flow through the occluded coronary vessel. Very prompt use (ie, within 3 hours of first symptoms) of t-PA in patients with ischemic stroke is associated with significantly better clinical outcomes. The thrombolytic agents are also used in cases of severe pulmonary embolism, severe DVTs, and ascending thrombophlebitis of the iliofemoral vein with severe lower extremity edema. Bleeding is the most important hazard of all the thrombolytic drugs. Cerebral hemorrhage is the most serious manifestation, and must be ruled out before therapeutic use.

DRUGS THAT FACILITATE CLOTTING

Inadequate blood clotting may result from vitamin K deficiency, inherited clotting factor disorders (eg, hemophilia), a variety of drug-induced conditions, or thrombocytopenia. Therefore, treatment may involve administration of vitamin K, preformed clotting factors, or antiplasmin drugs (Figure 11-2). Thrombocytopenia can be treated by administration of platelets.

Replacement Factors

The most important agents used to treat hemophilia are fresh plasma and human blood-clotting factors, especially factor VIII and factor IX, which are purified from blood products. Factor VIII is used to treat classic hemophilia (hemophilia A) and factor IX is used to treat Christmas disease (hemophilia B). These products are purified from human blood and carry the risk of infection and immunologic reactions. Donor screening and testing of blood products for infectious disease agents (eg, human immunodeficiency virus [HIV] and hepatitis B and C) has minimized contamination by blood-borne pathogens. However, these processes do not reduce the risk of prion-associated diseases. Products produced by recombinant DNA technology eliminate these risks, but are expensive. The recombinant factor VIII-Fc domain conjugate is **eloctate**; the recombinant coagulation factor IX-albumin conjugate is **idelvion**.

Vitamin K

Vitamin K is actually a group of chemically related fat-soluble vitamins including vitamin K_1 and a group of other compounds called vitamin K_2. Vitamin K deficiency is particularly common in newborns and in older individuals with abnormalities of fat absorption. The deficiency is readily treated with oral or parenteral **phytonadione** (vitamin K_1). Since 1961, all newborns in the United States receive an injection of vitamin K_1 because newborns have little vitamin K stores and are at risk for bleeding. Large doses of vitamin K_1 are also used to reverse the anticoagulant effect of excess warfarin.

Antiplasmin Drugs

Antiplasmin agents are valuable for the management of acute bleeding episodes in hemophiliacs and others with bleeding disorders. **Aminocaproic acid** and **tranexamic acid** are orally active agents that inhibit fibrinolysis by inhibiting activation of plasminogen (Figure 11-6).

REHABILITATION RELEVANCE

Drugs affecting the blood are prescribed for a broad spectrum of clinical conditions. These drugs have the potential to influence, both positively and negatively, rehabilitation outcomes in these patient populations. Common adverse effects include:

- **Myalgia** and **arthralgia** may occur as a result of bleeding into muscles and joints in patients taking anticoagulant or antiplatelet drugs, or in those with bleeding disorders who are undermedicated. Pain may limit functional outcomes. Careful monitoring of appropriate laboratory values may help the clinician differentiate pain associated with exercise (eg, delayed-onset muscle soreness) from that associated with adverse drug effects and assist in prescribing the appropriate intensity of the rehabilitation protocol.
- **Ostealgia** may be associated with administration of the hematopoietic growth factors often used to treat neutropenia. As above, this pain may decrease patient function and adversely affect rehabilitation outcomes.

- Therapists must follow current and evolving guidelines for **when it is safe to mobilize patients after administration of an anticoagulant**. For example, in patients being treated for a lower extremity DVT, it is safe to mobilize within several hours after treatment with LMW heparins, fondaparinux, or the oral direct thrombin inhibitors and direct factor Xa inhibitors. Delaying mobilization for more than 48 hours is recommended after treatment with unfractionated heparin. With warfarin, mobilization should not occur until the INR is between 2 and 5.
- **Increased bleeding of integumentary wounds** may occur as a result of anticoagulants and antiplatelet drugs. Certain chronic wound debridement options such as conservative sharps debridement may be contraindicated.
- **Decreased exercise tolerance** may occur in patients with anemia. Patients receiving erythropoiesis-stimulating agents are treated to a maximum hemoglobin range of 10-12 g/dL. Thus, these individuals are still considered anemic even when being successfully treated with these drugs. As such, these patients may have minimal exercise reserve.
- Falls in patients taking both anticoagulants and antiplatelet drugs carry an **increased risk of increased intracranial bleeding** if they impact their head during the fall. Some types of subdural hemorrhage may take days to clinically manifest. If a patient states that he or she has had a previously unreported fall that potentially impacted the head, referral to other healthcare professionals should be considered.

CASE CONCLUSION

The pain in S.R.'s shoulders and knees may be related to restarting the conditioning program following the 1-week abstinence. However, the circumferential bruise at the wrist, combined with the other manifestations, and the client's lack of knowledge of his current anticoagulation level, should prompt concern about excessive anticoagulation with warfarin. S.R. commented about the absence of vegetables in his diet the previous week while visiting his grandchildren. As the vitamin K from his diet decreased, the anticlotting effects of warfarin (a vitamin K antagonist that prevents formation of many clotting factors) were increased. Immediate referral to the prescribing healthcare professional is recommended. As an additional note, patients may misinterpret the dietary instructions regarding vitamin K consumption while taking warfarin. Many patients mistakenly assume that they should avoid foods like green leafy vegetables that are rich sources of vitamin K. Patients are actually advised to eat *consistent* amounts of dietary vitamin K or anticipate that seasonal adjustments of warfarin dosage is sometimes necessary for consistent anticoagulation.

CHAPTER 11 QUESTIONS

1. Which of the following drugs would *not* be used to treat anemia due to renal failure?

   a. Darbepoetin alfa
   b. Folic acid
   c. Iron
   d. Pegfilgrastim

2. A deficiency in which of the following would result in both megaloblastic anemia and neurologic defects?

   a. Folic acid
   b. Cyanocobalamin
   c. Iron
   d. Niacin

3. Which of the following drugs is orally administered for thrombocytopenia?

   a. Romiplostim
   b. Epoetin alfa
   c. Sargramostim
   d. Eltrombopag

4. Which of the following drugs is an orally effective direct-acting thrombin inhibitor?

   a. Argatroban
   b. Enoxaparin
   c. Dabigatran
   d. Warfarin

5. Which of the following drugs irreversibly inhibits cyclo-oxygenase in platelets?

   a. Aspirin
   b. Clopidogrel
   c. Vorapaxar
   d. Dipyridamole

6. Which of the following is a common adverse effect to antiplatelet drugs and anticoagulants?

   a. Headache
   b. Tachycardia
   c. Rash
   d. Bleeding

7. Which of the following is a monoclonal antibody that is the reversal agent for dabigatran?

   a. Abciximab
   b. Idarucizumab
   c. Protamine
   d. Aminocaproic acid

8. Which of the following would have the greatest inhibitory effect on the anticoagulant actions of warfarin?

   a. Spinach
   b. Eggs
   c. Cheese
   d. Fish

9. Which of the following would be used to treat hemophilia type A?

   a. Iron
   b. Idelvion
   c. Eloctate
   d. Romiplostim

10. Which of the following drugs enzymatically converts plasminogen to plasmin?

   a. Streptokinase
   b. Abciximab
   c. Tranexamic acid
   d. Tenecteplase

Introduction to the Pharmacology of Central Nervous System Drugs

Drugs acting in the central nervous system (CNS) were among the first to be discovered by humans and are still the most widely used group of pharmacologic agents. In addition to their use in therapy, many drugs acting on the CNS are used without prescription to increase one's sense of well-being.

The mechanisms by which various drugs act in the CNS have not always been clearly understood. Since the causes of many of the conditions for which these drugs are used (eg, schizophrenia, anxiety) are themselves poorly understood, it is not surprising that in the past much of CNS pharmacology has been purely descriptive. However, dramatic advances in the methodology of CNS pharmacology have made it possible to study the action of a drug on individual cells and even on single ion channels within synapses. This information has provided the basis for several major developments in studies of the CNS.

Nearly all drugs with CNS effects act on specific receptors that modulate synaptic transmission, either directly by affecting the receptors themselves or indirectly through various second-messenger coupling systems, ion channels, or other mechanisms. Drugs are also among the most important tools for studying all aspects of CNS physiology, from the mechanism of convulsions to the laying down of long-term memory. Synthetic agonists that mimic natural transmitters (and in many cases are more selective than the endogenous substances) and antagonists are extremely useful in such studies. Unraveling the actions of drugs with known clinical efficacy has led to some of the most fruitful hypotheses regarding the mechanisms of disease. For example, information about the action of antipsychotic drugs on dopamine receptors has provided the basis for important hypotheses regarding the pathophysiology of schizophrenia. Studies of the effects of a variety of agonists and antagonists on gamma-aminobutyric acid

(GABA) receptors have resulted in new concepts pertaining to the pathophysiology of several diseases, including anxiety and epilepsy.

This chapter provides an introduction to the functional organization of the CNS and synaptic transmitters as a basis for understanding the actions of the drugs described in the following chapters.

ION CHANNELS AND NEUROTRANSMITTER RECEPTORS

Most drugs that act on the CNS appear to do so by changing ion flow through transmembrane channels of nerve cells. Neuronal membranes contain two types of ion channels: *voltage gated* and *ligand gated*. These channels are defined on the basis of the mechanisms that control their gating (opening and closing). Voltage-gated (or, voltage-sensitive) channels open and close in response to changes in membrane potential (Figure 12–1A). In neurons, voltage-gated sodium channels are concentrated at the axon initial segment. Activation of voltage-gated sodium channels is responsible for the fast action potential that transmits the electrical signal from the cell body to the axon terminal. There are also many types of voltage-sensitive calcium and potassium channels on the cell body, dendrites, and initial segment, which act on a slower time scale and modulate the rate at which the neuron discharges. Ligand-gated channels (also called *ionotropic receptors*) open in response to binding of a neurotransmitter (ie, ligand) to the receptor-channel complex (Figure 12–1B). The channel, formed by transmembranous protein subunits, is an

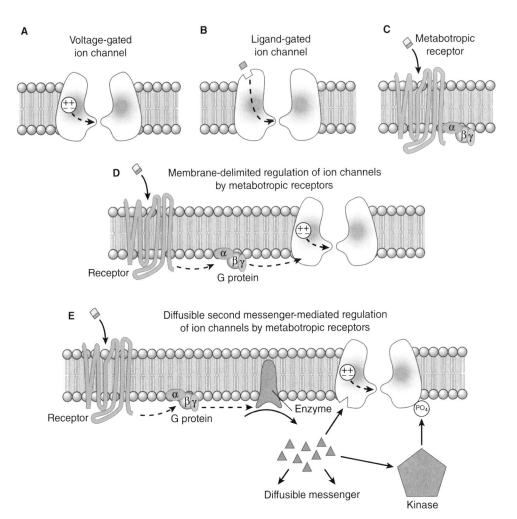

FIGURE 12-1 **Types of ion channels and neurotransmitter receptors in the CNS. A** shows a voltage-gated ion channel in which a voltage sensor controls the gating (broken arrow) of the channel. **B** shows a ligand-gated ionotropic channel in which binding of the neurotransmitter (blue rectangle) controls gating of the channel. **C** shows a G protein-coupled (metabotropic) receptor, which when bound by the neurotransmitter, activates the heterotrimeric G protein. **D** and **E** show two ways that metabotropic receptors regulate ion channels. In **D**, a subunit of the activated G protein directly modulates the ion channel. In **E**, the activated G protein activates an enzyme that generates a diffusible second messenger (eg, cAMP) that can interact with the ion channel or can activate a kinase that phosphorylates and modulates the ion channel.

integral part of the receptor-channel complex. Ligand-gated channels are insensitive or only weakly sensitive to changes in membrane potential. Activation of these channels, which are found on both the presynaptic and postsynaptic sides of synapses, typically results in a brief (few milliseconds to tens of milliseconds) opening of the channel. Ligand-gated channels are responsible for fast synaptic transmission typical of hierarchical pathways in the CNS (see below).

Neurotransmitters also exert their effects on neurons by binding to metabotropic receptors (Figure 12-1C). In contrast to ligand-gated channels, the binding of neurotransmitter to metabotropic receptors does not result in *directly* gating an ion channel. Instead, neurotransmitter binding activates a seven-transmembrane G protein-coupled receptor. This process often leads to the modulation of voltage-gated channels via a membrane-delimited pathway or via the generation of diffusible second messengers. In the membrane-delimited pathway, a portion of the activated G protein itself interacts

directly with the voltage-gated ion channel (Figure 12-1D). Two types of voltage-gated ion channels are involved in this type of signaling: calcium channels and potassium channels. When G proteins interact with calcium channels, they inhibit channel function. This mechanism accounts for the presynaptic inhibition that occurs when presynaptic metabotropic receptors are activated. In contrast, when these metabotropic receptors are postsynaptic, they open potassium channels, resulting in a slow postsynaptic inhibition. Stimulation of some metabotropic receptors activates a G protein-coupled receptor that mediates the production of diffusible intracellular second messengers such as cyclic adenosine monophosphate (cAMP), which can interact with the ion channel, or can activate a kinase that subsequently phosphorylates and modulates the channel (Figure 12-1E).

An important consequence of the involvement of G proteins in receptor signaling is that, in contrast to the brief effect of transmitters on ionotropic receptors, the effects of metabotropic receptor activation can last tens of seconds to minutes. Metabotropic receptors predominate in the diffuse neuronal systems in the CNS.

THE SYNAPSE AND SYNAPTIC POTENTIALS

In most cases, communication between neurons in the CNS occurs through chemical synapses. An action potential in the presynaptic fiber propagates into the axon terminal, opening voltage-sensitive calcium channels. The resulting increase in intraterminal calcium concentration promotes the fusion of synaptic vesicles with the presynaptic membrane. The neurotransmitter contained in the vesicles is released into the synaptic cleft and diffuses to the receptors on the postsynaptic membrane. Binding of the transmitter to its receptor causes a brief change in membrane conductance (permeability to ions) of the postsynaptic cell either directly or indirectly (as described above).

Binding of the neurotransmitter to the postsynaptic membrane can result in either an excitatory or an inhibitory postsynaptic potential. Excitatory postsynaptic potentials (EPSPs) are usually generated by the opening of sodium or calcium channels. In some synapses, depolarizing potentials result from the *closing* of potassium channels. When a sufficient number of excitatory synapses are activated on a neuron, the EPSP may reach threshold and generate an action potential in the postsynaptic cell. Inhibitory postsynaptic potentials (IPSPs) are usually generated by the opening of potassium or chloride channels. For example, opening of potassium channels in the postsynaptic cell causes K^+ to leave, resulting in a hyperpolarization that makes the cell less likely to fire an action potential. Opening of chloride channels does not cause significant hyperpolarization because the equilibrium potential for Cl^- is close to the neuron's resting membrane potential. However, opening of chloride channels makes the neuron more "leaky." This shunting effect makes it more difficult to change the membrane potential. Functionally, this means that the neuron is less likely to be impacted by incoming EPSPs. Another type of inhibition is *presynaptic* inhibition, which can occur via a decrease in calcium influx elicited by activation of presynaptic metabotropic receptors.

BLOOD-BRAIN BARRIER

The blood-brain barrier (BBB) is a functional separation that limits penetration of certain substances (such as drugs) within circulating blood into the extracellular fluid of the CNS. The BBB is anatomically formed by tight junctions between the endothelial cells of the capillaries and the end-feet of astrocytes that surround the capillaries. While water, some gases, and lipid-soluble molecules can cross the BBB via passive diffusion, circulating nutrients such as glucose and the essential amino acids must utilize specific transporters to move across the BBB.

In order to enter the CNS, drugs must either be highly lipophilic (eg, anesthetics) or employ specific transport mechanisms.

For example, second-generation antihistamines are far less sedating because they were intentionally developed to be much more polar than first-generation agents. In the treatment of Parkinson's disease (Chapter 17), oral **levodopa** (**L-DOPA**), a precursor to dopamine, is used to enhance central dopamine levels because dopamine cannot cross the BBB. L-DOPA can cross the BBB by utilizing an amino acid transporter.

SITES OF DRUG ACTION

Virtually all of the drugs that act in the CNS produce their effects by modifying some step in chemical synaptic transmission. Figure 12-2 illustrates some of the presynaptic and postsynaptic steps that can be altered. Drugs acting on the synthesis, storage, metabolism, and release of neurotransmitters fall into the presynaptic category. Synaptic transmission can be depressed by blocking transmitter synthesis or storage (Figure 12-2, sites 2 and 3). For example, **reserpine** depletes monoamine synapses by interfering with their intracellular storage. Blockade of transmitter catabolism within the axon terminal (Figure 12-2, site 4) can increase transmitter concentration and has been reported to increase the amount of transmitter released per impulse. Drugs can also alter the release of transmitter (Figure 12-2, site 5). For example, the stimulant **amphetamine** induces the release of catecholamines (dopamine, epinephrine, norepinephrine) from adrenergic nerve endings, while **botulinum toxin** blocks the release of acetylcholine. After a transmitter has been released into the synaptic cleft, its action is terminated either by uptake or degradation (Figure 12-2, sites 6 and 7, respectively). For many neurotransmitters, there are uptake mechanisms into the synaptic terminal and also into surrounding neuroglia. **Cocaine** blocks the uptake of catecholamines at adrenergic synapses and thus potentiates the action of these amines. In contrast, the action of acetylcholine is not terminated by uptake from the synapse, but rather by enzymatic inactivation within the synapse by acetylcholinesterase. Anticholinesterase drugs (used in the treatment of Alzheimer's disease; Chapter 5) block the degradation of acetylcholine and thereby prolong its action. No uptake mechanism has been found for any of the numerous CNS peptides, and it has yet to be demonstrated whether specific enzymatic degradation terminates the action of peptide transmitters.

In the postsynaptic region, the transmitter receptor is the primary site of drug action (Figure 12-2, site 8). Drugs can act either as neurotransmitter agonists, such as opioids that mimic the action of endogenous peptides such as β-endorphin, or as neurotransmitter antagonists that block receptor function. Drugs can also act directly on the ion channel of ionotropic receptors (Figure 12-2, site 9). For example, barbiturates can enter and block the channel of many excitatory ionotropic receptors. In the case of metabotropic receptors, drugs can act at any of the steps downstream of the receptor. Perhaps the best example is provided by the methylxanthines (such as **caffeine**), which can modify neurotransmitter responses mediated through the second-messenger cAMP. At high concentrations,

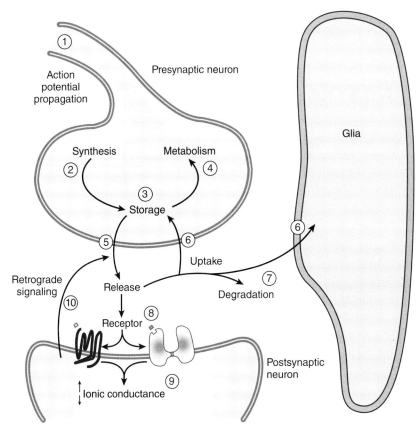

FIGURE 12-2 **Steps at which drugs can alter synaptic transmission.** (1) Action potential in presynaptic fiber; (2) synthesis of transmitter; (3) storage; (4) metabolism; (5) release; (6) reuptake into the nerve terminal or uptake into a proximal glial cell; (7) degradation; (8) receptor for the transmitter; (9) receptor-induced increase or decrease in ionic conductance; (10) retrograde signaling.

the methylxanthines increase the concentration of cAMP by blocking its catabolism, thereby prolonging its action in the postsynaptic cell. Last, synapses may also generate signals that feed back onto the presynaptic terminal to modify neurotransmitter release (Figure 12-2, site 10). Endocannabinoids demonstrate such retrograde signaling in which postsynaptic activity causes synthesis and release of endocannabinoids that then bind to receptors in the presynaptic terminal.

The *selectivity* of CNS drug action is based almost entirely on two factors. First, different transmitters are usually released by different groups of neurons. Furthermore, these transmitters are often segregated into neuronal systems that subserve different CNS functions. Second, each neurotransmitter has a number of distinct receptor subtypes that often have differential distribution throughout the neuraxis. These factors allows for the development of drugs that selectively target particular receptors and CNS functions.

CELLULAR ORGANIZATION OF THE BRAIN

Most of the neuronal systems in the CNS can be divided into two broad categories: hierarchical systems and nonspecific or diffuse neuronal systems.

Hierarchical Neuronal Systems

These systems include all of the pathways directly involved in sensory perception and motor control. Generally, the pathways are clearly delineated anatomically and contain large myelinated, rapidly conducting fibers. The information is typically phasic (ie, dependent on the frequency of action potential firing), and processed sequentially at each successive relay nucleus on the way to its destination. A lesion at any link will incapacitate the system. Within each nucleus and in the cortex, there are two types of cells: relay or projection neurons and local circuit neurons (Figure 12-3A). Projection neurons form interconnecting pathways transmitting signals over long distances. The cell bodies are relatively large and their axons are long. These neurons are excitatory, typically releasing glutamate that acts at ionotropic receptors. The responses tend to be very short-lived.

Local circuit neurons are typically smaller than projection neurons, and their axons arborize in the immediate vicinity of the cell body. The vast majority of these neurons are inhibitory, and they release either GABA or glycine. They synapse primarily on the cell body of the projection neurons, but can also synapse on the dendrites of projection neurons as well as with each other. Common communication pathways for local circuit neurons include recurrent feedback pathways and feed-forward pathways (Figure 12-3A). In the spinal cord,

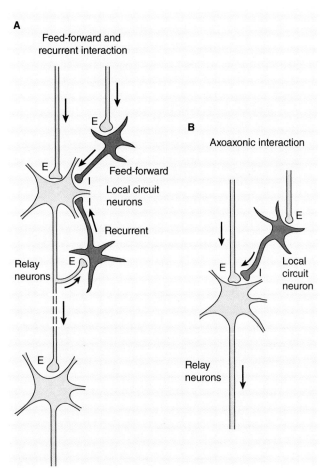

FIGURE 12-3 **Hierarchical communication in the CNS.**
A shows parts of 4 excitatory (E) relay neurons (blue) and 2 inhibitory (I) local circuit neurons (gray), forming recurrent and feed-forward pathways. **B** shows presynaptic axoaxonic inhibition in which the axon of a local circuit neuron synapses on the axon terminal of an excitatory relay fiber.

some local circuit neurons presynaptically inhibit release of excitatory neurotransmitter by forming axoaxonic synapses on the terminals of sensory axons (Figure 12-3B). Although a great variety of synaptic connections exist in these hierarchical systems, the fact that a limited number of transmitters are utilized by these neurons indicates that any major pharmacologic manipulation of this system will have a profound effect on the overall excitability of the CNS.

Diffuse Neuronal Systems

Diffuse systems are broadly distributed, with single neurons frequently sending processes to many different areas of the brain. These systems differ in fundamental ways from the hierarchical systems. The axons of these neurons are very fine, unmyelinated, and slowly conducting. The axons branch repeatedly and diverge into many brain regions. Branches from the same neuron can innervate several functionally different parts of the CNS. The axons commonly have periodic enlargements (called varicosities) that contain transmitter vesicles.

Transmitters released in diffuse systems include acetylcholine, the monoamines, and neuropeptides. They act primarily on metabotropic receptors and, therefore, initiate long-lasting synaptic effects. Based on all of these observations, the diffuse neuronal systems cannot convey specific topographic or highly transient types of information. Instead, activation of these systems affects large areas of the CNS at the same time and in a rather uniform way. Thus, drugs that affect these diffuse systems have dramatic effects on such global functions as sleeping and waking, attention, appetite, and emotional states.

CENTRAL NEUROTRANSMITTERS

To be accepted as a neurotransmitter, a candidate chemical must: (1) be present in higher concentration in the synaptic area than in other areas (ie, must be localized in the appropriate areas), (2) be released by electrical or chemical stimulation via a calcium-dependent mechanism, and (3) produce the same type of postsynaptic response that is seen with physiologic activation of the synapse (ie, must exhibit synaptic mimicry) and application of a selective antagonist should block the response. Broadly, the central neurotransmitters can be classified into amino acids (glutamate, GABA, and glycine), acetylcholine, monoamines (dopamine, norepinephrine, serotonin, histamine), neuropeptides, and other signaling substances. Table 12-1 lists the most important chemicals currently accepted as neurotransmitters in the CNS.

Glutamate (Glutamic Acid)

Most neurons in the brain are excited by glutamate. A vesicular glutamate transporter (VGLUT) within synaptic terminals ensures that there is a high concentration of glutamate within synaptic vesicles. Once glutamate is released, the neurotransmitter activates both ionotropic and metabotropic receptors. The ionotropic receptors are further divided into three subtypes based on the action of selective agonists: α-amino-3-hydroxy-5-methylisoxazole-4-propionate (AMPA), kainate (KA), and *N*-methyl-*D*-aspartate (NMDA). The AMPA- and KA-activated channels are often referred to as non-NMDA channels and are permeable to Na^+ and K^+. **Domoic acid**, produced by algae, is a potent agonist at kainate and AMPA receptors. Consumption of shellfish that have accumulated this neurotoxin causes illness in animals and humans.

NMDA receptors are just as abundant as AMPA receptors. In contrast to AMPA and kainate receptors, all NMDA receptors are highly permeable to Ca^{2+}, as well as Na^+ and K^+. There are three requirements for the opening of the NMDA receptor channel: (1) glutamate must bind the receptor; (2) glycine must bind a separate site of the receptor, and (3) the neuronal membrane must already be depolarized to expel the Mg^{2+} that blocks the NMDA receptor pore. When the NMDA receptor channel opens, the rise in intracellular Ca^{2+} causes a long-lasting increase in synaptic strength termed long-term potentiation (LTP). LTP is one form of synaptic plasticity that is a critical cellular mechanism underlying learning and memory.

TABLE 12-1 Select summary of neurotransmitter pharmacology in the CNS.

Transmitter	Major Receptor Subtypes	Receptor Agonists *Receptor Antagonists*	Receptor Mechanisms
Acetylcholine (ACh)	Muscarinic (M$_1$)	Muscarine *Pirenzepine, atropine*	Excitatory: ↓ K$^+$ conductance; ↑ IP$_3$, DAG
	Muscarinic (M$_2$)	Muscarine, bethanechol *Atropine*	Inhibitory: ↑ K$^+$ conductance; ↓ cAMP
	Nicotinic (N)	Nicotine *a-bungarotoxin*	Excitatory: ↑ cation conductance
Dopamine	D$_1$-like (D$_1$ and D$_5$)	Dihydrexidine *Phenothiazines*	Excitatory: ↑ cAMP
	D$_2$-like (D$_2$, D$_3$, and D$_4$)	Bromocriptine *Phenothiazines, haloperidol*	Inhibitory (presynaptic): ↓ Ca^{2+} conductance Inhibitory (postsynaptic): ↑ K$^+$ conductance; ↓ cAMP
Endocannabinoids	CB$_1$	Anandamide, 2-arachidonylglycerol *Rimonabant*	Inhibitory (presynaptic): ↓ Ca^{2+} conductance; ↓ cAMP
GABA	GABA$_A$	Muscimol, benzodiazepines, zolpidem, alcohol, barbiturates *Bicuculline, picrotoxin*	Inhibitory: ↑ Cl$^-$ conductance
	GABA$_B$	Baclofen *2-OH saclofen*	Inhibitory (presynaptic): ↓ Ca^{2+} conductance Inhibitory (postsynaptic): ↑ K$^+$ conductance
Glutamate	NMDA	NMDA *Phencyclidine, ketamine, memantine*	Excitatory: ↑ cation conductance, especially Ca^{2+}
	AMPA	AMPA *NBQX*	Excitatory: ↑ cation conductance
	Kainate	Kainate, domoic acid *ACET*	Excitatory: ↑ cation conductance
	Metabotropic	ACPD, quisqualate *MCPG*	Inhibitory (presynaptic): ↓ Ca^{2+} conductance; ↓ cAMP Excitatory (postsynaptic): ↓ K$^+$ conductance; ↑ IP$_3$ and DAG
Glycine	GlyR	Taurine *Strychnine*	Inhibitory: ↑ Cl$^-$ conductance
Histamine	H$_1$	2(*m*-fluorophenyl-histamine) *Mepyramine*	Excitatory: ↓ K$^+$ conductance; ↑ IP$_3$, DAG
	H$_2$	Dimaprit *Ranitidine*	Excitatory: ↓ K$^+$ conductance; ↑ cAMP
Norepinephrine	α$_1$	Phenylephrine *Prazosin*	Excitatory: ↓ K$^+$ conductance; ↑ IP$_3$, DAG
	α$_2$	Clonidine *Yohimbine*	Inhibitory (presynaptic): ↓ Ca^{2+} conductance Inhibitory (postsynaptic): ↑ K$^+$ conductance; ↓ cAMP
	β$_1$	Isoproterenol *Atenolol*	Excitatory: ↓ K$^+$ conductance; ↑ cAMP
	β$_2$	Albuterol *Butoxamine*	Excitatory: may involve ↑ in electrogenic sodium pump; ↑ cAMP
Opioid peptides	Mu (μ)	β-Endorphin *Naloxone*	Inhibitory (presynaptic): ↓ Ca^{2+} conductance; ↓ cAMP
	Delta (δ)	Enkephalin *Naloxone*	Inhibitory (postsynaptic): ↑ K$^+$ conductance; ↓ cAMP
	Kappa (κ)	Dynorphin *Naloxone*	Inhibitory (postsynaptic): ↑ K$^+$ conductance; ↓ cAMP

(continued)

TABLE 12-1 Select summary of neurotransmitter pharmacology in the CNS. (*Continued*)

Transmitter	Major Receptor Subtypes	Receptor Agonists *Receptor Antagonists*	Receptor Mechanisms
Serotonin	5-HT$_{1A}$	Eptapirone *Metergoline, buspirone (partial agonist)*	Inhibitory: ↑ K$^+$ conductance; ↓ cAMP
	5-HT$_{2A}$	LSD *Ketanserin, clozapine, risperidone, and olanzapine*	Excitatory: ↓ K$^+$ conductance; ↑ IP$_3$ and DAG
	5-HT$_3$	2-methyl-5-HT *Ondansetron*	Excitatory: ↑ cation conductance
	5-HT$_4$	Cisapride *Piboserod*	Excitatory: ↓ K$^+$ conductance
Tachykinins	NK$_1$	Substance P methylester *Aprepitant*	Excitatory: ↓ K$^+$ conductance; ↑ IP$_3$ and DAG
	NK$_2$	Neurokinin A *Saredutant*	Excitatory: ↓ K$^+$ conductance; ↑ IP$_3$ and DAG
	NK$_3$	Neurokinin B *Osanetant*	Excitatory: ↓ K$^+$ conductance; ↑ IP$_3$ and DAG

However, *excessive* activation of NMDA receptors after neuronal injury may be responsible for cell death. Excitotoxic activation of neurons via NMDA receptors has been postulated as a contributory factor in the etiology of Alzheimer's disease. **Memantine**, a noncompetitive NMDA receptor antagonist, has shown modest efficacy in the treatment of moderate-to-severe Alzheimer's dementia.

At least eight metabotropic glutamate receptors have been identified based on structure and physiological activity. Unlike the ionotropic receptors, activation of metabotropic receptors does not *directly* open an ion channel. Instead, binding results in activation of biochemical cascades such as G protein-coupled activation of phospholipase C or inhibition of adenylate cyclase that modifies other proteins (which may include ion channels; Figure 12-1D and E). Depending on the subtype activated, these receptors can initiate a slow postsynaptic excitation or a presynaptic inhibition.

GABA and Glycine

GABA and glycine are inhibitory neurotransmitters that are usually released from interneurons. GABA is the primary inhibitory neurotransmitter in the brain, but it is also important in the spinal cord. Glycine is the primary inhibitory neurotransmitter in the spinal cord and brainstem. Glycine receptors are selectively permeable to Cl$^-$. By selectively blocking glycine receptors, **strychnine** is a potent spinal convulsant.

For GABA, there are two types of receptors: ionotropic GABA$_A$ receptors and metabotropic GABA$_B$ receptors. In many areas of the brain, IPSPs include a fast and a slow component. The *fast* component is attributed to GABA$_A$ receptor activation that triggers opening of a chloride ion-selective pore, which hyperpolarizes the cell. The *slow* component of the IPSP is attributed to activation of GABA$_B$ receptors that are coupled to G proteins that either activate potassium channels or inhibit calcium channels. Commonly used drugs that influence GABA$_A$ receptors include the sedative-hypnotics (Chapter 13) such as benzodiazepines, barbiturates, and **zolpidem** used to treat anxiety, muscle spasms, and insomnia. **Baclofen**, which activates GABA$_B$ receptors, is a very useful drug for decreasing muscle spasticity (Chapter 33) due to upper motor neuron lesions such as cerebral palsy and spinal cord injury.

Acetylcholine

Approximately 5% of brain neurons have receptors for acetylcholine (ACh). The two major cholinergic receptor subtypes are nicotinic and muscarinic, named after their selective agonists nicotine and muscarine, respectively. Nicotinic receptors are less common in the CNS than muscarinic receptors. There are five subtypes of G protein-coupled muscarinic receptors (M$_1$-M$_5$), but most CNS responses to ACh are mediated by M$_1$ receptors that lead to slow excitation when activated. The ionic mechanism of slow excitation involves a *decrease* in membrane permeability to K$^+$. At a few sites, ACh causes slow inhibition of the neuron by activating the M$_2$ subtype of receptor, which opens potassium channels.

A number of CNS nuclei contain ACh, including neurons in the neostriatum, the medial septal nucleus, and the reticular formation. Cholinergic pathways play an important role in cognitive functions, especially memory. Presenile dementia of the Alzheimer's type is reportedly associated with a profound loss of cholinergic neurons. However, the specificity of this loss has been questioned since the levels of other putative transmitters, for example, somatostatin, are also decreased. Drugs affecting the activity of cholinergic systems in the brain include the acetylcholinesterase inhibitors used in Alzheimer's disease (eg, **donepezil**, **rivastigmine**) and the muscarinic receptor antagonists used in parkinsonism (eg, **benztropine**).

Dopamine

The major pathways containing dopamine are the projections linking the substantia nigra in the basal ganglia to the neostriatum and those linking the ventral tegmental area to limbic structures, particularly the limbic cortex. Dopaminergic neurons in the ventral hypothalamus also play an important role in regulation of pituitary function. All five identified dopamine receptors (D_1-D_5) are metabotropic. The D_1-like receptors (D_1 and D_5) are coupled to a G protein that activates adenylate cyclase, thus increasing the intracellular concentration of cAMP. In contrast, the D_2-like receptors (D_2, D_3, D_4) are coupled to a G protein that inhibits adenylate cyclase and the formation of cAMP. Dopamine typically exerts a slow inhibitory action on CNS neurons. The D_2 receptor is the main receptor subtype in basal ganglia neurons, and it is widely distributed at the supraspinal level. Drugs that increase dopaminergic activity in the brain include CNS stimulants such as amphetamine and the commonly used antiparkinsonism drug levodopa. Older antipsychotics such as **chlorpromazine** and **haloperidol** decrease the activity of dopaminergic pathways by antagonizing D_2 receptors.

Norepinephrine

Noradrenergic neuron cell bodies are mainly located in the brainstem (locus ceruleus) and the lateral tegmental area of the pons (reticular formation). These neurons diverge to provide most regions of the CNS with diffuse noradrenergic input. All noradrenergic receptor subtypes are metabotropic. Excitatory effects are produced by activation of α_1 and β_1 receptors, whereas inhibitory effects are produced by activation of α_2 and β_2 receptors. Excitatory effects are produced by both direct and indirect mechanisms. The direct mechanism involves the blockade of a potassium conductance that normally slows neuronal discharge. The indirect mechanism involves disinhibition; that is, inhibitory local circuit neurons are inhibited. Facilitation of excitatory synaptic transmission is in accordance with many of the behavioral processes thought to involve noradrenergic pathways (eg, attention and arousal). CNS stimulants, monoamine oxidase inhibitors, and tricyclic antidepressants *enhance* the activity of noradrenergic pathways.

Serotonin

Most serotonin (5-hydroxytryptamine, 5-HT) pathways originate from cell bodies in the raphe or midline regions of the pons and upper brainstem; these pathways contain unmyelinated fibers that innervate most regions of the CNS. More than a dozen 5-HT receptor subtypes have been identified and, with the exception of the 5-HT$_3$ subtype, all are metabotropic.

In most areas of the CNS, 5-HT has a strong *inhibitory* action. This action is mediated by 5-HT$_{1A}$ receptors and is associated with membrane hyperpolarization caused by an increase in potassium conductance. The 5-HT$_{1A}$ receptors and GABA$_B$ receptors activate the same family of potassium channels. At a very limited number of sites in the CNS, the ionotropic 5-HT$_3$ receptor exerts a rapid excitatory action. Serotonin can exert both excitatory and inhibitory actions on the same neuron, depending on the receptor subtypes that are activated. Serotonin has been implicated in many brain functions, including mood, anxiety, pain, sleep, appetite, and neuroendocrine regulation. Given the structural diversity of 5-HT receptors and the CNS roles for this neurotransmitter, it is not surprising that many therapeutic agents target the 5-HT system. For example, most drugs used in the treatment of major depressive disorders (Chapter 19) enhance serotonergic transmission (eg, tricyclic antidepressants, selective serotonin reuptake inhibitors [SSRIs]). The actions of some CNS stimulants and newer antipsychotic drugs (eg, **olanzapine**) may also be mediated via effects on serotonergic transmission.

Histamine

In the CNS, histamine is only made by neurons in one nucleus in the posterior hypothalamus. However, these histaminergic projections extend widely throughout the brain and spinal cord. Histamine is involved in arousal, attention, memory, and feeding behavior. All four identified receptors (H$_1$-H$_4$) are metabotropic. First-generation centrally acting antihistamines (eg, **diphenhydramine**) have sedative properties. Antagonism of H$_1$ receptors is a common adverse effect of many drugs including some tricyclic antidepressants and antipsychotics.

Neuropeptides

Many peptides have been identified in the CNS, and some meet most or all of the criteria for acceptance as neurotransmitters. These peptides include opioid peptides (endorphins, enkephalins, dynorphins), neurotensin, substance P, somatostatin, cholecystokinin, vasoactive intestinal polypeptide, neuropeptide Y, orexin, and thyrotropin-releasing hormone. As in the peripheral autonomic nervous system, peptides often coexist with a conventional nonpeptide transmitter in the same neuron. Peptide transmitters differ from nonpeptide transmitters in that (1) the peptides are synthesized in the cell body and transported to the nerve ending via axonal transport, and (2) no reuptake or specific enzyme mechanisms have been identified for terminating their actions. Most neuropeptide receptors are metabotropic. Because most neuropeptides were initially discovered in the periphery, the names reflect their peripheral functions and are often unrelated to their CNS roles. Neuropeptides typically serve modulatory roles in diverse CNS actions such as arousal, pain, appetite, social behaviors, reward, reproduction, learning, and memory.

The best-defined peptide transmitters are the opioid peptides (β-endorphin, met- and leu-enkephalin, and dynorphin), which are distributed at all levels of the neuraxis. The most important therapeutic actions of opioid analgesics (eg, **morphine**) are mediated by receptors for these endogenous opioids. Substance P, a peptide contained in and released from unmyelinated primary sensory neurons in the spinal cord and brainstem, causes slow EPSPs in target neurons involved in nociceptive sensory pathways. While substance P receptor antagonists modify responses to certain types of pain, these agents do not block the response. Glutamate, which is co-released with substance P from these synapses, likely plays an important role in transmitting nociceptive information.

Endocannabinoids

The primary psychoactive ingredient in marijuana is Δ^9-tetrahydrocannabinol (Δ^9-THC), which affects the brain mainly by activating a specific cannabinoid receptor, CB_1 (Chapter 21). Several brain lipid derivatives (eg, 2-arachidonyl-glycerol and anandamide) have been identified as endogenous ligands for CB_1 receptors. Unlike classic neurotransmitters, endocannabinoids are not stored. Rather, they are rapidly synthesized in response to depolarization and consequent Ca^{2+} influx or activation of metabotropic receptors (eg, by Ach and glutamate). Endogenous cannabinoids are released post-synaptically, but act presynaptically on CB_1 receptors (retro-grade transmission, Figure 12-1, site 10) to decrease transmitter release. Suppression of transmitter release may be transient or long lasting, depending on the pattern of activity. Cannabinoids may affect memory, cognition, and pain perception by this mechanism.

Nitric Oxide

Nitric oxide (NO) gas is synthesized in many tissues in response to a variety of stimuli. The CNS contains a substantial amount of nitric oxide synthase (NOS) within certain classes of neurons. Neuronal NOS is an enzyme activated by calcium-calmodulin. Activation of NMDA receptors, which increases intracellular calcium, results in the generation of NO. While a physiologic role for NO has been clearly established for *peripheral* vascular and erectile smooth muscle, its role in synaptic transmission and synaptic plasticity remains controversial.

Purines

Purines such as adenosine triphosphate (ATP), uridine triphosphate (UTP), and uridine diphosphate (UDP) are found throughout the body, including the CNS. For example, ATP is co-released from catecholaminergic synaptic vesicles. In the extracellular environment, ATP may get converted to adenosine. In the CNS, adenosine acts on metabotropic A_1 receptors. Activation of presynaptic A_1 receptors can inhibit release of amino acid and monoamine neurotransmitters. ATP co-released with other neurotransmitters binds to P2X nonselective ligand-gated cation channel receptors and to P2Y metabotropic receptors. Implicated roles of co-released ATP include broad functions in memory, wakefulness, and appetite.

REHABILITATION RELEVANCE

Drugs acting in the CNS are the most widely used group of pharmacologic agents. These drugs can provide a wide range of therapeutic benefit, but, because of the organization of the CNS, they can also produce a wide range of adverse drug reactions. Drugs acting in the CNS can have effects (both positive and negative) at all levels of the International Classification of Functioning, Disability and Health (ICF) model. For example, a benzodiazepine such as **diazepam** can be a useful sleeping (hypnotic) agent and skeletal muscle relaxant, but it can also impair motor function and decrease the ability to carry out activities of daily living. On the other hand, a dopamine antagonist (eg, **clozapine**) when used to treat schizophrenia, can have profoundly positive effects on an individual's ability to participate in his or her own responsibilities in life situations.

CHAPTER 12 QUESTIONS

1. Which of the following neurotransmitters does *not* act primarily as an inhibitory neurotransmitter?

   a. Glutamate
   b. Glycine
   c. Dopamine
   d. GABA

2. Which of the following actions would result from activation of metabotropic receptors?

   a. Direct opening of an ion channel
   b. Direct closing of an ion channel
   c. Activation of a G protein that can modulate an ion channel
   d. Fast IPSPs in the brain

3. Which of the following neurotransmitters is *not* a monoamine and therefore will not be susceptible to breakdown by monoamine oxidase?

   a. Dopamine
   b. Norepinephrine
   c. Acetylcholine
   d. Serotonin

4. Which of the following chemicals does *not* meet criteria for a neurotransmitter?

   a. Dopamine
   b. Acetylcholine
   c. Glycine
   d. Cyclic AMP

5. In the central nervous system, which of the following chemicals is co-released with a traditional neurotransmitter?

   a. Histamine
   b. Substance P
   c. Glutamate
   d. Dopamine

6. Which of the following receptors activates the same family of potassium channels as the 5-HT$_{1A}$ receptors?

    a. GABA$_B$ receptors
    b. Dopamine D$_1$ receptors
    c. Muscarinic M$_1$ receptors
    d. Noradrenergic α$_1$ receptors

7. Which of the following is a property of hierarchical neuronal systems?

    a. Release of neuropeptides
    b. Axons with wide and diffuse projections throughout the brain
    c. Actions primarily mediated by glutamate and GABA in the brain
    d. Actions primarily mediated by metabotropic receptors

8. Retrograde synaptic signaling has been demonstrated for which of the following neurotransmitters?

    a. Glutamate
    b. Endocannabinoids
    c. GABA
    d. Norepinephrine

9. Which of the following is a true statement regarding neurotransmitter receptors?

    a. Ligand-gated channels open and close in response to changes in membrane potential.
    b. Voltage-gated channels open and close in response to changes in membrane potential.
    c. Binding of neurotransmitter to metabotropic receptors typically results in directly altering the gating of an ion channel.
    d. Binding of neurotransmitter to metabotropic receptors typically results in effects that are phasic and short-lasting.

10. Cyclic adenosine monophosphate (cAMP) is a diffusible second messenger that is increased after activation of which of the following?

    a. β$_1$ and β$_2$ adrenoceptors
    b. Glycine receptors
    c. GABA$_A$ receptors
    d. GABA$_B$ receptors

Sedative-Hypnotic Drugs

CASE STUDY

D.H. is a 72-year-old man with a primary diagnosis of lumbar strain that was the result of lifting a large generator during an electricity outage due to a recent tropical hurricane. The patient was initially seen in an urgent care facility. He followed up with an orthopedic physician who recommended spinal imaging, which was negative for any bony abnormalities. The orthopedic physician recommended physical therapy for evaluation and treatment as indicated. On initial examination, the physical therapist noted that the patient demonstrated a forward flexed posture with limited trunk range of motion in all planes with pain at end ranges. Upon palpation, D.H.

had tenderness in the low back paraspinal musculature. The patient had significant pain with bed mobility, sit-to-stand transfers, and stair negotiation. D.H. was also unable to assist with the post-hurricane cleanup of his home and property. D.H. stated that he felt useless because he had to rely on others to take care of these issues. This made him very anxious and unable to sleep at night. He stated he has been taking diazepam (10 mg) occasionally at night to help him sleep and have a restful night. The urgent care physician prescribed this benzodiazepine for his back spasms, but D.H. found that it helped him sleep.

REHABILITATION FOCUS

The prevalence of the use of sedative-hypnotics is high in patients undergoing rehabilitation. With the exception of diazepam that is prescribed as a skeletal muscle relaxant, sedative-hypnotics are not typically used to directly influence musculoskeletal disorders. Since this class of drugs is frequently used to decrease anxiety and insomnia, many patients involved in rehabilitation programs will be taking these agents. In all practice settings, patients may experience increased levels of anxiety related to their physical state of health and well-being. In hospitalized patients or those in long-term care facilities, sedative-hypnotics may also be used for sleep disorders.

Use of these drugs as antianxiety agents can be beneficial during therapy sessions if they result in the patient being able to remain calm and relaxed. However, if their use produces significant central nervous system (CNS) depressant effects, therapy sessions requiring active participation and coordination such as gait training or motor control training may be unproductive and potentially hazardous. As a class, sedative-hypnotic drugs are associated with significant adverse outcomes such as motor vehicle accidents, falls, and fractures resulting in hospitalization. To emphasize this concern, most of the drugs within the sedative-hypnotics class are listed in Beers Criteria as potentially inappropriate medications for older adults.

BACKGROUND

Assignment of a drug to the sedative-hypnotic class indicates that it is able to cause sedation (with concomitant relief of anxiety) or encourage sleep (hypnosis). Because there is considerable chemical variation within the class, this drug classification is based on clinical uses rather than on similarities in chemical structure. Anxiety states and sleep disorders are common problems, and sedative-hypnotics are among the most commonly prescribed drugs worldwide. Drugs in this class include benzodiazepines, alcohols, barbiturates, carbamates, and several newer hypnotic agents (Figure 13-1).

An effective *sedative* (anxiolytic) agent should reduce anxiety and exert a calming effect. The degree of CNS depression caused by a sedative should be the minimum consistent with therapeutic efficacy. A *hypnotic* drug should produce drowsiness and encourage the onset and maintenance of a state of sleep. Hypnotic effects involve more pronounced depression of the CNS than sedation; this is achieved with most drugs in this class simply by increasing the dose. However, individual drugs differ in the relationship between the dose and the degree of CNS depression. Figure 13-2 shows two examples of such dose-response relationships. The linear slope for "Drug A" means an increase in dose above that needed for hypnosis may lead to a state of general anesthesia. At still higher doses, Drug A depresses respiratory and vasomotor centers in the medulla,

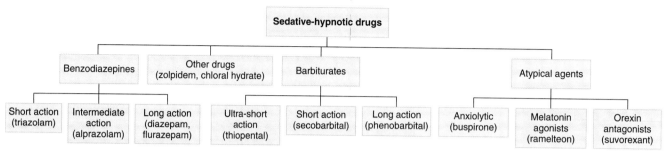

FIGURE 13-1 **The sedative-hypnotics are a chemically heterogeneous class of drugs almost all of which produce dose-dependent CNS depressant effects.** Major subgroups are the benzodiazepines and barbiturates. Other drugs such as carbamates, alcohols, and cyclic ethers are still in use. Newer Z-drugs used as hypnotics (zolpidem, zaleplon, eszopiclone) may be classified as nonbenzodiazepine benzodiazepine receptor agonists. Atypical agents include the anxiolytic buspirone and the novel drugs used in sleep disorders (melatonin agonists and orexin antagonists). Prototype drugs are in parentheses.

leading to coma and potentially death. In contrast, "Drug B" deviates from a linear dose-response relationship, meaning that proportionately greater dosage increments will be required in order to achieve CNS depression more profound than hypnosis.

PHARMACOKINETICS

After oral administration, sedative-hypnotic drugs are absorbed from the gastrointestinal (GI) tract, rapidly enter the blood, and have good distribution to the brain. The rates of oral absorption of individual agents differ depending on a number of factors. Oral absorption of **triazolam** and the newer hypnotics (eg, **eszopiclone, zaleplon, zolpidem**) is extremely rapid, and that of **diazepam** and the active metabolite of **clorazepate**

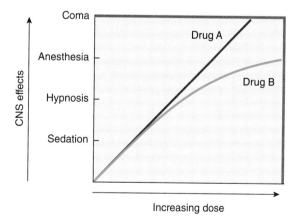

FIGURE 13-2 **Dose-response curves for 2 hypothetical sedative-hypnotics.** The linear slope for Drug A is typical of many older sedative-hypnotics, including barbiturates and alcohols. An increase in dose higher than that needed for hypnosis may lead to a state of general anesthesia. At higher doses, these sedative-hypnotics may depress medullary respiratory and vasomotor centers, leading to coma and death. Drug B deviates from a linear dose-response relationship. Proportionately greater dosage increments are required to achieve CNS depression more profound than hypnosis. This appears to be the case for benzodiazepines and certain newer hypnotics that have a similar mechanism of action.

(nordiazepam) is more rapid than other commonly used benzodiazepines (Table 13-1).

Lipid solubility plays a major role in determining the rate at which a particular sedative-hypnotic enters the CNS. This property is responsible for the rapid onset of CNS effects of triazolam, **thiopental** (see Chapter 15), and several of the newer hypnotics (eg, eszopiclone, zaleplon, zolpidem). All sedative-hypnotics cross the placental barrier during pregnancy. If sedative-hypnotics are given in the predelivery period, they may depress neonatal vital functions. Sedative-hypnotics are also detectable in breast milk and may exert depressant effects in the nursing infant.

For clearance of sedative-hypnotics from the body, biotransformation to more water-soluble metabolites is necessary. The microsomal drug-metabolizing enzyme systems of the liver are most important in this regard. Few sedative-hypnotics are excreted from the body in unchanged form, so elimination half-life depends mainly on the rate of metabolic transformation. The half-lives of common sedative-hypnotics and their major active metabolites are presented in Table 13-1. Although the metabolic rates and pathways vary, many benzodiazepines are initially converted to active metabolites with long half-lives. After several days of therapy with some drugs (eg, diazepam, **flurazepam**), accumulation of active metabolites can lead to excessive sedation. Cumulative and residual effects are less of a problem with **oxazepam** and **lorazepam**, which have shorter half-lives and are conjugated to form inactive metabolites. The barbiturates are also metabolized by hepatic enzymes. The exception is **phenobarbital**, which is excreted partly unchanged in the urine. The rate of hepatic metabolism depends on the individual drug, but is usually slow (with the exception of the thiobarbiturates). For example, the elimination half-lives of **secobarbital** and **pentobarbital** range from 18 to 48 hours in different individuals. In contrast, the half-life for phenobarbital is 4-5 days. Thus, it is evident that multiple dosing with these agents can lead to cumulative effects.

Newer hypnotics colloquially known as the "Z-drugs" (eszopiclone, zaleplon, zolpidem) are only approved for treating insomnia (ie, only as hypnotics). In general, these agents are metabolized more quickly than most other sedative-hypnotics.

TABLE 13-1 Pharmacokinetic properties of benzodiazepines and new hypnotics in humans.

Drug	$T_{max}{}^a$ (hours)	Elimination Half-Life^b (hours)	Comments
Alprazolam	1-2	12-15	Rapid oral absorption
Chlordiazepoxide	2-4	15-40	Active metabolites; erratic bioavailability from IM injection
Clorazepate	1-2 (nordiazepam)	50-100	Prodrug; hydrolyzed to active form in stomach
Diazepam	1-2	20-80	Active metabolites; erratic bioavailability from IM injection
Eszopiclone	1	6	Minor active metabolites
Flurazepam	1-2	40-100	Active metabolites with long half-lives
Lorazepam	1-6	10-20	No active metabolites
Oxazepam	2-4	10-20	No active metabolites
Temazepam	2-3	10-40	Slow oral absorption
Triazolam	1	2-3	Rapid onset; short duration of action
Zaleplon	< 1	1-2	Metabolized by aldehyde dehydrogenase
Zolpidem	1-3	1.5-3.5	No active metabolites

IM, intramuscular.
^{a}Time to peak blood level.
^{b}Includes half-lives of major metabolites.

Zolpidem and zaleplon are rapidly metabolized to inactive metabolites by the liver and have very short elimination half-lives of 1.5-3.5 hours and 1-2 hours, respectively. Eszopiclone is metabolized a bit more slowly, with a half-life of 6 hours. Dosage reductions of zolpidem and zaleplon are recommended for individuals with hepatic dysfunction, older adults, and in those taking cimetidine, a drug taken for frequent heartburn that may inhibit hepatic metabolism of the Z-drugs. In contrast, the activity of certain hepatic drug-metabolizing enzymes (cytochrome P450 isoforms) may be *increased* in persons exposed to barbiturates (especially phenobarbital) and **meprobamate**. This latter effect may increase the drug's own hepatic metabolism as well as that of other drugs metabolized by the same cytochrome P450 (CYP) isoform, potentially decreasing their bioavailability and therapeutic efficacy. Benzodiazepines and the Z-drugs do not alter hepatic CYP activity with continuous use.

PHARMACODYNAMICS

Gamma-aminobutyric acid (GABA) is the major inhibitory neurotransmitter in the CNS (Chapter 12). Benzodiazepines, barbiturates, and the Z-drugs bind to particular subunits of the $GABA_A$ receptor. The $GABA_A$ receptor is an ionotropic receptor and ligand-gated chloride ion channel that is widely distributed throughout the CNS. Figure 13-3 illustrates the structure of the $GABA_A$ receptor that is assembled from five protein subunits (each with four membrane-spanning domains) selected from multiple polypeptide classes (α, β, γ, δ, ε, π, ρ, etc). Multiple subunits of several of these classes have been characterized (eg, six different α, four β, and three γ).

Ligand binding to the α1 subunits of $GABA_A$ receptors has been proposed to mediate the sedative, amnesic, and ataxic effects of benzodiazepines, whereas binding to α2 and α3 subunits mediates their anxiolytic and muscle-relaxant actions. It has been proposed that binding to the α5 subunit is involved in at least some of the anterograde memory impairment caused by benzodiazepines.

$GABA_A$ receptors in different areas of the CNS consist of various combinations of the essential subunits. A major isoform of the $GABA_A$ receptor in many regions of the brain consists of two α1 subunits, two β2 subunits, and one γ2 subunit. In this isoform, the two binding sites for GABA are located between adjacent α1 and β2 subunits, whereas the binding pocket for benzodiazepines (known as the BZ site) is between an α1 and the γ2 subunit (Figure 13-3). However, benzodiazepines bind to many $GABA_A$ receptor isoforms, including receptor isoforms containing α2, α3, and α5 subunits. The Z-drugs are often called nonbenzodiazepine benzodiazepine receptor agonists because they appear to exert their CNS effects via interaction with certain BZ binding sites on $GABA_A$ receptors. However, zolpidem, zaleplon, and eszopiclone bind more selectively than the benzodiazepines because these drugs interact only with $GABA_A$-receptor isoforms that contain α1 subunits. Barbiturates also bind to multiple isoforms of the $GABA_A$ receptor, but at different sites than benzodiazepines.

Many other drugs with CNS effects modify the function of $GABA_A$ receptors. These include alcohol and certain intravenous anesthetics (etomidate, propofol) in addition to thiopental. For example, etomidate and propofol (Chapter 15) appear to act selectively at $GABA_A$ receptors that contain α2 and α3 subunits. $GABA_A$ receptors are also thought to be targets for

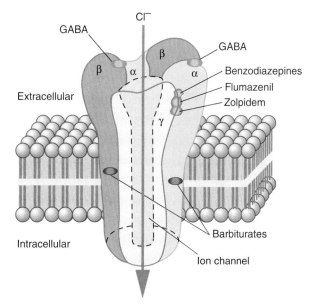

FIGURE 13-3 **Model of the GABA$_A$ receptor-chloride ion channel macromolecular complex.** The complex consists of 5 or more membrane-spanning glycoprotein subunits. Multiple forms of α, β, and γ subunits are arranged in different pentameric combinations so that GABA$_A$ receptors exhibit molecular heterogeneity. GABA appears to interact at two sites between α and β subunits, triggering chloride channel opening with resulting membrane hyperpolarization. Binding of benzodiazepines and the Z-drugs such as zolpidem occurs at a single site between α1 and γ2 subunits, facilitating the process of chloride ion channel opening. The benzodiazepine antagonist flumazenil also binds at this site and can reverse the clinical effects of benzodiazepines and the Z-drugs. Note that these binding sites are distinct from those of the barbiturates.

some of the actions of volatile anesthetics such as halothane (Chapter 15). Most of these agents facilitate or mimic the action of GABA. However, it has not been shown that all these drugs act *exclusively* by this mechanism. The heterogeneity of GABA$_A$ receptors may constitute the molecular basis for the varied pharmacologic actions of benzodiazepines and related drugs. In contrast to GABA itself, benzodiazepines and other sedative-hypnotics have a low affinity for GABA$_B$ receptors, which are activated by the spasmolytic drug baclofen (Chapter 33).

Benzodiazepines

Benzodiazepines (generic drug names end in "-pam" or "-lam") do not directly activate GABA$_A$ receptors or open the associated chloride channels. Rather, benzodiazepines appear to augment GABA's effects as allosteric enhancers (Chapter 2). The interaction of benzodiazepines with GABA increases the *frequency* of channel-opening events, thus enhancing chloride ion conductance and facilitating the inhibitory actions of GABA. Benzodiazepines potentiate GABAergic inhibition throughout all levels of the neuraxis where GABA$_A$ receptors are distributed, including the spinal cord, hypothalamus, hippocampus, substantia nigra, cerebellar cortex, and cerebral cortex.

As noted above, the Z-drugs are selective agonists at the BZ sites on GABA$_A$ receptors that contain an α1 subunit. *Endogenous* agonist ligands for the BZ binding sites have also been proposed, because benzodiazepine-like chemicals have been isolated from brain tissue of animals that have never been exposed to these drugs. Nonbenzodiazepine molecules that have affinity for BZ sites on the GABA$_A$ receptor have also been detected in human brain.

The benzodiazepine derivative **flumazenil** competitively blocks the actions of benzodiazepines and the nonbenzodiazepine Z-drugs, but does not antagonize the actions of barbiturates, opioids, meprobamate, or ethanol. Flumazenil is the only benzodiazepine receptor antagonist available for clinical use. Flumazenil is approved for reversing the CNS depressant effects of benzodiazepine overdose and to hasten recovery following use of these drugs in anesthetic and diagnostic procedures. While flumazenil reverses the sedative effects of benzodiazepines, its effect on benzodiazepine-induced respiratory depression is less predictable. When given intravenously, flumazenil acts rapidly but has a short half-life (0.7-1.3 hours) due to rapid hepatic clearance. Since all benzodiazepines have a longer duration of action than flumazenil, sedation commonly *recurs*, requiring repeated administration of the antagonist. Adverse effects of flumazenil include agitation, confusion, seizures, dizziness, and nausea. Flumazenil may also cause a severe precipitated abstinence syndrome in patients who have developed physical dependence to benzodiazepines (see below).

Barbiturates

The sedative actions of barbiturates are less selective than benzodiazepines, though these drugs also facilitate the actions of GABA at multiple sites in the CNS. In contrast to benzodiazepines that increase the frequency of GABA-gated chloride channel openings, barbiturates appear to increase the *duration* of their openings. At high concentrations, the barbiturates may also be GABA-mimetic, directly activating chloride channels. These barbiturate effects involve a binding site or sites distinct from the benzodiazepine binding sites, as their actions are *not* antagonized by the benzodiazepine receptor antagonist flumazenil. Barbiturates also depress the actions of the excitatory neurotransmitter glutamate by acting as an antagonist at the α-amino-3-hydroxy-5-methyl-4-isoxazolepropionic acid (AMPA) receptor. In addition to their effects on GABA and glutamate neurotransmission, barbiturates exert nonsynaptic membrane effects. This multiplicity of sites of action of barbiturates may be the basis for their ability to induce full surgical anesthesia (Chapter 15) and for their more pronounced CNS depressant effects (Figure 13-2, Drug "A") compared with benzodiazepines and the Z-drugs (Figure 13-2, Drug "B").

Organ Level Effects

The CNS effects of most sedative-hypnotics depend on dose (Figure 13-2). These effects range from sedation and relief of anxiety (anxiolysis), through hypnosis (facilitation of sleep), to anesthesia and coma. Depressant effects are additive when two or more drugs are given together. The steepness of the dose-response curve varies among drug groups; those with flatter curves, such as the benzodiazepines, are safer for clinical use.

Sedation

Benzodiazepines, barbiturates, and other older sedative-hypnotic drugs exert calming effects with concomitant reduction of anxiety at relatively low doses. In most cases, the anxiolytic effects are accompanied by some depressant effects on psychomotor and cognitive functions. In experimental animal models, benzodiazepines and older sedative-hypnotic drugs are able to disinhibit punishment-suppressed behavior. This disinhibition has been equated with the antianxiety effects of sedative-hypnotics. For example, disinhibition is not a characteristic of all drugs that have sedative effects (eg, tricyclic antidepressants, antihistamines). However, the disinhibition of previously suppressed behavior may be more related to behavioral disinhibitory effects of sedative-hypnotics, including euphoria, impaired judgment, and loss of self-control, which can occur at dosages in the range of those used for management of anxiety. The benzodiazepines also exert dose-dependent anterograde amnesic effects (inability to remember events occurring during the drug's duration of action), an effect associated with use of these drugs in date rape situations.

Hypnosis

By definition, all of the sedative-hypnotics, except **buspirone**, induce sleep if high enough doses are given (Table 13-2). The effects of sedative-hypnotics on the stages of sleep depend on several factors, including the specific drug, the dose, and the frequency of its administration. The general effects of benzodiazepines and older sedative-hypnotics on patterns of normal sleep are as follows: (1) the latency of sleep onset (time to fall asleep) is decreased; (2) the duration of stage 2 NREM (nonrapid eye movement) sleep is increased; (3) the duration of REM (rapid eye movement) sleep is decreased; and, (4) the duration of stage 4 NREM slow-wave sleep is decreased. Among the newer hypnotics, zolpidem decreases REM sleep, but has minimal effect on slow-wave sleep. Zaleplon decreases the latency of sleep onset with little effect on total sleep time, NREM, or REM sleep. Eszopiclone increases total sleep time, mainly via increases in stage 2 NREM sleep, and at low doses has little effect on sleep patterns. At the highest recommended dose, eszopiclone decreases REM sleep. **Suvorexant** is an orexin antagonist (discussed below) that decreases time to persistent sleep and increases total sleep time.

More rapid onset of sleep and prolongation of stage 2 NREM sleep are presumably clinically useful effects. However, the significance of older sedative-hypnotic drug effects on REM and slow-wave sleep is not clear. Deliberate interruption of REM sleep causes anxiety and irritability followed by a rebound increase in REM sleep at the end of the experiment. A similar pattern of "REM rebound" can be detected following abrupt cessation of drug treatment with older sedative-hypnotics, especially when drugs with short durations of action (eg, triazolam) are used at high doses. With respect to the Z-drugs, there is little evidence of REM rebound when these drugs are discontinued after use of recommended doses. However, rebound insomnia occurs with both zolpidem and zaleplon if used at higher doses. Despite possible reductions in slow-wave sleep, there are no reports of disturbances in the secretion of pituitary or adrenal hormones when either barbiturates or benzodiazepines are used as hypnotics. The use of sedative-hypnotics for more than

TABLE 13-2 Dosages of drugs used commonly for sedation and hypnosis.

Sedation		Hypnosis	
Drug	**Dosage**	**Drug**	**Dosage (at bedtime)**
Alprazolam	0.25-0.5 mg, 2-3 times daily	Chloral hydrate	500-1000 mg
Buspirone	5-10 mg, 2-3 times daily	Estazolam	0.5-2 mg
Chlordiazepoxide	10-20 mg, 2-3 times daily	Eszopiclone	1-3 mg
Clorazepate	5-7.5 mg, twice daily	Lorazepam	2-4 mg
Diazepam	5 mg, twice daily	Quazepam	7.5-15 mg
Halazepam	20-40 mg, 3-4 times daily	Secobarbital	100-200 mg
Lorazepam	1-2 mg, once or twice daily	Suvorexant	10 mg
Oxazepam	15-30 mg, 3-4 times daily	Temazepam	7.5-30 mg
Phenobarbital	15-30 mg, 2-3 times daily	Triazolam	0.125-0.5 mg
		Zaleplon	5-20 mg
		Zolpidem	2.5-10 mg

1-2 weeks leads to some tolerance (see below) to their effects on sleep patterns.

Anesthesia

High doses of certain sedative-hypnotics depress the CNS to the point known as stage III general anesthesia (Chapter 15). However, the suitability of a particular agent as an adjunct in anesthesia depends mainly on the physicochemical properties that determine its rapidity of onset and duration of effect. Among the barbiturates, thiopental and **methohexital** are very lipid-soluble, penetrating brain tissue rapidly following intravenous administration, a characteristic favoring their use for the induction of anesthesia. Rapid tissue redistribution, not rapid elimination, accounts for the short duration of action of these drugs, a feature useful in recovery from anesthesia.

Diazepam, lorazepam, and **midazolam** are benzodiazepines used intravenously in anesthesia, often in combination with other agents. Not surprisingly, benzodiazepines given in large doses as adjuncts to general anesthetics may contribute to a persistent postanesthetic respiratory depression. This is probably related to their relatively long half-lives and the formation of active metabolites. However, such depressant actions of the benzodiazepines are usually reversible with the benzodiazepine antagonist flumazenil.

Anticonvulsant Effects

Most sedative-hypnotics are capable of inhibiting the development and spread of epileptiform electrical activity in the CNS. Some selectivity exists in that some members of the group can exert anticonvulsant effects without marked CNS depression, although psychomotor function may be impaired. Of the benzodiazepines, **clonazepam**, **nitrazepam**, lorazepam, and diazepam are sufficiently selective to be clinically useful in the management of seizures (Chapter 14). Of the barbiturates, phenobarbital and **metharbital** (which is converted to phenobarbital in the body) are effective in the treatment of generalized tonic-clonic seizures, though they are not the drugs of first choice. The Z-drugs lack anticonvulsant activity, presumably because of their more selective binding to specific $GABA_A$ receptor isoforms.

Muscle Relaxation

Certain drugs in the sedative-hypnotic class, particularly members of the carbamate and benzodiazepine groups, exert inhibitory effects on polysynaptic reflexes and interneuron transmission. At high doses, these agents may also depress transmission at the skeletal neuromuscular junction. Somewhat selective actions of this type that lead to muscle relaxation can be readily demonstrated in animals and have led to claims of usefulness for relaxing muscle spasms. The Z-drugs do not have muscle relaxant properties.

Effects on Respiration and Cardiovascular Function

At hypnotic doses in healthy individuals, the effects of sedative-hypnotics on respiration are comparable to changes during natural sleep. However, in individuals with pulmonary disease, even therapeutic doses of sedative-hypnotics can produce significant respiratory depression. Effects on respiration are dose related, and depression of the medullary respiratory center is the usual cause of death due to overdose of sedative-hypnotics.

At doses up to those that induce hypnosis, there are no significant effects on the cardiovascular system in healthy people. However, in hypovolemic states, heart failure, and other diseases that impair cardiovascular function, normal doses of sedative-hypnotics may cause cardiovascular depression, probably due to actions on the medullary vasomotor centers. At toxic doses, central and peripheral actions of these agents may depress myocardial contractility and vascular tone, leading to circulatory collapse. These effects may be due to facilitation of the actions of adenosine. Respiratory and cardiovascular effects are more marked when sedative-hypnotics are given intravenously, or if comorbidities affecting these systems exist in the patients taking these drugs.

Tolerance, Dependence, and Addiction

Tolerance is decreased responsiveness to a drug following repeated exposure. Tolerance is a common feature of sedative-hypnotic use and may result in the need for an increase in the dose required to maintain symptomatic improvement or to promote sleep. The physical therapist should also recognize that *partial* cross-tolerance occurs between sedative-hypnotics agents and also with ethanol, as explained below. The mechanisms responsible for tolerance to sedative-hypnotics are not well understood. In the case of chronic administration of barbiturates, metabolic tolerance—an increase in the rate of drug metabolism—may be partly responsible. However, pharmacodynamic tolerance is of greater importance for most sedative-hypnotics. Pharmacodynamic tolerance refers to the changes in drug responsiveness. In the case of benzodiazepines, the development of tolerance in animals has been associated with down-regulation of benzodiazepine receptors in the brain. Tolerance has also been reported to occur with extended use of zolpidem, although minimal tolerance has been observed with the use of zaleplon over a 5-week period and eszopiclone over a 6-month period.

The perceived desirable properties of anxiety relief, euphoria, disinhibition, and promotion of sleep have led to the compulsive misuse of virtually all sedative-hypnotics. Because of their potential for abuse, most sedative-hypnotic drugs are classified as Schedule III or Schedule IV drugs for prescribing purposes. The consequences of abuse of these agents can be defined in both psychological and physical terms. The psychological component may initially parallel behavior patterns difficult to differentiate from those of the inveterate coffee drinker or cigarette smoker. When the pattern of sedative-hypnotic use becomes compulsive, *addiction* (often used to replace the older term of psychological dependence) can result, and more serious complications develop, including *dependence* (often used to replace the older term of physical dependence) and tolerance.

Dependence may be described as an altered physiological state that requires continuous drug administration to prevent an abstinence or withdrawal syndrome. In the case of sedative-hypnotics, the withdrawal syndrome is characterized by states of increased anxiety, insomnia, and CNS excitability that may progress to convulsions. Most sedative-hypnotics—including benzodiazepines—are capable of causing dependence when used on a long-term basis. However, the severity of withdrawal symptoms differs among individual drugs and depends also on the magnitude of the dose used immediately before cessation of use. When higher doses of sedative-hypnotics are used, abrupt withdrawal leads to more serious withdrawal signs. Differences in the severity of withdrawal symptoms resulting from individual sedative-hypnotics relate in part to half-life, since drugs with long half-lives are eliminated slowly enough to accomplish gradual withdrawal with few physical symptoms. The use of drugs with very short half-lives used for hypnotic effects may lead to signs of withdrawal even between doses. For example, triazolam, a benzodiazepine with a half-life of about 4 hours, has been reported to cause daytime anxiety when used to treat sleep disorders. Abrupt cessation of the Z-drugs may also result in withdrawal symptoms, though usually of less intensity than those seen with benzodiazepines.

CLINICAL USES

Treatment of Anxiety States

The psychological, behavioral, and physiologic responses that characterize anxiety can take many forms. Typically, the psychic awareness of anxiety is accompanied by enhanced vigilance, motor tension, and autonomic hyperactivity. Anxiety is often secondary to disease states—acute myocardial infarction, angina pectoris, GI ulcers, etc—which themselves require specific therapy. Another type of secondary anxiety state is called situational anxiety. Situational anxiety results from circumstances that may have to be dealt with only once or a few times, such as anticipation of medical or dental procedures, family illness, or other stressful event. Short-term use of sedative-hypnotics may be appropriate for the treatment of both situational anxiety and certain disease-associated anxiety states. Similarly, the use of a sedative-hypnotic as premedication prior to surgery or some unpleasant medical procedure is rational and proper.

Excessive or unreasonable anxiety about life circumstances (generalized anxiety disorder, GAD), panic disorders, and agoraphobia are also amenable to drug therapy, sometimes in conjunction with psychotherapy. Because of their relatively fast onset of action, benzodiazepines continue to be widely used for the management of *acute* anxiety states and for rapid control of panic attacks. However, they are used less commonly in the long-term management of GAD and panic disorders, conditions in which antidepressants such as selective serotonin reuptake inhibitors (SSRIs) and serotonin-norepinephrine reuptake inhibitors (SNRIs) are more effective and safer because they do not cause anterograde amnesia and are not associated with the

tolerance and dependence of benzodiazepines (see Chapter 19). Many benzodiazepines may relieve anxiety symptoms, but it is not always easy to demonstrate the superiority of one drug over another. The choice of benzodiazepines for anxiety is based on several sound pharmacologic principles: (1) a rapid onset of action; (2) a relatively high therapeutic index (Figure 13-2, Drug B), plus availability of flumazenil for treatment of overdose; (3) a low risk of drug interactions based on liver enzyme induction; and, (4) minimal effects on cardiovascular or autonomic functions.

Disadvantages of the benzodiazepines include the risk of dependence, CNS depression, and amnestic effects. In addition, the benzodiazepines exert additive CNS depression when administered with other drugs, including ethanol. Patients should be warned of these effects and to avoid performing any task requiring mental alertness and motor coordination (eg, driving a motor vehicle).

To minimize adverse effects, sedative-hypnotics should be used with several appropriate cautions. A dose should be prescribed that does not impair mentation or motor functions during waking hours. Some people may tolerate the drug better if most of the daily dose is given at bedtime, with smaller doses during the day. Prescriptions are typically written for short periods (2 months or less) since there is little justification for long-term therapy. Combinations of antianxiety agents should be avoided, and people taking sedatives should be cautioned against the consumption of alcohol and the concurrent use of over-the-counter medications containing antihistaminic (Chapter 35) or anticholinergic drugs (Chapter 5).

Beta blockers (eg, propranolol) may be used as anxiolytic agents in situations such as performance anxiety. Beta blockers appear to relieve the over-activity of the sympathetic nervous system associated with anxiety, and may also slightly improve some of the nonsomatic components of anxiety. Adverse effects of propranolol include lethargy, vivid dreams, and a decreased cardiac response to exercise.

Treatment of Sleep Problems

Sleep disorders are common, especially in older adults. Most often, sleep disorders result from inadequate treatment of underlying medical conditions or psychiatric illness. True primary insomnia—persistent problems falling and/or staying asleep—is rare. Nonpharmacologic therapies (collectively called "sleep hygiene") that are useful for insomnia include regular sleeping habits and limiting or avoiding naps, avoiding stimulants before retiring, ensuring a comfortable sleeping environment, and retiring at a regular time each night. In some cases, however, the individual may need and should be given a sedative-hypnotic for a limited period. Abrupt discontinuance of many sedative-hypnotics can lead to rebound insomnia.

Benzodiazepines can cause a dose-dependent decrease in both REM and slow-wave sleep, though to a lesser extent than the barbiturates. The Z-drugs are less likely than the benzodiazepines to change sleep patterns. However, so little is known about the clinical impact of these effects that statements about the desirability of a particular drug based on its effects on sleep architecture have more theoretical than practical significance. Clinical criteria of efficacy in alleviating a particular sleeping problem are more useful. The drug selected should be one that provides sleep of fairly rapid onset (decreased sleep latency) and sufficient duration, with minimal "hangover" effects such as drowsiness, dysphoria, and mental or motor depression the following day. Older drugs such as **chloral hydrate**, secobarbital, and pentobarbital continue to be used, but benzodiazepines, and the Z-drugs are generally preferred. Daytime sedation is more common with benzodiazepines that have slow elimination rates, and those that are biotransformed to active metabolites (Table 13-1). If benzodiazepines are used nightly, tolerance can occur, which may lead to dose increases by the patient to produce the desired effect. Anterograde amnesia occurs to some degree with all benzodiazepines used for hypnosis.

Eszopiclone, zaleplon, and zolpidem have efficacies similar to those of the hypnotic benzodiazepines in the management of sleep disorders. Favorable clinical features of the Z-drugs include rapid onset of activity and modest day-after psychomotor depression with few amnestic effects. Zolpidem, one of the most frequently prescribed hypnotic drugs in the United States, is available in a biphasic release formulation that provides sustained drug levels for sleep maintenance. Zaleplon acts rapidly, and because of its short half-life, the drug appears to have value in the management of individuals who awaken early in the sleep cycle. At recommended doses, zaleplon and eszopiclone (despite its relatively long half-life) appear to cause less amnesia or day-after somnolence than zolpidem or benzodiazepines. Suvorexant (see below) is a hypnotic agent that—unlike the benzodiazepines and the Z-drugs—does not bind to $GABA_A$ receptors. Suvorexant is approved for treatment of both sleep-onset and sleep-maintenance insomnia.

Table 13-2 summarizes the drugs (and recommended dosages) commonly used for hypnosis. Finally, if insomnia does not remit after 7-10 days of treatment, the person should be evaluated for the presence of a primary psychiatric or medical illness.

Other Therapeutic Uses

Table 13-3 summarizes several other important clinical uses of sedative-hypnotic drugs. Drugs used in the management of seizure disorders and as intravenous agents in general anesthesia are discussed in Chapters 14 and 15. For sedative and possible amnestic effects during medical or surgical procedures such as endoscopy and bronchoscopy—as well as for premedication prior to anesthesia—oral formulations of shorter-acting drugs are preferred. Long-acting drugs such as **chlordiazepoxide** and diazepam and, to a lesser extent, phenobarbital are administered in progressively decreasing doses to patients during withdrawal from physical dependence on ethanol or other sedative-hypnotics. Parenteral lorazepam is used to suppress the symptoms of delirium tremens (see Chapter 21).

TABLE 13-3 Clinical uses of sedative-hypnotics.

Relief of anxiety
Insomnia
Sedation and amnesia before medical and surgical procedures
Treatment of epilepsy and seizure states
As a component of balanced anesthesia (intravenous administration)
Control of ethanol or other sedative-hypnotic withdrawal states
Muscle relaxation in specific neuromuscular disorders
As diagnostic aids or for treatment in psychiatry

The benzodiazepines, particularly diazepam, have frequently been used as skeletal muscle relaxants, though evidence for general efficacy *without* accompanying sedation is lacking. However, diazepam may be useful in treating muscle spasticity of central origin (Chapter 33).

Psychiatric uses of benzodiazepines other than treatment of anxiety states include the initial management of mania and the control of drug-induced hyperexcitability states (eg, phencyclidine intoxication). Sedative-hypnotics are also used occasionally as diagnostic aids in neurology and psychiatry.

ATYPICAL SEDATIVE-HYPNOTICS

Buspirone

Buspirone has selective anxiolytic effects, and its pharmacologic characteristics are different from those of other drugs described in this chapter. Buspirone relieves anxiety without causing marked sedative, hypnotic, or euphoric effects. Unlike benzodiazepines, the drug has no anticonvulsant or muscle relaxant properties. Buspirone does not interact directly with GABAergic systems. It may exert its anxiolytic effects by acting as a partial agonist at brain serotonin $5-HT_{1A}$ receptors, but it also has affinity for brain dopamine D_2 receptors. Buspirone-treated patients show no rebound anxiety or withdrawal signs on abrupt discontinuance. The drug is not effective in blocking the acute withdrawal syndrome resulting from abrupt cessation of use of benzodiazepines or other sedative-hypnotics. Buspirone has minimal abuse liability. In marked contrast to the benzodiazepines, the anxiolytic effects of buspirone may take 3-4 weeks to become established, making the drug unsuitable for management of acute anxiety states. The drug is used in generalized anxiety states but is less effective in panic disorders.

Buspirone is rapidly absorbed orally but undergoes extensive first-pass metabolism. The major metabolite, which has α_2-adrenoceptor-blocking actions, enters the CNS and reaches higher levels than the parent drug. Whether the metabolite plays a role in the central actions of buspirone is unknown. The elimination half-life of buspirone is 2-4 hours, and liver dysfunction may slow its clearance.

Melatonin Receptor Agonists

The suprachiasmatic nucleus (SCN) within the hypothalamus is considered the master circadian clock in the brain. Melatonin, a hormone involved in the sleep-wake cycle, acts on melatonin MT_1 and MT_2 receptors in the SCN. Two agonists at these receptors are available to treat individuals with specific sleep-wake disorders. These drugs have no direct effects on GABAergic neurotransmission. **Ramelteon** is a hypnotic drug prescribed specifically for people who have difficulty *falling* asleep (sleep onset insomnia). Ramelteon reduces the latency of persistent sleep with no effects on sleep architecture and the drug produces no rebound insomnia or significant withdrawal symptoms. The drug is rapidly absorbed after oral administration and undergoes extensive first-pass metabolism, forming an active metabolite with a longer half-life (2-5 hours) than the parent drug. Concurrent use with the antidepressant fluvoxamine increases the peak plasma concentration of ramelteon over 50-fold. Ramelteon should be used with caution in patients with liver dysfunction. **Tasimelteon** is approved specifically for treating non-24-hour sleep-wake disorder in people who are blind.

Orexin Receptor Antagonists

Orexin A and B are peptides found in specific hypothalamic neurons that are involved in the control of wakefulness. Orexin levels increase in the day and decrease at night. Consistent with the hypothesis that orexins promote wakefulness, loss of orexin neurons is associated with narcolepsy, a disorder characterized by daytime sleepiness and cataplexy. Suvorexant is an antagonist at orexin receptors. Suvorexant both decreases time to persistent sleep and increases total sleep time and is thus used to treat both sleep onset and sleep maintenance insomnia.

ADVERSE EFFECTS

Many of the common adverse drugs reactions (ADRs) of sedative-hypnotics result from dose-related depression of the CNS. Relatively low doses may lead to drowsiness, impaired judgment, and diminished motor skills, sometimes with a significant impact on driving ability, job performance, and personal relationships. Sleep driving and other somnambulistic behavior with no memory of the event have occurred with the sedative-hypnotic drugs used to treat sleep disorders. Benzodiazepines may cause a significant dose-related anterograde amnesia; they can significantly impair ability to learn new information, particularly that involving effortful cognitive processes, while leaving the retrieval of previously learned information intact. The criminal use of many sedative-hypnotics in cases of "date rape" is based on their dose-dependent amnestic effects.

A "hangover syndrome" characterized by daytime sedation and drowsiness is not uncommon following use of hypnotic drugs with long elimination half-lives. Anxiolytic drugs that act through non-GABAergic systems (eg, buspirone) might

have a reduced propensity for such actions. Because older adults are more sensitive to the effects of sedative-hypnotics, doses approximately half of those used in younger adults are safer and usually as effective. Overuse of sedative-hypnotics is the most common reversible cause of confusional states in the elderly. All benzodiazepines increase the risk of delirium, cognitive impairment, falls, fractures, and motor vehicle accidents in older adults. Use of the newer nonbenzodiazepine Z-drugs carry many of the same risks in this population. Accordingly, benzodiazepines and the Z-drugs as well as many barbiturates are included in the updated Beers Criteria for potentially inappropriate medications for use in older adults. At higher doses of sedative-hypnotics, toxicity may present as lethargy or a state of exhaustion or, alternatively, as gross symptoms equivalent to those of ethanol intoxication. Increased sensitivity to sedative-hypnotics is more common in older adults and in individuals with cardiovascular disease, respiratory disease, or hepatic impairment. Sedative-hypnotics can exacerbate breathing problems in patients with chronic pulmonary disease and in those with symptomatic sleep apnea.

The atypical sedative-hypnotics and anxiolytics have a lower frequency and/or different adverse effect profile. Buspirone causes less psychomotor impairment than benzodiazepines and does not affect driving skills. The drug does not potentiate effects of conventional sedative-hypnotic drugs, ethanol, or tricyclic antidepressants. In addition, older adults do not appear to be more sensitive to buspirone's actions. Nonspecific chest pain, tachycardia, palpitations, dizziness, nervousness, headache, tinnitus, GI distress, paresthesias, and a dose-dependent pupillary constriction may occur. Blood pressure may also be significantly elevated in patients receiving monoamine oxidase (MAO) inhibitors. Buspirone may be used during pregnancy, though risk of teratogenicity is based on limited human data. For ramelteon, ADRs include dizziness, somnolence, fatigue, and endocrine changes. For suvorexant, the most common adverse effect is next-day somnolence.

Adverse effects of the sedative-hypnotics that are *not* related to their CNS actions occur infrequently. Hypersensitivity reactions, including skin rashes, occur only occasionally with most drugs in this class. Reports of teratogenicity leading to fetal deformation following use of certain benzodiazepines justify caution in the use of these drugs during pregnancy. Barbiturates may also precipitate acute intermittent porphyria in susceptible patients.

OVERDOSAGE

Sedative-hypnotics are the drugs most frequently involved in deliberate overdoses, in part because of their availability as very commonly prescribed drugs. Overdosage can cause severe respiratory and cardiovascular depression. These potentially lethal effects are more likely to occur with alcohols, barbiturates, and carbamates than with benzodiazepines because the latter have flatter dose-response curves (Figure 13-2). Management of intoxication requires maintenance of a patent airway and ventilatory support. Flumazenil may reverse CNS depressant effects of benzodiazepines or the Z-drugs, but has no beneficial action in overdosage with other sedative-hypnotics. However, flumazenil's duration of action is short, its antagonism of respiratory depression is unpredictable, and there is a risk of precipitation of withdrawal symptoms in long-term users of benzodiazepines. Consequently, the use of flumazenil in benzodiazepine overdose remains controversial and must be accompanied by adequate monitoring and support of respiratory function.

ALTERATIONS IN DRUG RESPONSE AND WITHDRAWAL

Depending on the dosage and the duration of use, tolerance occurs in varying degrees to many of the pharmacologic effects of sedative-hypnotics. It should not be assumed that the degree of tolerance achieved is identical for all pharmacologic effects. However, there is evidence that the lethal dose range is not altered significantly by chronic use of sedative-hypnotics. Cross-tolerance between the different sedative-hypnotics, including ethanol, can lead to an unsatisfactory therapeutic response when standard doses of a drug are used in a person with recent history of excessive use of these agents. However, there have been a few reports of tolerance development when zolpidem or zaleplon was used for even less than 4 weeks.

With chronic use of sedative-hypnotics, especially if doses are increased, a state of dependence can occur. Dependence may develop to a degree unparalleled by any other drug group, *including the opioids*. Withdrawal from a sedative-hypnotic in a dependent person can have severe and life-threatening manifestations. Withdrawal symptoms range from restlessness, anxiety, weakness, and orthostatic hypotension to hyperactive reflexes and generalized seizures. The severity of withdrawal symptoms depends to a large extent on the duration and dosage range used immediately prior to discontinuance but also on the particular drug. Symptoms of withdrawal are usually more severe following discontinuance of sedative-hypnotics with *shorter* half-lives. The Z-drugs appear to be exceptions to this, because despite their short half-lives, withdrawal symptoms are minimal following abrupt discontinuance of these newer agents. Symptoms are less pronounced with the long-acting drugs, which may partly be accomplished by their own "tapered" withdrawal simply by the virtue of their slow elimination. Cross-dependence, defined as the ability of one drug to suppress abstinence symptoms from discontinuance of another drug, is quite marked among sedative-hypnotics. This provides the rationale for therapeutic regimens in the management of withdrawal states. That is, longer-acting drugs such as chlordiazepoxide, diazepam, and phenobarbital can be used to alleviate withdrawal symptoms of shorter-acting drugs, including ethanol.

DRUG INTERACTIONS

The most common drug interactions involving sedative-hypnotics are interactions with other CNS depressant drugs, leading to additive effects. If not anticipated, such interactions can lead to serious consequences, including enhanced CNS depression. Additive effects can be predicted with concomitant use of alcoholic beverages, opioid analgesics, anticonvulsants, and certain antipsychotics. Less obvious—but just as important—is enhanced CNS depression with a variety of antihistamines, antihypertensive agents, and tricyclic antidepressants.

REHABILITATION RELEVANCE

As CNS depressants, sedative-hypnotics may affect patients' ability to achieve rehabilitation goals. Summarized below are common ADRs and potential strategies to limit their impact on physical therapy interventions.

- **Sedation**, **psychomotor delay**, and **decreased cognitive function** are common ADRs of barbiturates or benzodiazepines, especially those with long half-lives. "Hangover" effects may increase risk of falls and decrease the patient's ability to learn new therapy activities. Complex activities of daily living (ADLs) such as driving or making financial decisions may be impaired. If the medications are given at night to facilitate sleep, consider therapy sessions later in the day when drug plasma levels will be at their lowest. If these effects continue throughout the day, consult the referring healthcare professional.

- **Memory loss** following medication (anterograde amnesia) is a problem with many barbiturates or benzodiazepines that are used to treat sleep disorders. This effect prevents retention of newly learned cognitive and motor information. Anterograde amnesia may also result in individuals conducting complex ADLs without memory of the events. If this type of memory loss is suspected, the therapist should contact the referring healthcare provider immediately. The anterograde amnestic property of these drugs has also been exploited in their use in "date rape" crimes. If this is suspected, appropriate legal authorities should be contacted immediately so that blood samples for detection of the drug may be obtained. Remember that 95% of the drug is eliminated from the body after approximately 5 half-lives, therefore there is a limited time to detect the drug in the blood.

- **Confusion**, **lethargy**, or **exhaustion** may be clinical manifestations with overuse or near toxic levels of barbiturates or benzodiazepines, especially in older adults. Effects of participation in the rehabilitation program should be differentiated from ADRs of these drugs. If lethargy or exhaustion appears inappropriate from that normally observed with a specific therapy program, the therapist should alert the healthcare team or the referring provider.

- **Tachycardia**, **chest pain**, and **palpitations** are observed with buspirone. The therapist should differentiate these manifestations of the drug from those anticipated as a result of participation in an aerobic therapy program or those that may indicate a potential cardiac event. If a potential cardiac event is suspected, emergent assistance is imperative. The therapy program should be terminated until the underlying cause of these manifestations is determined.

CASE CONCLUSION

D.H. began physical therapy interventions consisting of modalities, manual therapy, and therapeutic exercise. On several occasions, the physical therapist noted that when D.H. came to therapy early in the morning, he was less attentive to his exercise regimen and seemed very tired. The therapist also noted that D.H. required more time to answer questions and seemed confused at times. Concerned, the physical therapist questioned him about this behavior. D.H. stated that he felt sleepy and it was difficult for him to concentrate. The therapist questioned him again regarding the medications he was taking. It became apparent that on the occasions that D.H. had these signs and symptoms, he had taken diazepam the night before to help him sleep. With multiple dosing, the active metabolite of diazepam, desmethyldiazepam, may have a half-life of up to 80 hours. The therapist hypothesized that D.H. was having a hangover effect due to the long half-life of the active metabolite, which may be even longer given the patient's age. The therapist encouraged D.H. to consult his regular physician regarding his current sleep problems. In the meantime, the therapist encouraged D.H. to try to reduce or eliminate taking this medication at night for sleep because of the potential that the benzodiazepine was causing morning hangover effects such as the ones he was experiencing and that these effects could cause serious consequences since he was driving himself to therapy. The therapist also provided D.H. with verbal and written education on basic principles of sleep hygiene. D.H. contacted his regular physician who instructed him not to take diazepam for sleeping at night and reinforced practicing the nonpharmacologic sleep hygiene practices. If his back pain was interfering with falling asleep, the physician advised D.H. to take an over-the-counter analgesic such as ibuprofen or acetaminophen prior to retiring. D.H. followed the recommendations and reported that he was able to get a restful night's sleep and had no more episodes of confusion or lethargy in the morning. D.H. continued his rehabilitation and was eventually discharged from physical therapy with all goals achieved.

CHAPTER 13 QUESTIONS

1. Which of the following drugs does *not* have a mechanism of action that involves activation of the $GABA_A$ ionotropic receptor?

   a. Ramelteon
   b. Pentobarbital
   c. Diazepam
   d. Zolpidem

2. A next day "hangover effect" would be *least* likely with which of the following drugs?

   a. Flurazepam
   b. Triazolam
   c. Alprazolam
   d. Secobarbital

3. In an overdose situation, flumazenil would *not* reverse the respiratory depression of which of the following drugs?

   a. Diazepam
   b. Clorazepate
   c. Phenobarbital
   d. Eszopiclone

4. Which of the following conditions would *not* exacerbate the pharmacologic effects of benzodiazepines?

   a. Chronic obstructive pulmonary disease
   b. Heart failure
   c. Hepatic cirrhosis
   d. Peptic ulcer

5. Which of the following is *not* a clinical use of the sedative-hypnotics?

   a. Narcolepsy
   b. Presurgical adjuvant
   c. Anxiolytic
   d. Ethanol detoxification

6. Which of the following describes the action of zolpidem on the $GABA_A$ receptor?

   a. Direct-acting agonist
   b. Allosteric enhancer
   c. Direct-acting antagonist
   d. Allosteric inhibitor

7. Which of the following describes the ability of a drug to encourage sleep?

   a. Anesthesia
   b. Coma
   c. Hypnosis
   d. Sedation

8. Which of the following drugs has its clinical hypnotic effect via direct receptor antagonism?

   a. Buspirone
   b. Phenobarbital
   c. Flumazenil
   d. Suvorexant

9. Which of the following drugs has no clinical hypnotic effect?
   a. Buspirone
   b. Suvorexant
   c. Halazepam
   d. Zaleplon

10. Which of the following is *not* a manifestation of an abstinence syndrome resulting from abrupt termination of diazepam after 6 months of use?
    a. Somnolence
    b. Anxiety
    c. Hyperreflexia
    d. Tachycardia

Antiseizure Drugs

14

CASE STUDY

C.M. is a 60-year-old man that experienced a right cerebrovascular accident 15 months ago, with resultant left hemiplegia. He initially received rehabilitation in an acute inpatient facility for 4 weeks and was transferred to a long-term cognitive rehabilitation facility for approximately 8 weeks. C.M. made significant improvements in his cognitive and speech abilities, but he was still nonambulatory when he was discharged to home. Home health providers felt he had potential for additional functional return and referred him for outpatient physical therapy. C.M. is medically stable living at home with his wife. His medications include escitalopram (antidepressant), pantoprazole (proton pump inhibitor), amlodipine (calcium channel blocker), warfarin (anticoagulant), valproic acid (antiseizure drug), and lamotrigine (antiseizure drug). C.M. told the outpatient physical therapist that he developed a seizure disorder poststroke and was initially treated only with valproic acid. However, he had breakthrough seizures and lamotrigine was added. C.M. reported that he had his blood levels of warfarin and valproic acid checked every 3 months. After 2 months of outpatient therapy, the physical therapist observed that C.M. was much more lethargic on several consecutive sessions. He began to require multiple rest periods during treatment sessions. Communication with the patient was difficult as his speech was soft and muffled. Notably, there were no new sensory or motor neurologic signs that might suggest another stroke.

BACKGROUND

Epilepsy and seizures are not the same. Epilepsy is a *chronic* disorder of the brain that is characterized by unpredictable and recurrent seizures. Approximately 1% of the world's population has epilepsy, making it the fourth most common neurologic disorder after migraine, stroke, and Alzheimer's disease. Seizures are transient alterations in behavior, sensation, and/or consciousness that result from finite episodes of abnormal, synchronized electrical discharges in the brain. Most seizures are the result of some damage to the brain such as a tumor, head trauma, stroke, infection, or developmental lesion such as a cortical or vascular malformation. In some individuals, the cause of seizures may be due to genetic factors, though a single gene defect is rarely identified.

In 2017, the International League Against Epilepsy (ILAE) revised its classification of seizures types to assist with accurate diagnosis, appropriate pharmacological treatment, and prognosis. Seizures are classified into two broad categories based on how and where they begin in the brain. Focal onset seizures (formerly known as "partial" or "partial onset") have their onset in a focal or local cortical site. Generalized onset seizures begin in *both* brain hemispheres. Table 14-1 provides a list of the ILAE's major seizure types with their corresponding clinical descriptions. Many of the frequently recognized older terms used to describe seizures have been replaced in this new classification.

Seizures can also occur in individuals that do *not* have epilepsy. Seizures may be caused by an underlying acute toxic or systemic metabolic disorder (eg, hypoglycemia, hypoxia, poisoning, high fever, meningitis), in which case appropriate therapy is usually directed toward the specific underlying abnormality. Seizures may also occur in the early period after a stroke, traumatic brain injury (TBI), or neurosurgery.

THERAPEUTIC STRATEGIES

In the treatment of epilepsy, the goal of antiseizure drugs is to prevent the occurrence of seizures. The choice of medication depends on the type of seizures that the patient exhibits or on the patient's seizure syndrome classification. A particular drug that is effective in one seizure type may be totally ineffective in others. In addition, owing to varying pharmacokinetic and pharmacodynamic factors, not all individuals with the same seizure type respond in the same manner to a given antiseizure medication. Thus, drug choice is usually based on established efficacy in the specific seizure state that has been diagnosed, the prior responsiveness of the patient, and the anticipated toxicity of the drug. Figure 14-1 outlines the medications used to treat the primary seizure types.

TABLE 14-1 International League Against Epilepsy classification of seizure types.

Seizure Type	Clinical Presentation
Focal Onset (Formerly Partial Onset) Seizures	
Focal aware seizure (formerly *simple partial*)	Consciousness preserved (person is awake, alert, and able to recall events *during* the seizure) Typically lasts < 2 min
Focal impaired awareness seizure (formerly *complex partial*)	Impaired consciousness (person loses awareness and stares blankly) May be preceded by focal aware seizure Typically lasts 1-2 min
Focal-to-bilateral tonic-clonic seizure (formerly *partial seizure secondarily generalized*, or *grand mal seizure*)	Seizure starts in one side or part of the brain and spreads to both sides May be preceded by focal aware seizure Abrupt loss of consciousness and fall to floor with muscle rigidity (tonic phase) followed by jerks (clonic phase) Breathing can be temporarily impaired Lip or tongue biting and fecal and urinary incontinence may occur Tonic-clonic convulsions usually last < 3 min, but followed by a postictal period of confusion and tiredness of variable duration A tonic-clonic seizure lasting > 5 min is a medical emergency
Generalized Onset Seizures	
Generalized tonic-clonic seizure (formerly *primary generalized tonic-clonic*, or *grand mal seizure*)	Same presentation as focal-to-bilateral tonic-clonic seizure; distinction is that the origin of seizure is on both sides of the brain
Generalized absence seizure (formerly *petit mal*)	Brief changes in awareness or unconsciousness (4-20 sec, usually <10 sec) with immediate resumption of consciousness (no postictal abnormality) Some may have automatic or repeated movements such as lip smacking Most common in children 4-14 yr of age; may be mistaken for daydreaming or not paying attention
Myoclonic seizure	Brief, shock-like jerks of a muscle or group of muscles with no awareness impairment Occurs in several epilepsy syndromes[a] (eg, juvenile myoclonic epilepsy, Lennox-Gastaut syndrome, Dravet syndrome)
Atonic seizure (drop attack or astatic seizure)	Sudden drop or loss of muscle tone affecting head, trunk or whole body, which can result in fall to floor Typically lasts <15 sec with partial lack of awareness during event Occurs in some epilepsy syndromes[a] (eg, Lennox-Gastaut syndrome, Dravet syndrome)

[a]Lennox-Gastaut syndrome, Dravet syndrome, and juvenile myoclonic epilepsy are epilepsy syndromes in which there are multiple different seizure types.

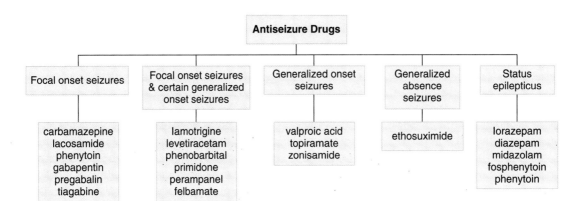

FIGURE 14-1 **Common antiseizure medications categorized by their use in specific seizure types.** Individual agents may be used in more than one seizure type; drugs are listed under the seizure type that they are most commonly used to treat.

In roughly two-thirds of those with epilepsy, appropriately chosen medications provide adequate seizure control. Use of a single drug is preferred. However, for patients with hard-to-control seizures, the simultaneous use of multiple drugs may be necessary following the principle of adding known effective agents if the preceding drugs have not provided adequate seizure control. Individuals who have not achieved seizure control after many trials with two or more appropriate drugs are considered "pharmacoresistant." The basis for pharmacoresistance is not understood. In certain cases, attempts to control epileptic seizures include surgical resection of the affected brain region or use of electrical stimulation devices (eg, vagus nerve stimulator).

Although seizures are usually self-limiting, even in the absence of drug therapy, their uncontrolled recurrence is not desirable because it is believed that uncontrolled seizures may cause further damage to already injured neurons and may even harm previously healthy neurons. Certain types of seizures can also lead to personal injury or even death due to impairment or loss of consciousness during driving or activities of daily living (eg, bathing, cooking). At the least, seizures may be personally embarrassing and socially disabling. Consequently, a comprehensive effort is made to find an effective drug regimen to adequately control or eliminate seizures without causing too many adverse effects.

The antiseizure drugs discussed in this chapter are typically used chronically to prevent the occurrence of seizures in people with epilepsy. These drugs are also used to prevent seizures in situations where seizures are more likely such as in meningitis, or soon after neurosurgery or TBI. In addition, certain antiseizure drugs are used to terminate ongoing seizures such as in status epilepticus (see end of chapter), prolonged febrile seizures, or after exposure to seizure-inducing nerve toxins. The terms *antiseizure drugs, antiepileptic drugs (AEDs),* and *anticonvulsants* are often used interchangeably. However, antiseizure drugs is most appropriate to describe these medications because not every seizure is due to epilepsy nor does every seizure result in convulsions.

Although people with epilepsy often need to take antiseizure drugs chronically, this does not mean that everyone with epilepsy must take antiseizure drugs indefinitely. For children who are seizure-free for longer than 2-4 years while on anti-epileptic drugs 70% will remain so when medications are withdrawn. The risk of recurrence depends on the seizure syndrome. For example, resolution of seizures is common for generalized absence epilepsy, but not for juvenile myoclonic epilepsy. Other risk factors for seizure recurrence include abnormal EEG, presence of neurologic deficits, or when seizure control had been difficult to achieve. For seizure-free adults, there is little information on withdrawal or discontinuation of antiseizure drugs. Discontinuation is thought to be more successful in those with generalized epilepsies who exhibit a single seizure type. Risk factors for seizure recurrence include longer duration of epilepsy, abnormal neurologic examination, abnormal EEG, and certain epilepsy syndromes. Because abrupt cessation may be associated with a seizure and risk of status epilepticus, antiseizure drugs are usually slowly withdrawn over a 1- to 3-month period or even longer. For barbiturates and benzodiazepines, there is a well-recognized risk of rebound seizures with abrupt withdrawal.

MECHANISMS OF ACTION OF ANTISEIZURE DRUGS

Regardless of the inciting cause, seizures are generated when there is an imbalance favoring excitation over inhibition, which can be due to excessive neuronal excitation or decreased neuronal inhibition, or both. Thus, to effectively suppress the repetitive, high frequency action potentials from epileptic foci in the brain, antiseizure medications either *inhibit excitation* or *enhance inhibition*. Inhibition of excitation can be produced by altering intrinsic firing mechanisms in excitatory neurons (eg, sodium channel blockers) or by decreasing excitatory synaptic transmission, which can be accomplished by decreasing release of the excitatory neurotransmitter glutamate (eg, levetiracetam, retigabine) or its postsynaptic actions (eg, perampanel). Enhancement of inhibition can be produced by increasing availability of the inhibitory neurotransmitter GABA (eg, tiagabine, vigabatrin) or increasing activation of $GABA_A$ receptors that mediate inhibition in cortical areas involved in seizures (eg, benzodiazepines, phenobarbital). For some antiseizure drugs, there is no consensus regarding the specific molecular target (eg, zonisamide, valproic acid) or there may be multiple targets (eg, topiramate, felbamate). Figure 14-2 illustrates the molecular sites on excitatory and inhibitory neurons where currently available antiseizure drugs are thought to exert their actions.

PHARMACOKINETICS

Antiseizure drugs are commonly used over long durations and adequate drug exposure must be continuously maintained. These drugs are predominantly taken orally and multiple daily dosing is typically required. In general, antiseizure drugs are well absorbed orally and have good bioavailability. Most antiseizure drugs are metabolized by hepatic enzymes, and, in some cases, active metabolites are formed. Resistance to antiseizure drugs may involve increased expression of drug transporters at the level of the blood-brain barrier.

Consideration of pharmacokinetic properties is especially important because many antiseizure drugs have a narrow therapeutic window and significant drug-drug interactions. The pharmacokinetic behavior of most antiseizure drugs varies markedly from patient to patient so that dosing must be individualized for optimum therapy. Established reference ranges for therapeutic blood levels are available for most of the older antiseizure drugs. Assessment of an individual's blood drug level may be used (1) to guide dose adjustments, (2) when breakthrough seizures occur, (3) when an interacting medication is added to or removed from a patient's regimen, (4) during pregnancy, (5) to establish an individual therapeutic concentration range when a patient is in remission, (6) to assist in determining if adverse effects relate to excessive levels of a specific drug, and (7) to assess medication adherence.

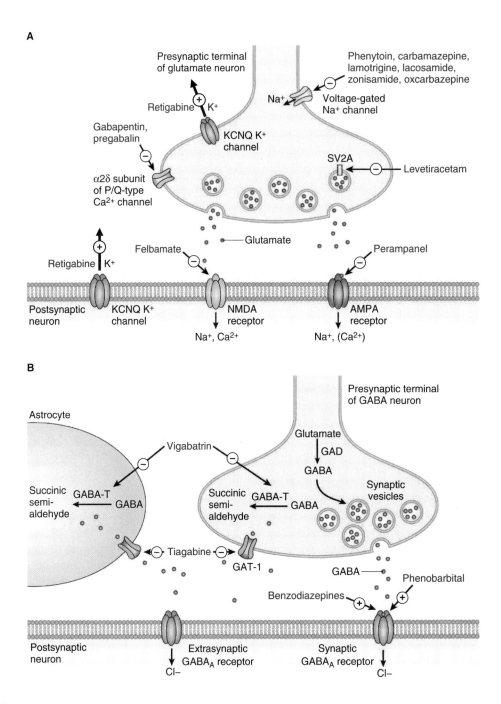

FIGURE 14-2 Molecular targets for antiseizure drugs at an excitatory glutamatergic synapse (A) and an inhibitory GABAergic synapse (B). Presynaptic targets that decrease glutamate release include voltage-gated sodium channels (carbamazepine, phenytoin, lamotrigine, and lacosamide); voltage-gated potassium channels (retigabine [ezogabine]), and the α2δ subunit of P/Q type calcium channels (gabapentin, pregabalin). Postsynaptic targets at excitatory synapses include AMPA receptors (perampanel), and voltage-gated potassium channels (retigabine [ezogabine]). At inhibitory synapses (and in astrocytes), vigabatrin inhibits GABA-transaminase (GABA-T) and tiagabine blocks the GABA transporter 1 (GAT-1). Blockade of GABA-T results in high GABA levels that may act on extrasynaptic GABA$_A$ receptors. Phenobarbital, primidone, and benzodiazepines act as positive allosteric modulators of synaptic GABA$_A$ receptors.

Pharmacokinetic drug interactions are very common with antiseizure drugs. Two notable exceptions are gabapentin and pregabalin, which are not known to have drug interactions. Drugs that inhibit drug metabolism (eg, cimetidine) or displace antiseizure drugs from plasma protein binding sites (eg, nonsteroidal anti-inflammatory drugs) may increase plasma concentrations of antiseizure agents to toxic levels. On the other hand, drugs that induce hepatic drug-metabolizing enzymes (eg, rifampin) may result in plasma levels of the antiseizure agents that are inadequate for seizure control. Antiseizure drugs can also interact with other medications. For example, some antiseizure drugs (eg, perampanel, topiramate, eslicarbazepine acetate) may reduce plasma levels of oral contraceptives. To avoid a failure of birth control, alternative modes of contraception may be recommended for women taking certain antiseizure medications. Last, several antiseizure drugs, especially carbamazepine and phenytoin, are also capable of inducing their own hepatic metabolism.

DRUGS USEFUL FOR FOCAL ONSET SEIZURES

The most popular drugs used in the treatment of focal onset seizures are **carbamazepine**, **lacosamide**, **phenytoin**, **lamotrigine**, and **levetiracetam**. If cost is a consideration, **phenobarbital** may be used. Due to their adverse effect profile, **felbamate** and **vigabatrin** are third-line agents.

Carbamazepine

Carbamazepine is tricyclic compound that is structurally similar to imipramine and similar antidepressants. However, since carbamazepine does not inhibit monoamine (serotonin and norepinephrine) transporters with high affinity, it is not used as an antidepressant. Carbamazepine blocks voltage-gated sodium channels responsible for the rising phase of the neuronal action potential. Carbamazepine and other sodium channel blockers such as phenytoin and lamotrigine preferentially bind to the channel in the inactivated state, *stabilizing* this state. Sodium channel blockers are also voltage dependent, thus blocking channels at more depolarized potentials. This use dependence and voltage dependence results in preferential inhibition of high-frequency repetitive neuronal firing such as occurs during seizure discharges. In addition, sodium channel blockers act presynaptically to decrease excitatory transmission (Figure 14-2A). Because these drugs are less likely to interfere with ordinary action potential firing, they are thought to prevent seizures without causing unacceptable neurologic impairment.

Carbamazepine is effective for the treatment of focal onset and focal-to-bilateral tonic-clonic seizures. Although the drug may be effective for generalized tonic-clonic seizures, caution must be used because it can exacerbate myoclonic and absence seizures. **Oxcarbazepine**, a derivative of carbamazepine, is sometimes used because it induces hepatic enzymes to a lesser extent than carbamazepine, which minimizes drug interactions. An alternative to oxcarbazepine is **eslicarbazepine acetate**. A potential advantage of this drug is that its long half-life enables once-daily dosing.

An important clinical advantage of carbamazepine, oxcarbazepine, and eslicarbazepine acetate is that they are not sedative in the usual therapeutic ranges. More common (and dose-dependent) adverse effects include mild gastrointestinal distress, dizziness, blurred vision, diplopia, and ataxia.

Lacosamide

Lacosamide is widely prescribed for focal onset seizures. The drug is a sodium channel blocker, but has slower binding kinetics than other sodium channel blockers. Lacosamide does not induce cytochrome P450 (CYP) enzymes, so drug interactions are minimal. Adverse drug reactions (ADRs) include dizziness, headache, nausea, and diplopia.

Hydantoins

Drugs in this class include phenytoin, **fosphenytoin**, **ethotoin**, and **mephenytoin**, though the latter two agents are rarely used. Phenytoin is a sodium channel-blocking agent that acts in a similar way to carbamazepine. Phenytoin is the oldest nonsedative drug used to treat seizures, and remains one of the most frequently prescribed despite its adverse effects and potential difficulty in consistently achieving therapeutic levels.

Phenytoin is effective for preventing focal onset seizures and tonic-clonic seizures, whether they are focal-to-bilateral tonic-clonic seizures, or seizures that occur in the setting of an idiopathic generalized epilepsy syndrome. Phenytoin may worsen seizures in primary generalized epilepsies, absence epilepsy, juvenile myoclonic epilepsy, and Dravet syndrome. **Fosphenytoin** is a more water-soluble prodrug of phenytoin that is used exclusively for intravenous administration to treat status epilepticus (see end of chapter).

There is significant inter-individual variability in the oral bioavailability of phenytoin due to differences in first-pass metabolism and serum albumin levels. Phenytoin binds extensively to plasma proteins (97-98%). Thus, free phenytoin plasma levels are increased by drugs that compete for albumin binding (eg, warfarin, valproic acid) or by low plasma albumin (such as in liver disease). These factors can result in abnormally high free concentrations and toxicity. Phenytoin, like many other antiseizure drugs (eg, carbamazepine, phenobarbital, primidone) is also a major CYP inducer that stimulates the rate of metabolism of many coadministered antiseizure drugs.

Early adverse effects of phenytoin include nystagmus and loss of smooth extraocular pursuit movements. Diplopia and ataxia are common dose-related ADRs that require dosage adjustments. Sedation usually only occurs at much higher dosages. Phenytoin use is associated with potential cosmetic problems including gingival hyperplasia, coarsening of facial features, and hirsutism. Long-term use can cause mild peripheral neuropathy manifested as diminished deep tendon reflexes in the lower extremities. Dysregulation of vitamin D metabolism, leading to osteomalacia, may also occur. Distal to the phenytoin injection site, a purplish-black discoloration ("black glove syndrome") with accompanying edema and pain can occur. Though this ADR is rare, the condition may progress and carries a potential risk for amputation. This phenomenon has been proposed to be due to the low water solubility of phenytoin with resulting intravascular crystallization and blood flow disruption distal to the injection site. This ADR is minimized by injection of fosphenytoin, which is more water soluble.

Gabapentin and Pregabalin

Gabapentin and **pregabalin** are known as "gabapentinoids." Despite their structural similarity to GABA, the effects of these agents are *not* mediated via actions on GABA receptors or any other mechanism related to GABA-mediated neurotransmission. Instead, the gabapentinoids strongly bind to a protein subunit (α2δ) on voltage-dependent P/Q-type calcium channels (Figure 14-2A). The mechanism by which these drugs protect against seizures is not precisely known. However, binding may decrease glutamate release at excitatory synapses.

The gabapentinoids are considered less effective than other antiseizure drugs for treating focal onset seizures. There is no evidence that they are effective in generalized epilepsies; gabapentin may aggravate absence seizures and myoclonic seizures. Both gabapentinoids are relatively well tolerated. The most common ADRs—which often resolve with continued dosing—are sedation, dizziness, ataxia, headache, and tremor. Both drugs can cause weight gain and peripheral edema.

Tiagabine

Tiagabine inhibits GABA uptake in both neurons and glia, thus prolonging the inhibitory action of GABA in the synaptic cleft (Figure 14-2B). Tiagabine is highly selective for the GAT-1 GABA transporter expressed in the brain, and has little to no effect on other GABA transporters. Tiagabine is a second-line treatment for focal seizures. Its use is contraindicated in generalized onset seizures. Limited efficacy and adverse effects have limited its use. Minor dose-related ADRs include nervousness, dizziness, tremor, difficulty concentrating, and depression. Excessive confusion, somnolence, or ataxia may require discontinuation. Psychosis occurs rarely.

Retigabine (Ezogabine)

In the United States, **retigabine** is called ezogabine. The drug's antiseizure mechanism of action is opening the KCNQ subtype of potassium channels. As positively charged cations move out, the neuron becomes more hyperpolarized and less likely to fire action potentials (Figure 14-2A). Because of its adverse effect profile, retigabine is a third-line option for treating focal seizures. While several of the dose-dependent ADRs (dizziness, somnolence, blurred vision, confusion, dysarthria) are not unique to this agent, retigabine also causes blue pigmentation in the skin, lips, palate, and retina. Due to reports of adverse ophthalmologic reactions including macular abnormalities and decreases in visual acuity, use of retigabine is only recommended in cases where other antiseizure drugs are not effective or tolerated.

DRUGS USEFUL FOR FOCAL ONSET SEIZURES AND CERTAIN GENERALIZED ONSET SEIZURE TYPES

The drugs in the previous section effectively treat focal onset and focal-to-bilateral tonic-clonic seizures. The antiseizure drugs covered in this section are effective for treating focal

onset seizures and *certain* generalized onset seizures. Correct diagnosis is absolutely critical because some of these drugs can exacerbate certain generalized seizure types.

Lamotrigine

Lamotrigine produces a voltage- and use-dependent inhibition of presynaptic sodium channels that results in suppression of rapidly firing neurons (Figure 14-2A). Lamotrigine is effective as monotherapy for focal seizures. The drug has also been shown to be effective in treatment of generalized tonic-clonic seizures (in idiopathic generalized epilepsy) and generalized absence seizures. Although less effective than **ethosuximide** and **valproic acid** (discussed below) for absence seizures, lamotrigine may be preferentially prescribed because of its better adverse effect profile. In addition, lamotrigine may be chosen for females of childbearing age because it has fewer fetal risks than valproic acid. Adverse effects include sedation and paradoxical insomnia, ataxia, nausea, dizziness, headache, and diplopia. There is a potential for a life-threatening rash (especially in children), which may be diminished by starting with slow and low drug dosing.

Levetiracetam

Levetiracetam is one of the most commonly prescribed drugs for a broad spectrum of seizure types. Several advantages include a favorable adverse effect profile, wide therapeutic window, favorable pharmacokinetic properties, and lack of drug-drug interactions. Levetiracetam selectively binds to SV2A, a synaptic vesicle membrane protein thought to function as a regulator of action potential-dependent glutamate release (Figure 14-2A). The drug's antiseizure mechanism of action is the reduction of glutamate vesicle release during high-frequency firing.

Levetiracetam is used to treat focal seizures in adults and children, primary generalized tonic-clonic seizures, and myoclonic seizures of juvenile myoclonic epilepsy. The most common ADRs are somnolence, dizziness, ataxia, asthenia, and infection (colds). Less common, but more troublesome adverse effects are mood and behavioral changes. These include irritability, anger, aggression, anxiety, apathy, depression, and emotional lability.

Brivaracetam, a drug structurally similar to levetiracetam, has recently been approved for treating focal onset seizures. No evidence is available at this time to determine if this analog will have the broad-spectrum activity of levetiracetam.

Phenobarbital

Phenobarbital is the oldest of the currently available antiseizure drugs. Originally introduced as a sleeping aid in 1912, this barbiturate was found to be useful in treating epilepsy. In the developed world, phenobarbital is no longer a first-line choice because of its significant sedative properties and many drug interactions. However, the drug is inexpensive and still useful for treating neonatal seizures.

Phenobarbital increases the effect of GABA by increasing the average duration that the GABA$_A$ receptor chloride channel is open (Figure 14-2B). The drug exerts other actions on intrinsic neuronal excitability and synaptic function. Although phenobarbital is equally effective as phenytoin and carbamazepine in controlling focal seizures and generalized tonic-clonic seizures, its significant sedative effects lead to more frequent discontinuation. Phenobarbital is not the first drug of choice for juvenile myoclonic seizures, but it can be useful. The drug may worsen absence seizures and infantile spasms. Long-term administration causes physical dependence; thus, the drug must be discontinued gradually over many weeks to avoid recurrence of seizures or status epilepticus.

Primidone

Primidone is metabolized to phenobarbital and phenylethylmalonamide, another active antiseizure metabolite. Primidone is effective against focal onset seizures and generalized tonic-clonic seizures. Primidone was introduced for treating epilepsy in the 1950s, but use of the drug has decreased primarily because of its adverse effects. Acute toxicities (drowsiness, dizziness, ataxia, nausea, and vomiting) may be mitigated by slow titration. At effective doses, sedation still occurs.

Perampanel

Perampanel is used to treat focal seizures and primary generalized tonic-clonic seizures in idiopathic generalized epilepsies. Perampanel is a noncompetitive antagonist of the glutamate ionotropic AMPA receptor (Figure 14-2A). At therapeutic concentrations, the drug's ability to partially block AMPA receptors reduces seizure occurrence because AMPA receptors are critical in local generation of seizure activity as well as the spread of neuronal excitation. Common ADRs include dizziness, somnolence, and headache. Perampanel is often associated with dose-dependent adverse behaviors such as aggression, hostility, irritability, and anger. These unwanted behaviors occur more frequently in younger individuals and in those with learning disabilities or dementia. Alcohol use may exacerbate the level of anger.

Felbamate

Felbamate is an adjunct antiseizure agent with severe ADRs that ultimately limit its clinical use. Felbamate appears to have more than one antiseizure mechanism of action. The drug produces a use-dependent block of *N*-methyl-D-aspartate (NMDA) receptors that decrease excitatory neurotransmission. In addition, felbamate potentiates GABA$_A$ receptor responses in a similar fashion to barbiturates. The drug is used in the treatment of focal seizures and in Lennox-Gastaut syndrome (severe form of epilepsy with multiple different type of seizures that appears during infancy or early childhood). However, because felbamate can cause aplastic anemia and severe hepatotoxicity at unexpectedly high rates, its use is reserved for patients with seizures that respond poorly to other medications.

DRUGS USEFUL FOR GENERALIZED ONSET SEIZURES

For individuals with generalized onset seizures, **valproic acid** is a first-line antiseizure drug. Because of its adverse effect profile and teratogenicity, other frequently used agents that have broad activity in generalized epilepsy are **topiramate** and **zonisamide**.

Valproic Acid

Valproic acid was originally introduced as a primary agent in the treatment of generalized seizures, but it has proven to be one of the most broad-spectrum and effective antiseizure medications. The drug is effective against all types of generalized onset seizures, including tonic-clonic, generalized absence, myoclonic, and atonic. Valproic acid is also used to treat focal onset seizures, though it may not be as effective as carbamazepine or phenytoin. Intravenous formulations can be used to treat status epilepticus.

Valproic acid is well absorbed after an oral dose, with peak blood levels within a couple hours. The active form of the drug is the valproate ion, which is highly bound to plasma proteins. At doses nearing the upper end of the therapeutic range, protein binding becomes saturated, which increases the plasma free fraction of valproate, and an apparent increase in total valproate clearance.

The mechanisms for valproate's antiseizure actions are not definitively known. Because the time course of the drug's actions poorly correlates with blood or tissue levels of valproic acid, there is some speculation regarding the active species.

The most common dose-related ADRs of valproic acid include gastrointestinal distress such as nausea, abdominal pain, vomiting, and heartburn. Slow titration of the drug can minimize these symptoms. Other reversible ADRs include increased appetite, weight gain, hair loss, and lethargy. At higher doses, individuals present with a fine tremor. Rarely, valproic acid causes hepatotoxicity that may be severe and has been fatal. This risk is higher in children under 2 years of age and those taking multiple medications. Because valproic acid is a teratogen, the drug should not be used in women of reproductive potential without effective contraception.

Topiramate

Topiramate likely has several antiseizure mechanisms of action including blockade of voltage-gated sodium channels, potentiation of GABA (acting at a site different from benzodiazepine and barbiturate sites on the GABA$_A$ receptor channel complex), and blockade of excitatory amino acid receptors.

Topiramate is effective in focal onset and generalized tonic-clonic seizures. The drug may also be used in the treatment of

Lennox-Gastaut syndrome, juvenile myoclonic epilepsy, infantile spasms, Dravet syndrome, and childhood absence seizures.

A frequent reason for discontinuation of topiramate is adverse cognitive effects, the incidence of which increases in a dose-dependent manner. Affected patients report a general slowing of cognitive processing with specific impairments in language function and verbal memory. These effects often occur without sedation or mood alteration and represent a more unique ADR profile compared to other antiseizure drugs. Other dose-related adverse effects that occur more often in the first 4 weeks of therapy include paresthesias, somnolence, fatigue, dizziness, and nervousness. Some individuals (more commonly children) taking topiramate may experience decreased sweating and impaired thermoregulation in hot weather. Long-term therapy is associated with a low risk of kidney stones and a high risk of weight loss. In clinical trials, 85% of adults receiving topiramate lost, on average, 5% of mean baseline body weight.

Zonisamide

Zonisamide blocks voltage-gated sodium channels and probably has other actions that contribute to its antiseizure activity. Zonisamide is another broad-spectrum antiseizure drug effective for treating focal onset and generalized tonic-clonic seizures in adults and children. The drug may also be effective in some myoclonic epilepsies and infantile spasms. Zonisamide's adverse effects include drowsiness, cognitive impairment, kidney stones, and potentially serious skin rashes. Like topiramate, zonisamide is associated with weight loss.

DRUGS USEFUL FOR GENERALIZED ABSENCE SEIZURES

Ethosuximide is a first choice option for treating generalized absence seizures. The drug can be used as monotherapy; if generalized tonic-clonic seizures are also present, valproic acid is preferred, or ethosuximide is combined with another drug effective against generalized tonic-clonic seizures. Ethosuximide increases the seizure threshold and limits the spread of electrical activity in thalamocortical neurons by reducing low-threshold calcium currents. Ethosuximide's most common dose-related ADR is gastrointestinal distress, including pain, nausea, and vomiting. Other dose-related adverse effects include lethargy and fatigue. Less commonly, headache, dizziness, hiccups, and euphoria occur. Behavioral changes are usually in the direction of improvement.

OTHER ANTISEIZURE DRUGS

Benzodiazepines

As discussed in Chapter 13, benzodiazepines increase the inhibitory effects of GABA by augmenting the frequency of $GABA_A$ receptor chloride channel opening. Two properties of benzodiazepines limit their usefulness in chronic epilepsy.

First, these agents produce significant sedation. In children, they may cause paradoxical hyperactivity. Second, benzodiazepines produce tolerance such that seizures may respond initially, but recur within a few months. Due to these limitations, only a few benzodiazepines (**clonazepam**, **clorazepate**, **clobazam**) are used infrequently in the chronic treatment of epilepsy. Clonazepam is a long-acting drug with documented efficacy against absence, atonic, and myoclonic seizures. Clorazepate is occasionally used to treat focal onset seizures. Clobazam is also widely used to treat focal seizures, though in the United States, its use is limited to treating seizures associated with Lennox-Gastaut syndrome in children 2 years of age or older. Somnolence and sedation are dose-dependent adverse effects. Withdrawal symptoms may occur with abrupt discontinuation. Certain benzodiazepines are first-line treatment for acute repetitive seizures (seizure clusters) or in status epilepticus (see below).

Vigabatrin

Vigabatrin is an irreversible inhibitor of GABA transaminase (GABA-T), the enzyme responsible for the degradation of GABA (Figure 14-2B). The drug apparently produces a sustained increase in extracellular GABA that paradoxically inhibits $GABA_A$-mediated responses, but also prolongs the activation of extrasynaptic $GABA_A$ receptors that mediate tonic inhibition. Vigabatrin is useful in the treatment of infantile spasms and focal seizures, but not generalized seizures. However, use is typically reserved for patients with seizures that are refractory to other treatments because vigabatrin may cause irreversible loss of vision that can occur within weeks, months, or years of treatment initiation. Other ADRs include headache, somnolence, dizziness, and weight gain.

STATUS EPILEPTICUS

Status epilepticus is defined as abnormally prolonged or repetitive seizures. The condition can present in different forms. In *convulsive* status epilepticus, the person exhibits repeated generalized tonic-clonic seizures and demonstrates depressed neurologic function between seizures. In *nonconvulsive* status epilepticus, the person does not exhibit motor signs, but demonstrates a persistent alteration in behavior or mental processing with continuous epileptiform EEG. Last, in *focal status epilepticus*, the person may or may not have altered awareness. Convulsive status epilepticus is a life-threatening emergency. Because most seizures self-terminate in 2-3 minutes and persistent seizures are believed to cause permanent neuronal damage, it is generally accepted that treatment should begin when seizure duration reaches 5 minutes for generalized tonic-clonic seizures and 10 minutes for focal seizures with or without impairment of consciousness.

The initial treatment of choice is a benzodiazepine, either intravenous **lorazepam** or **diazepam**, although intramuscular **midazolam** may be equally effective. If these options are not available (eg, in settings outside of the hospital), rectal diazepam, intranasal midazolam, or buccal midazolam are alternative first treatments. If seizures continue, a second intravenous therapy (fosphenytoin, phenytoin, valproate, or levetiracetam) is administered. Phenobarbital may be used, but its long half-life causes long-lasting adverse effects (eg, sedation, respiratory depression, hypotension). If the second antiseizure drug is not effective at stopping seizure activity, an additional second-line agent is often tried. Refractory status epilepticus occurs when seizures continue or recur at least 30 minutes after treatment with first and second therapy agents. Refractory status epilepticus is treated with general anesthesia. If status epilepticus continues or recurs 24 hours or more after the onset of anesthesia, the condition is considered super-refractory. Super-refractory status epilepticus is typically recognized when anesthetics are withdrawn and seizures recur. There are no established therapies for super-refractory status epilepticus other than to reinstitute general anesthesia. Treatment of focal status epilepticus is similar to therapy for convulsive status epilepticus, although in some cases simply instituting oral antiseizure drug therapy is sufficient.

TERATOGENICITY

Most women with epilepsy who become pregnant still require antiseizure drug therapy for seizure control. No antiseizure drug is known to be completely safe for the developing embryo or fetus. If possible, valproic acid, phenobarbital, and topiramate should be avoided in women of childbearing potential because these drugs present the highest risk of major congenital malformations. Lamotrigine or levetiracetam have the lowest risks of major congenital malformations. Polytherapy may increase the risk of neurodevelopmental deficits, particularly when one of the drugs is valproic acid.

OTHER CLINICAL USES FOR ANTISEIZURE DRUGS

Several drugs originally intended as antiseizure drugs have demonstrated usefulness in treating different conditions. Valproic acid, carbamazepine, and lamotrigine are effective as mood stabilizers in bipolar disorder. Carbamazepine and oxcarbazepine are drugs of first choice for trigeminal neuralgia. Gabapentin and pregabalin are frequently used in the treatment of neuropathic pain, including postherpetic neuralgia and painful diabetic neuropathy. Pregabalin has been approved for the treatment of fibromyalgia. Valproic acid and topiramate are used as prophylactic medications for migraine. Primidone is used in the treatment of essential tremor.

REHABILITATION RELEVANCE

The need for physical therapists to take a thorough medical history is never more relevant than for individuals who have a history of seizures and are taking antiseizure medications. In many instances, patients will be receiving rehabilitation services for a condition unrelated to their epilepsy (eg, orthopedic

condition) and should be identified for the potential risk of a seizure during therapy. If a patient is receiving therapy for a diagnosis directly related to seizure activity (eg, stroke, brain tumor, head trauma), the therapist may help determine the acute efficacy of the antiseizure drug therapy. The primary goal of drug therapy is to control seizure activity without serious adverse effects. The physical therapist may play a vital role in this process by monitoring patient response to medication and informing the medical team of any abnormal findings. In some cases, the drug regimen may adequately control seizure activity, but result in significant adverse effects such as sedation, dizziness, ataxia, and gastric disturbances that negatively impact participation and functional improvement in rehabilitation. Finally, some people with epilepsy are sensitive to environmental stimuli such as loud sounds, flashing lights, and specific odors. Every attempt should be made to reduce these stimuli during therapy sessions. Physical therapists should be alert for any changes in behavior or functional status (eg, increase in seizures or increase in adverse reactions) in patients taking antiseizure drugs and report these changes to the appropriate medical personnel. Listed below is a summary of ADRs more commonly associated with particular antiseizure drugs.

- **Sedation**, **somnolence**, and **drowsiness**: carbamazepine (at high doses), gabapentin, pregabalin, tiagabine, retigabine, lamotrigine, levetiracetam, perampanel, primidone, vigabatrin, topiramate, zonisamide, ethosuximide, and all benzodiazepines
- **Dizziness**: carbamazepine, lacosamide, gabapentin, pregabalin, tiagabine, retigabine, lamotrigine, levetiracetam, perampanel, primidone, vigabatrin, topiramate, and ethosuximide (less common)
- **Ataxia**: carbamazepine, gabapentin, pregabalin, phenytoin, levetiracetam, and primidone
- **Tremor**: tiagabine; gabapentin and pregabalin (though usually resolve with continued dosing); valproic acid (at higher doses)
- **Headache**: lacosamide, gabapentin, pregabalin, lamotrigine, perampanel, and vigabatrin
- **Weight gain**: gabapentin, pregabalin, valproic acid, vigabatrin, and carbamazepine (rarely)
- **Visual disturbances**: diplopia (carbamazepine, lacosamide, retigabine, lamotrigine, phenytoin); blurred vision (carbamazepine, retigabine); nystagmus and loss of smooth extraocular pursuit movements (phenytoin); macular abnormalities (retigabine); acute myopia and angle-closure glaucoma (topiramate); permanent bilateral concentric visual field constriction (vigabatrin)
- **Peripheral neuropathy**: phenytoin
- **Osteomalacia**: phenytoin
- **Gastrointestinal disturbances (nausea, vomiting)**: carbamazepine, lacosamide, lamotrigine, primidone; valproic acid and ethosuximide (and abdominal pain)
- **Peripheral edema**: gabapentin and pregabalin
- **Cognitive changes**: tiagabine (difficulty concentrating, excessive confusion); retigabine (confusion); topiramate

(expressive language dysfunction, impaired verbal memory, slow cognitive processing); zonisamide (cognitive impairment). However, most individuals taking any of the antiseizure drugs experience some degree of mental slowing.

- **Skin changes**: rash (zonisamide; tiagabine, though rarely); potentially fatal Stevens-Johnson syndrome (lamotrigine); blue pigmentation (retigabine)

- **Urinary changes**: retention, hesitation, dysuria (retigabine); urolithiasis (topiramate and zonisamide)
- **Mood changes**: aggression or irritability (perampanel, clobazam, levetiracetam); anxiety, apathy, depression, emotional lability (levetiracetam)
- **Hepatotoxicity**: felbamate and valproic acid

CASE CONCLUSION

The therapist questioned the patient's wife about C.M.'s energy level; she confirmed that he was much less active at home. When the therapist asked the patient's wife when C.M.'s blood levels were last checked, she stated that it was almost time to do so. The therapist contacted the patient's physician to discuss C.M.'s current functional status. The physician scheduled blood work to be done that day. The physician reported that the patient's blood concentration of valproic acid was elevated above therapeutic levels, which could have accounted for C.M.'s lethargy because valproic acid significantly increases the half-life of lamotrigine. The physician subsequently lowered the patient's daily dose of valproic acid. After several days, C.M. began to return to his previous mental and physical status and continued with his therapeutic intervention without further problems.

CHAPTER 14 QUESTIONS

1. Which of the following is *not* a mechanism of action for drugs with antiseizure activity?

   a. Positive modulation of $GABA_A$ receptors
   b. $GABA_A$ receptor antagonism
   c. Blockade of glutamatergic AMPA receptors
   d. Inhibition of voltage-gated sodium channels

2. Which of the following statements is true regarding the pharmacological treatment of seizures?

   a. In some people, simultaneous use of multiple drugs may be necessary to provide adequate seizure control.
   b. Since most seizures are self-limiting, drugs are only used when an individual has a seizure that lasts more than 5 minutes.
   c. In those with epilepsy, antiseizure drugs are typically only taken for a short time after the occurrence of a seizure.
   d. Once an individual starts taking an antiseizure medication, continuous use must occur for the person's lifetime.

3. Which of the following drugs does *not* have its antiseizure effect by blocking sodium channels?

   a. Phenytoin
   b. Carbamazepine
   c. Lamotrigine
   d. Levetiracetam

4. Which of the following antiseizure drugs does *not* tend to have a sedative effect at usual therapeutic doses?

   a. Tiagabine
   b. Phenobarbital
   c. Carbamazepine
   d. Levetiracetam

5. Use of which of the following antiseizure drugs has been associated with cognitive slowing, particularly in the verbal realm?

   a. Gabapentin
   b. Topiramate
   c. Valproic acid
   d. Carbamazepine

6. Which of the following statements is true regarding the use of benzodiazepines in the treatment of seizures?

   a. Certain benzodiazepines are first-line agents to treat generalized onset seizures.
   b. Certain benzodiazepines are first-line agents to treat focal onset seizures.
   c. Certain benzodiazepines are first-line agents to treat generalized absence seizures.
   d. Certain benzodiazepines are first-line agents to treat status epilepticus.

7. Which of the following antiseizure drugs is associated with weight loss?

   a. Carbamazepine
   b. Zonisamide
   c. Vigabatrin
   d. Valproic acid

8. Which of the following antiseizure drugs has the lowest risk of teratogenicity?

   a. Valproic acid
   b. Phenobarbital
   c. Lamotrigine
   d. Topiramate

9. Which of the following is considered a first-line agent in the treatment of focal onset seizures?

a. Carbamazepine
b. Felbamate
c. Gabapentin
d. Retigabine

10. Aggression is a recognized adverse effect of all of the following drugs, except:

a. Perampanel
b. Clobazam
c. Phenytoin
d. Levetiracetam

General Anesthetics

A.F. is a 72-year-old woman who sustained a right proximal femoral fracture secondary to a fall down eight concrete stairs outside a medical office building. She was on her way to see her physician for an annual checkup and lost her balance while stepping onto the top step. A.F. was transported and emergently admitted to the hospital for an open reduction internal fixation (ORIF) of the right femur. Physical therapy evaluation was initiated 24 hours after surgery. Upon chart review, the therapist noted that the operation report was unremarkable and the surgeon established non-weightbearing status on the right lower extremity. The anesthesia report showed the patient received balanced anesthesia of inhaled nitrous oxide for induction followed by desflurane and intravenous anesthetics including midazolam and fentanyl. Postoperatively, A.F. is receiving pain medications as needed. Upon evaluation, the therapist noted that A.F. was extremely difficult to arouse and very lethargic. Nursing reported that the patient had a restful evening and that she had not requested additional pain medication. The therapist made several unsuccessful attempts to sit A.F. at the edge of the bed. The therapist, with the assistance of three aides, transferred the patient dependently to a cardiac chair for slow mobilization to an upright posture. During this activity, A.F. was somnolent and unable to carry on a conversation with the therapist. The patient was transferred back to bed with the ceiling lift. After reading the therapist's initial evaluation, the hospital discharge planner shared with the therapist that she felt that A.F. should likely be discharged to a skilled nursing facility. The therapist requested that any recommendation about discharge destination be deferred by at least one day.

REHABILITATION FOCUS

Adverse effects from general anesthetics that often interfere with early therapeutic interventions include sedation and muscle weakness. Older adults or individuals with impaired drug metabolism and elimination mechanisms may continue to show physical and cognitive deficits such as hypotension, respiratory depression, ataxia, and confusion for several days after discontinuance of anesthetic agents. General anesthetics also depress mucociliary clearance, resulting in increased bronchial secretions and pooling of mucus in the lungs. This obstruction may result in atelectasis and respiratory infections. Pulmonary hygiene and early therapeutic activities that increase respiration depth and rate may help offset these effects. By providing early mobilization along with functional and balance activities, therapists may assist in the recovery of patients who have received general anesthesia.

Physical therapy practice has expanded to include rehabilitation in healthcare areas not previously encountered. Because of changing healthcare policies and current advances in surgical procedures, many patients undergoing minor surgery go home that same day. This can be problematic, especially when the patient requires physical therapy for immediate mobilization (crutch training, upright activity, etc). In addition, physical therapy is being conducted on patients in the intensive care unit (ICU), resulting in decreased hospital stays and improved physical function outcomes. As such, physical therapists need to understand the physical and cognitive effects of these drugs in order to set appropriate goals and safely provide services for these patients.

BACKGROUND

Drugs used as general anesthetics are central nervous system (CNS) depressants with actions that can be induced and terminated more rapidly than those of conventional sedative-hypnotics (Chapter 13). A general anesthetic produces three principal actions: immobility, amnesia, and unconsciousness. Immobility is the easiest anesthetic end point to measure. Anesthetic-induced immobility is mediated primarily by neural inhibition within the spinal cord, but may also include inhibited nociceptive transmission to the brain. Amnesia is the ablation of memory and arises from actions within several locations in the CNS. These areas include the hippocampus, amygdala, prefrontal cortex, and regions of the sensory and motor cortices. Any *specific* awareness as well as any *unconscious* acquisition of information is inhibited when individuals are at surgical levels of general anesthesia. Finally, general anesthetics produce unconsciousness, which is a lack of personal awareness. Consciousness involves the cerebral cortex, thalamus, and reticular activating system. Neural pathways emanating from these regions seem to interact as a cortical system to produce the mental state in which humans are awake, aware, and perceiving. The capacity of anesthetic drugs to abolish consciousness requires actions at these anatomic locations.

MECHANISM OF ACTION

Original research that aimed at understanding the mechanism of action of general anesthetics focused on the unitary theory, which attempted to identify a *single* biologic site where these drugs had their effect. Current research presents a more complex picture of multiple molecular targets throughout the CNS. Anesthetics affect neurons at various cellular locations, but the primary focus has been on the synapse. A presynaptic action may alter the release of neurotransmitters, whereas a postsynaptic effect may change the frequency and/or amplitude of impulses of the postsynaptic neuron. The cumulative effect of anesthetic actions may produce strengthened inhibition (Figure 15-1, panel A) or diminished excitation (Figure 15-1, panel B) within key areas of the CNS. Studies on isolated spinal cord tissue have demonstrated that anesthetics impair excitatory transmission more strongly than they potentiate inhibitory effects. Major inhibitory receptors considered legitimate candidates of anesthetic action include chloride channels (gamma-aminobutyric acid-A [GABA$_A$] receptors and glycine receptors) and potassium channels. Anesthetics also inhibit excitatory ion channel receptors, including nicotinic and muscarinic cholinergic receptors, glutamatergic AMPA, kainate, and NMDA receptors, and serotonergic 5-HT$_2$ and 5-HT$_3$ receptors.

TRADITIONAL GENERAL ANESTHETICS

Older and slower-acting anesthetics produce four stages of increasing depth of CNS depression. In Stage 1 (Analgesia), the patient has decreased awareness of pain, sometimes with amnesia. Consciousness may be impaired, but is not lost. In Stage 2 (Disinhibition), the patient appears to be delirious and excited. Amnesia occurs, reflexes are enhanced, and respiration is typically irregular; retching, vomiting, and incontinence may occur. For these reasons, efforts are made to limit the duration and severity of this stage, which ends with the reestablishment of regular breathing. In stage 3 (Surgical Anesthesia), the patient is unconscious and immobile

with no pain reflexes; respiration is very regular, and blood pressure is maintained. Stage 4 (Medullary Depression) is characterized by severe respiratory and cardiovascular depression that requires mechanical and pharmacologic support. Without full circulatory and respiratory support, death rapidly ensues.

MODERN GENERAL ANESTHETICS

Clinically, general anesthetics not only produce immobility (relaxation of skeletal muscles), unconsciousness and amnesia, but also analgesia and inhibition of autonomic reflexes. An *ideal* anesthetic drug would also induce rapid and smooth loss of consciousness, be rapidly reversible upon discontinuation, and possess a wide margin of safety. No single currently available anesthetic agent can satisfactorily achieve all five of these desired effects. Therefore, the modern practice of anesthesia relies on the use of a combination of drugs, often including both inhaled and intravenous drugs for what is called *balanced anesthesia*. General anesthetics can broadly be defined by method of administration into inhaled agents and intravenous agents, with subgroups within each class (Figure 15-2).

INHALED ANESTHETICS

There is a clear distinction between volatile and gaseous anesthetics, both of which are administered by inhalation. *Volatile* anesthetics include **halothane**, **desflurane**, **enflurane**, **isoflurane**, and **sevoflurane**. Volatile anesthetics have low vapor pressures and high boiling points. Thus, volatile anesthetics are liquids at room temperature (20°C) and sea level ambient pressure (760 mm Hg), but are easily vaporized. These characteristics make it necessary to administer volatile anesthetics using precision vaporizers. In contrast, *gaseous* anesthetics are gases at room temperature (having high vapor pressures and low boiling points). Because the standard pressure of the total inhaled mixture is atmospheric pressure, the partial pressure may also be expressed as a percentage. Thus, 50% **nitrous oxide** in the inhaled air would have a partial pressure of 380 mm Hg (ie, 50% × 760 mm Hg).

Speed of Induction

The speed of induction of anesthesia is a very important characteristic of anesthetic drugs. Speed of induction depends on both the drug's properties and the patient's clinical condition. Relevant properties include drug solubility, inspired gas partial pressure, ventilation rate, pulmonary blood flow, and arteriovenous concentration gradient.

One of the most important factors influencing the transfer of an anesthetic from the lungs to the arterial blood is the solubility of the drug. The blood:gas partition coefficient is used to describe the solubility of inhaled anesthetics. This ratio is

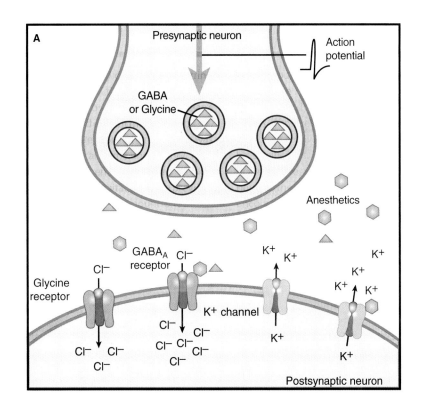

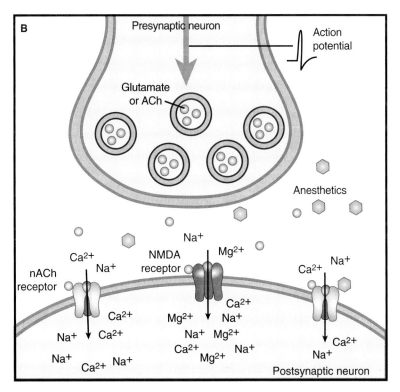

FIGURE 15-1 **Putative targets of anesthetic action. Anesthetic drugs may (A) enhance inhibitory synaptic activity or (B) diminish excitatory activity.** In panel **A**, the anesthetic drugs increase the activity of inhibitory synaptic activity by binding to and opening the channels directly, or binding to the receptor and enhancing the action of the natural ligand for the receptor. Binding of anesthetic increases the flow of positive K^+ ions out of the neuron or increases the flow of negative Cl^- ions into the neuron. The result of either of these processes is hyperpolarization of the postsynaptic neuron. In panel **B**, the anesthetic drugs inhibit opening of excitatory channels by either competitive inhibition with the natural ligand or by allosteric inhibition. Binding of the anesthetic (far right) decreases the flow of positive ions into the postsynaptic neuron. ACh, acetylcholine; GABA, γ-aminobutyric acid; nACh, nicotinic acetylcholine.

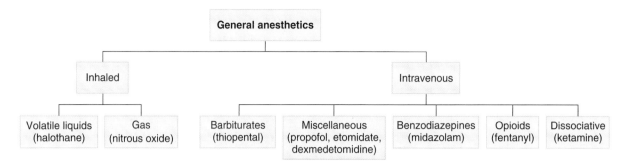

FIGURE 15-2 **General anesthetics are divided into two major subgroups based on route of delivery.** Subclasses of inhaled and intravenous agents are listed with prototype agents in parentheses.

the concentration of the drug in the blood to its concentration in the gas that is in contact with the blood when the partial pressure in both compartments is equal. The more rapidly the drug equilibrates with blood, the more quickly the drug passes into the brain to produce anesthetic effects. Figure 15-3 illustrates that drugs with low blood:gas partition coefficients (eg, nitrous oxide) equilibrate more rapidly than those with higher blood solubility (eg, halothane). Thus, anesthetic drugs with lower blood:gas partition coefficients will have a more rapid onset of action as well as rate of recovery (see below) compared to those with higher coefficients. Table 15-1 shows partition coefficients for inhalation anesthetics.

A high partial pressure of the gas in the lungs results in more rapid achievement of anesthetic levels in the blood. This effect can be exploited by initially administering gas concentrations higher than those required for maintaining anesthesia in order to increase the rate of anesthesia induction by increasing the rate of transfer into the blood. For inhaled anesthetics that have a relatively slow onset (such as halothane or isoflurane), a

higher percent concentration (3-4%) is administered initially to increase the rate of induction and then reduced (to 1-2%) for maintenance when adequate anesthesia is achieved. Adding these agents in combination with an even less soluble agent such as nitrous oxide will further reduce the time required for loss of consciousness.

The greater the ventilation rate, the more rapid is the rise in alveolar and blood partial pressure of the agent and the onset of anesthesia. High ventilation rates can be achieved by mechanical or assisted ventilation via an endotracheal tube (intubation).

At high pulmonary blood flows, the gas partial pressure in the blood rises at a slower rate because a larger volume of blood is exposed to the anesthetic gas in the lungs; thus, the onset of anesthesia is delayed. At low pulmonary blood flow rates, the rate of rise of arterial tension of inhaled anesthetics is increased and onset of anesthesia is faster.

The last variable that affects the speed of anesthetic induction is the arteriovenous concentration gradient. Uptake of

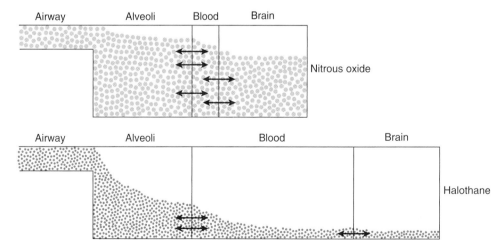

FIGURE 15-3 **Why induction of anesthesia is slower with more soluble anesthetic gases.** In this schematic diagram, solubility in blood is represented by the relative size of the blood compartment (the more soluble, the larger the compartment). Relative partial pressures of the agents in the compartments are indicated by the degree of filling of each compartment. For a given concentration or partial pressure of the two anesthetic gases in the inspired air, it will take much longer for the blood partial pressure of the more soluble gas (halothane) to rise to the same partial pressure as in the alveoli. Since the concentration of the anesthetic agent in the brain can rise no faster than the concentration in the blood, the onset of anesthesia will be slower with halothane than with nitrous oxide (the less soluble gas).

TABLE 15-1 Properties of some inhaled anesthetics.

Anesthetic	Blood: Gas Partition Coefficient[a]	Minimal Alveolar Concentration (MAC%)[b]	Comments
Halothane	2.30	0.75	Medium rate of onset and recovery
Isoflurane	1.40	1.4	Medium rate of onset and recovery
Enflurane	1.80	1.7	Medium rate of onset and recovery
Sevoflurane	0.69	2.0	Rapid onset and recovery; unstable in soda-lime
Desflurane	0.42	6.5	Low volatility; poor induction agent; rapid recovery
Nitrous oxide	0.47	> 100	Incomplete anesthetic; rapid onset and recovery

[a]Partition coefficients (at 37°C) are from multiple literature sources.
[b]MAC is the anesthetic concentration that produces immobility in 50% of patients exposed to a noxious stimulus such as a surgical incision.

soluble anesthetics into highly perfused tissues may decrease gas tension in mixed venous blood. This can influence the rate of onset of anesthesia because achievement of equilibrium is dependent on the difference in anesthetic tension between arterial and venous blood. The greater the difference in anesthetic tensions between arterial and venous blood, the more has been taken up by viscera, muscle, etc, and the more time it will take to achieve equilibrium with brain tissue.

Dose-Response Characteristics

The potency of inhaled anesthetics is best measured by the minimum alveolar anesthetic concentration (MAC). The MAC is defined as the alveolar concentration required to eliminate the response to a standardized painful stimulus (eg, surgical incision) in 50% of patients. The higher the MAC of a given anesthetic, the *lower* its potency. Each inhaled anesthetic has a defined average MAC (Table 15-1), though this value varies depending on the patient's age and cardiovascular status, as well as use of adjuvant drugs. MACs for infants and older adults are lower than those for adolescents and young adults. When several anesthetic agents are used simultaneously, their MAC values are additive.

Termination of Inhaled Anesthetic Action

Inhaled anesthetics are primarily terminated by redistribution of the drug from the brain to the blood followed by elimination of the drug through the lungs. Like induction of anesthesia, the rate of recovery from anesthesia is faster with drugs with low blood:gas partition coefficients (ie, low blood solubility) than with anesthetics with high partition coefficients. This important property has led to the introduction of several newer inhaled anesthetics such as desflurane and sevoflurane that, because of their low blood:gas partition coefficients, are characterized by considerably shorter recovery times than older agents. Some volatile liquids such as halothane are also partly eliminated by metabolism in the liver. While metabolism has only a minor influence on the speed of recovery, it can play a significant role in the toxicity of these anesthetics.

Pharmacodynamics

Organ system related effects of inhaled anesthetics are dependent upon the drug and the system. In the CNS, inhaled anesthetics decrease brain metabolic rate and generally decrease blood flow within the brain. Volatile anesthetics reduce vascular resistance. The ultimate effect on cerebral blood flow is dependent upon the anesthetic concentration delivered. Nitrous oxide does not reduce vascular resistance and may increase cerebral blood flow, which can increase intracranial pressure. High concentrations of enflurane may cause spike-and-wave activity and muscle twitching, but this effect is unique to this drug. Although nitrous oxide has low anesthetic potency (ie, a high MAC), it exerts marked analgesic and amnestic actions when provided as a gas mixed 50/50 with oxygen.

In the cardiovascular system, halothane, enflurane, isoflurane, desflurane, and sevoflurane all depress normal cardiac contractility. All inhaled volatile anesthetics decrease mean arterial pressure (MAP) in direct proportion to their alveolar concentration. For enflurane and halothane, the decrease in MAP is related to their myocardial depression. In contrast, isoflurane, desflurane, and sevoflurane decrease MAP by peripheral vasodilation. Nitrous oxide is less likely to lower blood pressure than other inhaled anesthetics. Halothane, and to a lesser extent other volatile anesthetics, may sensitize the myocardium to the arrhythmogenic effects of catecholamines. Most inhaled agents also decrease blood flow to the liver and kidney.

In the respiratory system, all volatile anesthetics cause varying degrees of bronchodilation, yet they may also cause airway irritation. Nitrous oxide causes minimal airway irritation. With the exception of nitrous oxide, all inhaled anesthetics increase respiratory rate, but cause a dose-dependent decrease in tidal volume and minute ventilation. This leads to an increase in arterial carbon dioxide (CO_2). Because volatile anesthetics reduce the ventilatory response to increased CO_2 blood levels and raise the apneic threshold, these agents raise both the $PaCO_2$ required for CO_2-driven respiratory stimulation and decrease the ventilatory response to hypoxia. Inhaled anesthetics also depress mucociliary function, resulting in mucus pooling and plugging that may develop into postoperative respiratory complications.

Adverse Effects

All inhaled anesthetics can produce some carbon monoxide (CO) from their interaction with strong bases in dry carbon dioxide absorbers. Desflurane produces the most CO. Carbon monoxide binds to hemoglobin with an affinity 230 times that of oxygen, reducing the ability of red blood cells to deliver oxygen to peripheral tissues.

In susceptible individuals exposed to volatile anesthetics while undergoing general anesthesia, malignant hyperthermia is a rare but serious hazard. Malignant hyperthermia is an inheritable genetic disorder that results in uncontrolled calcium release from the sarcoplasmic reticulum in skeletal muscle when there is exposure to some triggering agent. This hypercatabolic state presents as tachycardia, fever, rigid muscles, and metabolic acidosis. Use of the depolarizing muscle relaxant **succinylcholine** (Chapter 5) with volatile anesthetics is a common trigger for malignant hyperthermia. Treatment includes administration of **dantrolene** (Chapter 33) to reduce calcium release from the sarcoplasmic reticulum and decrease skeletal muscle contractions and hyperthermia.

A small subset of individuals previously exposed to halothane may develop fulminant hepatic failure (severe hepatic necrosis in the absence of preexisting liver disease). The mechanisms underlying halothane hepatotoxicity remain unclear, but may include the formation of reactive metabolites that either cause direct hepatocellular damage or initiate immune-mediated responses.

Last, prolonged exposure to nitrous oxide decreases methionine synthase activity, which could cause megaloblastic anemia.

INTRAVENOUS ANESTHETICS

Intravenous nonopioid anesthetics play an essential role in the practice of modern anesthesia. They are used to facilitate rapid induction of anesthesia and have replaced inhalation as the preferred method of anesthesia induction in most settings except for pediatric anesthesia. However, similar to the inhaled agents, the currently available intravenous anesthetics are not ideal drugs in the sense of producing *all and only* the five desired effects of anesthesia (immobility, unconsciousness, amnesia, analgesia, and inhibition of autonomic reflexes). Consequently, balanced anesthesia is generally used to minimize unwanted effects. Intravenous anesthetics used for induction of general anesthesia are lipophilic and therefore preferentially partition into highly perfused lipophilic tissues (brain, spinal cord), which accounts for their rapid onset of action. Regardless of the extent and speed of their metabolism, termination of the effect of a single bolus is determined by redistribution of the drug into less perfused and inactive tissues such as skeletal muscle and fat. Thus, all drugs used for induction of anesthesia have a similar duration of action when administered as a single bolus dose despite significant differences in their metabolism. Characteristics of selected intravenous anesthetics are summarized in Table 15-2.

Barbiturates

Historically, barbiturates played a critical role as anesthetic agents. Now, the use of **thiopental** and **methohexital** for induction of general anesthesia and for short surgical procedures has

---

TABLE 15-2 Characteristics of intravenous anesthetics.

Drug	Induction and Recovery	Comments
Dexmedetomidine	Rapid onset and recovery	Resembles physiologic sleep Bradycardia and hypotension
Etomidate	Rapid onset and moderately fast recovery	Minimal change in cardiac function or respiratory rate No analgesic properties
Ketamine	Rapid onset and recovery	Cardiovascular stimulation Increased cerebral blood flow Emergence reactions impair recovery
Methohexital	Rapid onset and rapid recovery	Respiratory and circulatory depressants
Midazolam	Rapid onset and recovery Flumazenil reversal available	Marked amnestic, anxiolytic, and sedative effects
Propofol	Rapid onset and rapid recovery	Hypotension Useful antiemetic action

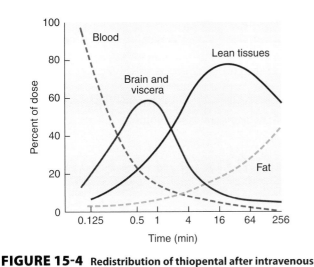

FIGURE 15-4 Redistribution of thiopental after intravenous bolus injection. Induction of anesthesia occurs following distribution of the drug from the blood to the central nervous system (CNS) and termination occurs following redistribution of the drug from the CNS to other tissues. Redistribution curves for bolus administration of other intravenous anesthetics are similar. Note that the time axis is not linear. The order of distribution into the tissues during the accumulation phase parallels the loss of the drug from these tissues during the elimination phase. Drug disappears from the blood, then the brain and viscera, next the lean tissues, and finally the fat. Individuals with lower lean body mass to body fat ratios have larger volumes of distribution and longer half-lives for these drugs. Thus, elimination of these drugs may be longer for individuals with higher fat percentages.

mostly been replaced by **propofol** (see below). Thiopental and methohexital have high lipid solubility, which promotes rapid entry into the brain and results in surgical anesthesia in one circulation time (< 1 minute). Their anesthetic effects are terminated by redistribution from the brain to other highly perfused tissues (Figure 15-4), but hepatic metabolism is required for elimination from the body. Barbiturates are respiratory and circulatory depressants. Because they depress cerebral blood flow, they can also decrease intracranial pressure. Finally, barbiturate-induced histamine release is occasionally observed. Barbiturates are discussed in greater detail in Chapter 13.

Propofol

In most countries, propofol has largely replaced barbiturates as the most frequently administered drug for induction of anesthesia. Propofol produces anesthesia as rapidly as the intravenous barbiturates, and recovery is more rapid. Propofol has antiemetic actions, and recovery is not delayed after prolonged infusion. The drug is a common component of balanced anesthesia and as an anesthetic in outpatient surgery. Propofol is also effective in producing prolonged sedation in patients in critical care settings to mitigate the pain and stress of uncomfortable procedures such as tracheal intubation and physical restraint.

Propofol may cause marked hypotension during induction of anesthesia, and is a respiratory depressant. Total body clearance of propofol is greater than hepatic blood flow,

suggesting that its elimination includes other mechanisms besides metabolism by liver enzymes. **Fospropofol,** a water-soluble prodrug form, is broken down in the body by alkaline phosphatase to form propofol. However, onset and recovery are both slower than propofol. Although fospropofol appears to cause less pain at injection sites than propofol, many patients experience paresthesias.

Benzodiazepines

Benzodiazepines commonly used in the perioperative period include **midazolam, lorazepam,** and less frequently, **diazepam.** Midazolam is widely used adjunctively with inhaled anesthetics and intravenous opioids. The onset of its CNS effects is slower than that of thiopental, and it has a longer duration of action. Cases of severe postoperative respiratory depression have occurred. Administration of **flumazenil,** a selective antagonist at the benzodiazepine recognition site on the $GABA_A$/benzodiazepine receptor complex, can terminate the actions of all benzodiazepines. Benzodiazepines are discussed in Chapter 13.

Opioids

Opioids, such as **fentanyl** and **morphine,** are routinely used as postoperative analgesic agents, but these drugs are distinct from general anesthetics and hypnotics. Even when high doses of opioids are administered, recall cannot be reliably prevented (ie, amnesia is not produced) unless hypnotic agents such as benzodiazepines are also used. As part of a balanced anesthesia regimen, opioids are used intraoperatively, which may be especially helpful in high-risk patients less likely to survive a full general anesthetic. Fentanyl may be combined with **droperidol** and nitrous oxide to provide "neuroleptanesthesia," a state of analgesia and amnesia. Newer opioids related to fentanyl have been introduced for intravenous anesthesia. **Alfentanil** and **remifentanil** have been used for induction of anesthesia. Recovery from remifentanil is faster than recovery from other opioids used in anesthesia because of its rapid metabolism by blood and tissue esterases. The actions of all opioids can be terminated by administration of the opioid antagonist **naloxone.** Opioids are discussed in Chapter 20.

Etomidate

Etomidate affords rapid induction with minimal change in cardiac function or respiratory rate and has a short duration of action. The drug has hypnotic, but not analgesic effects. Its primary advantage is in induction of anesthesia for patients with limited cardiac or respiratory reserve. Etomidate may cause pain and myoclonus on injection and nausea postoperatively. Prolonged administration may cause adrenal suppression.

Dexmedetomidine

Dexmedetomidine is a centrally acting α_2-adrenergic agonist that has analgesic and hypnotic actions when used intravenously. The drug is rapidly cleared, resulting in a short elimination half-life. Dexmedetomidine's sedative effect has a different quality than that produced by other intravenous anesthetics in that it more completely resembles a physiologic sleep state through activation of endogenous sleep pathways. This drug is used mainly for short-term sedation of intubated and ventilated patients in ICU settings. When used in general anesthesia, dexmedetomidine decreases dosage requirements for both inhaled and intravenous anesthetics.

Ketamine

Ketamine produces a state of "dissociative anesthesia" or a cataleptic state in which the patient's eyes remain open with a slow nystagmic gaze. Ketamine is a chemical variant of the psychotomimetic agent **phencyclidine** (PCP). Though its exact mechanisms of action are unknown, the drug's major effects are likely due to inhibition of NMDA receptor-mediated glutamate transmission. Ketamine is a cardiovascular stimulant, and this action may lead to an increase in intracranial pressure. Emergence reactions from ketamine-induced anesthesia can include disorientation, excitation, and hallucinations. These effects can be lessened by preoperative use of benzodiazepines.

CLINICAL USE OF ANESTHETICS

The choice of anesthetic technique is determined by the type of diagnostic, therapeutic, or surgical intervention that the patient needs. For minor surgeries or invasive diagnostic procedures, oral or parenteral sedatives can be combined with local anesthetics (Chapter 16) in a technique termed "monitored anesthesia care." These techniques provide profound analgesia, but retain the patient's ability to maintain a patent airway and to respond to verbal commands. One approach to monitored anesthesia care is "conscious sedation," a technique that produces alleviation of anxiety and pain with less alteration to the level of consciousness by using smaller doses of sedative medications. Therapists working in certain critical care settings may work with patients under conscious sedation. For example, it is not uncommon in burn units for conscious sedation (sometimes also referred to as procedural sedation) to be induced to minimize the patient's pain and awareness solely for the purpose of range of motion of affected body segments.

"Deep sedation" is similar to a light state of general anesthesia characterized by decreased consciousness from which the patient is not easily aroused. The transition from deep sedation to general anesthesia is fluid and can be difficult to define. Because deep sedation is accompanied by loss of verbal responsiveness, protective airway reflexes, and the ability to maintain a patent airway, it may be indistinguishable from general anesthesia. A specialized form of sedation is occasionally required in the ICU, when patients are under severe stress and require mechanical ventilation for prolonged periods. In this situation, sedative-hypnotic drugs and low doses of intravenous anesthetics may be combined. For more invasive surgical procedures, anesthesia may begin with a preoperative

sedative (Chapter 13), be induced with an intravenous anesthetic agent, and then be maintained with a combination of inhaled and/or intravenous anesthetics. In summary, the choice of the particular agents used vary depending on each patient case, with the ultimate goal to produce the depth of anesthesia needed and to achieve this safely despite frequent medical problems and comorbidities.

REHABILITATION RELEVANCE

Therapists are not usually involved in working directly with patients under general anesthesia. However, therapists must have a basic understanding of anesthetic agents' mechanisms of action, subsequent residual effects, and how these drugs may influence rehabilitation outcomes for several days *after* their use.

- Following any procedure with general anesthesia, **sedation** and **confusion** are predictable consequences that can decrease patient participation in therapy and increase fall risk due to delayed psychomotor responses. Goals for initial sessions should be adjusted accordingly. Over time, the influence of anesthetic agents should dissipate. However, older individuals and those with more body fat are more likely to take longer to recover from anesthetic effects. Due to the higher frequency of outpatient surgeries and shorter hospital stays, postsurgical instructions and task goals should be discussed with patients prior to surgery, if possible.
- **Asthenia** may occur following administration of these drugs and/or the surgical procedure. As above, goals should be adjusted accordingly and patients should be assessed for fall risk.
- **Amnesia** following general anesthesia may decrease patients' ability to remember instructions provided by healthcare professionals. Anticipate and provide frequent reminders for critical information such as the necessity of using a call button to request assistance, weightbearing status, or activity precautions.
- Following exposure to any of the inhaled volatile general anesthetics, **hypoxemia** may result from increased CO in the blood, which decreases oxygen-carrying capacity of red blood cells. Individuals with pulmonary or cardiac comorbidities should be monitored closely for cyanosis or activity intolerance because pulse oximetry is inaccurate and unreliable in this situation. Aerobic goals should be decreased until the condition has been appropriately managed.
- **Decreased aerobic capacity** may result from cardiac and pulmonary depression. Several anesthetic agents increase the apneic threshold, resulting in hypercapnia and hypoxemia. Aerobic goals should be appropriately modified and oxygen saturation closely monitored. If patients desaturate at rest or with activity, therapists should alert the medical team.
- **Malignant hyperthermia** is rare, but may be triggered by certain general anesthetics. A rapid rise in body temperature with sweating, flushed skin, muscle rigidity, and tachycardia requires immediate medical attention because this is a life-threating condition.

- **Hypertension** and **tachycardia** may result from ketamine. Careful monitoring of vital signs should be conducted at initial evaluation if this intravenous anesthetic was used.
- Unpleasant **emergence reactions** are possible following recovery when ketamine is used as an intravenous anesthetic. These reactions may cause the patient to be fearful and confused. Additional manifestations include hallucinations and distorted auditory, visual, or tactile sensations. If the patient presents with any of these manifestations, a nurse or physician should be contacted immediately.

CASE CONCLUSION

The physical therapist documented in the initial evaluation that the patient was difficult to arouse and had limited ability to follow commands due to profound sedation. On postoperative day two, A.F. was alert and actively participated in out-of-bed activities and gait training with the therapist. The patient stated that she did not remember any interactions with the therapist the previous day. The therapist reassured the patient and concluded that she had still been recovering from the effects of anesthesia. Several factors contributed to A.F.'s reduced physical and cognitive function during the initial physical therapy session. These include the type of balanced anesthesia regimen she received, prolonged elimination time due to her age, and the trauma associated with major orthopedic surgery. By the end of today's therapy session, the patient required minimal assistance to get out of bed, transfer to standing in a front-wheeled walker, and ambulate 50 ft within her non-weightbearing precautions. The therapist documented the patient's progress and followed up with the discharge planner to recommend that the patient be discharged home with home health services.

CHAPTER 15 QUESTIONS

1. Which of the following is an inhaled general anesthetic that carries the highest risk of carbon monoxide exposure?

   a. Desflurane
   b. Propofol
   c. Etomidate
   d. Halothane

2. Which of the following is an intravenous general anesthetic that has no analgesic properties?

   a. Propofol
   b. Etomidate
   c. Midazolam
   d. Enflurane

3. Which of the following is an intravenous general anesthetic that is an agonist at α_2 receptors within the central nervous system?

   a. Midazolam
   b. Methohexital
   c. Dexmetomidine
   d. Sevoflurane

4. Which of the following is the stage of general anesthesia in which pulmonary and cardiovascular depression occurs?

   a. Disinhibition
   b. Medullary depression
   c. Surgical anesthesia
   d. Analgesia

5. Based on the blood:gas partition coefficient, which of the following is a general inhaled anesthetic with the *slowest* onset for anesthesia?

   a. Isoflurane (1.40)
   b. Nitrous oxide (0.47)
   c. Enflurane (1.80)
   d. Desflurane (0.42)

6. The minimum alveolar concentration (MAC) represents which of the following?

   a. Concentration at which 50% of the population loses consciousness
   b. Concentration at which 50% of the population demonstrates amnesia
   c. Concentration at which 50% of the population demonstrates analgesia
   d. Concentration at which 50% of the population remains immobile to noxious stimulus

7. Which of the following is *not* an adverse effect associated with inhaled general anesthetics?

   a. Sedation
   b. Hypertension
   c. Asthenia
   d. Confusion

8. Which of the following is an intravenous general anesthetic whose mechanism of action is proposed to be inhibition of NMDA receptors?

   a. Ketamine
   b. Propofol
   c. Halothane
   d. Thiopental

9. The combination of inhaled and intravenous general anesthetics to provide the desired clinical effect is defined as which of the following?
    a. Neuroleptanesthesia
    b. Dissociative anesthesia
    c. Conscious sedation
    d. Balanced anesthesia

10. Which of the following adverse events presents as hyperthermia and tachycardia with increased muscle rigidity and is reversed by dantrolene?
    a. Malignant hyperthermia
    b. Emergence reaction
    c. Asthenia
    d. Hallucination

Local Anesthetics

CASE STUDY

K.P. is a 71-year-old retired accountant who had a right total knee arthroplasty (TKA) yesterday afternoon. To optimize pain control and promote early mobilization, the hospital follows a multimodal analgesia protocol in the perioperative period for individuals undergoing joint replacements. This protocol involves nonsteroidal anti-inflammatory drugs and acetaminophen, femoral nerve block with bupivacaine, and opiates as needed for additional pain control. On postoperative day one, the physical therapist enters the patient's room to initiate an evaluation. She finds K.P. seated at the edge of the bed and attempting to stand with the front-wheeled walker. The therapist asks the patient to permit her to assist, but to first allow her to don the knee immobilizer. The patient gets upset and states that he urgently needs to use the bathroom and does not want to waste time. The therapist explains that if he were to attempt standing without the knee immobilizer, he would risk a fall to the floor because of the femoral nerve block that was administered.

REHABILITATION FOCUS

Local anesthetics have applications in many different clinical settings. These drugs share a similar mechanism of action and their generic drug names end in "-caine." These drugs may be applied topically to relieve pain from minor skin injuries or irritations. Local anesthetics such as lidocaine may be infiltrated locally prior to suturing wounds. These drugs are used for inpatient and outpatient day surgeries as the sole form of anesthesia, in combination with general anesthesia, and/or to provide postoperative analgesia. When administered via portable infusion pumps, local anesthetics may be used in ambulatory patients with various chronic pain states. Physical therapists may also directly apply local anesthetics either topically or transdermally for pain management in musculoskeletal disorders (eg, tendonitis, bursitis).

Use of local anesthetics for acute and chronic pain is increasing because they have demonstrated increased pain control and improved functional outcomes under many different clinical scenarios. These drugs are being substituted for opioids in both acute and chronic pain control because local anesthetics have minimal abuse potential. Physical therapists should be aware that patients with postsurgical indwelling spinal catheters delivering a local anesthetic could have temporary motor and sensory loss in the affected extremities. Before attempting rehabilitation interventions, thorough motor and sensory assessment is vital to ensure safe outcomes. Because of the seriousness of systemic adverse effects associated with local anesthetics, therapists should also be alert for signs and symptoms of central nervous system (CNS) effects in patients receiving these drugs.

BACKGROUND

Local anesthetics block sensory transmission from a specific area of the body to the CNS. Their primary use is to temporarily and reversibly block the sensation of pain, although all peripheral sensations are blocked. Local anesthesia differs from general anesthesia, which is delivered to the systemic circulation in order to depress the CNS. With local anesthesia, the drug is delivered directly to the target organ—*not* to the systemic circulation. The systemic circulation serves only to decrease and terminate the effect of local anesthetics. Local anesthetics are chemically similar agents that block the sodium channels of excitable membranes. Because these drugs can be administered by topical application or by injection into the target area, the anesthetic effect can be fairly well restricted to a localized area (eg, cornea, foot). Even when these drugs are given in the vicinity of the spinal cord (eg, epidural block), the anesthesia is still considered local because impulse transmissions from only a specific spinal cord level are blocked. Figure 16-1 categorizes local anesthetics based on their chemical structure and duration of clinical effect.

Chemistry and Pharmacokinetics

Local anesthetics in clinical use are esters or amides, meaning that the bond linking the lipophilic group to the hydrophilic

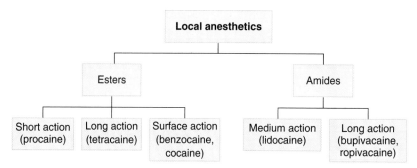

FIGURE 16-1 **Local anesthetics classified by chemical class (ester or amide) and duration of action.** Common agents are in parentheses.

group is either an ester (carbon-oxygen) or an amide (hydrogen-nitrogen-carbon) linkage. These drugs are weak bases that are formulated into salts to increase solubility and stability. Thus, these drugs exist in one of two states, an uncharged base or a cation, based on their pK$_a$. As described below, both states are important in their mechanism of action. Local anesthetics have varying degrees of lipid solubility. More lipid-soluble drugs, such as **tetracaine** and **ropivacaine**, are more potent, have a longer duration of action, and require more time to achieve analgesia or anesthesia compared to more water-soluble drugs such as **lidocaine** or **procaine**. Many short-acting local anesthetics are readily absorbed into the blood from the injection site after administration.

Lipid solubility and local blood flow at the application site determine the elimination half-lives (eg, 1.6 hours for lidocaine and up to 4.2 hours for ropivacaine) of local anesthetics. These drugs have a longer clinical effect when blood flow to the region of interest is *lower*. Thus, a vasoconstrictor (usually an adrenergic α-receptor agonist such as epinephrine or phenylephrine) is often administered with the local anesthetic agent to prolong

the anesthetic effect. The vasoconstrictor also retards systemic absorption of the anesthetic from the injection site and may reduce the potential for systemic toxicity. The longer-acting agents (eg, ropivacaine and **bupivacaine**) are less dependent on the coadministration of vasoconstrictors. **Cocaine**, a surface action local anesthetic, has intrinsic vasoconstrictive activity and thus is not administered with a vasoconstrictor. Amide-based local anesthetics undergo hepatic metabolism, whereas ester-based drugs are metabolized in the plasma. All local anesthetics are metabolized to more water-soluble compounds for excretion in the urine.

Mechanism of Action

Local anesthetics block voltage-dependent sodium channels and reduce the influx of sodium ions, thereby preventing depolarization of the membrane and blocking conduction of the action potential. Figure 16-2 illustrates how local anesthetics gain access to their receptors from the cytoplasmic surface or from within the plasma membrane. In its uncharged form, the

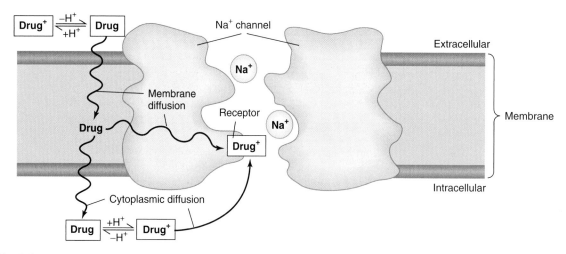

FIGURE 16-2 **Schematic diagram of the sodium channel in an excitable membrane (eg, an axon) and paths by which a local anesthetic molecule (Drug/Drug⁺) may reach the receptor.** The local anesthetic diffuses through the plasma membrane in its uncharged form (Drug). In the aqueous extracellular and intracellular spaces, the charged form (Drug⁺) is also present. The local anesthetic may reach the receptor within the sodium channel either by diffusion through the membrane to the inside of the sodium channel, or through the cytoplasm after becoming charged. The charged form is the more effective channel blocking entity.

drug diffuses within the membrane to the receptor site where the drug ionizes into a cation (Drug$^+$) and blocks the receptor. Alternatively, the drug may enter the cytoplasm, become charged, then diffuse to and block the receptor within the channel. In either scenario, the more lipid-soluble (uncharged) form reaches effective intracellular concentrations more rapidly than the charged form. Once inside the cytoplasm of the axon, the charged form of the drug is the more effective blocking entity. Thus, both the uncharged and the charged forms play important roles—the first in reaching the receptor site and the second in causing the effect. When the drug is bound to the receptor site on the sodium channel, the channel is maintained in a blocked condition. By blocking a sufficient number of sodium channels, the local anesthetic prevents action potential propagation along the affected portion of the axon. The affinity of the receptor site for the local anesthetic is also a function of the state of the sodium channel, whether it is resting, open, or inactivated, and therefore follows the same rules of use dependence and voltage dependence that were described for the sodium channel-blocking antiarrhythmic drugs (Chapter 10). If other factors are equal, rapidly firing fibers are usually blocked before slowly firing fibers because the drug has increased access to rapidly opening channels. Other ions can influence local anesthetic action by their effect on the membrane potential. High extracellular K$^+$ concentration enhances local anesthetic activity. In contrast, elevated H$^+$ concentration (as would occur in an abscess) or increased extracellular Ca^{2+} concentration inhibits the effect of local anesthetics.

Factors Affecting Block

Nerve fibers have different sensitivities to local anesthetics depending on their firing rate, diameter, myelination, and anatomic location (Table 16-1). Sensory fibers are usually blocked more than motor fibers since they fire more rapidly. Because nociceptive transmission along A delta and C fibers is typically at higher frequency, local anesthetics may block these fibers earlier and at lower concentrations. In general, smaller diameter fibers are blocked more readily than larger diameter fibers, and myelinated fibers are blocked more easily than unmyelinated fibers. Fibers located in the periphery of a thick nerve bundle are blocked sooner than those within the core because they are exposed earlier to higher concentrations of the anesthetic.

Methods of Administration and Clinical Uses

Local anesthetics may be administered in a number of ways for conditions ranging from minor skin irritations to surgical procedures (Table 16-2). Topically, these drugs are available in formulations such as creams, sprays, or ointments to relieve pain or itching from minor burns, insect bites, or rashes. The 5% lidocaine adhesive patch (Lidoderm) is FDA-approved for the treatment of postherpetic neuralgia (pain after shingles). Physical therapists are more likely to encounter patients wearing lidocaine patches (which may be worn up to 12 hours per day) for their off-label use to decrease pain due to chronic musculoskeletal or postsurgical pain. Despite being called a patch, the lidocaine patch is actually a topical (not transdermal) medication, meaning that there is theoretically limited drug penetration to the tissues and circulation below the skin. In an effort to optimize therapeutic efficacy, mixtures of topical local anesthetics have been developed. The term "eutectic" refers to a mixture of components that has a lower melting temperature than the individual components—thus the *intention* is to enhance the flux of the drugs to the target area. EMLA (eutectic mixture of local anesthetics) is a mixture of lidocaine and **prilocaine** that is applied topically to numb unbroken skin prior to certain procedures (eg, venipuncture or placement of intravenous catheters in children). Finally, topical local anesthetics are used to anesthetize the cornea and oral tissue for procedures in optometry and dentistry, respectively. Cocaine's use is largely restricted to topical anesthesia

TABLE 16-1 Relative size and susceptibility of different types of nerve fibers to local anesthetics.

Fiber Type	Function	Diameter (µm)	Myelination	Conduction Velocity (m/s)	Sensitivity to Block
Type A					
Alpha	Proprioception, motor	12-20	Heavy	70-120	+
Beta	Touch, pressure	5-12	Heavy	30-70	++
Gamma	Muscle spindles	3-6	Heavy	15-30	++
Delta	Pain, temperature	2-5	Heavy	5-25	+++
Type B	Preganglionic autonomic	< 3	Light	3-15	++++
Type C					
Dorsal root	Pain	0.4-1.2	None	0.5-2.3	++++
Sympathetic	Postganglionic	0.3-1.3	None	0.7-2.3	++++

TABLE 16-2 Methods of administration and clinical uses of local anesthetics.

Method of Administration	Description	Clinical Uses
Topical	Drug applied directly to skin, mucous membrane, cornea, and other regions to produce analgesia	Minor surface irritation or injury (minor burn, abrasion, insect bite) Minor surgical procedures (wound cleansing, piercing, circumcision)
Transdermal	Drug applied to skin with the goal for the drug to be absorbed into underlying tissues May be enhanced by use of electrical current (iontophoresis) or ultrasound (phonophoresis)	Painful subcutaneous structures (tendons, bursae, soft tissue) Dermatological surgeries
Infiltration anesthesia	Drug injected directly into selected tissue and allowed to diffuse to sensory nerve endings within that tissue	Suturing of lacerated skin
Peripheral nerve block	Drug injected close to or within the nerve trunk so that transmission along the peripheral nerve is interrupted	Dental procedures Total joint arthroplasties Minor surgical procedures Some chronic conditions (eg, interstitial cystitis) Specific nerve pain (eg, brachial plexus)
Central nerve blockade	Drug injected within spaces surrounding the spinal cord (epidural) or within the spinal cord (spinal or intrathecal block)	Obstetric procedures Alternative to general anesthesia for lumbar surgery and hip or knee arthroplasty Relief of acute or chronic pain
Sympathetic block	Selective interruption of sympathetic efferent discharge (not used to provide analgesia)	Complex regional pain syndrome (CRPS)
Intravenous regional anesthesia (Bier Block)	Anesthetic injected into peripheral distal vein in selected arm or leg with a proximally placed tourniquet to isolate the limb circulation	Short surgical procedures (< 45 min) such as those involving distal upper or lower extremity open or closed reductions

for the ear, nose, and throat. While its ability to vasoconstrict has the advantage of decreasing bleeding during minor procedures, its use has declined due to its abuse potential and status as a controlled substance (Chapter 21).

Transdermal delivery of local anesthetics can be enhanced using iontophoresis or phonophoresis to provide an analgesic effect at sites that are not anatomically deep to the application site. Novel systems are in development that use ultrasound to trigger release of local anesthetics encapsulated into liposomes, though concern regarding potential tissue or systemic toxicity needs to be resolved.

A peripheral nerve block is a form of regional anesthesia that involves injection of local anesthetics into or near a nerve supplying the area of interest. Two of the most frequently used peripheral nerve blocks are femoral nerve blocks and brachial plexus blocks. Given as a single injection, multiple injections, or continuous infusions, nerve blocks are common in many surgical procedures ranging from tooth extractions and orofacial laceration repair to total joint replacements. A peripheral nerve block may also be used to treat pain conditions that are specific to one nerve. For example, a trigeminal nerve block can provide temporary hemifacial anesthesia as a component of treatment for trigeminal neuralgia.

Central nerve blockade is another form of regional anesthesia that includes both epidural and spinal blocks (Figure 16-3). When local anesthetics are injected *extradurally*, it is referred to

as an epidural block. When these drugs are injected *intrathecally* into the cerebrospinal fluid (CSF), it is referred to as a spinal block. Epidural and spinal anesthesia are used for a wide variety of gastrointestinal, gynecological, urological, and orthopedic surgical procedures. Postoperatively, slow epidural infusions of local anesthetics at low concentrations have been used successfully for postoperative analgesia (similar to epidural opioid infusions; Chapter 20). However, repeated epidural injection in anesthetic doses may lead to a quickly diminishing response (tachyphylaxis). Epidural administration of local anesthetics also blunts perioperative stress responses and decreases inflammation and platelet aggregation.

Though not as common, *systemic* administration of local anesthetics has limited clinical applications. The use of lidocaine as an antiarrhythmic drug was discussed in Chapter 10. In addition, systemic delivery of local anesthetics is sometimes used to suppress pain processing, which may be especially helpful in the treatment of chronic pain. These drugs may suppress ectopic neuronal discharges at concentrations an order of magnitude *lower* than that required for blockade of action potential propagation in normal nerves. At escalating doses, local anesthetics appear to exert the following systemic actions: (1) low concentrations may preferentially suppress ectopic impulse generation in chronically injured peripheral nerves; (2) moderate concentrations may suppress central sensitization, which would explain therapeutic benefit that may extend beyond the

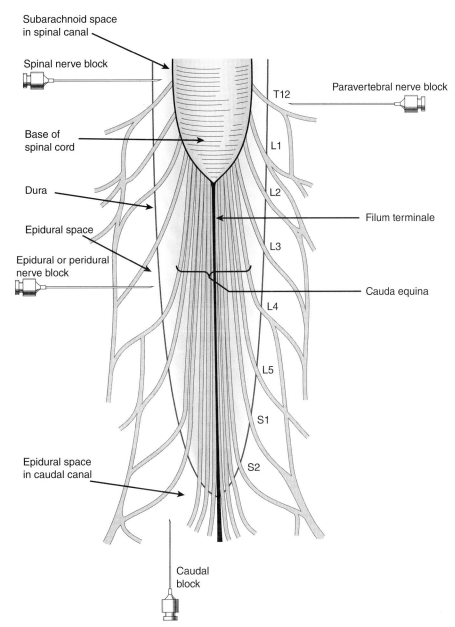

FIGURE 16-3 **Schematic diagram of typical injection sites of local anesthetics in and around the spinal canal.** When local anesthetics are injected extradurally, it is referred to as an epidural block. A caudal block is a specific type of epidural block in which a needle is inserted into the caudal canal via the sacral hiatus. Injections around peripheral nerves are known as perineural blocks (eg, paravertebral block). Injection into the cerebrospinal fluid in the subarachnoid (intrathecal) space is referred to as a spinal block.

anesthetic exposure; and (3) higher concentrations will produce general analgesic effects and may culminate in serious toxicity. At clinically relevant concentrations, local anesthetics demonstrate low affinity for sodium channels, but these drugs also bind and inhibit a multitude of other ion channels. Binding to additional channels may account for their clinical effectiveness that goes beyond analgesia and anesthesia.

Adverse Effects

The intended effect of any administered local anesthetic is to produce a regional response by affecting specifically targeted

nerves. However, these drugs can be absorbed into the general circulation and have effects on other tissues and organs. Systemic effects are most likely to occur if an excess of drug is used, if there is greater absorption of the drug than anticipated, or if the drug is unintentionally injected into the systemic circulation.

The most important toxic effects are in the CNS. All local anesthetics are capable of producing a spectrum of central effects, including light-headedness, sedation, restlessness, confusion, agitation, and nystagmus. At very high doses, tonic-clonic convulsions can occur, which may be followed by coma with respiratory and cardiovascular depression. Spinal anesthesia, especially continuous spinal anesthesia in which a subarachnoid catheter is used to infuse repetitive doses of local anesthetics, has the potential to initiate neuronal injury that is not related to the blockade of sodium channels. Lidocaine has been identified in the majority of these cases. The resulting neuronal injury may result in prolonged or permanent alterations in proprioception, touch, temperature, and muscle weakness. Additionally, transient neurologic syndrome (TNS), which presents as pain and abnormal sensations (dysesthesia) without motor weakness, has been identified with lidocaine use for spinal anesthesia.

High plasma levels of local anesthetics may cause heart block or other cardiac electrical dysfunction in individuals with preexisting cardiac disease. These adverse effects may result in decreased heart rate, decreased force of contraction, and decreased cardiac excitability. Local anesthetics (except cocaine) cause vasodilation, though any drug-induced hypotension may be opposed by baroreceptor reflex responses. **Bupivacaine** has been associated with severe cardiotoxicity, which led to the development of the two enantiomers **levobupivacaine** and ropivacaine that are slightly less cardiotoxic. Both **benzocaine** and prilocaine have the potential to cause methemoglobinemia, a condition in which hemoglobin contains ferric (Fe^{+3}) rather than ferrous (Fe^{+2}) iron, which decreases the oxygen-carrying capacity of red blood cells. Patients with preexisting comorbidities associated with decreased oxygen delivery to peripheral tissues (heart failure, obstructive pulmonary diseases, decreased ventilation capacity) should be monitored for manifestations of hypoxemia.

Finally, the topical application of local anesthetics such as lidocaine is often intended for cutaneous targets, rather than transcutaneous sites. However, low systemic concentrations of lidocaine (~ 3% of applied dose) and its major metabolite have been demonstrated following cutaneous application in normal volunteers. The extent of systemic absorption following cutaneous application depends on location and duration of cutaneous application, concentration of local anesthetic (regardless of whether formulated in a gel, patch, or ointment), and integrity of the skin at the application site.

REHABILITATION RELEVANCE

Although local anesthetics can provide dose-dependent analgesia and local anesthesia, multiple and diverse adverse effects require therapists to understand how these drugs may interfere with rehabilitation outcomes. The adverse effects relevant to rehabilitation depend in part on the specific drug, its method of administration, and its clinical application.

- **Sedation**, **nystagmus**, and **restlessness** may occur when these drugs are administered intrathecally (as a spinal block) or when systemic plasma concentrations achieve toxic concentrations. These effects may decrease cognitive function and increase fall risk. If observed, the therapist should alert appropriate healthcare professionals. If these effects are an expected outcome of their clinical application, the therapist should consider working with the patient at a later time point when drug plasma concentration (and their adverse effects) will be decreased.
- **Dysesthesia** (abnormal sensations) or **hyperesthesia** following spinal anesthesia with lidocaine is rare, but recognized. Physical therapy treatment should be terminated and appropriate healthcare professional contacted.
- Due to their vasodilatory effect, local anesthetics may cause **hypotension** if the drugs are systemically delivered or systemic concentrations reach toxic levels. These drugs have the **potential for cardiac toxicity**, resulting in decreased electrical conduction and stroke volume. Therapists should monitor vital signs and symptoms of activity or orthostatic intolerance closely.
- **Hypoxemia** may result with the use of benzocaine or prilocaine due to methemoglobinemia, which decreases oxygen-carrying capacity of red blood cells. Individuals with pulmonary or cardiac comorbidities should be monitored closely for cyanosis or activity intolerance because pulse oximetry is inaccurate and unreliable in patients with this condition. Aerobic goals should be decreased until the condition has been appropriately managed.
- Temporary **decreased proprioception** or **muscle weakness** may occur following local tissue infiltration of local anesthetics and peripheral or central nerve blocks. The therapist should assess and guard against fall risk in these patients.
- Very rarely, patients recovering from spinal anesthesia with lidocaine present with **prolonged pain (with or without dysesthesia), but without motor deficit**. If noted, the therapist should contact an appropriate healthcare professional as these symptoms may indicate transient neurologic syndrome.
- **Spinal headaches** may occur following intrathecal injection of local anesthetics. The headache is a result of the continued loss of CSF through the thecal membrane at the injection site. This loss of fluid results in pressure differences in the CSF when the patient is vertical, but not horizontal. A spinal headache presents as a severe headache that increases in intensity the longer the patient is standing or sitting, but subsides when the patient lays prone or supine. When identified, the therapist should immediately alert the nurse or physician.

CASE CONCLUSION

Current literature supports the use of femoral nerve blockade (FNB) after TKA because this strategy improves analgesia and significantly reduces intravenous opioid consumption postoperatively. Decreased opiate consumption is especially beneficial since patients experience fewer of the common opiate adverse effects such as nausea, hypotension, respiratory depression, and constipation that can all slow down rehabilitation. In the elderly population, reducing the opiate requirement is also a key component of delirium prevention. FNB can be performed as a one-time injection of a local anesthetic into the peripheral nerve sheath or as a continuous femoral nerve block (CFNB) via indwelling catheter. The local anesthetic temporarily interrupts nerve conduction in sensory nerves—which are more sensitive than motor nerves—producing localized anesthesia and analgesia. However, it has been proposed that the FNB may also reduce pain that is associated with reflex spasms of the quadriceps muscle after TKA. Optimal analgesia after TKA leads to early mobilization and maximization of range of motion, ambulation, return to normalized gait pattern, and reduced hospital length of stay. Though recognized as safe and effective for postoperative analgesia after joint replacements, falls due to quadriceps weakness can occur. Such falls have resulted in wound dehiscence and periprosthetic fractures (requiring reoperation) in patients undergoing TKA with FNB. All healthcare staff must recognize quadriceps weakness after FNB. As a component of fall prevention programs, many hospitals have suggested or mandated the use of knee immobilizers while femoral nerve catheters are in place or until the patient can independently perform a straight leg raise (which may take 1-2 days postsurgery with a single FNB injection). While the soft knee immobilizers are not designed to *prevent* knee buckling, it serves as a kinesthetic and visual reminder to the patient (and therapist) that the affected limb may not be able to support full weightbearing due to quadriceps weakness.

CHAPTER 16 QUESTIONS

1. Which of the following local anesthetics does *not* cause vasodilation?

   a. Cocaine
   b. Lidocaine
   c. Benzocaine
   d. Ropivacaine

2. Which of the following local anesthetics is most likely to cause hypoxemia?

   a. Lidocaine
   b. Prilocaine
   c. Tetracaine
   d. Cocaine

3. The patient is recovering from orthopedic day surgery with an intrathecal injection for local anesthesia. She complains of a headache when standing or sitting, and the headache is relieved when she lies down. The patient may be demonstrating which of the following manifestations?

   a. Migraine headache
   b. Hyperesthesia
   c. Nystagmus
   d. Spinal headache

4. Which form of the local anesthetic is responsible for sodium channel blockade in the plasma membrane?

   a. Nonionized base
   b. Nonionized acid
   c. Ionized base
   d. Ionized acid

5. A local anesthetic enters the sodium channel from which interface?

   a. Extracellular
   b. Intercellular
   c. Paracellular
   d. Cytoplasmic

6. Which nerve fiber type is the *least* susceptible to local anesthetics?

   a. Type B fiber
   b. Type A gamma fiber
   c. Type A alpha fiber
   d. Type C fiber

7. In which of the following states is the sodium channel *least* sensitive to the blockade effect of local anesthetics?

   a. Active state
   b. Resting state
   c. Inactive state
   d. Recovered state

8. Analgesia occurs prior to anesthesia due to the increased sensitivity of which of the following nerve fiber types?

   a. Type A beta fibers
   b. Type A gamma fibers
   c. Type A alpha fibers
   d. Type C fibers

9. The use of local anesthetics to provide anesthesia for suturing a cutaneous wound would be which of the following?

    a. Peripheral nerve block
    b. Transdermal administration
    c. Infiltration anesthesia
    d. Intravenous regional anesthesia

10. Which of the following is *not* an adverse effect associated with systemic administration of lidocaine?

    a. Sedation
    b. Dysesthesia
    c. Hyperesthesia
    d. Hypertension

Pharmacologic Management of Parkinson's Disease and Other Movement Disorders

CASE STUDY

L.S. is a 78-year-old man who was referred to physical therapy after a progressive reduction in his physical capabilities secondary to Parkinson's disease diagnosed 7 years ago. The patient stated that he did not require medication initially, but 6 months ago he was started on a combination of levodopa and carbidopa when his signs and symptoms had worsened and his neurologist felt it was time to begin medication. The patient's chief complaints are generalized stiffness, slow movement, and a resting tremor in his hands and arms. He also feels that he has gotten very weak over the last several months. During the initial evaluation, the physical therapist observed that the patient had a minimal stooped posture. L.S. also had limited passive and active range of motion in bilateral hips and upper extremities in flexion, abduction, and external rotation. His overall functional strength was diminished for his age and he had extremely poor endurance. Upon interview by the therapist, L.S. revealed that he had lost 25 lb over the last 6 months and that his appetite had diminished drastically.

REHABILITATION FOCUS

The major movement disorders include Parkinson's disease, Huntington's disease, Wilson disease, and Tourette syndrome. Table 17-1 defines terms used to describe different types of abnormal movements or signs that may be characteristic of particular movement disorders. Abnormal movements can also be caused by a variety of general medical conditions and certain drugs.

Many of the movement disorders have been attributed to disturbances of the basal ganglia, but the precise function of these anatomic structures is not yet fully understood, and it is not possible to relate individual symptoms or impairments to involvement at specific sites. Furthermore, clinicians must recognize that individuals with the same disease can present very differently in terms of physical manifestations and symptoms and may respond quite differently to drug and rehabilitative therapies.

PATHOPHYSIOLOGY OF PARKINSON'S DISEASE

Parkinson's disease is a common movement disorder that involves dysfunction in the basal ganglia and associated brain structures. Motor signs and symptoms include *r*igidity of skeletal muscles, *a*kinesia (or bradykinesia), *f*lat facies, and *t*remor at rest (mnemonic RAFT). There are also many nonmotor symptoms associated with the disease. These include affective disorders (anxiety or depression), cognitive impairment, personality changes, fatigue, autonomic dysfunction (eg, dysphagia or choking, blood pressure disturbances, sweating abnormalities), sleep disorders, and pain or other sensory complaints.

In Parkinson's disease, there is a slow, progressive degeneration of dopaminergic neurons in the basal ganglia. The resulting clinical signs and symptoms are thought to be due to an imbalance in neurotransmitter function as a result of this neuronal degeneration. The exact pathogenesis remains uncertain, but may be related to a combination of factors such as altered protein degradation, intracellular protein accumulation, oxidative stress (ie, free radical cellular damage), mitochondrial damage, inflammatory cascades, and apoptosis. Dysfunction is progressive, with increasing disability occurring more frequently from the fifth or sixth decade of life onward. There is no cure for Parkinson's disease, but treatment—both pharmacologic and rehabilitative—may delay the associated disability and improve quality of life for many years.

Degeneration of dopaminergic neurons in the substantia nigra in Parkinson's disease results in decreased inhibitory input (primarily via D_2 receptors) onto striatal GABAergic neurons (Figure 17-1). This pathologic reduction of dopaminergic

TABLE 17-1 **Types of abnormal movements.**

Movement	Description
Tremor	Rhythmic oscillatory movement around a joint (eg, fingers, wrist, jaw)
Resting tremor	Occurs in the absence of any intended movement
Postural tremor	Occurs while maintaining a particular posture
Intention tremor	Occurs during voluntary effort (eg, picking up a phone)
Chorea	Irregular, involuntary movements occurring in any part of the body. May involve facial grimacing or tongue movements and abnormal speech. Impairs voluntary activity.
Ballismus	Form of chorea involving proximal muscles in which a limb may move violently
Tics	Sudden, involuntary, and repetitive coordinated movements (eg, blinking, turning head, smacking lips)
Athetosis	Involuntary slow, writhing movements
Dystonia	Prolonged, sustained athetosis that resembles abnormal posture
Dyskinesia	Acute dystonia or muscle spasm, often caused by dopamine-blocking drugs
Akathisia	Inability to sit or stand still, motor restlessness; usually caused by dopamine-blocking drugs
Myoclonus	Sudden, rapid, twitch-like movements; may be localized or generalized

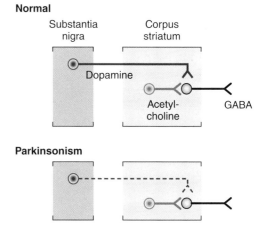

FIGURE 17-1 **Representation of the sequence of neurons involved in Parkinson's disease. Normal:** Dopaminergic neurons (red) originating in the substantia nigra normally inhibit GABAergic output from the striatum, whereas striatal cholinergic neurons (orange) exert an excitatory effect onto the GABAergic neurons (black). **Parkinsonism:** Selective loss of dopaminergic neurons (dashed, red) results in a relative increase in excitatory cholinergic input onto GABAergic neurons in the striatum.

DRUGS USED TO TREAT PARKINSON'S DISEASE

Figure 17-2 outlines the drugs used in Parkinson's disease. Treatment strategies involve restoring dopamine activity in the brain by either increasing the activity of dopamine already available or by providing exogenous dopamine. The benefits of dopaminergic drugs are mainly due to stimulation of the D_2 receptors that are located postsynaptically on striatal neurons as well as presynaptically on axons in the substantia nigra (dopamine receptors are discussed fully in Chapter 12). For maximal clinical benefit, activation of D_1 receptors may also be required. In addition, one new drug, **pramipexole**, is a D_3 agonist. Several treatment approaches have evolved to optimize dopaminergic therapy, including the combined use of **levodopa** (the precursor to dopamine) with agents to inhibit enzymatic breakdown of dopamine (monoamine oxidase-B inhibitors and catechol-O-methyltransferase [COMT] inhibitors) and dopamine receptor agonists. In an attempt to restore the normal balance of cholinergic and dopaminergic influences on the basal ganglia,

neurotransmission leads to excessive excitatory actions of cholinergic neurons on striatal GABAergic neurons; thus, the activity of dopamine and acetylcholine are out of balance in Parkinson's disease. The resulting excessive excitatory action onto inhibitory neurons appears to be responsible for the typical signs of bradykinesia and muscle rigidity.

Certain drugs that block dopamine receptors can cause *reversible* parkinsonian symptoms. Classic examples include the antipsychotic drugs haloperidol and the phenothiazines. At high doses, **tetrabenazine** causes similar symptoms, presumably by depleting brain dopamine. MPTP (1-methyl-4-phenyl-1,2,3,6-tetrahydropyridine), a by-product of the attempted synthesis of an illicit meperidine analog (a heroin-like drug), causes *irreversible* parkinsonism through destruction of dopaminergic neurons in the nigrostriatal tract.

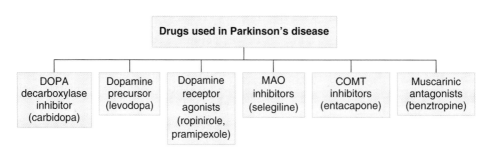

FIGURE 17-2 **Classification of drugs used in the treatment of Parkinson's disease.** Prototype drugs are in parentheses. COMT, catechol-O-methyltransferase; MAO, monoamine oxidase.

antimuscarinic drugs may be added to the drug regimen. In general, the dopaminergic agents (especially levodopa) are particularly effective at relieving bradykinesia, whereas the anticholinergic agents may improve the resting tremor and rigidity, but have little effect on bradykinesia.

Finding a drug regimen that works effectively without serious adverse effects over a period of time is difficult. Since Parkinson's disease is a progressive disorder, drug regimens must be closely monitored by all professionals involved in the care of the patient. An overview of drugs used in Parkinson's disease is shown in Table 17-2.

Levodopa

Dopamine does not cross the blood-brain barrier (BBB) and thus has no therapeutic effect in Parkinson's disease if given

as such. However, its precursor, L-dopa (levodopa), is transported across the BBB via an amino acid transporter into the brain, where it is rapidly converted to dopamine by L-amino acid decarboxylase (DOPA decarboxylase), an enzyme present in many body tissues including the brain. To prevent premature conversion of levodopa to dopamine in peripheral tissues, levodopa is usually given with a DOPA decarboxylase inhibitor such as **carbidopa**, which does not cross the BBB and thus prevents the conversion of levodopa to dopamine only in peripheral tissues. This levodopa-carbidopa combination reduces the daily requirements of levodopa by approximately 75% and results in fewer peripheral adverse effects (Figure 17-3). Combination treatment is typically started with small doses of levodopa that are increased gradually, but ultimately below a relatively low ceiling dose to reduce the risk of response fluctuations (see below). Levodopa is taken

TABLE 17-2 Drug therapy in Parkinson's disease.

Drug	Mechanism of Action	Comments
Levodopa	Converted to dopamine after crossing BBB to restore CNS dopamine levels	Effectively ameliorates motor signs of Parkinson's disease, especially bradykinesia Causes significant peripheral dopaminergic effects Use with carbidopa (to prevent conversion to dopamine in periphery and to decrease required dosage) is now standard treatment Use with MAO-B and COMT inhibitors prolongs duration of effect Responsiveness decreases with long-term use Decreases mortality rate Not always first drug used due to development of response fluctuations over time
Dopamine receptor agonists	Agonists at dopamine D_2 or D_3 receptors	Used as initial monotherapy or in combination with levodopa or anticholinergic drugs Helps smooth out on-off phenomenon May cause impulse control disorders
MAO-B inhibitors	Selectively inhibit MAO-B, the enzyme that metabolizes dopamine in the basal ganglia Enable dopamine to remain active for longer periods of time	Sometimes used as sole agent in newly diagnosed patients Adjunct to levodopa Should not be taken concurrently with meperidine, TCAs, or SSRIs because of risk of acute toxic interactions
COMT inhibitors	Inhibit COMT, the enzyme that converts levodopa to 3-OMD in peripheral tissues or 3-MT in the brain Allow more levodopa to reach the brain	Adjunct to levodopa-carbidopa administration May reduce levodopa dosage needed to improve symptoms Entacapone does not enter CNS, thus only inhibits COMT in periphery Tolcapone enters CNS, thus inhibits COMT in periphery and in brain
Antimuscarinic drugs	Antagonists at cholinergic muscarinic receptors Inhibit excessive acetylcholine influence on cells in the striatum	May improve tremor and rigidity with little effect on bradykinesia Frequent peripheral adverse effects (eg, sedation, urinary retention, confusion)
Amantadine	Antagonist at glutamate NMDA receptors, which results in anticholinergic actions May potentiate dopaminergic function by increasing synthesis or release of dopamine or inhibiting its reuptake	May improve bradykinesia, rigidity, and tremor for only a limited time (weeks)

BBB, blood-brain barrier; CNS, central nervous system; COMT, catechol-*O*-methyltransferase; MAO, monoamine oxidase; NMDA, *N*-methyl-D-aspartate; SSRIs, selective serotonin reuptake inhibitors; TCAs, tricyclic antidepressants; 3-MT, 3-methyoxytyramine; 3-OMD, 3-*O*-methyldopa.

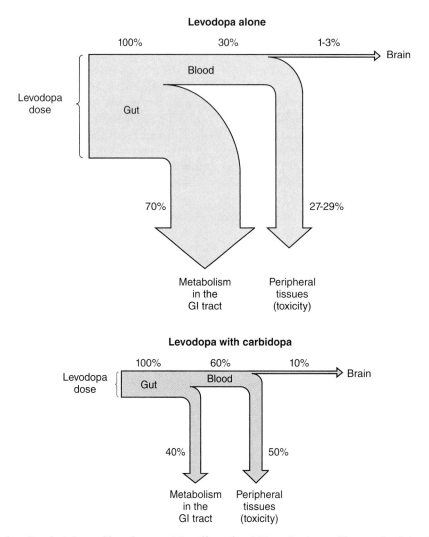

FIGURE 17-3 **Fate of orally administered levodopa and the effect of carbidopa (estimated from animal data).** The width of each pathway indicates the *absolute* amount of the drug present at each site, while the percentages shown denote the relative proportion of the administered dose. Benefits of coadministration of carbidopa include reduction in the amount of levodopa initially administered, reduction in the amount of levodopa diverted to peripheral tissues, and an increase in the fraction of levodopa dose that reaches the brain.

3 or 4 times daily and 30-60 minutes before meals. Ingestion of food delays the appearance of levodopa in the plasma. In particular, certain amino acids can compete with levodopa for absorption from the gut and for the transporter across the BBB. Plasma concentration of levodopa typically peaks 1-2 hours after an oral dose, and plasma elimination half-life is between 1 and 3 hours.

Levodopa can ameliorate all the clinical motor features of Parkinson's disease, but is particularly effective in relieving bradykinesia and its associated disabilities. While the response may be dramatic, the best results with levodopa are obtained in the first few years of treatment. In some patients, the decreased responsiveness to levodopa is due to the fact that the dose must be reduced over time to avoid adverse effects at doses that were previously well tolerated. For some patients, levodopa's decreased effectiveness may reflect progression of the disease process. Regardless of the initial therapeutic response, the benefits of levodopa begin to diminish after 3-4 years of therapy. Although levodopa does not stop

the progression of Parkinson's disease, early initiation of treatment with levodopa lowers the mortality rate.

After a period (usually months to years) of good or excellent clinical response, the response to levodopa may begin to fluctuate rapidly. These response fluctuations occur with increasing frequency as treatment continues and there may be several underlying factors. In some cases, clinical response fluctuations may be related to *timing* of levodopa dosing such that patients experience a wearing-off reaction or end-of-dose akinesia. Other response fluctuations—the so-called on-off phenomena—are *not* related to the timing of dosing. That is, at the *same* therapeutic dosage or drug plasma concentration, "off" periods of akinesia may alternate over a few hours with "on" periods of improved mobility, but often with dyskinesias. In patients with severe "off" periods, subcutaneously injected **apomorphine** (discussed below) may provide temporary relief of akinesia. The mechanism of the on-off phenomenon is unknown.

The likelihood of such response fluctuations can sometimes be reduced by alterations in the drug regimen. Controlled release carbidopa-levodopa formulations, an extended release carbidopa-levodopa formulation (**Rytary**), or COMT inhibitors used adjunctively may improve levodopa responses (see discussion below). While "drug holidays" (drug discontinuation for 3-21 days) were occasionally used to reduce toxic effects of levodopa, they rarely affect response fluctuations and are no longer recommended because of the associated risks of immobility accompanying severe Parkinson's disease (eg, aspiration pneumonia, deep vein thromboses).

Most adverse drug reactions (ADRs) associated with levodopa are dose dependent. Gastrointestinal (GI) effects such as anorexia (loss of appetite), nausea, and emesis occur in about 80% of patients when the drug is given without a peripheral decarboxylase inhibitor. These ADRs can be reduced by taking the drug in divided doses, with or immediately after meals, and by increasing the total daily dose very slowly. Tolerance to the emetic action of levodopa usually occurs after several months. Antiemetics such as phenothiazines should be avoided because they may reduce the antiparkinsonism effects of levodopa and exacerbate symptoms. When levodopa is given in combination with carbidopa to reduce its peripheral metabolism, adverse GI effects are much less common (<20% of cases), so patients can tolerate proportionally higher doses.

Among cardiovascular effects, orthostatic hypotension is common, especially in the early stage of treatment, but often is asymptomatic. Other cardiac effects include tachycardia and cardiac arrhythmias (rare). Hypertension may also occur, especially in the presence of nonselective monoamine oxidase inhibitors or when massive doses of levodopa are being taken.

Dyskinesias occur in up to 80% of individuals receiving levodopa therapy for long periods. Although the form and nature of dyskinesias vary widely, the character of the dyskinesia tends to remain constant in individual patients. Choreoathetosis of the face and distal extremities is the most common presentation. Chorea, ballismus, athetosis, dystonia, myoclonus, tics, and tremor may occur individually or in any combination in the face, trunk, or limbs. Development of dyskinesias is dose-related, but there is considerable individual variation in the dose required to produce them.

A wide variety of adverse mental effects have been reported including depression, anxiety, agitation, insomnia, somnolence, confusion, delusions, hallucinations, nightmares, euphoria, and other changes in mood or personality. Such ADRs are more common in individuals taking levodopa in combination with a decarboxylase inhibitor rather than levodopa alone, presumably because higher levels are reached in the brain. Atypical antipsychotic agents, such as clozapine and risperidone, may be helpful in counteracting the behavioral complications of levodopa. Levodopa is contraindicated in patients with a history of psychosis.

Rare adverse effects include various blood disorders; hot flushes; aggravation or precipitation of gout; abnormalities of smell or taste; brownish discoloration of saliva, urine, or vaginal secretions; priapism; and mydriasis (pupil dilation). Last, since levodopa is a precursor of melanin and could conceivably activate malignant melanoma, the drug should be used with care in individuals with history of melanoma.

Dopamine Receptor Agonists

Dopamine receptor agonists are often first-line therapy for Parkinson's disease. Although these agents provide less symptomatic benefit than levodopa, their use is associated with lower rates of response fluctuations and dyskinesias than occur with long-term levodopa therapy. In other cases, dopaminergic therapy is initiated with low dose carbidopa plus levodopa and then a dopaminergic agonist is added.

Figure 17-4 summarizes the pharmacologic strategies for dopaminergic therapy in Parkinson's disease. The dopamine agonists act directly on dopamine receptors and do not require enzymatic conversion to an active metabolite. These drugs are orally active and readily cross the BBB. The older dopamine agonists, **bromocriptine** and **pergolide**, are ergot derivatives. Because of their serious adverse effects, they are now rarely used in the treatment of Parkinson's disease. The newer nonergot agents, **pramipexole** and **ropinirole**, are selective D_3 and D_2 agonists, respectively, with efficacy similar to that of the older agents, but with a safer profile. Both drugs can be used as monotherapy in mild disease, or they can be added to levodopa regimens for those with more advanced disease and to help alleviate response fluctuations. Pramipexole may also have a neuroprotective effect because it has been reported to act as a scavenger for hydrogen peroxide in dopaminergic cell cultures.

Pramipexole and ropinirole are rapidly absorbed after oral administration, reaching peak plasma levels in approximately 2 hours. Pramipexole and ropinirole are usually dosed 3 times daily, starting with a smaller dose and building up to a therapeutic dose in approximately 3-4 weeks. Both agents are also available in extended release forms that permit once daily dosing. Pramipexole is excreted largely unchanged in the urine, whereas ropinirole is metabolized in the liver by CYP1A2, which also metabolizes other drugs such as warfarin and caffeine.

The last two dopamine receptor agonists are not given via oral administration. **Rotigotine** transdermal is a dopamine receptor agonist approved for treatment of early stage Parkinson's disease. The drug may provide more continuous dopaminergic receptor stimulation than oral formulations, but its efficacy in more advanced stages of the disease is unknown. Application site reactions may be serious. Apomorphine is injected subcutaneously. This drug has been approved for rescue treatment of severe acute immobility ("off periods") in Parkinson's disease. Apomorphine can provide rapid (within 10 minutes), but temporary relief (1-2 hours) of akinesia in patients optimized on dopaminergic therapy. Apomorphine necessitates pretreatment with antiemetic drugs to prevent severe nausea and vomiting. Other ADRs of apomorphine include dyskinesias, hypotension, sedation, and sweating.

As with levodopa, most of the ADRs associated with dopamine agonists are dose dependent and may be decreased by reducing the total dose of dopaminergic drugs. Common GI

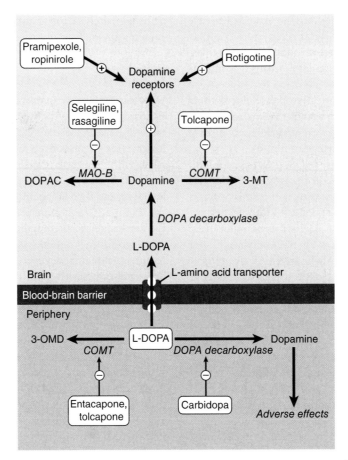

FIGURE 17-4 Pharmacologic strategies for dopaminergic therapy in Parkinson's disease. Actions of each of the drugs are described in the text. COMT, catechol-*O*-methyltransferase; DOPAC, dihydroxyphenylacetic acid; L-DOPA, levodopa; 3-MT, 3-methoxytyramine; 3-OMD, 3-*O*-methyldopa.

effects (anorexia, nausea, vomiting) are more pronounced with initial use and can be minimized by taking the medication with meals. Again, the most common cardiovascular effect is orthostatic hypotension, particularly at the initiation of therapy. If cardiac arrhythmias occur, this is an indication for discontinuing treatment. Peripheral edema has also been reported. Dyskinesias similar to those caused by levodopa may occur.

Behavioral and psychiatric effects (eg, confusion, hallucinations, and delusions) are more common with dopamine receptor agonists than with levodopa and tend to occur earlier in older patients. However, these effects may be also manifestations of advancing Parkinson's disease. The effects may respond to atypical antipsychotics (eg, clozapine, olanzapine). Finally, impulse control disorders such as gambling, shopping, and sexual activity have been noted in up to 25% of individuals with Parkinson's disease treated with dopamine agonists. These behaviors may occur either as an exaggerated previous tendency or as a new phenomenon. They may not be dose-dependent, but tend to resolve when the offending drug is withdrawn.

Monoamine Oxidase Inhibitors

In the nervous system, there are two forms of monoamine oxidase (MAO) that metabolize the monoamine transmitters.

MAO-A metabolizes norepinephrine, serotonin, and dopamine, whereas MAO-B selectively metabolizes dopamine. At normal doses, **selegiline** is a selective and irreversible inhibitor of MAO-B (at higher doses, the drug also inhibits MAO-A). By inhibiting the breakdown of dopamine, selegiline may increase brain dopamine levels (Figure 17-4). Selegiline is used as an adjunct to levodopa and has also been used as the sole agent in newly diagnosed patients. The drug may reduce mild "on-off" or wearing-off phenomena seen with levodopa therapy. When given alone, selegiline has only a minor therapeutic effect on Parkinson's disease. Hepatic metabolism results in the formation of desmethylselegiline (possibly neuroprotective owing to anti-apoptotic mechanisms) and small quantities of amphetamine.

Rasagiline and **safinamide** are newer MAO-B inhibitors. Rasagiline is a more potent irreversible inhibitor than selegiline and may be used as monotherapy for early treatment in mild Parkinson's disease. Rasagiline is also used adjunctively with carbidopa-levodopa to prolong their effects in those with advanced symptoms and response fluctuations. Safinamide is clinically used in a similar fashion as rasagiline, except that it is a reversible MAO-B inhibitor and not as effective as monotherapy for Parkinson's disease.

Adverse effects associated with MAO-B inhibitors include insomnia, mood changes, dyskinesias, GI distress, and orthostatic hypotension. These drugs should not be taken concurrently with meperidine, tricyclic antidepressants, or selective serotonin reuptake inhibitors because of the risk of acute toxic interactions (see Chapter 19).

Catechol-*O*-methyltransferase Inhibitors

Inhibition of dopa decarboxylase (by carbidopa) is associated with compensatory activation of other pathways of levodopa metabolism, especially catechol-*O*-methyltransferase (COMT), which results in 3-*O*-methyldopa (3-OMD). Increased plasma levels of 3-OMD are associated with poor therapeutic response to levodopa, partly because 3-OMD competes with levodopa for active transport across the intestinal mucosa and the BBB into the CNS. **Entacapone** and **tolcapone** are selective COMT inhibitors (Figure 17-4). COMT inhibitors prolong the action of levodopa by increasing the amount transported into the brain and diminishing its peripheral catabolism.

COMT inhibitors may be helpful in patients receiving levodopa who have developed response fluctuations, improving response and prolonging "on" time. They may also provide the option of reducing the total daily levodopa dose. Entacapone is generally preferred because tolcapone has been associated with hepatotoxicity (including acute liver failure) and requires routine monitoring of liver function tests. Several ADRs of both medications relate to increased levels of levodopa and include dyskinesias, orthostatic hypotension, confusion, and GI distress. Other adverse effects include sleep disturbances and orange discoloration of urine.

A newer combination agent (**Stalevo**) includes carbidopa, levodopa, and entacapone. This agent provides more symptomatic relief than carbidopa-levodopa alone. While this preparation simplifies the dosing regimen by enabling fewer tablets to be taken throughout the day, Stalevo may be associated with earlier occurrence and increased frequency of dyskinesia than with carbidopa-levodopa.

Amantadine

Amantadine, an oral antiviral agent (Chapter 28), was incidentally found to have weak antiparkinsonism properties. Amantadine inhibits the *N*-methyl-D-aspartic acid (NMDA) receptor-mediated stimulation of acetylcholine release in rat striatum. In addition to this anticholinergic effect, amantadine may enhance dopaminergic neurotransmission by increasing synthesis or release of dopamine or by inhibiting dopamine reuptake. Amantadine has limited but favorable influence on the bradykinesia, rigidity, and tremor of Parkinson's disease. The drug is less effective than levodopa and its benefits may last for only a few weeks.

Amantadine has a number of undesirable CNS effects such as restlessness, agitation, insomnia, confusion, and acute toxic psychosis, all of which can be reversed by discontinuing the drug. Peripheral edema is another complication, which

responds to diuretics. Livedo reticularis (a dermatologic reaction) sometimes occurs and usually clears within a month after the drug is withdrawn.

Acetylcholine-Blocking Drugs

These drugs decrease the excitatory actions of cholinergic neurons on cells in the striatum by blocking muscarinic receptors (Figure 17-1). Antimuscarinic drugs used in Parkinson's disease include **benztropine**, **orphenadrine**, **procyclidine**, and **trihexyphenidyl**.

Antimuscarinic drugs may improve the tremor and rigidity of Parkinson's disease, but have little effect on bradykinesia. Treatment is usually started with low doses and gradually increased until benefit occurs or adverse effects limit further increments. If a patient does not respond to one antimuscarinic drug, a trial with another drug in this class may prove more successful. Antimuscarinic agents are used as adjunctive agents in Parkinson's disease. These drugs also have value in attenuating the parkinsonism-like extrapyramidal ADRs of typical antipsychotic drugs such as haloperidol.

Antimuscarinic medications have both central and peripheral nervous system adverse effects (Chapter 5). In general, these agents are poorly tolerated by older adults or individuals with cognitive impairments. CNS toxicity includes drowsiness, inattention, confusion, delusions, and hallucinations. Peripheral nervous system ADRs include dry mouth, blurred vision, mydriasis, urinary retention, nausea, constipation, and tachycardia. These agents also exacerbate tardive dyskinesias that result from prolonged use of antipsychotic drugs. Withdrawal of medication should be accomplished gradually in order to prevent acute exacerbation of tremor.

OTHER THERAPEUTIC STRATEGIES USED IN PARKINSON'S DISEASE

In patients with advanced disease who no longer respond adequately to pharmacotherapy, surgical intervention may provide worthwhile benefit. Ablative surgical procedures (thalamotomy and pallidotomy) have been replaced by functional, reversible lesions induced by high-frequency deep-brain stimulation using implantable electrodes in the subthalamic or globus pallidus. In patients undergoing deep-brain stimulation, antiparkinsonian medications can often be reduced.

A number of different compounds are currently under investigation as potential neuroprotective agents that may slow Parkinson's disease progression. These include antioxidants, antiapoptotic agents, glutamate receptor antagonists, intraparenchymally administered glia-derived neurotrophic factor, and anti-inflammatory drugs. To date, none of these agents have been shown to be clinically effective. Earlier hopes that coenzyme Q10, creatine, pramipexole, and pioglitazone would be effective in Parkinson's treatment have not produced positive results.

DRUGS USED TO TREAT OTHER MOVEMENT DISORDERS

Table 17-3 outlines characteristics of nonparkinsonian movement disorders and key drugs used to treat each.

Physiologic and Essential Tremor

Physiologic and essential tremor are enhanced postural tremors that are accentuated by anxiety, fatigue, and particular drugs (eg, bronchodilators, tricyclic antidepressants). These tremors can be ameliorated by β-adrenergic receptor antagonists (Chapter 6) including **propranolol**, or the $β_1$-selective antagonist **metoprolol** for individuals with coexisting pulmonary disease. Notably, these agents are banned in particular sports such as archery, darts, and shooting, where relief of tremor would provide competitive advantage. For essential tremor, antiepileptic drugs (**primidone**, **topiramate**, **gabapentin**), **alprazolam** (a benzodiazapine), or intramuscular injection of **botulinum toxin** may also be used.

Huntington's Disease

Huntington's disease, an autosomal dominant inherited disorder, is characterized by progressive chorea and dementia that typically begins in adulthood. The development of chorea seems to result from a loss of GABA transmitter functions and enhanced dopaminergic activity. There may also be a cholinergic deficit because choline acetyltransferase is decreased in the basal ganglia of patients with this disease. Drug therapy involves the use of dopamine-depleting drugs (eg, tetrabenazine, **deutetrabenazine**) or dopamine receptor antagonists (eg, **haloperidol**). Pharmacologic attempts to enhance brain GABA and acetylcholine activities have not been successful in patients with Huntington's disease. Because the pharmacologic interventions to decrease chorea are those that interfere with dopamine activity, reduction of the unwanted abnormal movements may result in iatrogenic parkinsonism. When chorea occurs as a complication of general medical disorders or due to a specific drug, treatment is directed to the underlying cause or withdrawal of the offending substance, respectively.

Tourette Syndrome

Tourette syndrome is a disorder of unknown cause that is characterized by chronic multiple involuntary tics involving sudden violent or repetitive movements and loud, obscene, or hostile vocalizations. The disease often occurs in adolescence or young adulthood. If severe, the disorder may have a significant impact on the patient's life that requires symptomatic treatment. The most effective pharmacologic approach is the use of dopamine receptor antagonists or drugs that deplete dopamine stores, which decrease the frequency and intensity of tics by roughly 60%. **Pimozide**, a D_2 receptor blocker, is a first-line agent. **Fluphenazine**, tetrabenazine, and haloperidol are other options. Treatment is started with small dosages that

TABLE 17-3   Characteristics of movement disorders and their pharmacologic therapy.

Disorder	Etiology	Manifestations	Common Signs	Drug Therapy Options
Essential tremor and physiologic postural tremor	Unknown	Postural tremor typically involving hands, head, voice (less common in legs)	Difficulty eating and drinking Ataxia	Beta blockers (propranolol) for both Essential tremor: primidone and topiramate (antiepileptics), alprazolam (benzodiazepine), gabapentin
Restless legs syndrome	Unknown (dopamine deficiency?)	Unpleasant feeling in legs, at rest, especially at night	Symptoms decrease with movement	Dopamine agonists (ropinirole, pramipexole) Gabapentin
Tourette syndrome	Unknown (dopamine excess?)	Chronic and multiple motor tics	Involuntary twitches, vocalizations	Dopamine receptor antagonists (pimozide, haloperidol, aripiprazole) $α_2$-adrenoceptor agonists (clonidine, guanfacine)
Wilson disease	Congenital error in copper transport and binding	Rest and postural tremor, chorea, ataxia	Increased copper in brain and viscera	Copper-binding drugs (penicillamine, trientine hydrochloride)
Huntington's disease	Loss of GABAergic neurons in the basal ganglia; strong genetic component	Progressive chorea and dementia	Abnormal movements and dementia	None satisfactory. Dopamine blockers or depleting drugs may reduce abnormal movements

COMT, catechol-*O*-methyltransferase; MAOIs, monoamine oxidase inhibitors.

are then increased gradually. Adverse effects include extrapyramidal movement disorders, dry mouth, blurred vision, and GI distress. If these agents are not successful, other medications can be tried, including **aripiprazole** (antagonist at D_2 receptors and certain serotonin receptor subtypes), **carbamazepine** (sodium channel blocker), **clonazepam** (benzodiazepine that increases GABAergic transmission at $GABA_A$ receptors), and **clonidine** and **guanfacine** (α_2-adrenoceptor agonists).

Drug-Induced Dyskinesias

As discussed above, levodopa and dopamine agonists produce dose-dependent and reversible dyskinesias in individuals with Parkinson's disease. Antipsychotic agents such as phenothiazines can cause parkinsonian symptoms (by decreasing dopaminergic transmission). These symptoms are usually reversible by lowering drug dosage, changing the therapy to a drug that is less toxic to extrapyramidal function, or treating with a muscarinic blocker (benztropine). Levodopa and bromocriptine are not useful because the antipsychotic drugs are blocking dopamine receptors. Acute dystonias can also be treated with parenteral administration of an antihistamine (**diphenhydramine**) or a benzodiazepine (**diazepam**).

Tardive dyskinesias are a special form of movement disorders that develop as a complication of long-term therapy with traditional antipsychotic drugs. The pharmacological basis of these reactions is not clear, but these reactions are usually *irreversible*. Paradoxically, dose reduction of the offending drug (a dopamine receptor blocker) usually worsens the dyskinesia and an increase in dose may suppress it. Two new drugs that modulate dopamine release—deutetrabenazine and **valbenazine**—show promise for modifying tardive dyskinesias.

Restless Legs Syndrome

The cause of restless legs syndrome, in which individuals experience unpleasant sensations in the legs especially during relaxation, is unknown. Symptoms often delay sleep onset because of the urge to move around to decrease symptoms. If the individual has iron-deficiency anemia, correction of this disorder may resolve symptoms of restless legs syndrome. Long-acting dopamine receptor agonists (pramipexole, ropinirole, rotigotine) are the preferred therapy for restless legs syndrome. Gabapentin is effective at reducing symptom severity. For those with intermittent symptoms, clonazepam may be helpful. If opioids are required, those with low addictive potential are recommended.

Wilson Disease

Wilson disease is a recessively inherited disorder of copper metabolism that results in deposits of copper salts in many tissues, including the brain. Clinically, Wilson disease is characterized by hepatic and neurologic dysfunction, which may be severe or fatal. Neurologic signs include tremor, chorea,

rigidity, hypokinesia, dysarthria, and dysphagia. Treatment involves low dietary copper and the use of chelating agents (**penicillamine** and **trientine hydrochloride**) to remove the excess copper. Starting doses are initially high until remission occurs; then, lower doses are maintained indefinitely. Toxic effects of penicillamine include GI distress, myasthenia, optic neuropathy, and blood disorders. Trientine may be preferred because neurologic worsening has been observed in about 10% of those taking penicillamine. Trientine also appears to have fewer drug interactions than penicillamine and few ADRs other than mild anemia due to iron deficiency in a few patients.

REHABILITATION RELEVANCE

Rehabilitation is a very important component of the overall medical care of individuals with movement disorders, especially degenerative diseases such as Parkinson's disease. For individuals with Parkinson's disease, physical therapy can improve mobility, axial rotation, functional reach, flexibility, balance, strength, gait, and postural stability. Interventions include, but are not limited to traditional gait training (especially with auditory cueing), body weight-supported treadmill training, balance training (including Tai Chi), stretching, and resistance and aerobic training. For people with other general movement disorders, learning strategies for minimizing and managing their abnormal movements can mean tremendous improvements in daily quality of life and overall self-esteem. With our emerging understanding of the importance of maintaining the physiologic system (muscle force, muscle length, joint integrity, receptor integrity) in individuals with neurologic disorders, rehabilitative therapy may reduce the patient's need for rapid escalation of anti-Parkinson's disease medications. Evidence suggests there is a synergistic effect of early physical rehabilitation intervention and medication in providing improved functional outcomes across all levels of body function and structure, activity, and participation.

Most, if not all, patients receiving physical therapy for movement disorders are also taking medications to ameliorate the motor manifestations. Therapists working with this population must be aware of the adverse effects associated with these medications, potentially mitigating factors, as well as when to alert referring and prescribing healthcare providers.

- **Dyskinesias** are extremely common with dopaminergic therapy for Parkinson's disease. Development is dose-related and the character of the dyskinesia (type and body part affected) tends to remain constant in individual patients. Therapeutic rehabilitation interventions can improve mobility and help patients maximize function; however, such interventions *cannot* alleviate these dyskinesias. Therapists can educate and reassure patients that these reactions are anticipated adverse effects of dopaminergic therapy. If dyskinesias significantly impact functional mobility, the prescribing provider should be alerted to determine if dose alterations or changes in drug regimen might be made.

- A variety of undesirable **mental effects** are associated with levodopa and dopamine receptor agonists. Anxiety, somnolence, confusion, hallucinations, nightmares, and changes in mood or personality have been reported and tend to occur earlier in older patients. Therapists should be alert to patient-reported symptoms and encourage direct communication with the patient's neurologist because atypical antipsychotic agents (eg, clozapine) may be helpful in counteracting these complications.

- Therapists working with individuals with Parkinson's disease must recognize that response fluctuations occur with increasing frequency as dopaminergic therapy continues. Therapists should attempt to determine whether a patient is experiencing a wearing-off reaction or **end-of-dose akinesia**, which is related to *timing* of levodopa dosing. If this is the case, therapy sessions should be appropriately timed to coordinate rehabilitative therapy with the peak effects of drug therapy for maximum benefit. If response fluctuations appear related to meals, consultation with a registered dietitian nutritionist may be indicated because regulation of dietary protein intake may improve response fluctuations.

- For individuals with Parkinson's disease receiving dopaminergic therapy that experience the **on-off phenomenon**, therapists should appreciate that the mechanism of this phenomenon is unknown; thus, trying to predict the timing of "off" periods of akinesia and "on" periods of improved mobility is likely ineffectual.

- In patients with severe "off" periods, subcutaneously injected apomorphine may provide temporary relief of akinesia. **Emesis** may occur if patients have not taken antiemetic drugs prior to apomorphine.

- **Gastrointestinal distress** (eg, anorexia, nausea, and vomiting) is one of the most common ADRs associated with all dopaminergic therapy for Parkinson's disease. Strategies such as taking the drug in divided doses, with or immediately after meals, and slowly increasing the total daily dose may mitigate GI symptoms. However, if appreciable unintended weight loss occurs, the patient's primary care provider or neurologist should be notified. Consultation with a registered dietitian nutritionist may also be indicated.

- **Orthostatic hypotension** is the most common cardiovascular ADR of dopaminergic therapy, especially in early stage levodopa treatment. Although often asymptomatic, therapists should monitor vitals and symptoms, especially to determine if orthostatic intolerance may be a contributory factor to falls. Other cardiac effects include **tachycardia** and **cardiac arrhythmias**. If cardiac arrhythmias occur, these signs must be relayed to the prescribing provider as this is an indication for discontinuing the offending drug.

- Since levodopa is a precursor of melanin and could conceivably activate malignant melanoma, any **suspicious undiagnosed skin lesion** noted in a patient receiving levodopa must be reported to the primary care practitioner emergently.

- For individuals with Parkinson's disease receiving amantadine, therapists should be vigilant for several **undesirable CNS effects** such as agitation, confusion, and acute toxic psychosis because these can be reversed by discontinuing the drug.

- For individuals with Parkinson's disease receiving adjunctive antimuscarinic drugs, **adverse CNS** (drowsiness, confusion, hallucinations) **and peripheral nervous system** (blurred vision, urinary retention, tachycardia) **reactions** are common. In particular, these agents are poorly tolerated by older adults or individuals with cognitive impairments.

- Therapists should be alert to new or amplified **impulse control disorders** (eg, gambling, shopping, sexual activity) in individuals with Parkinson's disease receiving dopamine receptor agonists. If recognized or suspected, this information should be shared with the prescribing healthcare provider because these behaviors tend to resolve when the offending drug is withdrawn.

- Therapists treating individuals with Tourette syndrome should be aware that anti-dopaminergic therapy is the most effective pharmacologic approach for treatment to decrease the frequency and intensity of tics. However, anticipated ADRs are **extrapyramidal movement disorders**.

CASE CONCLUSION

The physical therapist hypothesized that the patient's weight loss was due to diminished appetite, as a result of levodopa. Although L.S. was taking levodopa with carbidopa, which has been shown to reduce the GI adverse effects associated with levodopa, he still had lost significant lean muscle mass. The physical therapist contacted the referring prescribing provider and informed him of the patient's physical status. The practitioner subsequently met L.S. and made a few changes in his drug regimen: lowering his dose of levodopa, adding pramipexole (a dopamine agonist), and advising the patient to take his medication immediately following meals. L.S. began a rehabilitative program consisting of neuromuscular reeducation, therapeutic exercise, and patient education concurrent with this new drug regimen. After several weeks, L.S. stated he felt stronger and the therapist noted that he had also made objective improvements in strength. L.S. also began to gain back some of the weight he had lost.

CHAPTER 17 QUESTIONS

1. Which of the following is an advantage of coadministration of carbidopa with levodopa?

   a. Increase in amount of levodopa administered for clinical benefit
   b. Increase in amount of levodopa diverted to peripheral tissues
   c. Decreased fraction of the levodopa dose that reaches the brain
   d. Increased fraction of the levodopa dose that reaches the brain

2. Which of the following is a pathological result of Parkinson's disease?

   a. Decreased excitatory dopaminergic input onto GABAergic cells in the striatum
   b. Decreased inhibitory dopaminergic input onto GABAergic cells in the striatum
   c. Decreased cholinergic input onto GABAergic cells in the striatum
   d. Decreased noradrenergic input onto GABAergic cells in the striatum

3. Which of the following is *not* an adverse effect associated with levodopa or dopamine receptor agonists?

   a. Anorexia
   b. Orthostatic hypotension
   c. Weight gain
   d. Dyskinesias

4. Which of the following drugs is *not* used in the treatment of tremors?

   a. Propanolol
   b. Metoprolol
   c. Reserpine
   d. Topiramate

5. Which of the following drugs is an acetylcholine-blocking drug used in the treatment of Parkinson's disease?

   a. Benztropine
   b. Levodopa
   c. Entacapone
   d. Ropinirole

6. Which statement is accurate regarding drug therapy in Parkinson's disease?

   a. Selegiline is a selective inhibitor of COMT.
   b. The primary benefit of antimuscarinic agents is their ability to relieve bradykinesia.
   c. Amantadine provides clinical benefits for 10 years.
   d. Levodopa causes gastrointestinal effects in the majority of patients when the drug is given without a peripheral decarboxylase inhibitor.

7. Which of the following drugs is used as rescue treatment of severe acute immobility ("off periods") in Parkinson's disease?

   a. Levodopa
   b. Apomorphine
   c. Selegiline
   d. Ropinirole

8. Which of the following drugs may increase the risk of impulse control disorders?

   a. Amantadine
   b. Benztropine
   c. Haloperidol
   d. Ropinirole

9. Which of the following drugs is *not* clinically used in the treatment of Tourette syndrome?

   a. Haloperidol
   b. Pramipexole
   c. Tetrabenazine
   d. Pimozide

10. Which of the following drugs is contraindicated in a patient with a history of psychosis?

    a. Haloperidol
    b. Tetrabenazine
    c. Aripiprazole
    d. Levodopa

Antipsychotic Agents and Lithium

CASE STUDY

M.M. is a 56-year-old man who was referred to rehabilitation by his physician after several falls and increasing balance problems as per his wife's observation. The patient has a history of schizophrenia that has been well controlled with medication. Recent imaging and clinical diagnostic tests have ruled out any neurological or structural central nervous system (CNS) pathology. M.M. is currently taking pantoprazole (a proton pump inhibitor) and quetiapine. During the patient interview, M.M. reported that his prescribing practitioner increased his dose of quetiapine after a psychotic episode 2 months ago. Hesitantly, M.M. also reported several recent episodes of lightheadedness. M.M. states that he has begun to feel extremely stiff at times and has had a hard time moving. During the physical therapy examination, M.M. appeared to be in no acute physical distress. When moving from sitting to standing, M.M. stated that he became slightly lightheaded with the edges of his vision blurring. The therapist confirmed orthostatic hypotension during a sit-to-stand transfer with a fall in systolic and diastolic blood pressure of 24 and 18 mm Hg, respectively. Although M.M. had normal range of motion and strength in all extremities, he displayed some postural rigidity evident by resistance to passive stretch that was more severe in the lower extremities. The patient did not demonstrate a resting tremor. M.M.'s performance on the Mini-BESTest revealed moderate impairments in dynamic balance.

REHABILITATION FOCUS

Over the last 50 years, antipsychotic drugs have had a major impact on psychiatric treatment—enabling many individuals to move from inpatient mental institutions to the community. For many, this shift has provided a better quality of life as a result of improved behavior and reality perception. Physical therapists may encounter individuals taking antipsychotic medications in several settings. Many psychiatric facilities employ physical and occupational therapists to provide direct care to their patients. More commonly, therapists treat individuals within the community taking antipsychotic medications who have been referred for rehabilitation for a diagnosis unrelated to their psychosis. Prescribers always weigh the risk of adverse effects with the benefits of antipsychotic drugs. Adverse effects such as sedation, dry mouth, and constipation are usually tolerated. However, the extrapyramidal effects—bradykinesia, tremor, and rigidity—of many antipsychotic drugs can impair activities of daily living and increase the potential for falls and injury. Therapists noting increasing impairments in balance, posture, or involuntary movements should report these to the prescribing healthcare professional. Finally, patients may be referred to physical therapy for the development of physical activity programs, as several of the newer drugs have the potential for weight gain. Figure 18-1

outlines the drugs discussed in this chapter that are used to treat both psychosis and bipolar disorders.

BACKGROUND

The term "psychosis" denotes a variety of mental disorders that are characterized by the inability to distinguish between what is real and what is not. Psychosis can include the presence of delusions (false beliefs), grossly disorganized thinking, and various types of hallucinations that are usually auditory or visual, but may be tactile or olfactory. The most common psychotic disorder is schizophrenia, which is characterized by a marked thinking and perceptual disturbance. Schizophrenia is present in only about 1% of the population, but is responsible for roughly half of long-term psychiatric hospitalizations. Psychosis is *not* unique to individuals with schizophrenia. In addition, psychosis is not present in all people with schizophrenia at all times.

Based on twin, adoption, and family studies, schizophrenia has been established as a genetic disorder with high heritability. Current theories involve *multiple* genes with common and rare mutations combining to produce variable clinical presentations and courses. Schizophrenia is considered a neurodevelopmental disorder, implying that structural and

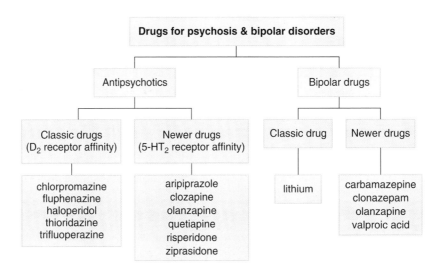

FIGURE 18-1   **Common drugs used to treat psychoses and bipolar disorder.** Antipsychotic drugs are broadly divided into two groups. The first-generation classic drugs have stronger affinity for the dopamine D_2 receptor than the newer second-generation drugs, which have stronger affinity for the serotonin 5-HT_2 receptor. Bipolar drugs include lithium, the first drug shown to be effective in treating bipolar disorder, and a diverse group of newer mood-stabilizing drugs.

functional changes in the brain are present in utero in some individuals, or that these changes develop during childhood and adolescence, or both.

NEUROTRANSMITTER/RECEPTOR HYPOTHESES OF SCHIZOPHRENIA

The Dopamine Hypothesis

Much evidence supports the hypothesis that *excessive* limbic dopaminergic activity plays a role in psychosis. First, many antipsychotic drugs strongly block central postsynaptic D_2 receptors, especially in the mesolimbic and striatal-frontal system; this includes partial dopamine agonists, such as **aripiprazole**. In contrast, drugs that increase dopaminergic activity (eg, levodopa, amphetamines, bromocriptine, apomorphine) either aggravate schizophrenia psychosis or produce psychosis de novo in some individuals. In postmortem studies, increased dopamine-receptor density has been found in the brains of schizophrenics who had not been treated with antipsychotic drugs. Some postmortem studies have reported increased dopamine levels and D_2-receptor density specifically in the nucleus accumbens, caudate, and putamen.

However, the hypothesis that schizophrenia is simply due to excessive limbic dopaminergic activity does not adequately explain all aspects of the disorder, especially the cognitive impairment. In fact, *diminished* cortical or hippocampal dopaminergic activity has been suggested to underlie the cognitive impairment and negative symptoms of schizophrenia (emotional blunting, social withdrawal, lack of motivation). This is supported by postmortem and in vivo imaging studies of schizophrenic subjects that have shown decreased dopaminergic activity in cortical, limbic, nigral, and striatal regions. Decreased dopaminergic innervation in the medial temporal cortex, dorsolateral prefrontal cortex, and hippocampus, and decreased levels of DOPAC (a metabolite of dopamine) in the anterior cingulate have also been reported.

Because several of the newer antipsychotic drugs have much less effect on D_2 receptors and yet are effective in treating schizophrenia, research has been redirected to the role of other dopamine receptors as well as nondopamine receptors. Serotonin receptors (especially the 5-HT_{2A}-receptor subtype discussed below) may mediate synergistic effects or protect against the extrapyramidal consequences of pharmacological blockade of the D_2 receptors. Research has changed to a greater focus on compounds that may act on several transmitter-receptor systems, such as serotonin and glutamate. The newer antipsychotic drugs share the property of *weak* D_2-receptor antagonism and more *potent* 5-HT_{2A}-receptor blockade.

The Serotonin Hypothesis

The hallucinatory effects of drugs such as LSD (lysergic acid diethylamide) and mescaline are due to stimulation of serotonin 5-HT_{2A} and possibly 5-HT_{2C} receptors. This pivotal discovery led to development of agents able that would be able to *block* these receptors. In the cortex, limbic region, and striatum, 5-HT_{2A} receptors modulate the release of many neurotransmitters (eg, dopamine, norepinephrine, glutamate, GABA, acetylcholine). Ultimately, stimulation of 5-HT_{2A} receptors leads to depolarization of glutamate neurons, but also stabilization of *N*-methyl-D-aspartate (NMDA) receptors on postsynaptic neurons. Antagonism of 5-HT_{2A} receptors is a key mechanism of action for the main class of newer second-generation antipsychotic drugs. **Clozapine** is the prototype in this class, which also includes aripiprazole, **melperone**, **olanzapine**, **quetiapine**, **risperidone**, and **ziprasidone**. These drugs do not act as direct antagonists at the $5\text{-}HT_{2A}$ receptor. Rather, they are inverse agonists, meaning that they block the *constitutive* endogenous activity of the $5\text{-}HT_{2A}$ receptor. By this mechanism, these drugs alter the release of many neurotransmitters in many parts of the cortex and limbic system. $5\text{-}HT_{2C}$ receptors also modulate dopamine in cortical and limbic areas. Stimulation of $5\text{-}HT_{2C}$ receptors leads to inhibition of cortical and limbic dopamine release. Clozapine and olanzapine are inverse agonists at both $5\text{-}HT_{2A}$ and $5\text{-}HT_{2C}$ receptors. $5\text{-}HT_{2C}$ agonists are currently being studied as antipsychotic agents.

The Glutamate Hypothesis

Glutamate is the major excitatory neurotransmitter in the brain (Chapter 12). Phencyclidine (PCP) and ketamine are noncompetitive inhibitors of the NMDA receptor. Both drugs exacerbate cognitive impairment and psychosis in patients with schizophrenia. In rodent and primate experiments, PCP increases locomotor activity and, acutely or chronically, increases a variety of cognitive impairments. The newer antipsychotic drugs are much more potent than D_2 antagonists in blocking these effects of PCP. These findings originated the hypothesis that *hypofunction* of NMDA receptors located on GABAergic interneurons leads to diminished inhibitory influences that contribute to schizophrenia. The diminished GABAergic activity can induce disinhibition of downstream glutamatergic activity, which can cause hyperstimulation of cortical neurons through non-NMDA receptors. The NMDA receptor is an ionotropic glutamate receptor that not only requires glutamate binding, but also requires glycine binding for full activation. It has been suggested that in patients with schizophrenia, the glycine site of the NMDA receptor is not fully saturated, contributing to decreased function of these receptors. However, trials of high doses of glycine have not been convincing.

ANTIPSYCHOTIC DRUGS

Antipsychotic drugs are able to reduce psychotic symptoms in a wide variety of conditions, including schizophrenia, bipolar disorder, psychotic depression, and psychoses associated with dementia or drugs. Antipsychotic drugs can improve mood and reduce anxiety and sleep disturbances, but they are not the treatment of choice when these symptoms are the primary disturbance in nonpsychotic patients. Neuroleptics is a term often used to represent the older classic antipsychotic drugs; the prototype neuroleptic is **haloperidol**. Neuroleptics produce a high incidence of unwanted extrapyramidal side effects (bradykinesia, rigidity, and tremor) at clinically effective doses. Today, the most widely used antipsychotic drugs are the newer or second-generation agents. In some patients, these newer drugs are more effective and less toxic than the older drugs. The second-generation agents appear to have lower affinity for the dopamine D_2 receptor, more selectivity in their pharmacological effects, and fewer adverse effects such as sedation and extrapyramidal effects. The newer drugs are much more costly than the classic antipsychotics, most of which can be prescribed as generic formulations. Table 18-1 lists several antipsychotic agents with their relative affinities for D_2 versus $5\text{-}HT_{2A}$ receptor affinity, clinical potencies, and severity of adverse effects.

Pharmacokinetics

Most antipsychotic drugs are well absorbed when given orally, though many undergo significant first-pass metabolism. Because they are highly lipid soluble, they readily enter the CNS and most other body tissues. Many are bound extensively (92-99%) to plasma proteins. Antipsychotic drugs tend to have large volumes of distribution (usually >7 L/kg). They generally have a much longer clinical action than would be estimated from their plasma half-lives. This is paralleled by prolonged occupancy of D_2 dopamine receptors in the brain by the classic

TABLE 18-1 Antipsychotic drugs: relationship of drug to potency and toxicities.

Drug	D_2/$5\text{-}HT_{2A}$ Ratio[a]	Clinical Potency	Extrapyramidal Toxicity	Sedative Action	Hypotensive Action
Chlorpromazine	High	Low	Medium	High	High
Fluphenazine	High	High	High	Low	Very low
Thiothixene	Very high	High	Medium	Medium	Medium
Haloperidol	Medium	High	Very high	Low	Very low
Clozapine	Very low	Medium	Very low	Low	Medium
Risperidone	Very low	High	Low[b]	Low	Low
Olanzapine	Low	High	Very low	Medium	Low
Quetiapine	Low	Low	Very low	Medium	Low to medium
Ziprasidone	Low	Medium	Very low	Low	Very low
Aripiprazole	Medium	High	Very low	Very low	Low

[a]Ratio of drug's affinity for D_2 receptors to its affinity for $5\text{-}HT_{2A}$ receptors.
[b]At dosages below 8 mg/day.

antipsychotic drugs. Most antipsychotic drugs are metabolized by hepatic cytochrome P450 enzymes. Metabolites are excreted in the urine weeks after the last dose of chronically administered drug. Parenteral forms of some agents are available for both rapid initiation of therapy and depot treatment. Depot treatment is the injection of a slow-release, slow-acting formulation that helps to improve medication adherence, a major problem for individuals who suffer from schizophrenia.

Pharmacodynamics

There are five dopaminergic systems or pathways that are important for understanding schizophrenia and the mechanism of action of antipsychotic drugs. The mesolimbic-mesocortical pathway is most closely related to behavior and psychosis. This pathway projects from cell bodies in the ventral tegmental area (VTA) to the limbic system and neocortex. The second pathway, which is critically involved in coordinating voluntary movement, is the nigrostriatal pathway that originates in the substantia nigra and projects to the dorsal striatum (ie, caudate nucleus and putamen). The third pathway is the tuberoinfundibular system that arises in hypothalamic neurons and releases dopamine into the pituitary portal circulation. The dopamine released by these neurons inhibits prolactin secretion from the anterior pituitary. The fourth dopaminergic system is the medullary-periventricular pathway, which consists of neurons in the motor nucleus of the vagus whose projections are not well defined. This system may be involved in eating behavior. Last, the incertohypothalamic pathway forms connections from the medial zona incerta to the hypothalamus and the amygdala. This pathway may be involved in regulating sexual behavior. However, it is not well defined in humans.

At present, five metabotropic dopamine receptor subtypes (D_1-D_5) consisting of two separate families—the D_1-like (D_1 and D_5) and D_2-like (D_2, D_3, D_4)—have been described. The D_1-like receptors are coupled to a G protein that activates adenylate cyclase, thus increasing intracellular concentration of cAMP. In contrast, the D_2-like receptors are coupled to a G protein that inhibits adenylate cyclase and the formation of cAMP. D_1 receptors are located mainly in the dorsal striatum and ventral striatum (nucleus accumbens and olfactory tubercle). The D_5 receptor is expressed more widely in the CNS than the D_1 receptor. D_5 receptors are found in the amygdala, frontal cortex, hippocampus, striatum, cerebellum, midbrain, thalamus, and hypothalamus. The therapeutic potency of antipsychotic drugs does *not* correlate with their affinity for binding to the D_1 receptor (in contrast to the D_2 receptor discussed below). In addition, a selective D_1 antagonist has not been shown to be an effective antipsychotic in individuals with schizophrenia.

Activation of the D_2-like receptors (D_2, D_3, D_4) decreases intracellular cAMP. This action inhibits calcium channels and opens potassium channels. The D_2 receptors are found both pre- and postsynaptically on neurons in the caudate-putamen, nucleus accumbens, and olfactory tubercle. The D_3 receptor is found primarily in limbic areas of the brain, and only at low levels in striatal regions. D_4 receptors are concentrated in the cortex. For most first-generation antipsychotic drugs (Figure 18-1), the D_2 receptor is the main target, with binding affinity strongly correlating with antipsychotic actions. The therapeutic antipsychotic efficacy of D_2 receptor inhibition is thought to be due (at least in part) to blocking the effect of dopamine in the mesolimbic system. Unfortunately, the blockade of D_2 receptors in the nigrostriatal pathway causes the unwanted extrapyramidal effects observed with clinical use of these drugs.

While all effective antipsychotic drugs block D_2 receptors, the degree of this blockade in relation to actions on *other* receptors varies considerably among drugs (Table 18-2). Some of the first-generation agents and *most* of the second-generation antipsychotic agents are at least as potent in inhibiting 5-HT_{2A} receptors as they are in inhibiting D_2 receptors. For example, aripiprazole is a partial agonist at D_2 and 5-HT_{1A} receptors, but is a strong antagonist at 5-HT_{2A} receptors. Varying degrees of antagonism of α_1 adrenoceptors occurs with risperidone, clozapine, olanzapine, quetiapine, and aripiprazole. Finally, most antipsychotic drugs, except haloperidol, also block histamine H_1 receptors.

Clinical Uses

Antipsychotic drugs have primarily been used in the treatment of schizophrenia. Table 18-3 lists the advantages and disadvantages of a representative group of antipsychotic drugs. Antipsychotic drugs reduce some of the positive symptoms of schizophrenia (hyperactivity, bizarre ideation, hallucinations, delusions). However, none of the older drugs have much effect on the negative symptoms of schizophrenia (emotional blunting, social withdrawal, lack of motivation). Most antipsychotic drugs cause unpleasant subjective effects in nonpsychotic individuals. In contrast, psychotic individuals may actually show improvement in their performance as the psychosis is alleviated. The ability of newer antipsychotic drugs to improve some domains of *cognition* in people with schizophrenia and bipolar disorder is controversial. Some individuals experience marked improvement. For that reason, cognition should be assessed in all patients with schizophrenia and a trial of a newer agent should be considered, even if positive symptoms are well controlled by first-generation agents.

In the last decade, the use of antipsychotics in the treatment of mood disorders such as bipolar disorder, psychotic depression, and treatment-resistant depression has eclipsed their use in the treatment of schizophrenia. The manic phase in bipolar affective disorder may require treatment with antipsychotic agents. Increasingly common clinical applications of antipsychotics include monotherapy for acute bipolar depression and as adjunctive therapy (with antidepressants; Chapter 19) in the treatment of unipolar depression. Antipsychotic drugs are also indicated for schizoaffective disorders, which share characteristics of both schizophrenia and affective disorders. Some of the intramuscular antipsychotics have been approved for the control of agitation associated with bipolar disorder and schizophrenia. Other indications for the use of

TABLE 18-2 Relative receptor-blocking actions of antipsychotic drugs.

Drug	D$_2$ Block	D$_4$ Block	α$_1$ Block	5-HT$_2$ Block	M Block	H$_1$ Block
Most phenothiazines (eg, chlorpromazine, thioridazine, fluphenazine) and thiothixene	++	—	++	+	+	+
Thioridazine	++	—	++	+	+++	+
Haloperidol	+++	—	+	—	—	—
Clozapine	—	++	++	++	++	+
Molindone	++	—	+	—	+	+
Olanzapine	+	—	+	++	++	+
Quetiapine	+	—	+	++	+	+
Risperidone	++	—	+	++	+	+
Ziprasidone	++	—	++	++	—	+
Aripiprazole[a]	+	+	+	++	—	+

D, dopamine; H, histamine; M, muscarinic.

+, blockade; —, no effect. The number of + signs indicates the intensity of receptor blockade.

[a]Partial agonist at D$_2$ and 5-HT$_{1A}$ receptors and antagonist at 5-HT$_{2A}$ receptors.

antipsychotics include Tourette syndrome and psychosis associated with Parkinsonism. In 2016, a new type of antipsychotic was approved for the treatment of psychosis in Parkinson's disease; **pimavanserin** is a selective serotonin inverse agonist. As such, it has no dopamine antagonist properties and is not associated with extrapyramidal adverse effects.

TABLE 18-3 Some representative antipsychotic drugs.

Drug	Advantages	Disadvantages
Classic Drugs		
Chlorpromazine	Generic, inexpensive	Many ADRs, especially autonomic
Thioridazine	Generic; slight extrapyramidal syndrome	800 mg/day limit; no parenteral form; cardiotoxicity
Fluphenazine	Depot form available (enanthate, decanoate)	Possible increased tardive dyskinesia
Thiothixene	Possible decreased tardive dyskinesia; parenteral form available	Uncertain
Haloperidol	Generic; parenteral form available	Severe extrapyramidal syndrome
Loxapine	Possible no weight gain	Uncertain
Newer Drugs		
Clozapine	May benefit treatment-resistant patients; little extrapyramidal toxicity	May cause agranulocytosis in up to 2% of patients; dose-related lowering of seizure threshold; not first-line drug
Risperidone	Broad efficacy; little or no extrapyramidal system dysfunction at low doses	Extrapyramidal system dysfunction; hypotension with higher doses
Olanzapine	Effective for treating negative and positive symptoms; little or no extrapyramidal system dysfunction	Weight gain; dose-related lowering of seizure threshold; not first-line drug
Quetiapine	Similar to olanzapine; *perhaps* less weight gain	May require high doses if there is associated hypotension; short half-life and twice-daily dosing
Ziprasidone	*Perhaps* less weight gain than clozapine; parenteral form available	QT$_c$ prolongation
Aripiprazole	Lower weight gain liability; long half-life, novel mechanism potential	Uncertain, novel toxicities possible

ADRs, adverse drug reactions; QT$_c$, QT interval that is corrected for heart rate on the electrocardiogram.

There are also a few nonpsychiatric indications for the use of antipsychotic drugs. Most first-generation antipsychotic drugs (with the exception of thioridazine) are strong antiemetics. This action is due to dopamine-receptor blockade, both centrally in the chemoreceptor trigger zone of the medulla, and peripherally on receptors in the stomach. Some drugs, such as **prochlorperazine**, are used solely for its antiemetic actions. **Promethazine** is used as preoperative sedative because of its significant inhibition of central histamine H_1 receptors. Low doses of some of these drugs, particularly quetiapine, are used to promote sleep onset and maintenance, although there is no approved indication for such usage.

Adverse Effects

Although it is has been difficult to identify the specific receptors responsible for the efficacy of antipsychotic drugs, it is relatively easy to explain most of their unwanted effects based on knowledge of their receptor affinity. For example, orthostatic hypotension is a more common adverse drug reaction (ADR) in antipsychotic drugs that cause α-adrenoceptor blockade (eg, chlorpromazine, clozapine; Table 18-2). Indeed, most ADRs associated with antipsychotics are extensions of their known pharmacologic actions (Table 18-1 and Table 18-4). A few are due to allergic and idiosyncratic reactions. For roughly 70% of individuals with schizophrenia, first- and second-generation antipsychotic drugs are equally effective for treating the positive symptoms of schizophrenia. However, evidence favors the use of second-generation drugs for their beneficial effects on negative symptoms and cognition. In addition, second-generation agents carry a lower risk of ADRs including tardive dyskinesia and other forms of extrapyramidal dysfunction as well as lower increases in prolactin levels.

Behavioral Effects

Because the older antipsychotic drugs cause unpleasant and potentially stigmatizing movement disorders, many individuals stop taking these drugs. Many adverse effects may be mitigated by giving small doses during the day and the major portion at bedtime. A "pseudodepression" that may be due to drug-induced akinesia occurs in some people. Confusional states may occur on very high doses of agents that have significant antimuscarinic actions (Table 18-2).

Extrapyramidal Symptoms

Extrapyramidal toxicity appears to be consistently associated with many of the first-generation antipsychotics that have high D_2 receptor affinity, such as haloperidol and fluphenazine (Tables 18-1 and 18-2). This drug-induced movement disorder may manifest as a Parkinson's-like syndrome (bradykinesia, rigidity, and tremor) and is common early during treatment with older agents. Other extrapyramidal symptoms include akathisia and dystonias. Akathisia manifests as a subjective sense of anxiety accompanied by uncontrollable restlessness such as pacing, rocking motions, and jitteriness. Acute dystonic reactions present as spastic retrocollis or torticollis. These extrapyramidal effects are dose-dependent and thus reversible by decreasing the dose of the D_2 antagonist or by treating the symptoms with conventional antiparkinsonism drugs of the antimuscarinic type (Chapter 17).

Tardive dyskinesia tends to develop after several years of antipsychotic drug therapy (but can appear as early as 6 months). This disorder is characterized by choreoathetoid movements of the muscles of the lips, tongue and jaw. It has been proposed that tardive dyskinesia is caused by a relative cholinergic deficiency secondary to supersensitivity of dopamine receptors in the caudate-putamen. Although the prevalence varies enormously, tardive dyskinesia is estimated to have occurred in 20-40% of chronically treated patients before the introduction of the newer antipsychotics. Early recognition is important, since advanced cases may be difficult to reverse. Newer antipsychotics with less D_2 antagonism reduce the risks of both extrapyramidal system dysfunction and tardive dyskinesia.

Neuroleptic Malignant Syndrome

This life-threatening disorder occurs in patients who are extremely sensitive to the extrapyramidal effects of antipsychotic agents. The initial symptom is marked muscle rigidity. If sweating is impaired, as it often is during treatment with anticholinergic drugs, fever may ensue, often reaching

TABLE 18-4 Adverse pharmacologic effects of antipsychotic drugs.

Type	Manifestations	Mechanism
Autonomic nervous system	Loss of accommodation, dry mouth, difficulty urinating, constipation	Muscarinic cholinergic receptor blockade
	Orthostatic hypotension, impotence, failure to ejaculate	α-adrenoceptor blockade
Central nervous system	Parkinson's syndrome, akathisia, dystonias	Dopamine receptor blockade
	Tardive dyskinesia	Supersensitivity of dopamine receptors
	Toxic-confusional state	Muscarinic cholinergic receptor blockade
Endocrine system	Amenorrhea-galactorrhea, infertility, impotence, insulin resistance	Dopamine receptor blockade resulting in hyperprolactinemia
Other	Weight gain, dyslipidemia	Possibly combined H_1 and 5-HT_2 blockade

dangerous levels. Autonomic instability, with altered blood pressure and pulse rate, is often present. Blood levels of muscle-type creatine kinase levels are usually elevated, reflecting muscle damage. This syndrome is believed to result from an excessively rapid blockade of postsynaptic dopamine receptors. After treatment and recovery, switching to an atypical drug is indicated.

Autonomic Effects

Autonomic effects result from blockade of peripheral muscarinic receptors and α adrenoceptors (Table 18-4). These are more difficult to manage in older adults. Tolerance to some of the autonomic effects occurs with continued therapy. Of the older antipsychotic agents, thioridazine has the strongest autonomic effects and haloperidol the weakest. Clozapine and most of the newer drugs have intermediate autonomic effects. Atropine-like effects (dry mouth, constipation, urinary retention, and visual problems) are often pronounced with the use of thioridazine and chlorpromazine. These effects also occur with most of the newer drugs, but not with **ziprasidone** or aripiprazole. Orthostatic hypotension caused by α-adrenoceptor blockade is a common manifestation of many of the older drugs, especially by low potency phenothiazines like chlorpromazine (Table 18-1). The newer drugs, especially clozapine and ziprasidone, also block α adrenoceptors and can cause orthostatic hypotension. Finally, the α-adrenoceptor blockade, especially caused by the phenothiazines and thioridazine, can cause a failure to ejaculate in men.

Cardiac Toxicity

Low-potency antipsychotic drugs such as chlorpromazine may decrease mean arterial pressure (MAP), peripheral resistance, and stroke volume—effects that are predictable from their autonomic actions (Table 18-4). Abnormal electrocardiograms (ECGs) have also been recorded, especially with thioridazine. Changes include prolongation of QT interval and abnormal configurations of the ST segment and T waves. Thioridazine is associated with torsades de pointes (a polymorphic ventricular tachycardic arrhythmia associated with a long QT interval on the ECG) and an increased risk of sudden death. Because of this latter ADR, the branded drug was removed from the market in 2005 and thioridazine is used as a second-line agent, only if other drugs have proven intolerable or ineffective. Among the newer drugs, ziprasidone carries the greatest risk of QT prolongation and therefore should not be combined with other drugs that prolong the QT interval. Although the newest antipsychotics may prolong the QT or QTc interval, there has not been evidence that this effect has manifested into increased incidence of arrhythmias. Clozapine is sometimes associated with myocarditis. If myocarditis occurs (symptoms such as chest pain, shortness of breath, arrhythmia, decreased exercise capacity), the drug must be discontinued. Sudden death due to arrhythmias is common in schizophrenia. These deaths are not always drug-related, and there are no studies that definitively show increased risk with specific drugs.

Metabolic and Endocrine Effects

Some newer antipsychotic drugs produce more weight gain and increases in plasma lipids than some first-generation drugs. This is especially true with clozapine and olanzapine, and requires monitoring of food intake, especially carbohydrates. Hyperglycemia may develop, but whether this is due to weight gain-associated insulin resistance or to other mechanisms is unknown. Hyperlipidemia may also occur. Thus, these drugs are associated with a metabolic syndrome that may increase the risk of coronary artery disease, stroke, and hypertension.

As a result of dopamine antagonism in the anterior pituitary, many older antipsychotics (and risperidone) increase prolactin secretion. Newer antipsychotics such as olanzapine, quetiapine, and aripiprazole cause no or minimal increases in prolactin. In women, hyperprolactinemia causes amenorrhea-galactorrhea syndrome and infertility; in men, loss of libido, impotence, and infertility may result. Hyperprolactinemia may also cause osteoporosis, particularly in women. If dose reduction is not indicated, or is not effective in controlling this pattern, patients may be switched to one of the newer agents that do not raise prolactin levels, a feature reflecting their diminished D_2 antagonism.

Additional Complications

In the brain, antipsychotic drugs produce shifts in the pattern of electroencephalographic (EEG) frequencies, usually slowing them and increasing their synchronization. These shifts may lead to an erroneous diagnosis of organic dysfunction. Some antipsychotic agents lower the seizure threshold and induce EEG patterns typical of seizure disorders.

A common complication of chlorpromazine therapy is formation of deposits in the anterior portions of the eye (cornea and lens) that may accentuate the normal aging process of the lens. Thioridazine is the only antipsychotic drug that causes retinal deposits, which in advanced cases may resemble retinitis pigmentosa. The deposits are usually associated with "browning" of vision. Agranulocytosis, cholestatic jaundice, and skin eruptions occur rarely with the high-potency antipsychotic drugs currently used. Although antipsychotic drugs appear to be relatively safe in pregnancy, a small increase in teratogenic risk may exist.

LITHIUM AND OTHER DRUGS USED IN BIPOLAR DISORDER

Bipolar affective disorder, formally known as manic-depressive disorder, affects roughly 1-3% of the adult population with the average age of diagnosis around 25 years. It is a psychiatric condition characterized by cyclic attacks of mania and depression. The manic phase is characterized by hyperactivity and decreased need for sleep, impulsivity, disinhibition, cognitive impairment, as well as symptoms of psychosis in some patients. The depressive phase appears similar to that of major depression, with psychotic symptoms that sometimes manifest. The mood swings, characteristic of bipolar disorder, are generally *unrelated* to life events. It is believed that there is an increase in catecholamine-related activity during the manic phase. This is supported by the fact that drugs that increase this activity tend to exacerbate mania, whereas those that reduce activity of dopamine or norepinephrine relieve mania. Acetylcholine or glutamate may also be involved. The nature of the abrupt switch from mania to depression experienced by some patients is uncertain. Bipolar disorder has a strong hereditary component. Genetic studies have identified at least three possible linkages to different chromosomes.

Lithium and a group of newer drugs from different pharmacologic classes are used to treat bipolar disorder (Figure 18-1). Lithium was the first agent that was *not* an antipsychotic drug shown to be useful in the treatment of the manic phase of bipolar disorder. Lithium continues to be started during the acute-phase illness, but is beneficial for prevention of recurrent manic and depressive episodes. However, antipsychotic drugs and a group of newer "mood-stabilizing" drugs— some of which are also anticonvulsants (Chapter 14)—have now become more widely used than lithium for most individuals with bipolar disorder. The mood-stabilizing drugs include, but are not limited to, **carbamazepine**, **clonazepam, olanzapine**, and **valproic acid**.

Pharmacokinetics

Table 18-5 shows the pharmacokinetics for lithium. Taken orally, lithium is absorbed rapidly and completely and is distributed throughout the body water. Lithium is not metabolized and is cleared by the kidneys. The drug's half-life is about 20 hours. Because major problems can arise if lithium accumulates within the body (see below), plasma levels should be monitored, especially during the first weeks of therapy, to establish a safe and effective dosage regimen. Plasma lithium levels may be altered by changes in body water. Thus, dehydration following prolonged exercise or treatment with thiazide

diuretics (but not loop diuretics) may result in an increase of plasma lithium to toxic levels. In contrast, caffeine and theophylline increase the renal clearance of lithium.

Pharmacodynamics

Despite considerable investigation, the biochemical basis for the efficacy of mood stabilizers—drugs that treat and prevent the manic and depressive phases characteristic of bipolar disorder—is not clearly understood. Potential mechanisms of action are listed in Table 18-6, and subsequently briefly described. Lithium, and potentially carbamazepine and valproic acid, may modulate second messenger systems. The major working hypothesis for lithium's therapeutic mechanism of action is that the drug affects the turnover or recycling of key enzymes. Specifically, lithium inhibits inositol monophosphatase (IMPase) and other important enzymes involved in the normal recycling of neuronal membrane phosphoinositides (Figure 18-2). This action may result in depletion of the second messenger source, phosphatidylinositol bisphosphate (PIP_2), which, in turn, decreases generation of the second messengers inositol trisphosphate (IP_3) and diacylglycerol (DAG). These second messengers are critical in amine neurotransmission, including that mediated by central adrenoceptors and muscarinic receptors. During a manic episode,

TABLE 18-5 Pharmacokinetics of lithium.

Absorption	Virtually complete within 6-8 hr; peak plasma levels in 30 min to 2 hr
Distribution	In total body water; slow entry into intracellular compartment. Initial volume of distribution is 0.5 L/kg, rising to 0.7-0.9 L/kg; some sequestration in bone. No protein binding.
Metabolism	None
Excretion	Virtually entirely in urine. Lithium clearance: ~ 20% that of creatinine. Plasma half-life: ~ 20 hr.
Target plasma concentration	0.6-1.4 meq/L

TABLE 18-6 Enzymes affected by therapeutic concentrations of lithium.

Enzyme	Enzyme Function and Action of Lithium
Inositol monophosphatase (IMPase)	Rate-limiting enzyme in inositol recycling; inhibited by lithium, resulting in depletion of substrate for IP_3 production (Figure 18-2)
Inositol polyphosphate 1-phosphatase	Involved in inositol recycling; inhibited by lithium, resulting in depletion of substrate for IP_3 production (Figure 18-2)
Bisphosphate nucleotidase	Involved in AMP production; inhibited by lithium; may be the target that results in lithium-induced nephrogenic diabetes insipidus
Fructose 1,6-bisphosphatase	Involved in gluconeogenesis; inhibition by lithium of unknown relevance
Phosphoglucomutase	Involved in glycogenolysis; inhibition by lithium of unknown relevance
Glycogen synthase kinase-3	Constitutively active enzyme that appears to limit neurotrophic and neuroprotective processes; lithium inhibits this enzyme

AMP, adenosine monophosphate; IP_3, inositol 1,4,5-trisphosphate.

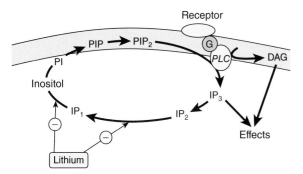

FIGURE 18-2 Postulated effect of lithium on the inositol trisphosphate (IP$_3$) and diacylglycerol (DAG) second messenger system. The diagram shows the synaptic membrane of a neuron in the brain. PI, PIP, PIP$_2$, IP$_2$, and IP$_1$, are intermediates in the production of IP$_3$. By interfering with recycling of neuronal membrane phosphoinositides, lithium may cause a use-dependent reduction of synaptic transmission. G, coupling protein; PLC, phospholipase C.

it is thought that activity of these pathways is markedly *increased* and lithium diminishes the activity in these circuits. The effects on specific isoforms of protein kinase C (that are downstream from the IP$_3$ and DAG second messengers) may be the most relevant. Changes in protein kinase C–mediated signaling alter gene expression and the production of proteins implicated in long-term neuroplastic events that could underlie long-term mood stabilization.

Lithium and valproic acid also inhibit glycogen synthase kinase-3 (GSK-3), a multifunctional protein kinase. GSK-3 is a component of diverse intracellular signaling pathways. Inhibition of GSK-3 may ultimately result in increased transcription of proteins that modulate energy metabolism, provide neuroprotection, and increase neuroplasticity. Lithium is also closely related to sodium and can substitute for sodium in generating action potentials and in Na$^+$-Na$^+$ exchange across the membrane. This activity may stabilize membrane potentials and possibly alter neurotransmitter release or postsynaptic excitation. Last, lithium also inhibits norepinephrine-sensitive adenylate cyclase by uncoupling the receptors from their G proteins. Such an effect could relate to both its antidepressant and its antimanic effects. Uncoupling of the vasopressin and thyroid-stimulating hormone (TSH) receptors from their G proteins may also be the cause of lithium's most common ADRs—polyuria and subclinical hypothyroidism.

Clinical Uses

Lithium carbonate continues to be used for the treatment of bipolar disorder, although other drugs including valproic acid and carbamazepine are equally effective. Maintenance therapy with lithium decreases manic behavior and reduces both the frequency and the magnitude of mood swings. Antipsychotic drugs and/or benzodiazepines (eg, clonazepam; Chapter 13) are commonly required at the initiation of treatment because both lithium and valproic acid have a slow onset of action. To treat the manic phase of bipolar disorder, aripiprazole, chlorpromazine, olanzapine, quetiapine, risperidone, and ziprasidone are used. For the depressive phase, olanzapine plus fluoxetine (a selective serotonin reuptake inhibitor) in combination and quetiapine are typically used. Although lithium has protective effects against suicide and self-harm, antidepressant drugs are often used concurrently during maintenance. Note that pharmacotherapy with antidepressants alone can precipitate mania in individuals with bipolar disorder.

There are additional clinical applications for lithium. Lithium may be used in recurrent clinical depression. The drug is also among the better-studied agents used to enhance the standard antidepressant response in acute major depression in individuals who have had inadequate response to monotherapy. Schizoaffective disorder, another condition characterized by a mixture of schizophrenic symptoms and depression or excitement, is treated with antipsychotic drugs alone or in conjunction with lithium. If depression is present, various antidepressants are added.

Adverse Effects

Many ADRs associated with lithium occur at varying times after treatment is started. Some are insignificant, but it is important to be alert to adverse effects that may signify impending serious toxic reactions. At therapeutic levels, the most common adverse neurologic effect of lithium is tremor. Other ADRs include choreoathetosis, motor hyperactivity, ataxia, dysarthria, and aphasia. At toxic concentrations, psychiatric disturbances generally include mental confusion and withdrawal. As discussed above, two of lithium's most common ADRs are subclinical hypothyroidism and polyuria. Thyroid enlargement may occur, but hypothyroidism is rare. Polyuria and polydipsia often occur at therapeutic drug levels, and result from the loss of sensitivity of vasopressin receptors in the kidney to the hormone. Edema, due to sodium retention, is also common. "Sick sinus" syndrome (bradycardia, tachycardia, or an alternating combination of these arrhythmias) is a definite contraindication to the use of lithium because the lithium ion further depresses the sinus node. Recent analyses suggest that the teratogenic risk of lithium is low, but its use requires special monitoring in nursing mothers due to transfer to the infant. Finally, acneiform skin eruptions occur early in therapy, and leukocytosis is always present.

REHABILITATION RELEVANCE

When treating individuals with certain psychiatric diagnoses, therapists must recognize that drugs taken for these conditions are usually taken on a chronic basis. Therapists must therefore adjust therapy to account for the pharmacologic effects of these drugs that may alter outcomes or goals.

- **Sedation**, **psychomotor delay**, and **decreased cognitive function** are potential adverse effects of many antipsychotic drugs. Timing therapy sessions when drug plasma levels at their lowest—prior to the next dose—may decrease the impact of these effects on physical therapy interventions. Consider using pictures and simple written instructions in home exercise programs rather than complex verbal instructions. Complex activities of daily living such as driving, operating power equipment, or making financial decisions may be inhibited. If these effects continue or increase, contact the referring healthcare professional.

- **Bradykinesia**, **rigidity**, and **tremor** and other extrapyramidal symptoms may occur with the older potent antipsychotic drugs (eg, haloperidol) that have significant D_2 receptor affinity (Table 18-2). If these manifestations increase or begin to significantly impair daily functioning, consult the referring healthcare professional to determine whether dosage or medication changes are indicated.

- **Tardive dyskinesia** is a late and potentially irreversible adverse effect of chronic therapy with high potency antipsychotics such as haloperidol, but the condition can also occur with newer drugs (Table 18-3). If suspected, contact the referring healthcare professional immediately to prevent or limit permanent dysfunction.

- There is a potential for **increased fall risk** for many antipsychotic drugs, likely as the result of multiple factors including psychomotor delay and extrapyramidal effects. Several antipsychotics that have significant α_1-adrenoceptor antagonism (eg, clozapine; Table 18-2) also cause orthostatic hypotension. Appropriate fall prevention education, balance training and compensation, and gait training with assistive devices should be implemented as necessary. If fall risk is particularly high or increasing, consultation with the referring healthcare professional is indicated.

- First-generation antipsychotic drugs (and risperidone) that cause varying degrees of hyperprolactinemia may also cause **osteoporosis**, especially in women. In patients on such medications or who have had a history of taking these medications, weightbearing exercises and resistance training should be incorporated into the treatment plan.

- **Hyperthermia** may result during aerobic activities due to perspiration inhibition caused by the antimuscarinic effect of some antipsychotic drugs (Table 18-2). The risk of hyperthermia should be considered when developing a treatment plan. Aerobic activities should be conducted in cooler, well-ventilated areas.

- **Arrhythmias** are rare, but significant adverse effects associated with thioridazine and ziprasidone. Careful cardiac monitoring may be required.

- **Weight gain** and potentially **hyperglycemia** and **hyperlipidemia** are effects of several newer antipsychotic drugs (especially clozapine and olanzapine). Development and implementation of physical activity programs may help prevent or mitigate weight gain and decrease the risk of diabetes and cardiovascular disease. In diabetic individuals, blood glucose should be monitored prior to and after exercise interventions.

- **Mental confusion** may occur when plasma lithium level is above, but sometimes at, a therapeutic level. Because plasma lithium level may be altered by changes in body water, potential causes of increased plasma lithium include conditions that lead to dehydration such as prolonged aerobic exercise or diuretic therapy. If mental confusion is noted in individuals taking lithium, contact the primary healthcare professional immediately.

CASE CONCLUSION

The therapist called the patient's prescribing practitioner and summarized her findings after M.M.'s evaluation, including symptomatic orthostatic hypotension, rigidity, absence of resting tremor, and impaired balance with a predicted increased risk of falls on a validated outcome measure. In consultation with the patient's physician, it was determined that M.M. may be experiencing adverse effects associated with the use of quetiapine at higher doses. Because the increased quetiapine dose was effectively controlling M.M.'s psychosis, the physician was reluctant to make any abrupt changes in his medication. Therefore, the physical therapist educated M.M. and his wife about postural hypotension and strategies to prevent episodes of syncope. Physical therapy interventions were directed at functional balance and gait training. M.M. and his wife, the physical therapist, and the prescribing practitioner agreed to closely monitor the patient's symptoms and to reevaluate his condition in 3 months.

CHAPTER 18 QUESTIONS

1. Which of the following drugs is most associated with tardive dyskinesia as an adverse effect?

   a. Haloperidol
   b. Lithium
   c. Aripiprazole
   d. Valproic acid

2. Which of the following antipsychotic drugs has the most sedative action?

   a. Haloperidol
   b. Chlorpromazine
   c. Olanzapine
   d. Aripiprazole

3. Inhibition of which of the following receptors is most closely associated with Parkinson's-like adverse effects?

    a. Muscarinic receptors
    b. Serotonin 5-HT$_2$ receptors
    c. Dopamine D$_2$ receptors
    d. Glutamate receptors

4. The newer "second generation" antipsychotic drugs have a greater affinity for which of the following receptors as a hypothesized mechanism of action?

    a. Dopamine D$_1$ receptors
    b. Glutamate receptors
    c. Histamine H$_1$ receptors
    d. Serotonin 5-HT$_2$ receptors

5. Why was pimavanserin specifically developed to treat psychosis associated with Parkinson's disease?

    a. The drug has no dopamine receptor antagonism.
    b. The drug has no serotonin receptor antagonism.
    c. The drug has muscarinic receptor antagonism.
    d. The drug has no glutamate receptor antagonism.

6. Blockade of which of the following receptors by antipsychotic drugs would most likely be associated with orthostatic hypotension?

    a. Muscarinic receptors
    b. Adrenergic α$_1$ receptors
    c. Dopamine D$_2$ receptors
    d. Serotonin 5-HT$_1$ receptors

7. Which of the following is *not* considered a mechanism associated with the clinical effect of lithium?

    a. Inhibition of intracellular second messenger diacylglycerol
    b. Inhibition of intracellular second messenger inositol triphosphate
    c. Substitution for potassium in membrane action potentials
    d. Inhibition of glycogen synthase kinase-3

8. Which of the following neurotransmitters is hypothesized to be increased in schizophrenia?

    a. Glycine
    b. Norepinephrine
    c. Histamine
    d. Dopamine

9. Inhibition of which of the following receptors would most likely increase the risk of hyperthermia?

    a. Muscarinic receptors
    b. Dopamine D$_1$ receptors
    c. Serotonin 5-HT$_1$ receptors
    d. Glutamate receptors

10. Which of the following activities may precipitate neuroleptic malignant syndrome?

    a. Transcutaneous electrical nerve stimulation
    b. Aerobic exercise
    c. Ultrasound
    d. Joint mobilization

Antidepressant Agents

R.N. is a 44-year-old man with a primary diagnosis of right transtibial amputation secondary to trauma sustained in a motor vehicle accident. The amputation left the patient with an 8-inch residual limb distal to the knee. While in the hospital, R.N. received physical therapy, occupational therapy, and social services. He was discharged home and immediately began outpatient physical therapy for further amputation rehabilitation, including permanent prosthesis fitting and gait training. Upon initial examination, R.N. demonstrated moderate weakness in the right lower extremity with tenderness and increased sensitivity in the residual limb. He required contact guard assistance with sit-to-stand transfers and demonstrated independence with household distance ambulation with his prosthesis and a front-wheeled walker. R.N. stated that his primary limitation was significant pain in his right residual limb with all weight-bearing activities. R.N. is currently unable to work in his lawn

maintenance and landscaping business. He admits that this has made him very anxious and unable to sleep at night. He has occasionally been taking diazepam at night to help him sleep and tramadol to help alleviate the pain. Initial rehabilitation interventions included therapeutic exercises focused on bilateral lower extremities and pelvic and trunk musculature and progressive gait training. On several occasions, the therapist noted that R.N. complained of not being able to take a deep breath and a burning and "squeezing" feeling in his chest. Upon further questioning, R.N. stated that this happened almost every night in the early evening and occasionally during the day. He stated that he was having a hard time sleeping at night but did not like taking the diazepam because it made him feel "groggy" in the morning. With the patient's approval, the physical therapist contacted the patient's physician to inform her of R.N.'s major complaints.

REHABILITATION FOCUS

Major depression is one of the most common forms of mental illness in the United States with as many as 5% of the population depressed at any given moment (point prevalence), and an estimated 17% of people becoming depressed during their lifetime (lifetime prevalence). The symptoms of depression can be both psychological and physiological, including intense feelings of sadness and despair, sleep disturbances (too much or too little), anorexia, fatigue, somatic complaints, and suicidal thoughts. Often, symptoms can be subtle and unrecognized by patients and healthcare professionals.

Depression is a heterogeneous disorder that has been classified as (1) "reactive" or "secondary" depression (most common) that occurs in response to situational stimuli such as grief or illness; (2) "endogenous" depression or major depressive disorder (MDD), a genetically determined biochemical disorder of depressed mood without any obvious medical or situational causes, manifested by an inability to experience ordinary pleasure or to cope with ordinary life events;

and (3) depression associated with bipolar affective (manic-depressive) disorder.

Physical therapists may encounter patients taking antidepressant medications under a number of circumstances. Many patients who have experienced life-changing disabilities become depressed and may require medication for a limited time to control their depression. Other patients may be receiving long-term treatment for chronic depression that is unrelated to their therapy diagnosis. Drugs used in treating depressive disorders are highly effective in some patients but only modestly, or not at all, effective in others.

While depression is the primary indication for antidepressant drugs, these agents are used to treat a wide variety of conditions. Some of these conditions—panic disorder, post-traumatic stress disorder (PTSD), generalized anxiety disorder (GAD), and obsessive-compulsive disorder (OCD)—are significant comorbidities in rehabilitation patients. Other applications for antidepressant agents—such as neuropathic pain, fibromyalgia, and stress urinary incontinence—may be the primary reason individuals are seeking physical therapy.

PATHOPHYSIOLOGY OF MAJOR DEPRESSION

There are at least three main hypotheses regarding the pathophysiology of depression. The long-standing predominant hypothesis was the monoamine hypothesis, which postulates that brain amines, particularly norepinephrine (NE) and serotonin (5-HT), are functionally or quantitatively decreased in depression. The monoamine hypothesis is largely based on studies showing that drugs (such as **reserpine**) that deplete central amines cause depression, and that most drugs that enhance the actions of NE and 5-HT in central synapses alleviate the symptoms of major depression. Indeed, all available antidepressants (at the time of this writing) appear to have significant effects on the monoamine system (Figure 19-1). However, several facts highlight difficulties with the monoamine hypothesis of depression. These include: (1) postmortem studies do *not* reveal decreases in brain levels of NE or 5-HT in untreated patients suffering from endogenous depression; (2) although antidepressant drugs may cause biochemical changes in brain amine activity within hours, the clinical effects may require *weeks* to achieve; and, (3) with chronic use, most antidepressants ultimately cause a *down*-regulation of amine receptors.

Accumulating evidence in animal and human studies supports the neurotrophic hypothesis, which proposes that there is a deficiency in trophic support for neurons in key cortical regions involved in mood (Figure 19-2). Work on this hypothesis has focused primarily on brain-derived neurotrophic factor (BDNF), a growth factor in the adult brain that is essential in the regulation of neural plasticity and neurogenesis. Stress and pain are associated with a drop in BDNF levels; this loss of trophic support contributes to structural changes in the hippocampus and other limbic regions associated with emotion. Many (but not all) imaging studies have shown a 5-10% loss of volume in the hippocampus in individuals with major depression. In animal models, all classes of antidepressants are associated with an increase in BDNF levels with chronic (but not acute) administration, which is consistent with increased neurogenesis in the hippocampus. In humans, administration of antidepressant drugs also increases BDNF levels and may be associated with an increase in hippocampal volume in some patients.

Finally, depression is recognized to be associated with several hormonal abnormalities. The most significant endocrine system abnormality implicated in depression is overactivity of the hypothalamic-pituitary-adrenal (HPA) axis. This is supported by observations that patients with depression have chronically increased levels of corticotropin-releasing hormone (CRH), increased levels of circulating adrenocorticotropic hormone (ACTH), and increased urinary cortisol excretion. Although the significance of these abnormalities is unclear, they indicate dysregulation of the HPA stress axis. Thyroid hormone dysfunction may also play a role in depression. Most individuals with major depression do *not* have thyroid hormone dysfunction; however, up to 25% have abnormal thyroid function, so screening for hypothyroidism is indicated. Clinical hypothyroidism often presents with depressive

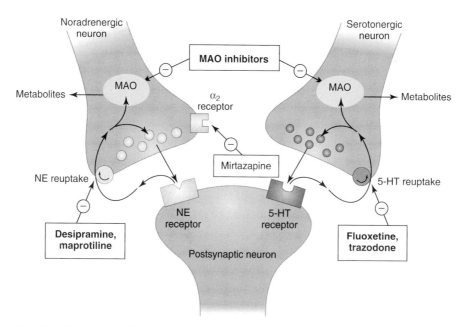

FIGURE 19-1 **Possible sites of action of antidepressant drugs.** Inhibition of neuronal reuptake of norepinephrine (NE) and serotonin (5-HT) increases the synaptic availability of these neurotransmitters. Inhibition of monoamine oxidase (MAO) increases presynaptic stores of both NE and 5-HT, which leads to increased neurotransmitter effects. Blockade of the presynaptic adrenergic α₂ autoreceptor prevents feedback inhibition of the release of NE, resulting in increased NE release. Note that these are *acute* actions of antidepressants.

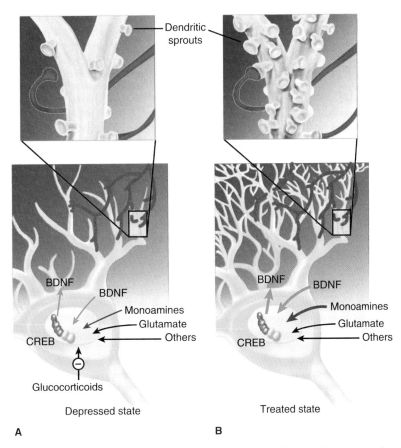

FIGURE 19-2 Neurotrophic hypothesis of depression. (A) In the depressed state, there are lower levels of trophic factors like brain-derived neurotrophic factor (BDNF), which results in a decrease in dendritic sprouting. **(B)** Successful treatment results in changes in levels of monoamines and BDNF. BDNF signaling results in downstream activation of cAMP response element-binding (CREB) proteins that ultimately results in changes in gene expression. (Reproduced with permission from Nestler EJ. Neurobiology of depression. *Neuron*. 2002;34[1]:13-25. Copyright Elsevier.)

symptoms that *resolve* with thyroid hormone supplementation. Thyroid hormones are also commonly used in conjunction with antidepressants to augment therapeutic effects of the latter. Last, sex steroids may be implicated in the pathophysiology of depression. This is primarily supported by the fact that hormone replacement therapy in hypogonadal men and women may be associated with an improvement in mood and depressive symptoms.

No *single* hypothesis provides a complete explanation or understanding of the etiology of depression. However, it is critical to recognize that none of the hypotheses are mutually exclusive. In fact, it is more likely that the monoamine, neurotrophic, and neuroendocrine systems act in an interrelated manner to regulate mood. For example, BDNF is reported to be a potent neurotrophic factor for both the NE and 5-HT neurotransmitter systems. Thus, BDNF could influence monoamine systems via actions at presynaptic sites (eg, increased function of monoamine neurons) and/or at postsynaptic sites (eg, increased response of the target neurons). One of the weaknesses of the original monoamine theory was that the maximum beneficial effects of antidepressants are not clinically seen for weeks—even though the amine levels

(NE and 5-HT) are increased almost immediately with antidepressant use. However, this delay of clinical antidepressant action can be reconciled if one considers that this timeframe may be required to synthesize the requisite neurotrophic factors in vital mood-regulating limbic regions. In fact, appreciable protein synthesis of products such as BDNF typically takes 2 weeks or longer.

DRUG CLASSIFICATION, PHARMACOKINETICS, AND PHARMACODYNAMICS

Figure 19-3 outlines the six main categories of antidepressant drugs based on their chemical structures or purported mechanisms of action: selective serotonin reuptake inhibitors (SSRIs), selective serotonin-norepinephrine reuptake inhibitors (SNRIs), tricyclic antidepressants (TCAs), 5-HT$_2$ receptor antagonists, tetracyclic and unicyclic antidepressants, and monoamine oxidase inhibitors (MAOIs).

All antidepressant drugs in current use appear to potentiate the neurotransmitter actions of NE, 5-HT, or both.

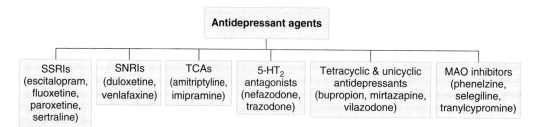

FIGURE 19-3 **Six major classes of antidepressants.** 5-HT, serotonin; MAO, monoamine oxidase; NE, norepinephrine; SSRIs, selective serotonin reuptake inhibitors; SNRIs, selective serotonin-norepinephrine reuptake inhibitors; TCAs, tricyclic antidepressants. Common agents are in parentheses.

Increased monoamine transmission ultimately results in altered protein synthesis. Production of key proteins—such as BDNF and glucocorticoid receptors—appears to bring about the clinical antidepressant action (as well as associated adverse effects).

Selective Serotonin Reuptake Inhibitors

The SSRIs are a chemically diverse class of drugs whose primary action is selective inhibition of the serotonin transporter (SERT), which blocks the reuptake of 5-HT without affecting reuptake of other amine neurotransmitters such as NE and dopamine (Figure 19-1). At therapeutic doses, roughly 80% of the activity of the SERT is inhibited. **Fluoxetine**, the prototype SSRI, is one of the most commonly prescribed drugs in medical practice. Though their primary indication is to treat depression, SSRIs are used to treat GAD, PTSD, OCD, panic disorder, premenstrual dysphoric disorder (PMDD), and bulimia. Currently, the SSRIs are the most popular antidepressants largely because of their relative tolerability, safety in overdose, broad spectrum of use, and lower cost (all are available in generic formulations).

All SSRIs require hepatic metabolism and have half-lives of 18-24 hours. However, fluoxetine forms an active metabolite with a half-life of several days (the basis for a once-weekly formulation). Other members of this group (eg, **sertraline**, **citalopram**, **escitalopram**, **fluvoxamine**, **paroxetine**) do not form long-acting metabolites.

Because of their selectivity for the 5-HT transporter, they produce fewer and less troublesome adverse effects than older classes of antidepressants such as the TCAs. Since SSRIs enhance serotonergic transmission throughout the body, increased serotonergic tone in the gut often causes gastrointestinal (GI) distress such as nausea and diarrhea. However, GI symptoms tend to improve after the first week of treatment. Extrapyramidal effects early in treatment may include akathisia ("jitteriness"), dyskinesias, and dystonic reactions. Jitteriness can be alleviated by starting with low doses or by adjunctive use of benzodiazepines. The SSRIs may also cause headache, anxiety, agitation, insomnia, and sexual dysfunction. Serotonin syndrome is a life-threatening cluster of autonomic (hyperthermia, cardiovascular instability), motor

(severe muscle rigidity), and mental status changes (agitation). The syndrome—first described for an interaction between fluoxetine and an MAOI—typically occurs when two or more serotonergic medications are used. Management of serotonin syndrome involves antiseizure medications and serotonin receptor antagonists. A withdrawal syndrome has been described for SSRIs that includes nausea, dizziness, anxiety, tremor, and palpitations.

Selective Serotonin-Norepinephrine Reuptake Inhibitors

The SNRIs bind to and inhibit both the serotonin transporter and the norepinephrine transporter (NET), thus increasing the synaptic availability of *both* neurotransmitters (Figure 19-1). The SNRIs include **venlafaxine**, its metabolite **desvenlafaxine**, **duloxetine**, **levomilnacipran**, and **milnacipran**. The SNRIs are chemically unrelated to each other and their affinity for the transporters varies. Venlafaxine weakly inhibits NET, whereas the other SNRIs are more balanced inhibitors of SERT and NET. In general, however, the affinity of most SNRIs is much greater for SERT than for NET. The SNRIs are used in the treatment of major depression, pain disorders including neuropathies and fibromyalgia, GAD, stress urinary incontinence, and vasomotor symptoms of menopause. Milnacipran is approved only for the treatment of fibromyalgia in the United States, though the drug is used to treat depression in other countries.

Although venlafaxine, desvenlafaxine, and duloxetine have relatively short half-lives, these drugs are available in once-daily dosage formulations. Milnacipran's half-life is shorter, requiring twice daily dosing. Venlafaxine and duloxetine undergo extensive oxidative metabolism in the liver, so hepatic impairment will alter plasma drug levels.

SNRIs have many of the serotonergic adverse effects associated with the SSRIs. In addition, SNRIs may cause noradrenergic effects such as increased heart rate and blood pressure and central nervous system (CNS) activation (eg, insomnia, agitation). In most patients, the hemodynamic effects are not problematic. However, cardiac toxicity (especially in overdose) may be more common with venlafaxine than with other SNRIs or SSRIs. In persons with liver damage, duloxetine is rarely associated with hepatotoxicity. The SNRIs have been associated with a discontinuation syndrome similar to that seen with SSRI discontinuation.

Tricyclic Antidepressants

Tricyclic antidepressants were the first successful antidepressants and the dominant class until the introduction of the SSRIs. The prototype TCA is **imipramine** along with its metabolite **amitriptyline**. The TCAs are structurally related to the phenothiazine antipsychotics and share certain of their pharmacologic effects.

The TCAs are well absorbed orally but may undergo first-pass metabolism. They have high volumes of distribution and are not readily dialyzable. Extensive hepatic metabolism is required for their elimination; plasma half-lives of 8-36 hours usually permit once-daily dosing. Most are dosed at night because of their sedating effects. Both amitriptyline and imipramine form active metabolites, **nortriptyline** and **desipramine**, respectively.

Similar to the SNRIs, the TCAs bind to and inhibit the SERT and NET and thus their antidepressant activity is thought to relate primarily due to inhibited uptake of 5-HT and NE (Figure 19-1). However, unlike the SNRIs, the TCAs have other effects due to their affinity at many receptors. As a class, the TCAs have anticholinergic, antihistaminergic, and α-adrenergic antagonistic properties. Anticholinergic effects are the most common (especially with imipramine and amitriptyline) and include dry mouth, constipation, blurred vision, urinary retention, and confusion. Orthostatic hypotension, a consequence of antagonism of α-adrenergic receptors, can be significant in older adults. Antihistamine effects of sedation and weight gain result from antagonism of central H_1 receptors. The TCAs can also cause cardiac conduction defects and severe arrhythmias. Discontinuation of TCAs results in a syndrome characterized by cholinergic rebound and flu-like symptoms. Overdosage with TCAs is extremely hazardous, and the ingestion of as little as a 2-week supply has been lethal. Manifestations of overdose include the characteristic "three Cs"—coma, convulsions, and cardiotoxicity.

Due to their adverse effect profile and lethality in overdose, TCAs are primarily used to treat depression that is resistant to more commonly used antidepressants such as the SSRIs or SNRIs. Other uses for TCAs include treatment of pain disorders, enuresis (involuntary urination), and insomnia.

5-HT$_2$ Receptor Antagonists

Nefazodone and **trazodone** act primarily as antagonists at the 5-HT$_{2A}$ receptor. This 5-HT receptor subtype is widely expressed near most of the serotonergic terminal rich areas throughout the neocortex. Inhibition of 5-HT$_{2A}$ receptors is associated with antianxiety, antipsychotic, and antidepressant effects. In contrast, activation of this receptor by lysergic acid (LSD) and mescaline often produces anxiety and hallucinations. Although antagonism of 5-HT$_{2A}$ receptors is implicated in the antidepressant actions of nefazodone and trazodone, both of these agents also weakly inhibit SERT and thus increase synaptic 5-HT (Figure 19-1). Nefazodone also weakly inhibits NET.

The half-lives of nefazodone and trazodone are quite short and usually require administration 2 or 3 times daily. Trazodone was frequently prescribed as an antidepressant until it was largely replaced by the SSRIs. Today, the main application of trazodone is as a hypnotic for insomnia because it is highly sedating and not associated with tolerance or dependence. For insomnia, trazodone is usually prescribed as a single dose at night in lower doses than those used in the treatment of depression.

Common adverse drug reactions (ADRs) associated with the 5-HT$_{2A}$ antagonists are sedation and GI disturbances. The GI effects are dose-related and less pronounced than those associated with SSRIs or SNRIs. Sexual effects are uncommon due to the more selective effect on the serotonergic system than the agents that affect the SERT. In some patients, both agents can induce a dose-related orthostatic hypotension. Nefazodone is not frequently prescribed because of a black box warning issued by the Food and Drug Administration implicating the agent in hepatotoxicity, including lethal cases of liver failure.

Tetracyclic and Unicyclic Antidepressants

Several antidepressants do not fit neatly into the other classes because they have varied structures, mechanisms of action, and adverse effect profiles. These agents include **bupropion**, **mirtazapine**, **amoxapine**, **maprotiline**, and **vilazodone**.

Bupropion, with a unicyclic chemical structure similar to amphetamine, also activates the CNS. The mechanism of action of bupropion is not completely understood. Bupropion has almost no direct effects on the serotonin system, but it does appear to increase the synaptic availability of NE and dopamine (to a smaller extent). Bupropion and mirtazapine are fairly unique in that they are not commonly associated with adverse sexual effects.

Mirtazapine, amoxapine, and maprotiline are the tetracyclic antidepressants. Mirtazapine has many pharmacological targets. The drug blocks presynaptic α$_2$-adrenergic autoreceptors, which augments the release of NE and 5-HT (Figure 19-1). Mirtazapine is also an antagonist at the histamine H_1 receptor and serotonin 5-HT$_2$ and 5-HT$_3$ receptors. Both amoxapine and maprotiline are potent NET inhibitors, but less potent SERT inhibitors. Because their adverse effect profiles are similar to the TCAs, use of amoxapine and maprotiline is typically reserved to treat major depression that is not responsive to other antidepressants. Vilazodone binds to the SERT, but not to the dopamine and NE transporters. Vilazodone also acts as a partial agonist of the 5-HT$_{1A}$ receptor. Partial agonists of this receptor such as **buspirone** have mild to moderate antidepressant and anxiolytic properties.

The pharmacokinetics of this group of drugs is also diverse. For most of these agents, the pharmacokinetics are similar to those of the TCAs. Bupropion has a significant first-pass effect and a two-phase elimination. Mirtazapine has a long half-life of 20-40 hours; a single dose is usually given in the evening because of its highly sedating effect. Vilazodone's long half-life (25 hours) also enables once-daily dosing; absorption is increased with a fatty meal. Vilazodone is associated with higher rates of GI symptoms (including diarrhea and nausea) than the SSRIs.

Monoamine Oxidase Inhibitors

The MAOIs are structurally related to amphetamines and are orally active. These drugs inhibit two forms of monoamine oxidases (MAO). By interfering with the metabolism of monoamines in the nerve endings, MAOIs increase brain amine levels due to an increase in the vesicular stores of NE and 5-HT (Figure 19-1). Inhibition of MAO-A (present in dopamine and NE neurons in the brain, liver, gut, and placenta) reduces the breakdown of primarily 5-HT, NE, and dopamine. Inhibition of MAO-B (present largely in the brain, liver, and platelets) primarily reduces the breakdown of dopamine and tyramine. MAOIs are classified according to their specificity for MAO-A or MAO-B and by whether their effects are reversible. **Phenelzine** and **tranylcypromine** are irreversible, nonselective MAOIs. At low doses, **selegiline** is an irreversible selective MAO-B inhibitor that is useful as an adjunctive treatment in Parkinson's disease because it inhibits the breakdown of dopamine (Chapter 17).

The MAOIs are well absorbed from the GI tract, though they have significant first-pass effects. When these agents inhibit MAO in the gut, the concentration of tyramine rises. Tyramine, a precursor for the synthesis of NE, cannot cross the blood-brain barrier. Thus, the result of MAO inhibition is an increase in NE in peripheral sympathetic nerve terminals. Increased NE release and subsequent vasoconstriction due to activation of α_1-adrenergic receptors can result in a hypertensive reaction. To avoid a hypertensive crisis, individuals taking MAOIs generally need to change their diets to limit or avoid foods containing tyramine (Table 19-1). Transdermal and sublingual MAOI formulations increase bioavailability and decrease the risk of food interactions.

Tranylcypromine has the quickest onset of action, but shorter duration of action (about 1 week) than other MAOIs (2-3 weeks). In spite of their prolonged action, the MAOIs are given daily. It is prudent to assume that drug effects will persist from 7 days (tranylcypromine) to 2 or 3 weeks (phenelzine) after *discontinuance* of the drug. MAOIs are also inhibitors of hepatic drug-metabolizing enzymes and cause many drug interactions.

Due to their toxicity and potentially lethal food and drug interactions, MAOIs are only used to treat depression that is unresponsive to other antidepressants. Nonselective MAOIs may also be used to treat panic disorder and social anxiety. In the absence of sympathomimetics, MAOIs typically lower blood pressure; overdosage with these drugs may result in shock, hyperthermia, and seizures. The most common ADRs of MAOIs that cause individuals to abandon treatment are

TABLE 19-1 Foods, beverages, and over-the-counter medications to avoid when taking monoamine oxidase inhibitors.

Meat and fish
Pickled herring
Liver
Cured meats (eg, salami, pepperoni, and dry-type summer sausages)
Smoked or processed meats (eg, hot dogs, bacon, bologna)
Vegetables
Broad beans (fava beans), snowpeas, soybeans (and soybean products)
Pickled or fermented foods (eg, sauerkraut, tofu, pickles, kimchi)
Dairy products
Aged or strong cheeses (cheeses from pasteurized milk such as cottage cheese, and cream cheese are allowed)
Yogurt and sour cream
Alcoholic beverages (especially tap beer, red wine, sherry, and liqueurs)
Alcohol-free and reduced-alcohol beer and wine products
Miscellaneous
Yeast extracts (eg, brewer's yeast, Marmite, sourdough bread)
Meat tenderizers
Excessive amounts of chocolate and caffeine
Spoiled or improperly refrigerated, handled, or stored protein-rich foods such as meats, fish and dairy products including foods that may have undergone protein changes by aging, pickling fermentation or smoking to improve flavor should be avoided
Over-the-counter medications
Cold and cough preparations (including those containing dextromethorphan)
Nasal decongestants (tablets, drops, or spray)
Hay fever medication
Sinus medications
Asthma inhalant medications
Antiappetite medications

weight gain and orthostatic hypotension. Irreversible and nonselective MAOIs are associated with the highest rates of sexual adverse effects (eg, anorgasmia) of all the antidepressant classes. As described above, serotonin syndrome is more likely to occur with the combined use of serotonergic drugs (eg, SSRI and MAOI). Last, some MAOIs cause insomnia and restlessness.

CLINICAL USES

The major indication for antidepressants is to treat depression, but a number of other uses have been established by clinical experience and controlled trials.

Depression

Most antidepressants are approved for both acute and chronic treatment of major depression. There is no overwhelming evidence that one antidepressant consistently demonstrates more effectiveness than another because patients with major depression typically vary in their responsiveness to individual agents. Because of more tolerable adverse effects and greater safety in overdose, the SSRIs are the most widely prescribed first-line drugs in the treatment of both depression and anxiety disorders. Other first-line agents for depression include the SNRIs, bupropion, and mirtazapine. Bupropion, mirtazapine, and nefazodone are often chosen because they have the least association with adverse sexual effects. Since mirtazapine is sedative, this drug is often given with a more activating antidepressant. The TCAs and MAOIs are second- or third-line agents for major depression usually reserved for patients who have been unresponsive to other drugs.

Antidepressants provide significant benefit for most individuals with depression. However, these drugs typically do not achieve maximal benefit for at least 1-2 months. Thus, a trial of a particular agent or agents may last 8-12 weeks at therapeutic doses. For 30-40% of individuals, this single trial of antidepressants improves depressive symptoms. If the person does not have a therapeutic response, the antidepressant agent is typically switched or supplemented with an additional antidepressant. About 70-80% of individuals achieve remission of symptoms with switching or supplementary regimens.

Anxiety Disorders

After major depression, anxiety disorders are the second most common indication for antidepressants. Imipramine, the prototype TCA, was first shown in 1962 to have a beneficial effect in acute episodes of anxiety that have come to be known as panic attacks. Now, SSRIs and SNRIs have largely replaced older antidepressants and sedative-hypnotics (eg, benzodiazepines) to treat panic disorder, PTSD, OCD, social anxiety disorder, and GAD. For *rapid* relief of anxiety and panic, benzodiazepines (Chapter 13) are more effective than any of the antidepressants. However, for *long-term* treatment of anxiety disorders, antidepressants are more effective and safer because they are not associated with the tolerance and dependence of benzodiazepines. For OCD, serotonergic antidepressants such as **clomipramine** and fluvoxamine (typically in combination with behavioral therapy) have been shown to be effective, whereas the noradrenergic agents have not been useful. Bupropion is not effective for treating anxiety disorders and may be poorly tolerated in anxious individuals.

Pain Disorders

Independent of their effects on mood, many antidepressants have analgesic properties. Decades ago, clinicians found TCAs to be useful for treating a variety of chronic pain and neuropathic pain conditions. Since then, it has been discovered that antidepressants that possess both NE and 5-HT reuptake blocking properties—the TCAs and SNRIs—are frequently helpful in treating pain disorders. One reason may be that a component of the endogenous analgesic system involves the ascending corticospinal monoamine pathways. Duloxetine,

an SNRI, is increasingly prescribed for chronic musculoskeletal pain, fibromyalgia, and diabetic neuropathic pain. In the United States, milnacipran is approved for the treatment of fibromyalgia. The SNRI desvenlafaxine indicated for treating major depression has also been investigated to treat chronic back pain and postherpetic neuralgia.

Other Clinical Uses

In addition to their uses described above, the SSRIs are used in the treatment of bulimia (but not anorexia), premenstrual dysphoric disorder (PMDD), vasomotor symptoms associated with menopause, and premature ejaculation. In PMDD, women experience more severe mood and physical symptoms than those associated with premenstrual syndrome. Treatment with SSRIs for 2 weeks of the month in the luteal phase may be as effective as continuous treatment. Antidepressants that modulate the serotonergic system may help perimenopausal or menopausal women with vasomotor symptoms (eg, hot flashes, night sweats). These drugs include the SSRIs, nefazodone, and especially the SNRIs desvenlafaxine and venlafaxine. Because SSRIs delay orgasm in some individuals, these agents are sometimes helpful to treat premature ejaculation.

In 1997, bupropion was approved as a treatment for smoking cessation. Bupropion appears to be as effective as nicotine patches, with roughly twice as many people treated with bupropion as with placebo having reduced urges to smoke. In the past, TCAs have been used in the treatment of enuresis, though this use is less frequent due to the ADRs of this class. For urinary stress incontinence, the SNRI duloxetine is approved for treatment in Europe. Last, the 5-HT$_2$ antagonist trazodone is frequently prescribed for insomnia.

ANTIDEPRESSANT USE IN PREGNANCY AND IN CHILDREN AND ADOLESCENTS

The Food and Drug Administration (FDA) has established a ranking system to indicate the potential of a drug to cause birth defects if used during pregnancy. For most antidepressants, animal studies have failed to demonstrate a risk to the fetus, but there are no adequate and well-controlled studies in pregnant women. A key exception is the SSRI paroxetine, which carries a risk of teratogenicity in the first trimester.

For all antidepressants, the FDA has issued a black box warning that there is an increased suicidality risk (suicidal ideation and gestures, but not completed suicides) in people younger than 25. In contrast, for those over the age of 25, there is either no increased risk of suicidal thoughts or even a reduced risk of these thoughts on antidepressants, especially in individuals over the age of 65. For this reason, parents, other family, and caregivers of children and adolescents being treated with antidepressants should be aware of potential warning signs such as agitation, irritability, unusual changes in behavior, and any other indicators of suicidal tendencies. Monitoring should be done on a daily basis and any changes should be reported to the prescribing practitioner immediately.

DRUG INTERACTIONS

Patients may have both pharmacodynamic and pharmacokinetic interactions when taking antidepressants with other drugs (Table 19-2). The most serious of these involve the MAOIs and, to a lesser extent, the TCAs. As noted earlier, a hypertensive crisis may occur in individuals taking MAOIs who consume foods that contain high concentrations of tyramine, an indirect sympathomimetic. The TCA interactions include additive CNS depression when taken with other central depressants, including ethanol, barbiturates, benzodiazepines, and opioids. The TCAs may also cause reversal of the antihypertensive action of guanethidine by blocking its transport into sympathetic nerve endings. Less commonly, TCAs may interfere with the antihypertensive actions of methylnorepinephrine (the active metabolite of methyldopa) and clonidine.

As discussed earlier, serotonin syndrome was first described for an interaction between an SSRI and an MAOI, though the syndrome is a predictable result of excess serotonin in the CNS. Symptoms can range from mild to severe with complications such as seizures and muscle breakdown. Drugs implicated in serotonin syndrome include MAOIs, TCAs, meperidine, and possibly illicit recreational drugs such as methylenedioxymethamphetamine (MDMA; "ecstasy"; Chapter 21). Antiseizure drugs, muscle relaxants, and 5-HT receptor antagonists have been used in the management of the syndrome.

Certain SSRIs are inhibitors of hepatic cytochrome P450 isozymes, an action that has led to increased activity of other drugs, including TCAs and warfarin. Of the SSRIs, citalopram and escitalopram cause fewer drug interactions. Both nefazodone and venlafaxine also inhibit cytochrome P450 isozymes.

Through this action, nefazodone enhances the action of many drugs including HMG-CoA reductase inhibitors (statins), TCAs, and carbamazepine.

REHABILITATION RELEVANCE

Therapists treating patients who have sustained a catastrophic injury or illness are likely to encounter the use of antidepressant agents to improve patients' mood and feelings of well-being. There is some evidence to suggest that use of these agents early in the rehabilitation process improves functional gains and outcomes. Treatment of depression—with both psychotherapy and antidepressant medication—is more effective than either strategy alone, but it is still a difficult clinical task. Even with appropriate psychological and pharmacological interventions, some patients do not respond. Treatment of 1 month or more may be required before the benefits of drug treatment are clinically apparent. The adverse effects of drug treatment also vary from individual to individual. ADRs must be monitored closely and relayed to the prescribing practitioner so that changes in the drug regimen may be made more efficiently in the search for the optimal drug for each individual. The ADRs inherent to particular drug classes are summarized below.

- **Gastrointestinal distress**—especially diarrhea and nausea—is associated with the SSRIs, SNRIs, 5-HT$_{2A}$ antagonists, and vilazodone. Symptoms tend to be dose-related and may improve with treatment duration. Vilazodone is associated with higher rates of GI symptoms, whereas the 5-HT$_{2A}$ antagonists cause less pronounced GI effects.
- **Sedation** is a common ADR of the TCAs, 5-HT$_{2A}$ antagonists (eg, trazodone), and mirtazapine. If sedation inhibits achievement of rehabilitation goals, this effect should be discussed with the patient and the prescriber.
- **Cardiac toxicities** range from orthostatic hypotension (with the TCAs, MAOIs, and 5-HT$_{2A}$ antagonists) to

TABLE 19-2 Drug interactions observed with antidepressants.

Antidepressant	Taken With	Consequence
Fluoxetine	Lithium, TCAs, warfarin	Increased blood level of second drug (dose may need to be decreased)
Fluvoxamine	Alprazolam, TCAs, theophylline, warfarin	Increased blood level of second drug (dose may need to be decreased)
MAOIs	SSRIs, sympathomimetics, tyramine-containing foods	Serotonin syndrome Hypertensive crisis
Nefazodone	Alprazolam, triazolam	Increased blood level of second drug (dose may need to be decreased)
Paroxetine	Procyclidine, TCAs, theophylline, warfarin	Increased blood level of second drug (dose may need to be decreased)
Sertraline	TCAs, warfarin	Increased effects of second drug (dose may need to be decreased)
TCAs	CNS depressants (eg, ethanol, sedative-hypnotics)[a] Clonidine, guanethidine, methyldopa	Additive CNS depression Decreased antihypertensive effects

CNS, central nervous system; MAOIs, monoamine oxidase inhibitors; SSRIs, selective serotonin reuptake inhibitors; TCAs, tricyclic antidepressants.
[a]Includes TCAs and antidepressants with sedative actions (eg, mirtazapine, nefazodone, and trazodone).

increased heart rate and blood pressure (with some SNRIs). The TCAs may also cause severe arrhythmias. While MAOIs can cause hypertensive reactions, this class tends to *lower* blood pressure in the absence of sympathomimetics. Abnormal resting vital signs and hemodynamic responses to exercise should be reported to the patient's primary practitioner and prescriber.

- General **CNS excitation** such as agitation (the "jitters") and insomnia is associated with the SSRIs, SNRIs, and some MAOIs. Starting with low doses may alleviate jitteriness. If these symptoms do not dissipate, the therapist should encourage the patient to relay these to the prescriber.
- **Extrapyramidal effects** such as dyskinesias and dystonic reactions may occur early in treatment with SSRIs. If persistent, report to the prescriber.
- **Anticholinergic effects** of the TCAs (especially with imipramine and amitriptyline) include dry mouth, constipation, blurred vision, urinary retention, and confusion. If these signs persistently inhibit the patient's function, inform the prescriber.
- **Weight gain** is associated with the TCAs, MAOIs, and mirtazapine. Although most of the SSRIs have been associated with weight loss with short-term use, they may cause weight gain when used over longer periods.
- Therapists should be aware that **discontinuation syndromes** are noted for the SSRIs, SNRIs, and TCAs. For the SSRIs and SNRIs, the withdrawal syndrome includes nausea, dizziness, anxiety, tremor, and palpitations. For the TCAs, discontinuation is associated with cholinergic rebound (nausea, vomiting, diarrhea) and flu-like symptoms.
- **Overdosage** of antidepressants is extremely hazardous for the TCAs and MAOIs. Therapists should be aware that ingestion of supplies that are potentially readily available to patients could be lethal. Manifestations of overdose include coma, convulsions, and cardiotoxicity for the TCAs and shock, hyperthermia, and seizures for the MAOIs. If therapists suspect potential overdose, emergent medical attention is necessary.
- Though not related to functional goals or outcomes, patients may report sexual issues to physical therapists. **Sexual dysfunction** (decreased libido, impotence, ejaculatory dysfunction) may be associated with depression, but these changes have also been reported with many antidepressants, including the SSRIs, MAOIs, and venlafaxine, with the highest rates being reported with the nonselective MAOIs. If these symptoms appear to be causing distress, therapists should encourage patients to discuss these with their prescribing practitioner.
- **Serotonin syndrome**, a potentially life-threatening cluster of autonomic, motor, and mental status changes, typically occurs when two or more serotonergic medications are used. The syndrome has been associated with the SSRIs and MAOIs. Suspicion of this syndrome must be managed as a medical emergency.

CASE CONCLUSION

R.N. subsequently had a complete cardiac work-up that proved negative. The patient's physician hypothesized that R.N. was suffering from secondary depression as a result of the car accident, traumatic loss of part of his limb, inability to perform his previous work, and the adjustment to all of these new circumstances. The physician prescribed paroxetine twice per day and esomeprazole (proton pump inhibitor) daily. R.N. tolerated this drug regimen with no major ADRs. He continued with rehabilitation therapy, and over the next several weeks, he reported improvement in his sleep pattern as well as a cessation of the burning and squeezing feeling in his chest. The therapist noted an improvement in R.N.'s attitude toward rehabilitation and compliance with his home exercise program and prosthetic training. R.N. was eventually discharged as independent with all functional activities, including sitting, kneeling, transferring from surfaces of varying heights, and negotiating stairs with his permanent prosthesis. He was eventually able to return to work.

CHAPTER 19 QUESTIONS

1. Dietary changes to reduce tyramine consumption are recommended for which of the following antidepressant classes?

    a. Serotonin receptor antagonists
    b. Monoamine oxidase inhibitors
    c. Selective serotonin reuptake inhibitors
    d. Selective serotonin-norepinephrine reuptake inhibitors

2. Overdosage of which of the following drugs can result in potentially fatal cardiotoxicity?

    a. Fluoxetine
    b. Duloxetine
    c. Mirtazapine
    d. Amitriptyline

3. Which of the following antidepressant drugs or classes is associated with the most pronounced sexual adverse effects?

   a. Selective serotonin reuptake inhibitors
   b. Mirtazapine
   c. Bupropion
   d. Monoamine oxidase inhibitors

4. Which of the following antidepressants would *not* be indicated for treating any type of anxiety disorder?

   a. Bupropion
   b. Imipramine
   c. Clomipramine
   d. Fluvoxamine

5. Which of the following is *not* a recognized hypothesis for the etiology of depression?

   a. Decreased amines in the brain
   b. Decreased neurotrophic factors in the brain
   c. Increased thyroid hormone levels
   d. Dysregulation of the hypothalamic-pituitary-adrenal axis

6. Which of the following drugs or drug classes would *not* be associated with serotonin syndrome?

   a. Bupropion
   b. Selective serotonin reuptake inhibitors
   c. Monoamine oxidase inhibitors
   d. Tricyclic antidepressants

7. Which of the following drugs or drug classes has been shown to be most effective at treating pain disorders?

   a. Monoamine oxidase inhibitors
   b. Selective serotonin reuptake inhibitors
   c. Bupropion
   d. Selective serotonin-norepinephrine reuptake inhibitors

8. Which of the following conditions is the main application for trazodone?

   a. Depression
   b. Insomnia
   c. Bulimia
   d. Pain disorders

9. Which of the following antidepressant drugs may be prescribed as an aid for smoking cessation?

   a. Mirtazapine
   b. Fluoxetine
   c. Bupropion
   d. Trazodone

10. Which of the following conditions is *not* an indicated use for selective serotonin reuptake inhibitors?

    a. Premenstrual dysphoric disorder
    b. Insomnia
    c. Vasomotor symptoms associated with menopause
    d. Anxiety disorders

Opioid Analgesics and Antagonists

CASE STUDY

S.F. is a 58-year-old woman with a long history of bilateral knee osteoarthritis. For the past several years, conservative treatment has included physical therapy and medications (oral cyclooxygenase-2 [COX-2] inhibitors and intra-articular triamcinolone acetonide injections). Because she has had progressively more pain and dysfunction over the past year, S.F. and her primary physician determined that it was time for bilateral total knee arthroplasties (TKA). The patient subsequently underwent bilateral TKA without complication. Postsurgical inpatient pain management includes oral oxycodone and a PCA pump with morphine sulfate for breakthrough pain. Early physical therapy interventions on postoperative days 1 and 2 focused on active and passive range of motion (ROM) of both lower extremities, transfer training, and upright mobility training. Prior to surgery, S.F. stated that her goal was to discharge from the hospital directly to her home. Her strong preference is not to be admitted to a skilled nursing facility, even for a short time. In line with this goal, S.F. has eagerly and actively participated in twice-daily physical therapy sessions. She has informed the nursing staff that she has a low tolerance for pain and asks for the oral pain medication 30-45 minutes before each therapy session. Initially, S.F. tolerated ROM exercises and limited mobility training well with this "pain premedication" regimen. However, upon standing and attempting gait training on postoperative day three, S.F. experienced dizziness, diaphoresis, and became very short of breath. On the second attempt to stand, the patient experienced syncope.

REHABILITATION FOCUS

Derivatives of the opium poppy have been used to relieve severe pain for hundreds (possibly thousands) of years. **Morphine**, the prototypic opioid agonist, does so with remarkable efficacy. This alkaloid (named after Morpheus, the Greek god of dreams) is extracted from crude opium, which is obtained from the opium poppy seedpod. Morphine remains the standard against which all drugs that have strong analgesic action are compared in terms of efficacy and potency. Opioids include the natural and semisynthetic alkaloid derivatives from opium, synthetic surrogates whose actions are blocked by the nonselective antagonist **naloxone**, and the endogenous peptides that interact with several opioid receptor subtypes. Although the term *narcotic* is often used interchangeably with *opioid*, use of the term narcotic originally referred to any sleep-inducing medication. In the United States, usage of the term narcotic has shifted more toward describing legal and regulatory scheduling of opioids.

Analgesic drug therapy and many physical therapy interventions are aimed at the same outcome: pain relief. Individuals participating in rehabilitative therapy are frequently taking analgesic drugs—especially nonsteroidal anti-inflammatory drugs (NSAIDs) and opioids. The NSAIDs (Chapter 34) have significantly lower maximal analgesic efficacy than the opioids, but have no addiction liability. While many NSAIDs are available over the counter for mild to moderate pain relief, opioids are usually prescribed to manage more severe or constant pain. For optimal pain relief and to achieve the most favorable patient outcomes, physical therapists must be familiar with the intended uses, duration of action, and common adverse effects of opioid analgesics. Healthcare professionals must understand that therapeutic dosages of opioid analgesics induce tolerance and physical dependence. Because of their potential for abuse, opioid medications are classified as controlled substances. Figure 20-1 outlines the major classes of opioids.

ENDOGENOUS OPIOID PEPTIDES

Opioids act on three major receptor subtypes: μ (mu), δ (delta), and κ (kappa) located throughout the neuraxis as well as on primary afferent nociceptive terminals. All three receptor subtypes appear to be involved in analgesic mechanisms (Table 20-1). However, activation of the μ receptor is responsible for the strongest analgesic effect (as well as a major role in the respiratory depressant effect) of opioids. At least three

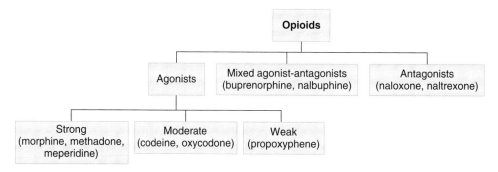

FIGURE 20-1 **Major classes of opioids based on their interaction with opioid receptors.** Opioid agonists may be classified as strong, moderate, or weak based on their ability to relieve pain. Prototype drugs are in parentheses.

families of endogenous opioid peptides have been described: **endorphins**, **enkephalins**, and **dynorphins**. Endorphins have the highest affinity for μ receptors, enkephalins for δ receptors, and dynorphins for κ receptors. These peptides are synthesized in neuronal cell bodies, transported to nerve endings, and stored in synaptic vesicles. Under the stress associated with pain or the anticipation of pain, painful stimuli evoke release of endogenous opioid peptides from nerve terminals and thus diminish the perception of pain. Whether these endogenous peptides function as classic neurotransmitters or as modulator neuropeptides remains unclear. Opioid peptides are also found in the adrenal medulla and the neural plexus of the gut (enteric nervous system).

DRUG CLASSIFICATION

Opioids may be classified in several ways. First, opioids can be subdivided according to major therapeutic uses: analgesics, antitussives, and antidiarrheals. Analgesic opioids are also classified according to their ability to relieve pain as strong, moderate, or weak agonists. Partial agonists are opioids that activate opioid receptors, but exert less analgesia than morphine, a strong (full) agonist at the μ receptor. Another clinically useful way to classify opioids is based on their ratio of agonist to antagonist effects. As such, opioid drugs may be classified as pure agonists (strong, moderate, or weak), pure antagonists (receptor blockers), or mixed agonist-antagonists. Mixed agonist-antagonists are drugs that activate some opioid receptor subtypes and block other subtypes. Table 20-2 uses this latter strategy to classify common opioid analgesics. The table also lists their routes of administration and duration of analgesic effect.

PHARMACOKINETICS

Opioids can be administered via almost every route, including oral, oral mucosal (lozenges or "lollipops"), injection (subcutaneous, intramuscular, intra-articular, epidural, intrathecal), rectal suppository, iontophoresis, nasal insufflation, and transdermal patch. A single transdermal patch can provide delivery of potent opioid analgesics over days. The epidural and intrathecal routes are usually used for postsurgical analgesia.

Most opioids are well absorbed when given by the oral route. However, because of extensive first-pass metabolism, the oral dose of some opioids such as morphine, **hydromorphone**, and **oxymorphone** may need to be much higher than the parenteral dose to elicit a therapeutic effect. Predicting an effective analgesic oral dose is also complicated due to the fact that there is significant inter-individual variability in first-pass metabolism of opioids. **Codeine** and **oxycodone** have reduced first-pass metabolism. Sustained-release oral forms of morphine and oxycodone are also available.

Opioid drugs are widely distributed to body tissues, but localize in highest concentrations in tissues that are highly

TABLE 20-1 **Opioid receptor subtypes, select functions, and endogenous opioid peptide affinity.**

Receptor Subtype	Functions	Endogenous Opioid Peptide Affinity
μ (mu)	Supraspinal and spinal analgesia Sedation Inhibition of respiration Slowed gastrointestinal transit Modulation of hormone and neurotransmitter release	Endorphins > enkephalins > dynorphins
δ (delta)	Supraspinal and spinal analgesia Modulation of hormone and neurotransmitter release	Enkephalins >> endorphins and dynorphins
κ (kappa)	Supraspinal and spinal analgesia Slowed gastrointestinal transit Psychotomimetic effects	Dynorphins >> endorphins and enkephalins

TABLE 20-2 Common opioid analgesics.

Generic Name	Route of Administration	Duration of Analgesia (hr)
Strong Agonists		
Morphine[a]	Oral, IM, IV, SQ	4-5
	Epidural, intrathecal	Up to 24
Hydromorphone	Oral, IM, IV, SQ	4-5
Oxymorphone	IM, IV, SQ, rectal	3-4
Methadone	Oral, IM, IV	4-6
Meperidine	Oral, IM, IV, SQ	2-4
Fentanyl	IM	1-2
	IV	0.5-1
Sufentanil	IV	1-1.5
Alfentanil	IV	0.25-0.75
Remifentanil	IV	0.05[d]
Levorphanol	Oral, IM, IV, SQ	4-5
Mild-to-Moderate Agonists		
Codeine	Oral, IM, SQ	3-4
Hydrocodone[b]	Oral	4-6
Oxycodone[a,c]	Oral	3-4
Partial Agonist		
Buprenorphine	Oral, IM, IV	4-8
Mixed Agonist-Antagonist		
Pentazocine	Oral	3-4
	IM, IV, SQ	2-3
Nalbuphine	IM, IV, SQ	3-6
Butorphanol	IM	3-4
	IV	2-4

IM, intramuscular; IV, intravenous; SQ, subcutaneous.
[a]Available in sustained-release forms: morphine (MS Contin) and oxycodone (OxyContin).
[b]Available in tablets containing acetaminophen (Norco, Vicodin).
[c]Available in tablets containing acetaminophen (Percocet) or aspirin (Percodan).
[d]Duration depends on context-sensitive half-life of 3-4 minutes.

perfused such as the brain, lungs, liver, kidneys, and spleen. Drug concentrations in skeletal muscle may be lower, but this tissue serves as the main reservoir because of its greater bulk. Even though blood flow to fatty tissue is much lower than to the highly perfused tissues, accumulation can be very important, particularly after frequent high-dose administration or continuous infusion of highly lipophilic opioids that are slowly metabolized (eg, **fentanyl**). Opioids cross the placental barrier and exert effects that can result in both respiratory depression and, with continuous exposure, physical dependence in neonates.

Opioids are primarily metabolized in the liver, although some degree occurs in the lungs, kidneys, and central nervous system (CNS). Hepatic enzymes usually metabolize opioids to *inactive* polar metabolites before their elimination by the kidney. However, there are two important *active* morphine metabolites. Morphine-3-glucuronide, the primary metabolite, has neuroexcitatory effects. Roughly 10% of morphine is metabolized to morphine-6-glucuronide, which has analgesic activity *exceeding* that of morphine. Because these polar metabolites are less able to cross the blood-brain barrier, single doses likely do not contribute to the CNS effects. However, individuals with accumulation of these metabolites (eg, renal failure, prolonged administration) may experience adverse effects such as seizures (due to accumulation of morphine-3-glucuronide) or sedation and respiratory depression (due to accumulation of morphine-6-glucuronide).

Many commonly prescribed opioids (eg, codeine, oxycodone, **hydrocodone**) are metabolized by a particular group of liver enzymes (CYP2D6) to form metabolites of *greater* potency than their parent compounds. This is clinically relevant because genetic polymorphisms in CYP2D6 are associated with inter-patient variations in analgesic and adverse effects. For example, some individuals may experience little to no analgesic effect after taking codeine (a moderate agonist at opiate receptors) because their CYP2D6 enzymes poorly metabolize the drug to morphine. In contrast, some individuals may have an exaggerated response to codeine because their CYP2D6 enzymes rapidly metabolize codeine to the strong agonist morphine, resulting in respiratory depression and profound sedation. One of the future hopes of personalized medicine is that prescribers will be able to identify particular opioids that effectively and safely manage pain based on an individual's pharmacogenomic profile.

PHARMACODYNAMICS

Mechanism of Action

Opioid agonists produce analgesia by binding to specific G protein-coupled receptors located primarily in the brain and spinal cord. Figure 20-2 illustrates key locations of opioid receptors in the ascending pathway for pain transmission (primary afferents and spinal cord transmission neurons) and in the descending pathway that functions in pain modulation (neurons in the midbrain and medulla). Other opioid receptors that may be involved in altering reactivity to pain are located on neurons in the basal ganglia, hypothalamus, limbic structures, and cerebral cortex.

Opioid analgesics *inhibit* synaptic activity partly through direct activation of opioid receptors and partly through release of endogenous opioid peptides (which then bind and activate opioid receptors). All three major opioid receptors are coupled to their effectors by G proteins and activate phospholipase C or inhibit adenylate cyclase. Figure 20-3 illustrates two direct actions that occur as a result of opioid receptor binding. Postsynaptically, activation of opioid receptors opens

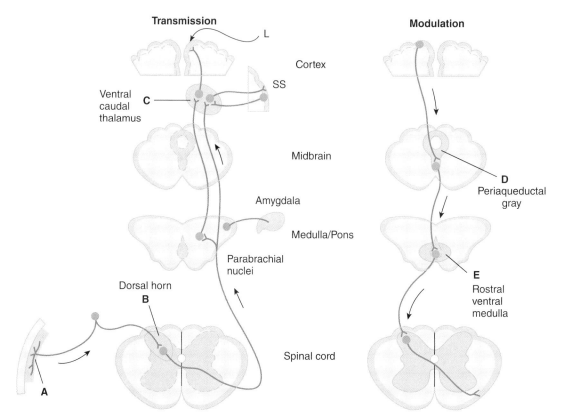

FIGURE 20-2 **Recognized sites of action of opioid analgesics.** The left side shows sites of action in the ascending pain transmission pathway from the periphery to higher centers. (A) Direct action of opioids on inflamed peripheral tissues. (B) Inhibition occurs in the spinal cord. (C) Possible sites of action in the thalamus that project to the somatosensory (SS) or limbic (L) cortex. Parabrachial nuclei (medulla/pons) project to the amygdala. On the right, sites of action in the descending pain modulation pathway are shown. Actions of opioids on neurons in the midbrain (D) and rostral ventral medulla (E) enhance descending inhibition to the spinal cord.

K^+ ion channels and hyperpolarizes the neuron. Presynaptically, activation of opioid receptors closes voltage-gated Ca^{2+} ion channels, which reduces neurotransmitter release. The presynaptic action—depressed transmitter release—has been demonstrated for a large number of neurotransmitters including glutamate, the principal excitatory amino acid released from nociceptive nerve terminals, as well as acetylcholine, norepinephrine, serotonin, and substance P.

Receptor Distribution and Neural Mechanisms of Analgesia

Most clinically available opioid analgesics act primarily at the μ-opioid receptor. Activation of μ-opioid receptors also results in euphoria, respiratory depression, and physical dependence. Efforts to develop opiate analgesics with a lower incidence of significant adverse effects such as respiratory depression and addiction potential have focused on compounds with higher affinity for κ receptors. For example, **butorphanol**—a mixed agonist-antagonist at μ receptors and a partial agonist at κ receptors—has had some success as an analgesic. However, butorphanol may also cause dysphoric reactions.

All three major opioid receptors are present in high concentrations in the dorsal horn of the spinal cord (Figure 20-2B). Receptors are present both on spinal cord pain transmission neurons and on the primary afferents that relay the nociceptive signal to them. Opioid agonists inhibit the release of excitatory transmitters from primary afferents and directly inhibit dorsal horn pain transmission neurons (Figure 20-3). Thus, opioids exert a powerful analgesic effect directly upon the spinal cord. This spinal action has been exploited clinically by direct application of opioid agonists to the spinal cord, which provides a regional analgesic effect while reducing the unwanted respiratory depression, nausea and vomiting, and sedation that often occur from the supraspinal actions of systemically administered opioids.

Under most circumstances, opioids are given systemically and thus act simultaneously at spinal and supraspinal sites to increase their overall analgesic efficacy. Opioid receptors are found in high concentration in areas of the brain implicated in ascending nociceptive transmission and descending pain modulation. Key opioid binding sites in pain-modulating descending pathways include the rostral ventral medulla, the locus ceruleus, and the midbrain periaqueductal gray area (Figure 20-2). Opioids *activate*

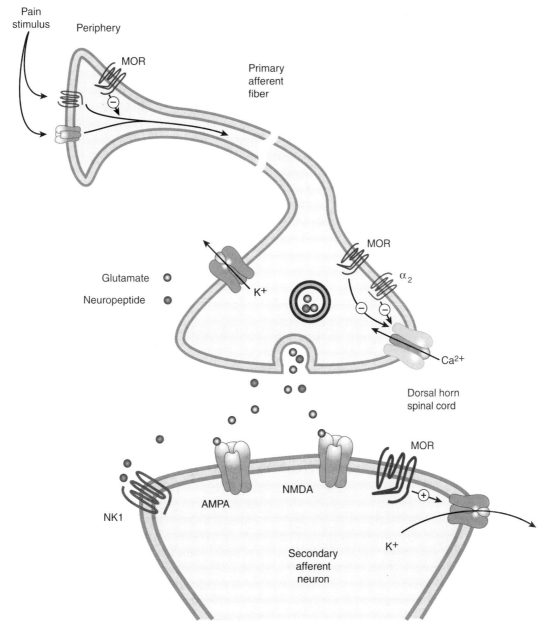

FIGURE 20-3 **Potential receptor-mediated mechanisms of analgesic drugs.** The primary afferent neuron (only the axon terminal is shown) originates in the periphery and transmits nociceptive signals via glutamate and neuropeptide transmitters onto the secondary neuron in the dorsal horn of the spinal cord. Under inflammatory conditions, painful stimuli can be attenuated in the periphery by opioids acting at μ-opioid receptors (MOR) or blocked in the afferent axon by local anesthetics (not shown; see Chapter 16). Opioids, calcium channel blockers (ziconotide), and α₂ agonists can attenuate input from nociceptive primary afferents by decreasing calcium influx into presynaptic terminals, which reduces transmitter release (often glutamate and excitatory neuropeptides). Postsynaptically, opioids hyperpolarize second-order pain transmission neurons by increasing K^+ conductance. AMPA and NMDA, glutamate receptors; NK1, tachykinin receptor that a group of neuropeptides including substance P binds to.

descending inhibitory neurons that send processes to the spinal cord and inhibit pain transmission neurons. This activation results from the inhibition of inhibitory neurons in several locations.

When pain-relieving opioid drugs are given systemically, they presumably act upon brain circuits normally regulated by endogenous opioid peptides. Part of the pain-relieving action of exogenous opioids involves the release of endogenous opioid peptides. An exogenous opioid agonist (eg, morphine) binds and acts primarily at the μ receptor, but this action may evoke the release of endogenous opioids that additionally act at δ and κ receptors. Thus, even a receptor-selective ligand can initiate a complex sequence of events involving multiple synapses, transmitters, and receptor subtypes.

Animal and human clinical studies demonstrate that both endogenous and exogenous opioids can produce opioid-mediated analgesia at sites *outside* the CNS. Pain associated with inflammation seems especially sensitive to these peripheral opioid actions. The identification of functional μ receptors on the peripheral terminals of sensory neurons supports this hypothesis. Furthermore, activation of peripheral μ receptors results in a decrease in sensory neuron activity and transmitter release. For example, intra-articular administration of opioids after arthroscopic knee surgery has shown some clinical benefit. With further development, opioids selective for a peripheral site would be useful adjuncts in the treatment of inflammatory pain (Box 20-1). Moreover, new peripherally acting dynorphins may provide a novel means to treat visceral pain.

Tolerance and Dependence

Tolerance is defined as a larger dose of a drug being necessary to reproduce the original response. Tolerance is a well-recognized, though poorly understood property of opioids. With frequently repeated administration of *therapeutic* doses of morphine or its surrogates, there is a gradual loss in effectiveness. Along with tolerance, physical dependence usually develops. Physical dependence (now simply called *dependence*; see Chapter 21) is defined as the occurrence of a characteristic withdrawal or abstinence syndrome when the drug is stopped abruptly. Withdrawal symptoms include rhinorrhea, lacrimation, chills, gooseflesh, muscle aches, diarrhea, yawning, anxiety, and hostility. A more intense state of precipitated withdrawal results when an opioid antagonist (eg, naloxone) is administered to a physically dependent individual (see discussion below in Opioid Antagonists).

Persistent activation of μ-opioid receptors (such as occurs with the treatment of severe chronic pain) appears to play a

---

BOX 20-1 Ion Channels and Novel Analgesics

Even the most severe acute pain (lasting hours to days) can typically be controlled—with significant but tolerable adverse effects—with currently available analgesics, especially the opioids. However, chronic pain (lasting weeks to months) and neuropathic (nerve injury) pain are *not* adequately managed with opioids. In chronic pain states, receptors on sensory nerve terminals contribute to increased excitability of sensory nerve endings (peripheral sensitization). The hyperexcitable sensory neuron bombards the spinal cord, leading to increased excitability and synaptic alterations in the dorsal horn (central sensitization). Such changes appear to be important in chronic inflammatory and neuropathic pain states.

Efforts to discover better analgesic drugs for chronic pain have focused on peripheral nociceptive synaptic transmission and sensory processing. Potentially important ion channels include members of the transient receptor potential family, especially the capsaicin receptor (TRPV1) that is activated by noxious stimuli such as heat and inflammatory products and the P2X receptor that is activated by purines released by damaged tissue. Certain subtypes of voltage-gated sodium channels are uniquely associated with nociceptive neurons in dorsal root ganglia. **Mexiletine** and **lidocaine**, which are useful in some chronic pain states, may act by blocking these channels. Transdermal patches and balms that deliver these drugs are aimed at inhibiting peripheral nociceptive transmission and transduction.

Many ion channels—especially several subtypes of calcium channels—are involved in central pain processing. **Ziconotide** antagonizes voltage-gated N-type calcium channels; this drug is approved for intrathecal analgesia in individuals with refractory chronic pain. **Gabapentin** and **pregabalin** bind to a particular subunit of voltage-gated calcium channels in the brain.

Though originally approved to treat partial seizures, these drugs have become increasingly popular because they have proven to be effective treatments for neuropathic pain.

Glutamate N-methyl-D-aspartate (NMDA) receptors appear to play an important role in central sensitization at spinal and supraspinal levels. Although certain NMDA antagonists have demonstrated analgesic activity (eg, **ketamine**), it has been difficult to find agents with an acceptably low profile of adverse effects. Low doses of ketamine improve analgesia and can reduce opioid requirements under conditions of opioid tolerance such as after major abdominal or spinal surgeries. GABA and acetylcholine (through nicotinic receptors) appear to control the central synaptic release of several transmitters involved in nociception. **Nicotine** itself and certain nicotine analogs cause analgesia; their use in postoperative analgesia is under investigation. Last, recent attention has focused on activation of cannabinoid receptors by **marijuana** and other cannabinoids to treat various types of pain. These agents have been used alone or with other analgesic drugs to treat cancer-related pain, chronic pain, and neuropathic pain.

As research improves our understanding of the peripheral and central transduction of pain, new therapeutic targets will be discovered, and new strategies to treat pain will become available. Now, a common therapeutic approach to treat pain is multimodal analgesia (Chapter 16). This approach involves the administration of multiple drugs that have complementary mechanisms of action to provide more effective pain relief than can be provided by a single drug. For example, using an NSAID, gabapentin, and an opioid may provide superior analgesia than any one of these agents alone with the added benefit of reducing opiate requirements.

primary role in the induction and maintenance of tolerance and dependence. Two main hypotheses for the development of tolerance—lack of opioid receptor recycling and opioid receptor uncoupling—have gained experimental support.

After *endogenous* opioid peptides activate μ-opioid receptors, the receptors undergo endocytosis and recycle to the plasma membrane, allowing resensitization. In contrast, morphine fails to induce endocytosis of μ receptors. On the other hand, **methadone**, a μ-receptor agonist used to treat opioid tolerance and dependence, induces receptor endocytosis. Thus, maintaining normal sensitivity of μ-opioid receptors may require reactivation by this process of endocytosis and recycling.

The second hypothesis for tolerance is the concept of receptor uncoupling. Under this hypothesis, tolerance is due to a dysfunction of structural interactions between the μ-opioid receptor and G proteins, second messenger systems, and their target ion channels. Moreover, the NMDA receptor for glutamate has been shown to play a critical role in tolerance development and maintenance because NMDA receptor antagonists such as ketamine can block tolerance development.

In addition to the development of tolerance, persistent administration of opioid analgesics may sometimes *increase* the sensation of pain. This paradoxical hyperalgesic response is another reason that the use of opioids for treating chronic pain is controversial. Opioid-induced hyperalgesia may be mediated by spinally derived dynorphin and activation of bradykinin and NMDA receptors.

ACUTE EFFECTS OF MORPHINE AND ITS SURROGATES

Central Nervous System Effects

The principal effects of opioid analgesics with affinity for μ receptors are in the CNS. Key effects include analgesia, euphoria, sedation, and respiratory depression. With repeated use, a high degree of tolerance occurs to all of these effects.

Analgesia

Opioids are the most powerful drugs available for the relief of pain, attenuating both the sensory and emotional (affective) aspects of the pain experience. In contrast, NSAIDs have no significant effect on the emotional component of pain. Strong agonists (ie, those with the highest analgesic efficacy, full μ-receptor agonists) include morphine, hydromorphone, oxymorphone, **meperidine**, fentanyl, **levorphanol**, methadone, and **heroin**.

Because of its adverse cardiac effects, meperidine has largely been replaced by fentanyl as one of the most commonly used synthetic opioids. Related drugs (**sufentanil**, **alfentanil**, and **remifentanil**) differ in potency and distribution. Sufentanil is more potent than fentanyl, while alfentanil is less potent than fentanyl. Alfentanil and remifentanil have very short durations of action, which make them useful in anesthesia.

Methadone is a strong μ-receptor agonist, but the drug also blocks NMDA receptors and monoaminergic (eg, serotonin, norepinephrine) reuptake transporters. These latter properties may contribute to methadone's ability to mitigate neuropathic and cancer pain, two pain syndromes in which morphine has largely failed. Methadone's oral bioavailability exceeds that of morphine, but the drug's highly variable pharmacokinetics and long half-life (25-52 hours) require close monitoring to avoid potentially harmful respiratory depression. Methadone's use in the treatment of opioid dependence and misuse is discussed later. Heroin is a fast-acting and potent agonist. Its use is prohibited in the United States (Schedule I) and Canada.

Codeine, hydrocodone, and oxycodone are partial agonists with mild to moderate analgesic efficacy. Often, hydrocodone and oxycodone are administered in formulations combined with acetaminophen. **Propoxyphene** is a very weak agonist with low analgesic efficacy. Propoxyphene has been withdrawn from use in the United States due to increasing incidence of death associated with its misuse.

Euphoria

Individuals who receive intravenous morphine typically experience a pleasant floating sensation with lessened anxiety and distress. However, dysphoria (unpleasant state characterized by restlessness and malaise) may occur. These effects can occur at doses below those required for maximum analgesia.

Sedation

Drowsiness and mental clouding are frequent opioid actions. There is little or no amnesia. Opioids induce sleep more frequently in older adults than in young, healthy individuals. Ordinarily, the patient can be easily aroused. However, the combination of morphine with other CNS-depressant drugs such as the sedative-hypnotics may result in very deep sleep. Marked sedation occurs more frequently with morphine, hydromorphone, and oxymorphone and less frequently with meperidine and fentanyl.

Respiratory Depression

All opioid analgesics depress brainstem respiratory mechanisms and decrease the ventilatory response to carbon dioxide challenge. Respiratory depression is dose-dependent, but may be seen at conventional analgesic doses with full agonists. This adverse effect is one of the biggest challenges in treating severe pain. Opioid-induced respiratory depression is strongly influenced by the degree of sensory input occurring at the time. For example, strongly painful stimuli may prevent opioid-induced respiratory depression, but once the stimuli are relieved, respiratory depression may suddenly become marked. Small to moderate decreases in respiratory function (as measured by elevated PCO_2) may be well tolerated in individuals without prior respiratory impairment. However, in individuals with asthma or chronic obstructive pulmonary disease, an opioid-induced decrease in respiratory function may not be tolerated.

Increased PCO_2 may cause cerebrovascular dilation, resulting in increased cerebral blood flow and increased intracranial pressure. In the case of death due to opioid overdose, the cause is respiratory depression.

Antitussive Actions

Individuals suffering from pathologic cough have long used codeine, though suppression of the cough reflex by opioids is not well understood. However, cough suppression by opioids may allow accumulation of secretions and thus lead to airway obstruction and atelectasis.

Miosis

Virtually all opioid agonists, except meperidine, cause pupillary constriction. Because little to no tolerance develops to this pharmacologic action (even in highly tolerant individuals), it is valuable in the diagnosis of opioid overdose. Miosis can be blocked by opioid antagonists such as naloxone. Miosis is mediated by parasympathetic pathways, which can be blocked by atropine.

Nausea and Vomiting

Opioid analgesics can activate the brainstem chemoreceptor trigger zone to produce nausea and vomiting. There may be a vestibular component of this effect because ambulation seems to increase the incidence of nausea and vomiting.

Truncal Rigidity

Via supraspinal actions, a number of opioids intensify the tone in the large trunk muscles. Truncal rigidity reduces thoracic compliance and thus interferes with ventilation. This effect is most apparent when high doses of very lipid-soluble opioids (eg, fentanyl, sufentanil, alfentanil) are rapidly administered intravenously. Truncal rigidity may be overcome by administration of an opioid antagonist, but this will also antagonize the analgesic effect. Preventing truncal rigidity while preserving analgesia requires the concomitant use of neuromuscular-blocking agents.

Peripheral Effects

Cardiovascular System

Most opioids have no significant direct effects on the heart and no major effects on cardiac rhythm (except bradycardia). Meperidine is an exception to this generalization because its antimuscarinic action may result in tachycardia. Blood pressure is usually well maintained in subjects receiving opioids unless the cardiovascular system is stressed, in which case hypotension may occur. This hypotensive effect is probably due to peripheral arterial and venous dilation, which has been attributed to a number of mechanisms including central depression of vasomotor-stabilizing mechanisms and release of histamine. No consistent effect on cardiac output is seen, and the electrocardiogram is not significantly affected.

However, caution should be exercised in patients with decreased blood volume, since the above mechanisms make these patients quite susceptible to hypotension. Opioid analgesics affect cerebral circulation minimally except when PCO_2 rises as a consequence of respiratory depression.

Gastrointestinal Tract

The constipating effects of opioids are mediated via actions in the CNS and the enteric nervous system. Tolerance does *not* develop to opioid-induced constipation. In the stomach, opioids may decrease motility (rhythmic contraction and relaxation), but increase tone (persistent contraction)—particularly in the central portion. In the large intestine, opioids decrease propulsive peristaltic waves and increase tone. This delays passage of fecal material and allows increased absorption of water, which leads to constipation. This powerful action is the basis for the clinical use of some of these drugs as antidiarrheal agents.

Smooth Muscle

Opioids (with the exception of meperidine) cause contraction of biliary tract smooth muscle, which may cause biliary colic or spasm. Therapeutic doses increase ureteral and bladder sphincter tone, which may lead to urinary retention especially in postoperative patients. Occasionally, ureteral colic caused by a kidney stone is made worse by the opioid-induced increase in ureteral tone. Opiates also reduce uterine tone, which may prolong labor.

Renal Effects

Opioids depress renal function (chiefly due to decreased renal plasma flow) and can decrease systemic blood pressure and glomerular filtration rate. In addition, μ-receptor agonists have an antidiuretic effect likely via CNS and peripheral mechanisms. Opioids also enhance renal tubular sodium reabsorption.

Endocrine Effects

Opioids have complex effects on hormonal release, stimulating release of antidiuretic hormone and growth hormone, but inhibiting release of luteinizing hormone. Chronic opioid therapy can lower testosterone, resulting in decreased energy and libido; women can experience dysmenorrhea or amenorrhea.

Pruritus

Therapeutic doses of opioid analgesics (especially morphine) produce flushing and warming of the skin sometimes accompanied by sweating and itching. This effect is mediated by both peripheral histamine release and CNS actions. Opioid-induced pruritus is more common when these drugs are administered parenterally, especially when given via spinal or epidural routes. In the latter case, the usefulness of opioids may be limited by intense pruritus over the lips and torso.

CLINICAL USES

Successful treatment of pain is a challenging task that begins with careful attempts to assess the source and magnitude of the pain. Clinicians try to quantify the degree of pain experienced by asking patients to rate their pain level. For adults, the most common tool is the 11-point numeric pain rating scale (NPRS) in which "0" represents no pain and "10" represents the worst pain imaginable. For children or those who cannot speak, the pain magnitude is often measured with the Wong-Baker FACES pain rating scale that depicts six faces (with corresponding numbers) ranging from smiling (no hurt) to crying (hurts worst). For both scales, the degree of pain may be considered mild (1-3), moderate (4-6), or severe (7-10).

In patients experiencing severe pain, the administration of an opioid analgesic is usually considered a primary part of the overall management plan. Determining the route of administration (oral, parenteral, spinal), duration of drug action, ceiling effect (maximal intrinsic activity), duration of therapy, potential for adverse effects, and the patient's past experience with opioids should all be addressed by the prescribing practitioner and monitored by all healthcare personnel involved in the patient's care. A key error made by practitioners is a failure to assess a patient's pain adequately and to match its severity with an appropriate level of drug therapy. Just as important is the principle of *reevaluating* the effectiveness of the therapeutic plan and modifying the plan if pain management is inadequate or adverse effects are excessive.

Use of opioid drugs in *acute* situations should be contrasted with their use in *chronic* pain management, where a multitude of other factors must be considered, including the development of tolerance, dependence, and addiction (see discussion below in Adverse Effects).

Analgesia and Anesthesia

Strong μ-opioid receptor agonists usually relieve severe, constant pain, but are not as effective for sharp, intermittent pain. The pain associated with cancer and other terminal illnesses must be treated aggressively and often requires a multidisciplinary approach for effective management. Such conditions may require continuous use of potent opioid analgesics and are associated with some degree of tolerance and dependence. However, there is incomplete cross-tolerance to the μ-receptor effects between various subclasses of opioids. This incomplete cross-tolerance provides the basis for "rotation" of different opioids in chronic pain management. If tolerance and dependence occurs, this should not be used as a barrier to providing patients with the best possible care and quality of life. Research in the hospice movement has demonstrated that fixed-interval administration of opioids (ie, regular dose at a scheduled time) is more effective in achieving pain relief than dosing on demand. New dosage forms of opioids that allow slower release of the drug are available (eg, sustained-release forms of morphine and oxycodone). Their purported advantage is a longer and more stable level of analgesia. However, there is little

evidence to support long-term (greater than 6 months) use of sustained-release opioids to manage chronic *noncancer* pain.

Prolonged analgesia, with some reduction in adverse effects, can be achieved with epidural administration of certain strong μ-receptor agonists (eg, fentanyl and morphine). If disturbances of gastrointestinal function prevent the use of oral sustained-release morphine, transdermal fentanyl (fentanyl patch) can be used over long periods. Administration of strong opioids by nasal insufflation has been shown to be efficacious, although few agents are currently available for this route. Opioid analgesics are often used during obstetric labor, but care must be taken to minimize neonatal depression because opioids cross the placental barrier and reach the fetus.

For less severe, but still chronic pain, moderate agonists are given by the oral route. Stimulants such as amphetamines have been shown to enhance the analgesic actions of opioids and thus may be useful adjuncts in the person with chronic pain. Other drug groups, such as various anticonvulsants (eg, gabapentin) and antidepressants (Chapter 19), are useful in managing chronic pain and should also be considered.

Opioids are frequently used before, during, and after many types of surgeries. As preoperative drugs, opioids are used because of their sedative, anxiolytic, and analgesic properties. Intraoperatively, opioids are adjunctive agents in balanced anesthesia protocols (Chapter 15) and in preparation for postoperative analgesia. High-dose intravenous opioids (eg, morphine, fentanyl) are often a primary component of the anesthetic regimen, most commonly in cardiovascular surgery and other types of high-risk surgery where a primary goal is to minimize the cardiovascular depression induced by most general anesthetics. In such situations, mechanical respiratory assistance must be provided.

Because opioids act directly on neurons in the dorsal horn of the spinal cord, epidural or intrathecal (subarachnoid) administration into the spaces of the spinal column can be used to provide regional analgesia. Long-lasting analgesia with minimal adverse effects can be achieved by epidural administration of 3-5 mg of morphine, followed by slow infusion through a catheter placed in the epidural space. Although it was initially assumed that epidural administration of opioids might selectively produce analgesia *without* impairment of motor, autonomic, or sensory functions other than pain, respiratory depression may occur after injection into the epidural space. Intrathecal and epidural opioid administration is common practice for postoperative analgesia. While these routes reduce the amount of systemic opioids and can reduce opioid-related adverse effects such as sedation and constipation, pruritus and nausea and vomiting are common with these methods of administration. Currently, the epidural route is favored because adverse effects are less common. If necessary, adverse effects may be reversed with naloxone. Another option to decrease the frequency of adverse effects is to use low doses of local anesthetics in combination with an opioid administered via a patient-controlled epidural pump. This strategy has the additional advantage of lowering the opioid dose requirements. In rare cases (chronic or cancer pain management), healthcare professionals may elect to surgically implant a programmable infusion pump connected to a spinal catheter for continuous infusion of opioids or other analgesic compounds.

Cough Suppression

Suppression of cough occurs at opioid doses lower than those needed for analgesia. However, the use of opioid analgesics (codeine and **dextromethorphan)** to allay cough has diminished because a number of effective synthetic compounds have been developed that are neither analgesic nor addictive (Chapter 35). The Food and Drug Administration (FDA) has banned the use of dextromethorphan for children younger than 6 years of age due to increasing reports of death in young children taking over-the-counter formulations. In addition, use of codeine is being reconsidered due to variations in its metabolism in young children (Chapter 3).

Treatment of Diarrhea

Diarrhea from almost any cause can be controlled with opioid analgesics, but if diarrhea is associated with infection, such use must not substitute for appropriate antimicrobial chemotherapy. **Diphenoxylate** and **loperamide** are used to treat diarrhea. These opioid preparations have more selective gastrointestinal effects and few or no CNS effects (Chapter 36).

Management of Acute Pulmonary Edema

Intravenous morphine dramatically reduces dyspnea due to the pulmonary edema associated with left ventricular failure. The mechanism is not clear, but probably involves reduced *perception* of shortness of breath and reduced patient anxiety as well as reduced cardiac preload (reduced venous tone) and afterload (decreased peripheral resistance). Morphine can also be particularly useful when treating the pain associated with myocardial ischemia in patients with acute pulmonary edema. However, other drugs with minimal or no respiratory depressant effects (diuretics) may also be used to manage acute pulmonary edema.

Opioid Dependence

There are two main reasons why methadone, a long-acting full μ-receptor agonist, has been used for both detoxification and maintenance of individuals with chronic relapsing heroin addiction. First, tolerance and dependence to methadone develop more slowly than with morphine. For detoxification of a heroin-dependent individual, low oral doses of methadone are given 2-3 times daily for a few days. Second, upon discontinuation of methadone, the individual experiences a less immediate and less severe (though more prolonged) withdrawal syndrome than that of heroin or morphine. In maintenance programs for opioid addiction, tolerance to oral methadone may be intentionally produced because cross-tolerance to heroin is also induced. This pharmacological property underpins one of the rationales

of methadone maintenance programs. By using methadone to block the euphoria-inducing and addiction-reinforcing effects of doses of shorter-acting opioids such as heroin and morphine, this helps remove the drive to illicitly obtain them, which reduces criminal activity, and makes the addicted individual more amenable to rehabilitative therapy. One hazard of maintenance methadone to persons addicted to heroin is increased risk of death due to respiratory arrest.

Buprenorphine, a partial μ-receptor agonist with a longer duration of action than methadone, has comparable efficacy to methadone. Buprenorphine is now considered the drug of choice for managing opioid withdrawal in most patients because its use is associated with a lower risk of death due to respiratory arrest and the drug does not need to be obtained through a licensed outpatient opioid treatment program. **Lofexidine**, a centrally acting α₂-adrenergic receptor agonist, is the first nonopioid FDA-approved drug for managing opioid withdrawal symptoms. For many years, **clonidine**, another centrally acting α₂-receptor agonist has been used off-label to reduce opioid withdrawal symptoms related to noradrenergic overactivity (eg, irritability, gastrointestinal symptoms). Lofexidine has similar efficacy to clonidine, but causes less hypotension. However, both lofexidine and clonidine can cause orthostatic hypotension, syncope, and bradycardia.

ALTERNATIVE ROUTES OF ADMINISTRATION

A popular type of pain management used in many hospitals is called patient-controlled analgesia (PCA). PCA permits the patient to control a parenteral (usually intravenous) infusion device by depressing a button to deliver a preprogrammed dose of the desired opioid analgesic. A lockout interval prevents administration of another dose for a programmable period of time. Clinical trials suggest that the use of PCA increases patient satisfaction, making this approach useful in postoperative breakthrough pain management. Overdosage secondary to misuse or improper programming of the PCA device must be guarded against because there is a risk of respiratory depression with hypoxia. Continuous pulse oximetry is recommended for individuals using opioid PCA devices. Risk of sedation is increased if patients are concurrently taking drugs with sedative properties (eg, benzodiazepines).

Rectal suppositories of morphine and hydromorphone have long been used when oral and parenteral routes are undesirable (eg, if vomiting precludes oral administration). Transdermal patches provide stable blood levels of drug and better pain control while avoiding the need for repeated parenteral injections. Fentanyl has been the most successful opioid in transdermal application; fentanyl is indicated for management of persistent unremitting pain. Introduction of an opioid transdermal patch is reserved for individuals with some degree of opioid tolerance. For example, the FDA recommends that the fentanyl patch only be initiated in persons with oral morphine requirements of at least 60 mg/day for at least 1 week.

Caution must be taken because peak drug effects may not occur until 24-48 hours after patch application. The intranasal route avoids the disadvantages of repeated drug injections and the first-pass metabolism of orally administered drugs. **Butorphanol** is the mostly widely used opioid currently available in the United States in a nasal formulation. Last, the buccal transmucosal route can be used as either a fentanyl citrate lozenge or a "lollipop" mounted on a stick.

ADVERSE EFFECTS

The direct adverse effects of opioid analgesics are extensions of their acute actions. These include respiratory depression, nausea, vomiting, and constipation. Other considerations include tolerance, dependence, addiction, diagnosis and treatment of opioid overdosage, and precautions and contraindications of opioid therapy. Table 20-3 lists common adverse effects of opioid analgesics.

Tolerance

Clinically, tolerance is observed as an increasing opioid dose requirement to produce the same level of analgesia that was experienced with the initial opioid administration. Tolerance development begins with the first dose of an opioid, but is not usually obvious until after 2-3 weeks of frequent exposure to ordinary *therapeutic* doses. Tolerance develops most readily when higher doses are given frequently. Tolerance is minimized by providing lower doses with longer latencies between each dose. Tolerance develops to varying degrees for different effects of opioid drugs. Marked tolerance is observed for analgesia, euphoria, sedation, respiratory depression, nausea and vomiting, and the antitussive effect. In contrast, minimal tolerance develops for miosis, constipation, and convulsions.

Cross-tolerance is an extremely important characteristic of opioids. Individuals tolerant to morphine also show a reduction in analgesic response to other opioid agonists. This is particularly true of drugs with primarily μ-receptor agonist activity. Morphine and its congeners exhibit cross-tolerance not only with respect to their analgesic actions but also to their euphoriant,

sedative, and respiratory effects. However, cross-tolerance among the μ-receptor agonists can often be partial or incomplete, which supports opioid rotation. For example, a patient who is experiencing less analgesia from morphine may be "rotated" to hydromorphone and subsequently experience improved analgesia at a reduced overall equivalent opioid dosage.

As discussed previously, the use of ketamine (an NMDA-receptor antagonist) is purported to prevent or reverse opioid tolerance. Ketamine has been shown to effectively reduce postoperative pain and opioid requirements in opioid-tolerant patients.

Dependence and Addiction

Dependence invariably develops along with tolerance to μ-receptor agonists. Table 20-4 lists the signs and symptoms of withdrawal or abstinence syndrome that occur upon abrupt discontinuation of a μ-receptor agonist. The number and intensity of these signs and symptoms depend on the degree of dependence and strength of the agonist. However, physical withdrawal has a definitive end point. Though some effects may persist for months, most disappear in less than a week. Opioid administration at this time almost immediately alleviates the effects associated with physical withdrawal. Because of its severity, opioid withdrawal syndrome is often treated with methadone replacement therapy to remove the drug from the system slowly with less severe withdrawal signs and symptoms (see discussion above in Clinical Uses). Management of opioid withdrawal symptoms without subsequent maintenance treatment for opioid use disorder is not recommended.

Psychologic dependence is now referred to as *addiction*. Addiction is strongly reinforced by the development of dependence. The euphoria, indifference to stimuli, and sedation caused by opioid analgesics tend to promote their compulsive use. The pleasurable effects of opioids promote the pathologic pursuit of reward and relief (avoidance of withdrawal syndrome) through continued use. Addiction is characterized by the inability to abstain consistently, impairment in behavioral control, craving, decreased recognition of significant problems

TABLE 20-3 Clinically important adverse effects of opioid analgesics.

Behavioral restlessness, tremulousness, hyperactivity (in dysphoric reactions)
Respiratory depression
Nausea and vomiting
Increased intracranial pressure
Postural hypotension accentuated by hypovolemia
Constipation
Urinary retention
Itching around nose, urticaria (more frequent with parenteral and spinal administration)

TABLE 20-4 Clinical presentation and timeframe of physical withdrawal syndrome.

Signs and Symptoms	Time Since Last Dose (strong μ-receptor agonist such as morphine or heroin)
Muscle aches	Initial: 6-10 hr
Rhinorrhea	Peak: 1.5-2 days
Lacrimation	Termination: ~ 5 days
Yawning	
Chills	
Fever	
Vomiting	
Diarrhea	
Anxiety	
Irritability/hostility	

with one's behaviors and relationships, and a dysfunctional emotional response. In contrast to dependence, addiction does *not* have a definitive end point. That is, individuals can continue to have cravings for opiates months and years beyond cessation of the dependence.

There are differences in severity of withdrawal effects and addiction. For example, withdrawal from dependence on a strong μ-receptor agonist (morphine) is associated with more severe withdrawal signs and symptoms than withdrawal from a mild or moderate agonist (hydrocodone). The potential and degree of dependence and addiction associated with the mixed agonist-antagonist opioids (eg, butorphanol) also appears to be less than that of the strong opioid agonists.

A transient, but dramatic withdrawal syndrome occurs upon administration of an opioid *antagonist* to an opioid-dependent person. Within a few minutes after injection of an opioid antagonist, signs and symptoms appear, peak in 10-20 minutes, and subside after about 1 hour.

The risk of inducing dependence and addiction is an important consideration in the therapeutic use of opioids. Despite this risk, pain relief should not be withheld because an opioid exhibits the potential for misuse or because legislative controls complicate the process of prescribing opioids.

Overdose

The triad of pupillary constriction (miosis), comatose state, and respiratory depression is characteristic of opioid overdose, with the latter being responsible for most fatalities. Diagnosis of overdosage is confirmed if intravenous injection of naloxone, an opioid receptor antagonist, results in prompt signs of recovery. Treatment of overdose involves the use of antagonists such as naloxone and other therapeutic measures, especially ventilatory support (see discussion below in Opioid Antagonists).

Drug Interactions

The most important drug interactions involving opioid analgesics are additive CNS depression with ethanol, sedative-hypnotics, anesthetics, antipsychotic drugs, tricyclic antidepressants, and antihistamines. Concomitant use of certain opioids (eg, meperidine) with monoamine oxidase inhibitors increases the incidence of hyperpyrexic coma. Meperidine has also been implicated in the serotonin syndrome when used with selective serotonin reuptake inhibitors.

Contraindications and Cautions in Therapy

Use of Pure Agonists With Weak Partial Agonists

As described in Chapter 2, a partial agonist behaves like an antagonist when given in the presence of a full agonist. Thus,

a weak partial μ-receptor agonist such as **pentazocine**, if given to a patient also receiving a full μ-receptor agonist (eg, morphine), may result in diminishing analgesia or even a state of withdrawal; such combinations should be avoided.

Use in Patients With Increased Intracranial Pressure

Respiratory depression caused by opioids causes carbon dioxide retention, which results in cerebral vasodilation. In patients with increased intracranial pressure (eg, acute head injury), further elevation in intracranial pressure may be lethal.

Use During Pregnancy

Chronic use of opioids during pregnancy may result in physical dependence in the fetus in utero and withdrawal symptoms in the neonate in the early postpartum period. Severe withdrawal syndrome in the infant may result in irritability, shrill crying, diarrhea, or even seizures. If withdrawal symptoms are judged to be relatively mild, drugs such as diazepam are given to control symptoms; with more severe withdrawal, small doses of opioids are often necessary.

Use in Patients With Impaired Pulmonary Function

Because opioids depress respiratory drive, their use in patients with borderline respiratory reserve may lead to acute respiratory failure.

Use in Patients With Impaired Hepatic or Renal Function

Most opioids are metabolized primarily in the liver and the metabolites are excreted in the urine. The half-lives of morphine and its congeners are, therefore, prolonged in patients with impaired hepatic or renal function. The parent drug and its metabolites may then accumulate; dosage should therefore be reduced in such patients.

Use in Patients With Endocrine Disease

Patients with adrenal insufficiency (Addison's disease) and those with severe hypothyroidism (myxedema) may have prolonged and exaggerated responses to opioids.

OPIOIDS WITH MIXED RECEPTOR EFFECTS

As stated above, administration of a partial agonist or drug with mixed opioid receptor actions to individuals receiving full μ-opioid receptor agonists should be avoided because decreased analgesia or even the precipitation of an explosive withdrawal syndrome (see later discussion) may occur.

The analgesic activity of partial μ-receptor agonists varies with the individual drug, but is *always* less than that of full μ-receptor agonists like morphine. Buprenorphine is a partial μ-receptor *agonist* (low intrinsic activity) and an *antagonist* at κ and δ opioid receptors. **Nalbuphine** and pentazocine are κ agonists, with weak μ-receptor antagonist activity. Thus, because these drugs have mixed receptor actions, they are referred to as mixed agonist-antagonists. Buprenorphine and nalbuphine afford greater analgesia than pentazocine, which is similar to codeine in analgesic efficacy. Buprenorphine binds strongly to μ receptors, providing a long duration of effect that is clinically useful to suppress withdrawal signs in opioid dependency. To deter diversion for illicit intravenous misuse, buprenorphine is available combined with naloxone.

The mixed agonist-antagonist drugs usually cause sedation at analgesic doses. Dizziness, sweating, and nausea may occur, and anxiety, hallucinations, and nightmares are also possible. Although respiratory depression may be less intense than that induced by pure μ-receptor agonists, it is not predictably reversed by naloxone. With chronic use, tolerance develops. However, it is less than the tolerance that develops to the pure μ-receptor agonists and there is minimal cross-tolerance. Dependence occurs, but the abuse liability of mixed agonist-antagonist drugs is less than that of the full μ-receptor agonists.

Miscellaneous

Tramadol is a moderately efficacious central-acting analgesic. Its complex mechanism of action involves enhanced serotonergic and noradrenergic neurotransmission. Tramadol also weakly binds to μ-opioid receptors. However, its analgesic effect is only partially antagonized by naloxone. Recommended oral dosing for analgesia is four times daily. However, the systemic concentration of tramadol and its analgesic effect depend on polymorphisms in the cytochrome P450 family responsible for its metabolism. Adverse effects include nausea and dizziness, but these symptoms typically decrease after several days of therapy. No clinically relevant effects on respiration or the cardiovascular system have been reported thus far. Seizures have been associated with use of tramadol. Therefore, tramadol is relatively contraindicated in patients with a history of epilepsy and for use with other drugs that lower the seizure threshold.

Tapentadol is an oral analgesic that significantly inhibits norepinephrine reuptake, but has less ability to inhibit serotonin reuptake than tramadol. While its binding to the μ-opioid receptor is higher than that of tramadol, its affinity is only modest. Tapentadol is as effective as oxycodone in treating moderate to severe pain, but is associated with fewer gastrointestinal adverse effects. Like tramadol, tapentadol carries the risk of seizures.

OPIOID ANTAGONISTS

Naloxone, **nalmefene**, and **naltrexone** are pure opioid receptor antagonists that have greater affinity for μ receptors than for other opioid receptors. Naloxone and nalmefene are primarily used for acute opioid overdose. Because a single injection of naloxone has a short duration of action (1-2 hours), multiple doses may be required to reverse the effects of severe opiate-induced respiratory depression. Due to the increase in

opioid-related deaths in the United States, more forms of naloxone including hand-held autoinjectors (for subcutaneous or intramuscular administration) and nasal sprays have become readily available. The intranasal formulation was developed for community use. Nalmefene is also used for opioid overdose, has a longer duration of action (8-12 hours), but is only available for intravenous administration.

Low doses of naloxone are increasingly being used in conjunction with therapeutic intravenous or epidural opioids to treat opiate-associated nausea, vomiting, and itching. Other opioid antagonists chemically related to naloxone and naltrexone are used in the treatment of opioid-induced constipation (**methylnaltrexone bromide**) and postoperative ileus after bowel resection (**naloxegol** and **alvimopan**). These opioid antagonists effectively relieve some of the common adverse effects of opioids while sparing the analgesia.

Because of its long elimination half-life, naltrexone has become valuable as a maintenance drug for individuals who are motivated to maintain opiate abstinence. After oral administration, naltrexone blocks the actions of strong opioid agonists for up to 48 hours. One dose of naltrexone given on alternate days blocks almost all the effects of a dose of heroin. Naltrexone also decreases the craving for alcohol and facilitates abstinence from cigarette smoking (with reduced weight gain).

If an opioid antagonist is given in the *absence* of an exogenous opiate agonist, there are almost no effects. However, when given to individuals taking opioids, the antagonist completely reverses the opioid's effects within 1-3 minutes. In acute opioid overdose, the antagonist normalizes respiration, consciousness, pupil size, bowel function, and awareness of pain. In opiate-dependent individuals who appear normal, administration of naloxone or naltrexone almost instantaneously precipitates a transient explosive abstinence syndrome with similar signs and symptoms to those seen after abrupt opiate discontinuation. However, this antagonist-precipitated withdrawal peaks in 10-20 minutes and mostly subsides after 1 hour.

REHABILITATION RELEVANCE

Use of opioid analgesics represents one of the most effective methods for treating moderate to severe pain. Opiates are rarely used alone, but rather as part of a multimodal treatment plan to reduce pain and improve quality of life. Physical therapists encounter patients using opioids recovering from trauma or following surgery (acute pain relief) and patients with terminal cancer or chronic pain (chronic pain relief). Pain relief afforded by opioids may allow for increased patient participation, progression of the rehabilitation program, and ultimate achievement of desired outcomes. When pain is a limiting factor to participation, therapists often try to coordinate therapy interventions with peak drug levels for maximum analgesic benefit. Although many clinicians have recommended therapy be initiated 45-60 minutes after oral opiate administration, it is especially difficult to predict peak analgesic effect because most opiates demonstrate significant inter-individual variability in first-pass metabolism. Thus, determination of peak analgesic effect is usually empirically determined for each patient. In the acute care setting, the length of stay may not be long enough to precisely establish the ideal time for the patient to be "premedicated" prior to therapy. Often, the option of parenteral administration provides more predictable and immediate analgesia to allow therapy interventions.

Physical therapists practicing in outpatient settings often treat individuals with chronic pain. In the United States, opiate prescriptions have decreased significantly over the past several years (after a peak in 2011) due to a combination of regulatory and legislative restrictions in response to the opioid epidemic. Still, opioids are commonly used for chronic pain. Professional organizations such as the American Pain Society and American Academy of Pain Medicine have published guidelines to help prescribers effectively use chronic opioid therapy for noncancer pain, while minimizing significant opioid adverse effects and outcomes related to their abuse potential. A key guideline includes educating patients that opioids are *not* first-line analgesics. That is, other pain-relieving interventions—including physical therapy and nonopioid analgesic medications—should be tried *before* prescribing opiates. Other guidelines include proper patient selection with regards to assessing the individual's risk for abuse (eg, personal or family history of substance abuse), establishing therapeutic goals (eg, starting with a short-term trial and limiting dosage), and keeping expectations realistic. The latter guideline refers to educating the patient that opioids are infrequently used as the sole strategy to reduce pain and that these drugs rarely provide complete pain relief. Rather, trials suggest that pain improvement averages less than 2-3 points on a 0-10 scale. Not only can physical therapists reinforce these realistic expectations, but they can also suggest or administer interventions that evidence supports may comparably reduce pain.

Below are common opiate-associated adverse effects and strategies to decrease their impact on rehabilitation. If adverse drugs reactions (ADRs) intervene with attaining goals, discuss potential alternatives with the prescribing practitioner.

- **Relevant pharmacokinetics**. Therapists should be aware that in older adults and individuals with more adipose tissue, multiple doses of opioids over time might result in progressively significant ADRs such as sedation and respiratory depression. Likewise, individuals with renal failure or those who have had prolonged administration of morphine may accumulate *active* morphine metabolites. ADRs such as seizures (due to accumulation of morphine-3-glucuronide) or sedation and respiratory depression (due to accumulation of morphine-6-glucuronide) can occur.
- **Sedation** or **mental clouding** negatively affects patient interventions that require active participation. If significant pain relief is the priority, physical therapy interventions should focus on enhancing analgesia via passive modalities or gentle manual therapy. Avoid providing complex directions (eg, surgical precautions) and anticipate that multiple

repetitions of patient education will be necessary. If sedation consistently limits mental and physical participation in therapy, alert the medical team to investigate alternative pain management strategies.
- To prevent falls or syncope that may result from **dizziness** or **orthostatic hypotension**, patients should be guarded closely during ambulation and be advised to slowly make positional changes.
- **Constipation** can be especially problematic in individuals with conditions that decrease gastrointestinal motility (eg, spinal cord injury, postabdominal surgery). Laxatives and stool softeners are often administered to minimize the risk of fecal impaction (and the associated pain) caused by opioids. Increasing the frequency of upright mobility (ie, sitting versus supine, walking versus sitting) facilitates bowel function. Often, increasing mobility to facilitate bowel movements can be used as an incentive to motivate individuals to participate in therapy in inpatient settings.
- **Respiratory depression** can lead to hypoxemia and the respiratory response to exercise may be blunted. Respiratory rate and pulse oximetry should be monitored; for individuals using opioid PCA devices, continuous pulse oximetry is recommended. If the patient demonstrates increased sedation with a significantly depressed respiratory rate, the medical team should be *immediately* alerted. Risk of sedation and respiratory depression is increased if patients are concurrently taking drugs with sedative properties (eg, benzodiazepines).
- **Nausea and vomiting** may limit participation in rehabilitation.
- **Tolerance and dependence** are anticipated physiological processes that occur at the cellular and molecular level in response to frequently repeated administration of *therapeutic* doses of opioids, especially strong μ-receptor agonists. Tolerance and dependence are distinct from addiction in that everyone will develop tolerance and dependence to opioids in response to frequent opioid administration, but not everyone develops an addiction to opiates. The withdrawal or abstinence syndrome when opiates are abruptly discontinued has a finite end point (typically ~ 1 week). In contrast, addiction to opioids may continue for months or years.
- Because of their **abuse potential**, opioid medications are classified as controlled substances. The pleasurable effects of opioids can promote addiction. Healthcare providers must be aware of drug-seeking behaviors and report concerns to the medical team and/or the prescribing provider.
- **Opioid withdrawal** may lead to muscle aches and pains. When patients are gradually weaned off opioid medications, they may experience withdrawal symptoms including diffuse muscle aches. Although muscle aches caused by opioid withdrawal are not due to a somatic disorder, physical agents such as heat and electrotherapy and manual techniques such as massage and relaxation may provide some relief from these somatic symptoms.

The physical therapist recognized that the patient's dizziness, shortness of breath, diaphoresis, and subsequent syncope could be due to the additional oral opioid analgesic she is taking prior to therapy sessions. Although the oxycodone helped mitigate the pain during ROM exercises and limited upright mobility, the adverse effects are limiting her upright tolerance and ability to initiate gait training. After the physical therapist spoke with the patient, nurse, and primary physician, it was determined that S.F. would receive gait and mobility training during the first part of each therapy session. She would then be given an oral dose of oxycodone prior to active and passive ROM exercises. Although the onset of analgesia would be somewhat delayed, it was felt that this drug regimen would allow her to get the maximal benefit from therapy to facilitate her goal of discharging directly home. This regimen was subsequently carried out and proved advantageous as long as the nursing staff was available to provide the oral medication at the time it was needed.

CHAPTER 20 QUESTIONS

1. Activation of which of the following receptors is responsible for the strongest analgesic effect?

   a. μ (mu) opioid receptor
   b. δ (delta) opioid receptor
   c. κ (kappa) opioid receptor
   d. α (alpha) adrenergic receptor

2. Which of the following opioids is a strong (full) agonist at the μ (mu) opioid receptor?

   a. Codeine
   b. Oxycodone
   c. Morphine
   d. Buprenorphine

3. Which of the following opioid actions is *not* mediated by the central nervous system?

   a. Decreased gastrointestinal motility
   b. Miosis
   c. Sedation
   d. Respiratory depression

4. Which of the following drugs used to treat diarrhea would have the fewest central nervous system effects?

   a. Codeine
   b. Dextromethorphan
   c. Loperamide
   d. Morphine

5. Which of the following is *not* a sign or symptom of opioid withdrawal?

   a. Muscle aches
   b. Constipation
   c. Chills
   d. Fever

6. Which of the following is *not* a characteristic of a morphine or heroin overdose?

   a. Pupillary dilation
   b. Comatose state
   c. Miosis
   d. Respiratory depression

7. Which of the following drugs is used to quickly reverse an acute opioid overdose?

   a. Naltrexone
   b. Alvimopan
   c. Naloxegol
   d. Naloxone

8. Which of the following drugs most readily induces tolerance and dependence?

   a. Codeine
   b. Nalbuphine
   c. Morphine
   d. Buprenorphine

9. Which of the following is *not* an adverse effect of opioid analgesics?

   a. Sedation
   b. Nausea
   c. Hypertension
   d. Constipation

10. Which of the following opioid analgesics is the strongest μ (mu) opioid receptor agonist?

    a. Hydrocodone
    b. Oxycodone
    c. Tramadol
    d. Hydromorphone

Drugs of Abuse

K.C. is a 54-year-old employee at an automotive assembly plant. Three weeks ago on the assembly line, he was rotating and bending when he felt a sudden pain in the left side of his low back. He was immediately taken to the emergency department, given a diagnosis of musculoskeletal strain, and provided Tylenol with codeine #3 (codeine and acetaminophen) with instructions to take on an as-needed basis for pain relief. K.C. was scheduled for evaluation and enrollment in a work-hardening program prior to return to full-time employment at the plant. Last week, K.C. was evaluated at the rehabilitation clinic. Relevant history during the initial assessment included intermittent exertional angina and an approximate 15 pack-year smoking history (half pack of cigarettes per day for 30 years). In addition to a daily baby aspirin, K.C. has been taking Tylenol #3 every day since his injury. For his first work-hardening therapy session, K.C. arrived for an early morning appointment. He admitted that he rushed to the clinic having only eaten a breakfast of "coffee and a couple of cigarettes" with Tylenol #3 about an hour ago. The clinic's work-hardening program includes a set of progressive aerobic activities designed to mimic the employees' activities at the plant in order to improve biomechanical function and reduce the incidence of workplace injuries. Within about 10 minutes of starting the session, K.C. complains of shortness of breath and pain along his left arm. The physical therapist instructs him to rest and measures his blood pressure and heart rate at 155/92 mm Hg and 99 bpm (with regular rhythm), respectively. The therapist continues monitoring the patient's vital signs and symptoms. Over the next 20 minutes, K.C.'s angina and dyspnea dissipate and blood pressure and heart rate decrease to 131/84 mm Hg and 83 bpm, respectively.

REHABILITATION FOCUS

As generally understood, drug abuse indicates the use of an illicit (illegal) drug or the excessive or nonmedical use of a licit drug. Often, drugs are abused for altering consciousness, but some are taken for other reasons such as enhancing muscle mass in bodybuilding. Drug abuse also includes the deliberate use of chemicals that are generally not considered drugs by the lay public (eg, inhalants), but may be harmful to the user. The motivation for the misuse or abuse of centrally acting drugs is usually the strong feelings of pleasure or altered perception that the drug induces. With chronic use, dependence occurs with most drugs of abuse. Thus, preventing a withdrawal syndrome reinforces continued drug abuse.

The term drug abuse connotes social disapproval and may have different meanings to different people. Some may also distinguish drug *abuse* from drug *misuse*. To misuse a drug might be to take it for the wrong indication, in the wrong dosage, or for too long a period. In the context of drug abuse, the drug itself is of less importance than the pattern of use. For example, taking 50 mg of diazepam (a benzodiazepine) to heighten the effect of a daily dose of methadone (an opioid) is an abuse of diazepam. On the other hand, taking an excessive daily dose of diazepam for its anxiolytic effect is misusing diazepam.

In the United States, it has been estimated that the abuse of tobacco, alcohol, and illicit drugs cost more than $740 billion annually in costs related to lost work productivity, crime, and healthcare. In 2013, the abuse and misuse of prescription opioids alone accounted for $78.5 billion in overall costs. Physical therapists will encounter patients in every setting and in every age group with problems of drug addiction. The addiction may or may not be acknowledged or recognized by the individual or by healthcare providers. Understanding drug addiction begins with clinicians having a working knowledge of the definitions and distinctions between dependence, tolerance, withdrawal, and addiction. This chapter also discusses the cultural considerations of such drug use, the neurobiological basis of addiction, and the major classes of these drugs. Figure 21-1 outlines the major classes of drugs of abuse and prototypic agents.

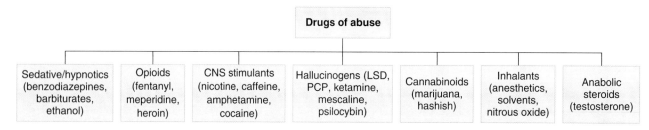

FIGURE 21-1   Major classes of drugs of abuse. LSD, lysergic acid diethylamide; PCP, phencyclidine. Prototype agents are in parentheses.

DEFINITIONS

The traditional term "physical dependence" is now referred to simply as "dependence" and the older term "psychological dependence" is now referred to as "addiction." *Dependence* refers to the biologic phenomena often associated with drug abuse. For example, when a chronic user is dependent on the drug, abrupt cessation results in a withdrawal or abstinence syndrome. The withdrawal syndrome is a combination of symptoms and signs that are frequently the opposite of those sought by the user. A traditional explanation for these manifestations is that the body adjusts to a new homeostasis during the period of drug use and reacts in opposite fashion when this equilibrium is disturbed. Alcohol withdrawal syndrome is perhaps the best-known example, but milder degrees of withdrawal may be observed in people who drink large amounts of coffee. Importantly, dependence is not a phenomenon exclusively associated with drugs of abuse. Dependence also occurs with nonpsychoactive drugs such as bronchodilators and sympathomimetic vasoconstrictors.

Repetitive exposure to many drugs of abuse often induces adaptive changes such as *tolerance*, in which a higher dose of the drug is needed to achieve the same effect as when the person first used it. Tolerance is closely associated with the phenomenon of dependence. Tolerance is largely due to compensatory responses that mitigate the drug's pharmacodynamic action. Metabolic tolerance due to increased disposition of the drug after chronic use is occasionally reported. Functional tolerance, which may be more common, is due to compensatory changes in receptors, effector enzymes, or membrane actions of the drug. Tolerance can be a serious problem because not all effects of a drug show the same *degree* of tolerance. For example, if morphine is used at short intervals—whether taken therapeutically to alleviate pain or recreationally for a euphoric "high"—the dose must be increased over the course of several days to maintain the analgesic or rewarding effects. However, with chronic use and escalating doses, the person increases the risk of potentially fatal respiratory depression because this particular effect of morphine does not show as much tolerance.

Addiction is manifested by a high motivation to seek out and compulsively use the drug, often despite negative consequences (eg, risks to health, criminal sanction, loss of job). Addiction has sometimes been described as "wanting without liking." Deprivation of the drug for a short period of time typically results in a strong desire or craving for it, especially in response to contextual cues. For example, a former smoker who successfully quit the habit for a period of months or even years may be overcome with very intense cravings for a cigarette when simply walking into a smoky bar to meet a group of friends that he/she formerly shared the habit with. Addiction is considered a disease that can—but does not always—result from repetitively taking drugs of abuse. In other words, a person can be dependent on a drug or have high tolerance to it, *without* being addicted to it. For instance, patients receiving opioid analgesics for weeks or months absolutely will develop tolerance and dependence; however, few of these patients will become addicts. In contrast, when taken for recreational purposes, opioids are highly addictive.

A number of experimental techniques have been devised to predict the ability of a drug to produce dependence and to assess its likelihood for abuse. Most of these techniques employ self-administration of the drug by animals. The rates of reinforcement can be altered to make the animal work harder for each dose of drug, providing a semiquantitative measure as well. Comparisons are made against a standard drug in the class; for example, morphine among the opioids. Withdrawal of dependent animals from drugs is done to assess the nature of the withdrawal syndrome and can be used to test drugs that might cross-substitute for the standard drug. Most agents with significant potential for dependence or addiction can be readily detected by these techniques. However, the relative risk for addiction (addiction liability) is difficult to predict since there are many variables. One variable getting more attention is the heritability of addiction. It has long been appreciated that there is large individual variation in vulnerability to substance-related addiction. Animal studies suggest that excessive anxiety or impulsivity may be critical traits that increase the risk for addiction. Observational studies in humans have shown that the heritability of addiction among twins is modest for cannabinoids, but very high for cocaine. The addiction liability of a drug correlates with its heritability, suggesting that what is being inherited may be the neurobiological basis of addiction common to all drugs.

There are some drugs of abuse that do not produce dependence or lead to addiction. The hallucinogens like lysergic acid diethylamide (LSD) and dissociative anesthetics (ketamine, phencyclidine [PCP]) alter sensory perceptions, but do not

TABLE 21-1 Schedules of controlled substances.

Schedule	Characteristics	Addiction Potential	Examples
I	No accepted medical use	Highest	Flunitrazepam (Rohypnol), heroin, LSD, marijuana (cannabis),[a] mescaline, MDMA (ecstasy), PCP
II	Approved for specific medical conditions	High	Amphetamines, cocaine, dextroamphetamine/amphetamine (Adderall), strong opioids (meperidine, oxycodone, fentanyl), nabilone, methylphenidate (Ritalin)
III	Medical use	Moderate to low	Anabolic steroids (testosterone), codeine, dronabinol, ketamine, moderate opioids (eg, buprenorphine), barbiturates (eg, butabarbital)
IV	Medical use	Low	Benzodiazepines, chloral hydrate, mild stimulants (eg, modafinil), most hypnotics (eg, zolpidem, zaleplon), weak opioids (eg, tramadol)
V	Medical use	Lowest	Pregabalin, preparations containing small amounts of certain opioids (eg, antitussives with < 200 mg codeine/100 mL); gabapentin[b]

LSD, lysergic acid diethylamide; MDMA, methylene dioxymethamphetamine; PCP, phencyclidine.
[a]Marijuana does not have high addiction potential, but is included in this schedule for historical and political reasons.
[b]Gabapentin is not a controlled substance at the federal level; however, several states have implemented legislative mandates requiring enhanced pharmacovigilance.

cause euphoria or reward. Unlike addictive drugs that primarily target the mesolimbic dopaminergic system, these agents target circuits in the thalamus and cortex. Even though these agents are not addictive, their use can still have negative short- and long-term effects.

CULTURAL CONSIDERATIONS

Current attitudes in the United States toward drugs that are claimed to have high abuse potential are reflected in the drug schedules made by the Food and Drug Administration (FDA) under the Controlled Substances Act (CSA) of 1970 (Table 21-1). The FDA drug schedule is quite similar to those published by international control bodies. Under the CSA, drugs, substances, and certain chemicals used to make drugs are classified into five categories ("schedules") depending upon the utility of the substance to be used as a medical product and the drug's abuse or addiction potential. The abuse rate is a determinate factor in the scheduling of the drug. For example, Schedule I drugs are stated to have no currently accepted medical purpose and have the highest abuse potential. These drugs can only be acquired with special permissions from the United States government. Drugs currently in Schedule I include heroin, ecstasy, PCP, and marijuana. As the drug schedule changes from Schedule II to Schedule V, so does the abuse potential, with Schedule V drugs representing the least potential for abuse. Such schedules affect law-abiding manufacturers and ethical prescribers of the drugs, but have little deterrent effect on illicit manufacturers or suppliers. Such schedules have been circumvented by the synthesis of "designer drugs" that make small modifications of the chemical structures of drugs with little or no change in their pharmacodynamic actions. Schedules are constantly revised to include new compounds not currently listed.

NEUROBIOLOGY OF DRUG ABUSE

Substantial progress has been made in elucidating the neurobiology of abused drugs and their effects. Most or all abused drugs act through neurotransmitter systems that involve norepinephrine (NE), dopamine (DA), gamma-aminobutyric acid (GABA), serotonin (5-HT), glutamate, endorphins, or enkephalins. However, regardless of the drug and the initial neurotransmitter, the final common pathway in addiction appears to be activation of the dopaminergic mesolimbic system. This system originates in a small group of dopaminergic neurons in the brainstem called the ventral tegmental area (VTA). These fibers project to the nucleus accumbens, amygdala, hippocampus, and prefrontal cortex. Activation of the mesolimbic pathway is widely implicated in drug and natural reward, pleasure, and positive reinforcement. Regardless of the role of dopamine under physiological conditions, all addictive drugs significantly increase dopamine concentration in target structures of the mesolimbic projections. Decades of research in animals and humans suggest that high levels of dopamine may actually be at the origin of adaptive changes that underlie dependence and addiction.

In the case of stimulants such as amphetamines and cocaine, the connection with dopamine-mediated effects is easily observed, since these drugs directly influence dopaminergic transmission. However, many other drugs of abuse do not directly increase dopaminergic transmission. For example, opioid analgesics mediate their direct effects by binding to μ-opioid receptors, which typically results in inhibition of the postsynaptic neuron. In the VTA, μ-opioid receptors are selectively expressed on GABA neurons. Thus, μ-opioid agonists inhibit GABAergic inhibitory interneurons, which eventually leads to disinhibition (ie, excitation) of dopamine neurons. Thus, while the receptors that addictive drugs bind are critical for their specific *acute* effects, as a general rule, all addictive drugs ultimately activate the mesolimbic dopamine system.

SEDATIVE-HYPNOTICS

The sedative-hypnotics include benzodiazepines, barbiturates, and ethanol. With the exception of ethanol, their medical uses are discussed in Chapter 13. Benzodiazepines are commonly prescribed drugs for anxiety, insomnia, and muscle spasms. Almost all benzodiazepines are Schedule IV drugs judged to have low abuse liability (Table 21-1). The notable exception is **flunitrazepam**, a potent and rapid-onset benzodiazepine, which is placed as Schedule I because it is considered to have no medicinal value. Short-acting barbiturates like **secobarbital** have high addiction potential and are classified as Schedule II (Table 21-1). Because barbiturates are rarely prescribed to individuals in outpatient settings, these agents constitute a less common prescription problem than benzodiazepines. Though not listed in schedules of controlled substances with abuse liability, alcohol (see below) is the most frequently abused drug in the world.

Sedative-hypnotics reduce inhibitions, suppress anxiety, and produce relaxation. All of these actions are thought to encourage repetitive use and the development of addiction. These drugs are central nervous system (CNS) depressants, and the depressant effects are enhanced by concomitant use of opioid analgesics, antipsychotic agents, marijuana, and any other drug with sedative properties.

Flunitrazepam (Rohypnol) is a rapidly acting benzodiazepine with marked amnestic properties that has been used in "date rape." Added to alcoholic beverages, **chloral hydrate** or **gamma-hydroxybutyrate** (**GHB;** sodium oxybate) also renders the victim incapable of resisting rape. Before causing sedation and coma, GHB induces euphoria, enhanced sensory perceptions, feelings of social closeness, and amnesia. These properties have made GHB a popular "club drug" used by teenagers and young adults at bars, nightclubs, and parties. Some of GHB's creative names include "liquid ecstasy," "liquid X," and "grievous bodily harm." GHB is odorless, colorless, and readily dissolves in beverages. After ingestion, GHB is rapidly absorbed and reaches maximal plasma concentration within 20-30 minutes. Importantly, *any* sedative-hypnotic, alone or in combination with other CNS depressants, may decrease an individual's ability to resist unwanted sexual advances.

Acute overdoses of sedative-hypnotics commonly result in death due to depression of the respiratory and cardiovascular centers in the medulla oblongata (Table 21-2). Management of overdose includes maintenance of a patent airway plus ventilatory support. **Flumazenil**, a GABA$_A$ receptor antagonist, can be used to reverse the CNS depressant effects of benzodiazepines, but there is no antidote for barbiturates or ethanol.

Benzodiazepine dependence is common and often unrecognized. Withdrawal occurs within days of the last dose and varies depending on the elimination half-life of the particular drug. Signs and symptoms of withdrawal are most pronounced with drugs that have half-lives of less than 24 hours. However, dependence may occur with any sedative-hypnotic, including the longer-acting benzodiazepines. The most important signs of withdrawal derive from excessive CNS stimulation (due to removal of the drug) and include anxiety, tremor, nausea and vomiting, delirium, and hallucinations (Table 21-2). Seizures are not uncommon, occur later in the withdrawal process, and may be life-threatening.

Treatment of sedative-hypnotic withdrawal involves administration of long-acting benzodiazepines such as **diazepam** or **chlordiazepoxide** to suppress the acute withdrawal syndrome, followed by gradual dose reduction. **Clonidine** or **propranolol** may also be used to suppress sympathetic overactivity. Discontinuance of long-term therapeutic sedative-hypnotics can also result in a syndrome of withdrawal. In addition to the classic withdrawal presentation (Table 21-2), this syndrome includes weight loss, paresthesias, and headache.

ETHANOL

Alcohol, primarily in the form of ethyl alcohol (**ethanol**), is a sedative-hypnotic drug with few medical applications. Its consumption in low to moderate amounts brings about feelings of well-being and even euphoria. However, its abuse is responsible for major medical and socioeconomic problems.

TABLE 21-2 Manifestations of overdose and withdrawal from selected drugs of abuse.

Drug	Overdose Effects	Withdrawal Signs and Symptoms
Barbiturates, benzodiazepines, ethanol[a]	Slurred speech, "drunken" behavior, dilated pupils, weak and rapid pulse, clammy skin, shallow respiration, coma, death	Anxiety, insomnia, delirium, tremors, seizures, death
Heroin; other strong opioids	Constricted pupils, clammy skin, nausea, drowsiness, respiratory depression, coma, death	Nausea, chills, sweats, cramps, lacrimation, rhinorrhea, yawning, hyperpnea, tremor
Amphetamines, methylphenidate, cocaine[b]	Agitation, hypertension, tachycardia, delusions, hallucinations, hyperthermia, seizures, death	Apathy, irritability, increased sleep time, disorientation, depression

[a]Ethanol withdrawal includes the excited hallucinatory state of delirium tremens (DTs).
[b]Cardiac arrhythmias, myocardial infarction, and stroke occur more frequently in cocaine overdose than with other CNS stimulants.

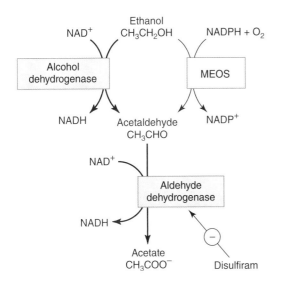

FIGURE 21-2 Metabolism of ethanol to acetaldehyde by alcohol dehydrogenase and microsomal ethanol-oxidizing system (MEOS). Aldehyde dehydrogenase metabolizes acetaldehyde to acetic acid, and is inhibited by disulfiram.

After ingestion, ethanol is rapidly and completely absorbed. Ethanol is then distributed to most body tissues, and its volume of distribution is equivalent to that of total body water (0.5-0.7 L/kg). Two enzyme systems metabolize ethanol to acetaldehyde (Figure 21-2). The first, alcohol dehydrogenase (ADH), is a cytosolic nicotinamide adenine dinucleotide (NAD)-dependent enzyme found mainly in the liver and gut. ADH accounts for the metabolism of low to moderate doses of ethanol. Because of the limited supply of the coenzyme NAD$^+$, the reaction has zero-order kinetics that results in a *fixed* capacity for ethanol metabolism of 7-10 g/hr. Gastrointestinal metabolism of ethanol is lower in women than in men, probably accounting for the greater sensitivity of women to equal intake of alcoholic drinks. Genetic variation in ADH affects the rate of ethanol metabolism as well as vulnerability to alcohol-use disorders. The second ethanol metabolic pathway is the microsomal ethanol-oxidizing systems (MEOS). This liver MEOS contributes little to ethanol metabolism at blood alcohol levels below 100 mg/dL. However, chronic alcohol consumption increases the activity of the MEOS and induces cytochrome P450 (CYP) enzyme synthesis. Increased MEOS activity may be partially responsible for the development of tolerance to ethanol. The primary CYP isoform that is induced by ethanol also converts acetaminophen to a hepatotoxic metabolite, accounting for the increased risk of acetaminophen toxicity in individuals with chronic alcohol exposure (Chapters 3 and 34).

Acetaldehyde that is formed from the oxidation of ethanol by either system is rapidly metabolized to acetate by aldehyde dehyrodenase, a mitochondrial enzyme found in the liver and many other tissues. Aldehyde dehydrogenase is inhibited by **disulfiram** (Figure 21-2) and other drugs, including **metronidazole**, oral hypoglycemics, and some **cephalosporins**. Certain persons, particularly of Asian descent, have a genetic deficiency of aldehyde dehydrogenase. In these individuals, consumption of even small quantities of ethanol may cause nausea and a flushing reaction from accumulation of acetaldehyde.

Acute Effects of Alcohol

In the CNS, the major acute effects of ethanol are dose-dependent, and include sedation, loss of inhibition, impaired judgment, slurred speech, and ataxia (Table 21-3). Impairment of driving ability is thought to occur at blood alcohol concentration (BAC) levels between 60 and 80 mg/dL. This serves as the physiological foundation for "drunk driving" laws that make it illegal to drive a motor vehicle with a BAC of ≥ 0.08% (80 mg/dL) in the United States where roughly 30-40% of all traffic accidents that result in a fatality involve at least one person with a BAC near or above the legal limits. Blood levels of 120-160 mg/dL are usually associated with gross drunkenness. Levels greater than 300 mg/dL may lead to loss of consciousness, anesthesia, and coma with occasional fatal respiratory and cardiovascular depression. Blood levels greater than 500 mg/dL are usually lethal. Although chronic alcoholics tolerant to the effects of ethanol can function almost normally at much higher blood levels than occasional drinkers, the lethal BAC is little changed. Additive CNS depression occurs with concomitant ingestion of a wide variety of CNS depressants (eg, sedative-hypnotics, opioids), as well as many drugs that block muscarinic and H$_1$ histamine receptors.

The molecular mechanisms underlying the complex CNS effects of ethanol are not fully understood. Specific receptors for ethanol have not been identified. Instead, ethanol appears to modulate the function of a number of signaling proteins. Ethanol facilitates the action of GABA at GABA$_A$ receptors, inhibits the ability of glutamate to activate *N*-methyl-D-aspartate (NMDA) receptors, and modifies the activities of adenylate cyclase, phospholipase C, and ion channels. "Blackouts" (periods of memory loss that occur with high levels of alcohol) may result from interference with activation of NMDA receptors.

TABLE 21-3 Blood alcohol concentration (BAC) and clinical effects in nontolerant individuals.

BAC (mg/dL)^a	Clinical Effect
50-100	Sedation, subjective "high," increased reaction times
100-200	Impaired motor function, slurred speech, ataxia
200-300	Emesis, stupor
300-400	Coma
> 500	Respiratory depression, death

^{a}In most of the United States, a BAC of ≥ 80 mg/dL (0.08%) for adults ≥ 21 years old is sufficient for conviction of "driving while under the influence, or DUI." The legal limit for commercial drivers is 0.04%. Many states also have lower limits (0.00%-0.02%) set for drivers under the age of 21.

Other organ systems are acutely affected by ethanol. Even at relatively low blood concentration, alcohol significantly depresses cardiac contractility. Ethanol is also a vasodilator due to both CNS effects (depression of vasomotor center) and direct effects of acetaldehyde on vascular smooth muscle. In cases of overdose, this may result in marked hypothermia in cold environments.

Effects of Chronic Alcohol Use

Consuming alcohol in high doses over long periods of time induces tolerance, dependence, and often addiction. In chronic drinkers, the mechanism underlying the observed tolerance to alcohol's intoxicating effects is not completely understood. However, both CNS and pharmacokinetic changes are involved. There is also cross-tolerance to sedative-hypnotic drugs that facilitate GABA activity (eg, benzodiazepines, barbiturates).

Ethanol has much lower potency than other drugs of abuse covered in this chapter. This means that it requires concentrations sometimes thousands of times *higher* than other drugs of abuse to produce its acute effects. Therefore, alcohol is consumed in much larger quantities than other pharmacologically active agents. Chronic alcohol consumption has significant negative effects on the functions of many organs, including the nervous, gastrointestinal, cardiovascular, and immune systems. Tissue damage induced by chronic alcohol intake is due to both the direct effects of ethanol and acetaldehyde and the consequences of metabolizing a heavy burden of an active substance.

The most common medical complication of chronic alcohol abuse is liver disease that can progress to irreversible hepatitis and liver failure. Women appear to be more susceptible to alcohol hepatotoxicity than men. Concurrent infection with hepatitis B or C increases the risk of severe liver disease. In the gastrointestinal system, chronic heavy alcohol ingestion causes inflammation, bleeding and scarring of the gut wall, which can cause significant nutrient malabsorption. Chronic alcohol abuse is also the most common cause of pancreatitis.

Peripheral neuropathy is the most common neurologic complication. However, if thiamine deficiency occurs in alcoholics, Wernicke-Korsakoff syndrome can result. This syndrome is a relatively uncommon but important entity characterized by paralysis of external eye muscles, ataxia, and a confused state that can progress to coma and death. The syndrome is rarely seen in the absence of alcoholism. Often, the ocular signs, ataxia, and confusion improve upon prompt administration of thiamine. However, most patients are left with a chronic disabling memory disorder known as Korsakoff's psychosis.

Chronic alcohol use has complex effects on the cardiovascular system. Excessive and long-term consumption is associated with dilated cardiomyopathy. Excessive drinking over several days ("binge" drinking) is associated with arrhythmias. In contrast, epidemiological studies have shown that moderate alcohol consumption may protect against coronary heart disease, likely due in part to ethanol's ability to raise serum high-density lipoprotein (HDL) levels.

Although ethanol is not a primary carcinogen, chronic alcohol consumption increases the risk of several cancers, including mouth, pharynx, esophagus, liver, and likely breast (in women).

Chronic maternal alcohol abuse is associated with several teratogenic effects, termed fetal alcohol syndrome (FAS). Because the fetus has little to no alcohol dehydrogenase, the fetus must rely on maternal and placental enzymes to metabolize alcohol. Key features of FAS include mental retardation, microcephaly, growth deficiencies, poor coordination, minor joint problems, and characteristic facial features.

Treatment of Acute Alcohol Intoxication and Alcohol Withdrawal Syndrome

Severe acute alcohol intoxication is managed by maintenance of vital signs and prevention of aspiration after vomiting. Correction of electrolyte imbalances is often required. Glucose administration may need to be given to reverse hypoglycemia and ketoacidosis. Thiamine is also administered to protect against the Wernicke-Korsakoff syndrome.

For chronic users of alcohol, abrupt discontinuation leads to a withdrawal syndrome characterized by insomnia, tremor, anxiety, and lowering of the seizure threshold. The severity of the withdrawal syndrome is typically proportionate to the degree and duration of alcohol abuse. Figure 21-3 illustrates the time course of events during alcohol withdrawal syndrome. In severe cases, life-threatening seizures can occur. Alcohol withdrawal is one of the most common causes of seizures in adults. Delirium tremens (DTs), a condition including diaphoresis, tremors, confusion, autonomic instability, and hallucinations, may follow. Delirium tremens is associated with 5-15% mortality. The primary goal of drug therapy in alcohol withdrawal syndrome is prevention of seizures, delirium, and arrhythmias. The withdrawal syndrome is usually managed by administration of thiamine, correction of electrolyte imbalance, and administration of benzodiazepines such as **lorazepam** or **diazepam**. Over several weeks, the dosage of benzodiazepines is gradually tapered.

Treatment of Alcoholism

Alcoholism (or, alcohol use disorder) is a complex sociomedical problem characterized by a high relapse rate. After alcohol detoxification, intensive (inpatient or outpatient) psychosocial therapy is the main treatment for alcoholism. Three drugs have FDA approval for adjunctive treatment of alcoholism: disulfiram, **naltrexone**, and **acamprosate**.

Disulfiram was the first FDA-approved drug for alcohol use disorder. Disulfiram inhibits aldehyde dehydrogenase, leading to the accumulation of acetaldehyde. Taken alone, disulfiram has little effect. However, if a person taking disulfiram consumes alcohol, acetaldehyde accumulation leads to nausea, headache, flushing, and hypotension. Effects may last

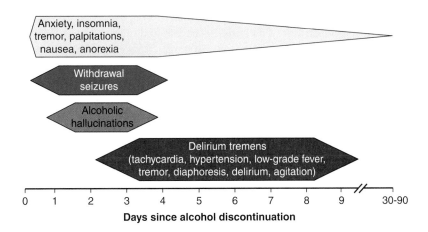

FIGURE 21-3 **Time course of signs and symptoms associated with alcohol withdrawal syndrome.** Early events include insomnia, anxiety, tremors, arrhythmias, nausea, and anorexia. In severe cases, hallucinations and seizures occur. Delirium tremens (DTs) usually develop 48-72 hours after abrupt alcohol discontinuation. Even several months after alcohol discontinuation, milder versions of early symptoms may persist.

30 minutes to several hours. Disulfiram therapy is rarely used due to low adherence and weak evidence for its effectiveness.

Many CNS neurotransmitter systems appear to be targets for drugs that may reduce the craving for alcohol. The opioid receptor antagonist naltrexone has been useful in this context, presumably through its ability to decrease the effects of endogenous opioid peptides in the brain (Chapter 20). When taken once daily (orally) or once every 4 weeks (intramuscularly), naltrexone decreases relapse rate and reduces alcohol craving in both short- and long-term trials and either alone or in combination with counseling. Acamprosate has actions on several neurotransmitter systems, but is well characterized as a weak glutamate NMDA receptor antagonist and positive allosteric GABA$_A$ receptor modulator. Acamprosate has shown mixed effectiveness in clinical trials in treating alcohol dependence.

Other drugs that have shown some efficacy in maintaining abstinence include certain antiseizure medications (eg, **topiramate**, **gabapentin**), a cholinergic nicotinic agonist for binge drinking (**varenicline**), selective serotonin reuptake inhibitors (SSRIs), and a 5-HT$_3$ receptor antagonist (**ondansetron**).

OPIOIDS

Chapter 20 discusses the medical uses of these drugs. Opioid analgesics are also among the most commonly abused drugs. The group includes a wide spectrum of scheduled drugs from **heroin** (Schedule I) to **propoxyphene** (Schedule IV), reflecting the differences in their addiction liability.

Over the past decade, healthcare practitioners and the general public have become increasingly aware of the "opioid epidemic" that has resulted in thousands of overdose deaths due to opioid abuse and misuse. The most frequently abused opioids are heroin, **morphine**, **codeine**, **oxycodone**, and,

among healthcare professionals, **meperidine**. **Kratom** is an illegal—though easily available—agent with opioid μ-receptor agonist activity. The drug, derived from leaves of a tree indigenous to Southeast Asia, is consumed in the form of pills or capsules, or the leaves are chewed or brewed in tea. Kratom is used for recreational purposes, but some users claim its benefit in managing chronic pain. As of 2018, the FDA has concluded that there is no evidence to support kratom's safety or efficacy for treating any condition.

All opioids cause tolerance and dependence, with more rapid development occurring with the stronger μ-opioid receptor agonists and with intravenous versus oral administration. Effects of intravenous administration of a strong μ-receptor agonist like heroin have been described as a "rush" or orgasmic feeling, followed by euphoria and then sedation. Opioid overdose leads to respiratory depression progressing to coma and death (Table 21-2). Overdose is managed with the opioid receptor antagonist **naloxone** (which can reverse opioid effects within minutes) and ventilatory support. As discussed in Chapter 20, naloxone provokes an explosive, but transient, precipitated withdrawal syndrome in an opioid-dependent person who has recently taken an opioid.

Deprivation of opioids in physiologically dependent individuals leads to an abstinence syndrome that includes lacrimation, rhinorrhea, yawning, sweating, weakness, gooseflesh or piloerection (basis for the phrase "quitting cold turkey"), nausea and vomiting, tremor, muscle jerks (basis for the phrase "kicking the habit"), and hyperpnea (Tables 20-4 and 21-2). Although extremely unpleasant, withdrawal from opioids is rarely fatal, unlike withdrawal from sedative-hypnotics. Treatment of opioid dependence often involves replacement of the illicit drug with a pharmacologically equivalent agent, such as **methadone**, followed by a slow dose reduction of the medication. In Canada and several European countries, medical heroin is used to substitute for street heroin. Chapter 20 discusses the use of other agents, including **buprenorphine**, a longer-acting partial μ-receptor agonist, and centrally acting α$_2$-adrenergic receptor agonists such as **lofexidine** and **clonidine** to suppress withdrawal symptoms. Neonates born to mothers physiologically dependent on opioids require special management of withdrawal symptoms.

CNS STIMULANTS

There are many CNS stimulants with a broad range of euphoria-producing capability. **Caffeine** and **nicotine** are the most commonly used mild licit stimulants, whereas illegal substances such as **amphetamines**, **ecstasy**, and **cocaine** are much more potent stimulants. Despite their similar behavioral effects, caffeine, nicotine, cocaine, and amphetamines have very different structures and sites of action in the brain.

Caffeine and Nicotine

Caffeine is a methylxanthine compound found at varying concentrations in many beverages (coffee, tea, soda). Caffeine appears to exert its central and at least some of its peripheral actions by blocking adenosine receptors. At higher concentrations, some of caffeine's effects may be due to inhibition of phosphodiesterase, the enzyme responsible for breaking down cyclic adenosine monophosphate (cAMP) and cyclic guanosine monophosphate (cGMP). Because caffeine does not act on dopaminergic brain structures related to reward and addiction, its abuse and dependence potential are quite small. However, psychologic dependence on caffeine has been recognized and recently, demonstration of abstinence signs and symptoms has provided evidence for physiologic dependence. Withdrawal from caffeine is accompanied by lethargy, irritability, and headaches. Perhaps surprisingly, withdrawal symptoms appear to occur in fewer than 3% of regular coffee drinkers. Acute toxicity from caffeine overdosage includes excessive CNS stimulation (tremor, insomnia, nervousness) and cardiac stimulation (arrhythmias). The morbidity associated with caffeine overdose is much less than the morbidity associated with other stimulants.

Nicotine (discussed at length in Chapter 5) contained within tobacco products is one of the most widely used licit drugs because it is heavily promoted and produces powerful dependence and addiction. Nicotine addiction exceeds all other forms of addiction, mostly in the form of smoking (cigarettes), but also in the chronic use of smokeless tobacco products, such as snuff and chewing tobacco. Electronic cigarettes (e-cigarettes, vapes) represent the most recent nicotine delivery system. "Vaping" has rapidly become the most commonly used form of tobacco among youth in the United States. Cigarette smoking is a major preventable cause of death, and is associated with a high incidence of cardiovascular, respiratory, and neoplastic diseases. In the United States, about 90% of cases of chronic obstructive pulmonary disease are linked to smoking.

The rewarding effects of nicotine are due to activation of nicotinic cholinergic receptors on dopamine neurons that project to the nucleus accumbens and prefrontal cortex. The anxiety and mental discomfort experienced from discontinuing nicotine are major impediments to quitting the habit.

Acute toxicity from overdosage of nicotine is similar to caffeine, and includes excessive CNS and cardiac stimulation, but can also include respiratory paralysis. Severe toxicity has been reported in small children who ingest discarded nicotine gum or nicotine patches, which are used as substitutes for tobacco products.

Nicotine withdrawal is characterized by irritability and sleep disturbance. However, the withdrawal is mild compared to opioid withdrawal. Nicotine is among the most addictive drugs and relapse after attempted cessation is very common. Treatment for nicotine addiction often includes administration of nicotine itself in forms that are slowly absorbed and remove the complications associated with toxic chemicals contained within tobacco smoke. Nicotine gum, lozenges, and transdermal patches slow the pharmacokinetics of the drug. Other drugs used to facilitate smoking cessation include **bupropion** (Chapter 19) and **varenicline**. Compared to placebo, bupropion appears to be as effective as nicotine patches in reducing urges to smoke. Its effectiveness is enhanced when combined with behavioral therapies. Varenicline, a partial agonist at nicotinic receptors, prevents nicotine from exerting its reinforcing action on dopaminergic neurons in the VTA. Varenicline has been associated with suicidal ideation and may impair the ability to drive.

Cocaine and Amphetamines

Cocaine is a plant product that has been used by natives of the South American Andes for more than a thousand years in the custom of chewing coca leaves. In contrast, amphetamine was synthesized in the late 1920s and has a large number of analogs. Cocaine is highly addictive in many forms. It can be injected or absorbed via mucosal membranes (eg, nasal snorting). When heated in an alkaline solution, cocaine is transformed into the free base called *crack* that is smoked. The euphoria, self-confidence, and mental alertness produced by cocaine are short-lasting and strongly reinforce its continued use. Users often lose their appetite, sleep little, and are hyperactive. Inhaled crack cocaine is very rapidly absorbed from the lungs and quickly enters the brain to produce an almost instantaneous "rush" or "high."

In the CNS, cocaine blocks the reuptake of dopamine, norepinephrine, and serotonin via their respective transporters. The rewarding effects of cocaine are attributed to its inhibition of the dopamine transporter (Figure 21–4). Inhibition of the norepinephrine transporter leads to cocaine's predictable acute activation of the sympathetic nervous system. Cardiac toxicity is partly due to this blockade of norepinephrine reuptake. Cocaine's local anesthetic action also contributes to the production of seizures due to its effect on sodium channels. In addition, the powerful vasoconstrictor action of cocaine may

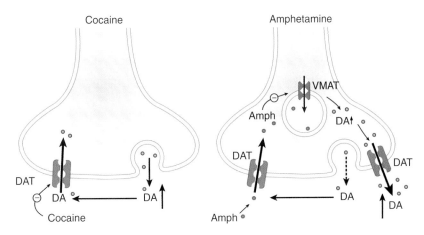

FIGURE 21-4 **Mechanism of action of cocaine and amphetamine at a central dopaminergic synapse. Left:** Cocaine inhibits the dopamine reuptake transporter (DAT). **Right:** Amphetamine (Amph) has several effects. Amph enters the nerve terminal via the DAT, then interferes with the vesicular monoamine transporter (VMAT) and hinders filling of synaptic vesicles. The result is that vesicles are empty and intracellular dopamine (DA) concentration increases, which causes reversal of the DAT and dopamine floods into the synapse.

lead to severe hypertensive episodes, resulting in myocardial infarctions and strokes. Overdoses with cocaine commonly result in fatalities from arrhythmias, seizures, or respiratory arrest (Table 21-2). No specific antidote is available. Infants born to mothers who abuse cocaine are often prematurely delivered, have low birth weights, and have smaller head circumferences. Decades ago, cocaine abuse during pregnancy was thought to result in a specific newborn syndrome called *crack-baby syndrome*. However, long-term follow-up of these children does not confirm a drug-specific deficit in cognition.

Although tolerance to cocaine may develop, some users experience a reverse tolerance in which they become more sensitive to smaller doses. The abstinence syndrome after withdrawal from cocaine (Table 21-2) includes severe depression of mood that strongly reinforces the compulsion to use the drug. Cravings for cocaine are very strong and to date, there are no pharmacologic interventions for cocaine addiction.

Amphetamines

Amphetamines are a group of synthetic sympathomimetic drugs that act indirectly to release amine neurotransmitters like norepinephrine and dopamine. Drugs in this class include **dextroamphetamine** and **methamphetamine** ("speed"), a crystal form ("ice") that can be smoked. These drugs cause a feeling of euphoria and self-confidence that contributes to the rapid development of addiction. These effects are exerted by the drugs' ability to *reverse* the action of amine (dopamine, norepinephrine, serotonin) transporters (Figure 21-4). First, amphetamines bind to the transporter and are taken up into the synaptic terminal. Once there, these drugs interfere with the vesicular transporter that is responsible for filling synaptic vesicles with the amine neurotransmitters. This results in depletion of synaptic vesicles, but increased levels of amine transmitters within the terminal itself. This concentration gradient drives the transporter in the opposite direction—that is,

releasing the amine into the synapse. Thus, normal vesicular exocytosis of transmitter decreases, but nonvesicular release increases.

Amphetamines are often called *club drugs* (along with GHB, ecstasy, LSD, and ketamine discussed later in chapter) because their use has been popular in nightclubs and "raves." Amphetamines differ from other club drugs in a couple key ways. First, amphetamines can be taken orally, but heavy users (especially of methamphetamine) often progress rapidly to intravenous administration. Second, addiction is far more common with amphetamines than with other club drugs.

Two common amphetamine derivatives are therapeutically used in the treatment of some children with attention deficit hyperactivity disorder (ADHD). The combination product **dextroamphetamine/amphetamine** (Adderall) and **methylphenidate** (Ritalin) enhance focus and learning in individuals with ADHD. However, these agents are used recreationally for their stimulant effects, and also misused or abused to enhance focus and attention for studying for exams. Individuals without ADHD have exploited the latter effect by taking these agents as purported "cognitive enhancers." The misuse and diversion of ADHD medications are common healthcare problems, with the prevalence highest among individuals aged 12-25 years. Past-year prevalence among college students has been reported as high as 35%. While studies have shown that some youth (without ADHD) demonstrate benefit in select cognitive domains, these agents can rapidly increase brain dopamine, which can lead to addiction.

Chronic high-dose abuse of amphetamines can lead to a psychotic state (thought to be due to effects on the dopamine system), with delusions and paranoia that may be difficult to differentiate from schizophrenia. Unlike many other abused drugs, amphetamines are neurotoxic and affect mainly serotonergic and dopaminergic neurons. Chronic abuse is also associated with the development of necrotizing arteritis that can lead to cerebral hemorrhage and renal failure. Tolerance can be marked, and an abstinence syndrome, characterized by increased appetite, sleepiness, exhaustion, and mental depression, can occur upon withdrawal. Antidepressant drugs may be indicated.

Symptoms of amphetamine overdose include agitation, restlessness, tachycardia, hyperthermia, hyperreflexia, and possibly seizures (Table 21-2). There is no specific antidote. Supportive measures are directed toward control of body temperature and protection against cardiac arrhythmias and seizures.

Ecstasy ("Molly") is actually the name of a *class* of drugs that includes several derivatives of the amphetamine compound **methylene dioxymethamphetamine** (MDMA). Taken orally, this popular club drug increases the activity of dopamine, norepinephrine, and serotonin. However, because MDMA has a preferential affinity for the serotonin transporter, the drug significantly increases synaptic serotonin concentration. Release is so profound that a single MDMA dose produces intracellular serotonin depletion for approximately 24 hours and repetitive use may cause *permanent* serotonin depletion. For roughly 3-6 hours after ingestion, ecstasy leads to feelings of increased energy, euphoria, and emotional empathy. The latter component is a significant reason that MDMA is abused. Specifically, ecstasy is purported to facilitate interpersonal communication and foster feelings of intimacy without cognitive impairment. MDMA has several acute toxic effects. The most serious is hyperthermia, which if combined with dehydration, can be fatal. After warnings of this effect became well known, users attempted to mitigate the hyperthermia by drinking excessive amounts of water. Cases of severe water intoxication, hyponatremia, and death have been reported. Other adverse effects include serotonin syndrome (Chapter 19) and seizures. Finally, ecstasy's ability to promote closeness and trust may encourage unsafe sexual behavior. Withdrawal from MDMA is characterized by depressed mood, irritability, increased impulsiveness, and aggressiveness that may last up to several weeks.

HALLUCINOGENS

Many agents fall under the category of hallucinogens because of their ability to alter consciousness such that the person senses things that are not present in reality. Hallucinogens induce a number of perceptual (eg, shape and color distortion) and somatic (eg, dizziness, nausea, paresthesias, blurred vision) symptoms, commonly referred to as a "trip." The components of a "trip" tend to be unpredictable. Some individuals also report "flashbacks" in which they re-experience a "trip" perhaps several years after the last drug exposure. Unlike most drugs described in this chapter that modulate dopaminergic pathways in the CNS, hallucinogens do not induce dependence or addiction; however, repetitive exposure leads to rapid tolerance (tachyphylaxis). Hallucinogenic agents modulate the activity of several different neurotransmitters. **Phencyclidine (PCP)** and **ketamine** are noncompetitive antagonists at

glutamate NMDA receptors, whereas **lysergic acid diethylamide (LSD)**, **psilocybin**, and **mescaline** modulate actions of serotonin. Almost all the hallucinogens are Schedule I controlled substances, except ketamine, which is Schedule III.

PCP and ketamine were originally developed as general anesthetics (Chapter 15). While ketamine (a structural congener of PCP) still has clinical uses as a dissociative anesthetic and analgesic, PCP has no clinical use and is probably the most dangerous of the currently popular hallucinogenic agents. In pure forms, PCP and ketamine are white powders, but they can be sold in different formulations to be snorted, ingested, injected, or smoked. The psychedelic effects of "angel dust" (PCP) or "Special K" (ketamine) last approximately an hour. Other effects include increased blood pressure, impaired memory function, and visual alterations. Psychotic reactions are common with PCP, and impaired judgment often leads to reckless behavior. Chronic exposure, especially to PCP, may lead to long-lasting psychosis that resembles schizophrenia, which may persist beyond drug exposure. Effects of overdosage with PCP include nystagmus (vertical and horizontal), marked hypertension, hyperthermia, and seizures, which may be fatal. Parenteral benzodiazepines (eg, diazepam, lorazepam) are used to curb excitation and protect against seizures. Although ketamine has clinical uses as an anesthetic and analgesic, its use is tightly restricted because of its illicit use.

Several other drugs with CNS effects that have been described as "psychedelic" or "mind-revealing" are serotonergic agonists and include LSD, mescaline, and psilocybin. LSD ("acid") is an ergot alkaloid that is typically sprinkled over blotter paper or sugar cubes. After swallowing, psychoactive effects usually appear after 30 minutes and can last 6-12 hours. Mescaline is a naturally occurring alkaloid in the peyote cactus, but the drug can also be synthesized; the drug can be swallowed as a liquid, consumed raw, or brewed into tea. Mescaline has similar psychoactive properties to LSD with claims of more unique characteristics including visual hallucinations of objects appearing geometrically altered. Psilocybin's common names "magic mushroom" and "shrooms" highlight this alkaloid's origin from certain types of mushrooms.

Hallucinogens impair rational judgment, which places the user at high risk of injury and accidents. Bizarre behaviors may prompt public health or law enforcement personnel intervention. Though not considered neurotoxic, LSD (like most ergot alkaloids) may cause strong uterine contractions that can induce abortion. Beyond the hallucinogenic effects of such drugs, short-term somatic effects that can be quite marked include nausea; alterations in blood pressure, temperature, heart rate; excessive sweating; weakness, and paresthesias. Panic reactions and paranoia ("bad trips") may also occur. Although there is little evidence that hallucinogen use leads to the development of dependence, some agents can be addictive.

For decades, the therapeutic value of some hallucinogens—particularly LSD and psilocybin—has been investigated for use in the treatment of several conditions such as anxiety or mood disorders and various addictions. Limited efficacy of psilocybin has recently been demonstrated for treatment-resistant depression, as indicated by the FDA's 2018 provision of a "Breakthrough Therapy" designation which indicates that clinical evidence supports that psilocybin may show substantial improvement over available therapy for treatment-resistant depression.

CANNABINOIDS

Endogenous cannabinoids include anandamide and 2-arachidonyl glycerol (2-AG). These chemicals are released post-synaptically, acting as retrograde messengers that inhibit the presynaptic release of classical neurotransmitters such as glutamate or GABA (Chapter 12). These very lipid-soluble endocannabinoids and exogenous cannabinoids found in marijuana ("grass" or "pot") mediate their CNS effects via activation of CB_1 receptors that have particularly high expression in the basal ganglia, limbic system, hippocampus, brainstem, cerebellum, and both ascending and descending pain pathways.

There are over 100 different cannabinoid compounds in the *Cannabis sativa* plant, but the primary psychoactive constituent is Δ^9-**tetrahydrocannabinol (THC)**. Another important compound in marijuana is **cannabidiol (CBD)**, which does *not* have the psychoactive properties of THC. Cannabidiol is increasing being used therapeutically for conditions such as anxiety, movement disorders, and pain as well as for rare, severe forms of epilepsy. Hashish is a partially purified material that is more potent.

The central psychoactive effects of marijuana (primarily due to THC) result in feelings of being "high." Effects include euphoria, disinhibition, relaxation, uncontrollable laughter, changes in perception, and achievement of a dream-like state. Mental concentration may be difficult. Vasodilation occurs, and heart rate is characteristically increased. Habitual users show reddened conjunctivae. The dangers of marijuana use are its impairment of judgment and reflexes, effects that are potentiated by concomitant use of sedative-hypnotics, including ethanol. In rare cases and in very high doses (eg, in hashish), visual hallucinations or frank psychotic episodes have been reported. Chronic marijuana use leads to dependence as indicated by a distinct, but mild withdrawal syndrome that includes restlessness, irritability, insomnia, nausea, and cramping.

Cannabinoids can be administered in a variety of routes. Marijuana can be inhaled by smoking (typically in the form of a "joint" that is hand-rolled and resembles a cigarette) or vaporizing (inhaled via a device such as a "bong"). The marijuana plant or its extracts can also be ingested via edible products (eg, baked into brownies, infused into oils or butter) or as synthesized THC in oral tablets. Currently, there are three FDA-approved cannabinoids: **dronabinol** (available as capsules and oral solution), **nabilone** (available as capsules), and **cannabidiol** (available as oral solution). The onset of effect varies dramatically depending on the agent's route of administration. Onset is quickest (within minutes) with inhalation and

slowest with edible products (~30-90 minutes). Effects may last only a few hours after inhalation, but as long as 12 hours after oral ingestion.

Therapeutic effects of marijuana and cannabinoids have been recognized for hundreds of years. Effects such as decreased intraocular pressure, increased appetite, chronic and neuropathic pain relief, and antiemetic actions have led to the use of cannabinoids to treat a variety of conditions. As of the writing of this chapter, 33 states and the District of Columbia in the United States have laws legalizing the uses of marijuana in *some* form. While the pace of legalization is increasing, this continues to be a controversial issue primarily due to fears that marijuana (and cannabinoids in general) may serve as "gateways" to consumption of "hard" drugs or induce schizophrenia in predisposed individuals. Reflecting that concern, marijuana itself still remains as a *federally* controlled Schedule I substance, indicating no currently accepted medical use and the highest abuse potential. Schedule I status severely restricts research into potential clinical benefits, impedes pharmacy stocking systems, and places patients (and potentially prescribers) at risk for criminal sanctions. Many professional organizations have called for a review of the federal Schedule I classification for marijuana.

The FDA-approved cannabinoids are still listed as controlled substances, indicating some potential for abuse and addiction. Dronabinol (Schedule III) is a synthetic formulation of THC that has been approved to combat chemotherapy-induced nausea and vomiting (CINV) and as an appetite stimulant for HIV/AIDS. Nabilone (Schedule II) is a THC formulation also used as an antiemetic for CINV. Cannabidiol (Schedule V), the most recently FDA-approved cannabinoid, is approved for treating rare forms of drug-resistant epilepsy. Though not yet FDA-approved in the United States, **nabiximols** (a *Cannabis* extract containing THC and cannabidiol in roughly equal proportion) is widely used to treat symptoms associated with multiple sclerosis.

INHALANTS

Certain gases or volatile liquids are abused because they provide a feeling of euphoria or disinhibition. These substances may be divided into three major groups: anesthetics, industrial solvents, and organic nitrites.

Anesthetic gases (discussed in Chapter 15) that are frequently abused include **nitrous oxide**, **chloroform**, and **diethyl ether**. These agents are hazardous because they affect judgment and induce loss of consciousness. Inhalation of nitrous oxide as the pure gas with no oxygen has caused asphyxia and death. Ether and chloroform sensitize the heart to arrhythmias. Also, ether is highly flammable.

Industrial and household solvents and a wide range of volatile compounds are in products such as gasoline, paint thinners, aerosol propellants, glues, rubber cement, and shoe polish. These substances are inhaled by "sniffing" (inhaling from an open container), "huffing" (breathing fumes from a cloth soaked in volatile solvent), or "bagging" (breathing from a paper or plastic bag filled with fumes). Because of their ready availability, these substances are most frequently abused by children and young teenagers. Active ingredients that have been identified include benzene, hexane, methylethylketone, toluene, and trichloroethylene. The exact mechanism of CNS action of most of these agents is unknown. However, many agents are toxic to the liver, kidneys, lungs, bone marrow, and peripheral nerves. White matter lesions in the CNS have been demonstrated after chronic exposure to the aromatic hydrocarbons (benzene, toluene).

Organic nitrites such as **amyl nitrite** and **isobutyl nitrite** are referred to as "poppers." These drugs cause smooth muscle relaxation and enhance erection. They are primarily used as sexual intercourse "enhancers." Though not addictive, inhalation causes dizziness, tachycardia, hypotension, and flushing. With the exception of methylglobinemia, few serious adverse effects have been reported.

ANABOLIC STEROIDS

The proper name for this group of synthetic or human-made variations of **testosterone** is anabolic-androgenic steroids. The anabolic function refers to the capacity of these drugs to increase muscle mass, whereas the androgenic function refers to the enhancement of male characteristics. Clinically, these steroids are used to treat conditions such as delayed puberty and conditions that cause profound muscle loss (cachexia) such as cancer and AIDS (Chapter 22). In many countries, including the United States, anabolic steroids are controlled substances (Schedule III) based on their potential for abuse. The effects sought by abusers are increased muscle mass and strength, rather than euphoria. However, excessive use can have adverse behavioral, cardiovascular, endocrine, and musculoskeletal effects. Premature closure of the epiphyses, masculinization in females, and severe acne are predictable androgenic adverse effects. Liver and kidney dysfunction have also been reported. The abuse of anabolic steroids may pose an increased risk of myocardial infarction due to cardiomyopathy, hypertension, and changes in cholesterol profile. Behavioral manifestations include increases in libido and aggression ("roid rage"), paranoid jealousy, and delusions. A withdrawal syndrome has been described as fatigue and depression of mood.

REHABILITATION RELEVANCE

The comorbidities associated with drugs of abuse are some of the most difficult problems facing healthcare professionals. These compounds are self-administered, often without divulging their use to healthcare professionals. The problem is further complicated by the fact that the clinical manifestations vary depending on which drugs are being abused. The most significant adverse effects that may affect rehabilitation treatments are those associated with the cardiovascular and the central nervous systems.

The use of illegal substances may be complicated by patient denial of their use. Therefore, clinicians need to recognize both the manifestations of the abuse of these illicit agents and the manifestations of withdrawal from such use. For CNS stimulants such as amphetamines and cocaine, the potential for adverse cardiovascular, thermoregulatory, or CNS adverse events occurs during the abuse stage, with a higher incidence for cocaine compared to amphetamines. Patients in withdrawal from CNS stimulants will often have the opposite clinical presentation: depressed and fatigued with delayed psychomotor responses, and possibly myalgia and arthralgia.

In contrast to abusers of CNS stimulants, those taking CNS depressants (including alcohol) present with depression and fatigue with delayed psychomotor responses during the abuse period. The risk for CNS adverse events such as seizures may occur during periods of abstinence.

For the hallucinogens, the incidence of morbidity and mortality is higher for PCP and ketamine compared to LSD and the other agents. The clinician should recognize the potential cardiovascular manifestations of PCP (hypertension and tachycardia) that interfere with therapy. Aggressive behavior may be associated with PCP intoxication.

Addiction is a chronic and frequently relapsing disease that is very difficult to treat. Even after successful withdrawal and long drug-free periods, addicted individuals have a high risk of relapsing. Relapse is typically triggered by stress, reexposure to the addictive drug, or a context that recalls prior use. Two of these common triggers are frequently encountered in the context of healthcare. The stresses of injury, illness, or progression of a chronic condition may trigger patients to relapse. Medical treatment and surgical intervention often involve the use of opioid analgesics. Patients with even a distant history of substance abuse may relapse into addiction during postoperative recovery. To assess the risk for abuse, current guidelines include an assessment of personal or family history of substance abuse prior to the prescription of opioid analgesics to prompt caution and closer monitoring. However, patients may not divulge current or previous substance abuse to healthcare professionals and the prescription of opioid analgesics to therapeutically treat post-surgical or post-trauma pain may set the stage for relapse.

Physical therapists have many distinct opportunities to provide support and education to help treat addiction. For example, since smoking is not allowed within the hospital, patients are often provided nicotine transdermal patches. Upon observation of a nicotine patch, the therapist can recognize this opportunity as a "teaching moment" to strategically employ the 5A's and 5R's for treating tobacco use and dependence. After identifying the patch, the therapist can confirm the patient's tobacco habit (*Ask*), provide a brief counseling session (*Advise*) to determine the patient's willingness to quit (*Assess*), offer to connect the patient with a smoking cessation counselor (*Assist*), and schedule a follow-up contact (*Arrange*) with the cessation counselor prior to hospital discharge. During physical therapy sessions, it is relatively easy to help the patient who may not be ready to make an attempt to quit now to identify why quitting smoking is *Relevant* at that time (eg, decrease dyspnea, improve exercise capacity) and the *Risks* of continued smoking (eg, delayed healing, readmission to hospital). By actively listening, the therapist can help the patient identify *Rewards* as well as *Roadblocks* to quitting (eg, reencountering triggers that stimulate cravings). The therapist can provide encouragement that smoking cessation is possible and explain that it often takes more than one intervention to quit (*Repetitions*).

Summarized below are adverse events likely to interfere with rehabilitation interventions or goals that may occur either during use of, or withdrawal from, drugs of abuse.

- With the exception of tobacco, alcohol is the cause of more **preventable morbidity and mortality** than all other drugs combined. Therapists can encourage patients to open a dialogue regarding alcohol abuse with their referring healthcare provider and/or refer patients to a therapeutic group (eg, Alcoholics Anonymous).
- **Decreased exercise capacity** results from smoking cigarettes (and to a lesser degree, marijuana) and increases the incidence of adverse events during therapy due to **increasing blood pressure and heart rate** and **sensitization of the heart to arrhythmias**. Smoking increases carbon monoxide and carboxyhemoglobin in the blood. Heavy smokers may have up to 9% of their hemoglobin as carboxyhemoglobin, which results in reduced oxygen-carrying capacity of the blood. Vitals during therapy should be closely monitored. Discussion of smoking cessation can be initiated using the 5A's and 5R's.
- CNS stimulants (eg, cocaine, amphetamines, ecstasy) and hallucinogens (eg, PCP, ketamine) are cardiovascular stimulants that can predispose the patient to **increased risk of hyperthermia**, **severe hypertension**, **seizures**, **cardiac arrhythmias**, **angina pectoris**, and **myocardial infarction**. Physical therapy during intoxication with these substances is not appropriate. Once the patient is medically stable, vital signs should be carefully monitored during progressive exercise interventions.
- Opioids and sedative-hypnotics (including alcohol) are respiratory depressants. Because respiratory drive is blunted,

decreased exercise capacity and **hypoxemia** are the clinical manifestations. Close monitoring of respiratory rate and oxygen saturation are warranted.
- Marijuana and organic nitrites can cause **orthostatic hypotension**, which may cause patients to faint when transferring from recumbent to more upright positions. Slower transfers and strategies to increase upright tolerance (eg, deep breaths, ankle pumps) should be employed.
- Hallucinogens, opioids, alcohol, marijuana, and CNS depressants can cause **cognitive changes** and **decreased psychomotor skills**, which increase the risk of falls and injury to both patient and therapist. These alterations also occur during withdrawal from CNS stimulants.
- Anabolic steroids and psychotomimetics (PCP, ketamine) can cause behavioral changes, including **increased aggressive behavior**. Therapists should take appropriate precautions that may include having other staff present during treatment sessions or discharging the patient from therapy.
- Withdrawal from CNS depressants and alcohol can result in **seizures**, **arrhythmias (especially tachycardia)**, **increased anxiety**, and **agitation**. In inpatient settings, alcohol withdrawal is not uncommon because the availability of alcohol is suddenly interrupted upon hospital admission. Physical therapists must be aware of patients who are at risk for alcohol withdrawal syndrome (AWS), and be vigilant of signs and symptoms of alcohol withdrawal. Inpatient therapists should be familiar with the Clinical Institute Withdrawal Assessment for Alcohol–Revised (CIWA–Ar), which is one of the most common tools used to assess the severity and manage AWS. Use of the CIWA–Ar helps guide pharmacological management (eg, symptom-based dosing strategy for benzodiazepines) of alcohol withdrawal. Nursing staff typically administers the CIWA-Ar prior to initial physical therapy examination. Therapists need to familiarize themselves with scoring of the CIWA–Ar (which determines severity of the AWS), determine whether physical therapy is appropriate at that time, and closely monitor vitals during treatment sessions, especially heart rate, because tachycardia at rest has been shown to be a strong predictor of the incidence of delirium tremens.

CASE CONCLUSION

On the morning of the work-hardening program, K.C. ingested two cardiovascular stimulants—nicotine and caffeine—at breakfast. Smoking also increased his carboxyhemoglobin concentration, effectively decreasing both the oxygen-carrying capacity of the blood and exercise tolerance. In addition, the opioid (codeine) contained in Tylenol #3 inhibited central respiratory drive. This combination of licit and prescribed drugs predisposed K.C. to exertional cardiac hypoxia, especially since he has a documented history of exertional angina. The therapist should contact the referring physician for approval of additional work-hardening participation prior

to the next scheduled appointment. The therapist should also recommend that the patient avoid smoking and drinking coffee prior to participating in the work-hardening program because of the potential of these agents to increase the likelihood of exertional angina. Administration of Tylenol #3 prior to the work-hardening program should be discussed with the referring healthcare provider. Finally, the referring healthcare provider should be notified that the patient is operating a motorized vehicle possibly under the influence of an opioid, to prompt a discussion of the legal ramifications of such action with the patient.

CHAPTER 21 QUESTIONS

1. Which of the following agents is a primary cannabinoid responsible for producing psychoactive effects?

   a. Cannabidiol
   b. Δ^9-tetrahydrocannabinol (THC)
   c. Dronabinol
   d. Heroin

2. Which of the following agents has *not* been used as an adjunctive treatment for alcoholism, or alcohol use disorder?

   a. Niacin
   b. Naltrexone
   c. Acamprosate
   d. Disulfiram

3. Which of the following agents would most likely be used in the treatment of acute alcohol ingestion to decrease the risk of seizures?

   a. Ondansetron
   b. Naltrexone
   c. Benzodiazepines
   d. Amphetamines

4. Which of these agents would *not* be used in the medical treatment of opioid dependence?

   a. Morphine
   b. Buprenorphine
   c. Lofexidine
   d. Clonidine

5. Which of the following drugs is abused in order to increase muscle mass?

   a. Amyl nitrite
   b. Isobutyl nitrite
   c. Testosterone
   d. Morphine

6. Which of the following drugs is a benzodiazepine associated with use in "date rape"?

   a. Flunitrazepam
   b. Diazepam
   c. Flumazenil
   d. Chlordiazepoxide

7. Which of the following is *not* an adverse effect of anabolic steroids?

   a. Severe acne
   b. Hypotension
   c. Cardiomyopathy
   d. Increased aggression

8. Which of the following drugs has been abused primarily in order to enhance sexual intercourse?

   a. Morphine
   b. Amyl nitrite
   c. Cannabidiol
   d. Chloroform

9. Which of the following statements regarding withdrawal is true?

   a. Abrupt cessation of benzodiazepines in tolerant individuals does not result in a withdrawal syndrome.
   b. Abrupt cessation of heavy alcohol ingestion in an individual with alcohol use disorder can result in delirium tremens.
   c. Abrupt cessation of opioids in tolerant individuals can result in delirium tremens.
   d. Abrupt cessation of marijuana in heavy users results in the most severe withdrawal syndrome.

10. Which of the following statements is true?

    a. Individuals who are dependent and tolerant to a drug will also be addicted to the drug.
    b. Tolerance only occurs with drugs of abuse.
    c. Individuals can be dependent and tolerant to a drug, but not be addicted to the drug.
    d. Addiction does not involve changes in the brain.

Growth, Thyroid, and Gonadal Pharmacology

CASE STUDY

The patient is a 56-year-old woman with a 10-year history of mild hypertension (stabilized with enalapril and hydrochlorothiazide/amiloride) and a 2-year history of bipolar disorder (stabilized with lithium). Three weeks ago, she was diagnosed with fibromyalgia and started working with a physical therapist to develop an exercise program to assist in pain relief. Weekly, she meets with the therapist to review and modify the exercise program and assess her fibromyalgia symptoms. Recent measurements of blood pressure and heart rate were 130/82 mm Hg

and 80 beats per minute, respectively. Last week, the patient was diagnosed with functional hypothyroidism likely resulting from the lithium treatment. She was prescribed levothyroxine and started taking the drug that day. Today, she told the physical therapist that over the past week she has experienced increased muscle weakness and shortness of breath that has made her unable to comfortably exercise on the stationary bicycle. The therapist measured her blood pressure at 142/86 mm Hg and heart rate at 96 beats per minute and irregular.

REHABILITATION FOCUS

The endocrine system integrates major organ systems with each other and with the nervous system. The endogenous ligands that the endocrine system uses to perform this integrative task are called hormones. Hormones released from specialized cells circulate in the blood and regulate physiologic processes in one or more target organs. In many endocrine systems, several hormones act in series to regulate organ function. The release of one hormone in the series regulates the release of the next hormone. This provides multiple levels of regulation and integration as well as the opportunity for negative feedback, in which the last hormone in the series can reduce the production of earlier hormones in the series and thereby regulate its own production. Feedback regulation is also critical to understand the pharmacologic treatments that affect endocrine systems.

While some endocrine drugs directly influence the practice of the physical therapist, other drugs influence the

patients' responses to the rehabilitation process. Many postmenopausal women use estrogens and progestins for hormone replacement therapy (HRT). A small percentage will experience cardiovascular events or develop breast or endometrial cancers, which are recognized adverse effects of HRT. Subsequently, these women may need rehabilitation. Androgen supplementation in older males with hypogonadism or decreased testosterone levels improves bone mineral density and exercise tolerance. However, abuse of androgens by athletes promotes abnormal distribution of cholesterol in serum lipoproteins and increases the risk of atherosclerosis and cardiovascular morbidities. Physical therapists should be aware of these adverse effects and counsel athletes appropriately. Drugs that affect endocrine function may also directly influence the response of the patient to rehabilitation. For example, excessive supplementation with levothyroxine can cause cardiovascular and respiratory dysfunction that may not appear at rest, but can be precipitated with exercise.

BACKGROUND

This chapter covers drugs that regulate three related endocrine systems. These are: (1) the hypothalamic-pituitary system, which exerts control over many integrative functions and other endocrine tissues and interacts directly with the nervous system, (chapter emphasis is on growth hormone); (2) the thyroid gland, an essential regulator of growth, development, and normal function of many organ systems; and (3) the gonadal system, which regulates the development and function of reproductive tissues. Other chapters focus on drugs that influence hormones produced by the adrenal gland (Chapter 23), hormones that regulate blood glucose (Chapter 24), and hormones involved with bone mineralization (Chapter 25). Figure 22-1 outlines the classic hypothalamic-pituitary-terminal organ series.

HYPOTHALAMIC HORMONES

Overall control of metabolism, growth, and reproduction is mediated by neural and endocrine systems in the hypothalamus and pituitary gland. The pituitary gland consists of an anterior lobe (adenohypophysis) and a posterior lobe (neurohypophysis). While the posterior pituitary is connected to the hypothalamus by a stalk of neurosecretory fibers, the anterior pituitary is connected to the hypothalamus by a unique portal venous system. The portal venous system carries small regulatory peptide hormones from the hypothalamus to the anterior pituitary. These hypothalamic hormones regulate release of anterior pituitary hormones, which subsequently regulate the release of hormones from target tissues throughout the body (Table 22-1). In contrast, hormones released from the posterior lobe of the pituitary (oxytocin and vasopressin) are synthesized in the hypothalamus and transported via neurosecretory fibers in the pituitary stalk to the posterior lobe from which they are released into the circulation.

Hypothalamic and pituitary hormones, and their synthetic analogs, have pharmacologic applications in three areas: (1) replacement therapy for hormone deficiency states, (2) antagonist therapy for diseases resulting from excessive production of, or response to, pituitary hormones, and (3) diagnostic tools for identifying specific endocrine abnormalities.

Growth Hormone–Releasing Hormone

Growth hormone–releasing hormone (GHRH) is a hypothalamic hormone that stimulates the release of growth hormone (GH) from the anterior pituitary. GH is required during childhood and adolescence for attainment of normal adult size. Throughout the lifespan, GH is an important regulator of macronutrient metabolism, lean body mass, and bone density. Two short synthetic peptides with activity similar to GHRH are available for clinical use. In normal individuals, these peptides produce a rapid increase in plasma GH concentrations. Occasionally, these agents are used as diagnostic tools in individuals with GH deficiency to determine whether the deficiency results from a problem in the hypothalamus, pituitary, or tissues targeted by GH.

Somatostatin

Whereas GHRH stimulates the release of GH from the anterior pituitary, somatostatin inhibits GH release from the anterior pituitary. Thus, somatostatin is also known as growth hormone–inhibiting hormone. Somatostatin is also found in other neuron populations, select pancreatic islet cells, and regions

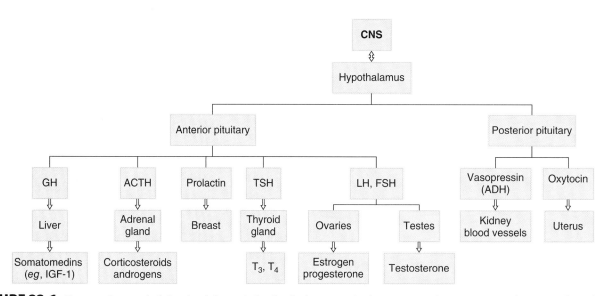

FIGURE 22-1 **Hormonal control of the classic hypothalamic-pituitary-terminal organ cascade.** In most cases, hormones from the terminal organ exert negative feedback effects upon release of hormones higher up in the cascade. ACTH, adrenocorticotropic hormone; ADH, antidiuretic hormone; CNS, central nervous system; FSH, follicle stimulating hormone; IGF-1, insulin-like growth factor-1; LH, luteinizing hormone; TSH, thyroid-stimulating hormone.

TABLE 22-1 Links among hypothalamic, pituitary, and target gland hormones.

Hypothalamic Hormone	Pituitary Hormone	Target Organ	Target Organ Hormone
Growth hormone–releasing hormone (GHRH)	Growth hormone (GH)	Liver	Somatomedins, especially insulin-like growth factor 1 (IGF-1)
Somatostatin[a]	Growth hormone (GH)	Liver	Somatomedins, especially IGF-1
Thyrotropin-releasing hormone (TRH)	Thyroid-stimulating hormone (TSH)	Thyroid	Thyroxine (T_4) Triiodothyronine (T_3)
Corticotropin-releasing hormone (CRH)	Adrenocorticotropic hormone (ACTH)	Adrenal cortex	Glucocorticoids Mineralocorticoids Androgens
Gonadotropin-releasing hormone (GnRH)	Follicle-stimulating hormone (FSH) Luteinizing hormone (LH)	Gonads	Estrogen Progesterone Testosterone
Prolactin-inhibiting hormone (PIH; dopamine)	Prolactin (PRL)	Anterior pituitary	
Oxytocin	None	Smooth muscle, especially uterus	
Vasopressin (also called anti-diuretic hormone, ADH)	None	Renal tubule Smooth muscle in blood vessels	

[a]Inhibits GH and TSH release. Also found in gastrointestinal tissues; inhibits release of gastrin, glucagon, and insulin.

of the gastrointestinal system. Somatostatin not only inhibits the release of GH, but also inhibits the release of glucagon, insulin, and gastrin. Somatostatin itself has little clinical value because of its short duration of action. **Octreotide**, a synthetic somatostatin analog with a longer duration of action, inhibits GH release much more potently than somatostatin. Octreotide is used to reduce symptoms caused by hormone-secreting tumors such as GH-secreting tumors that cause acromegaly, carcinoid tumors, gastrinoma, insulinoma, and glucagonoma. Regular octreotide must be administered subcutaneously 2-4 times daily. Once a brief course has been demonstrated to be effective and tolerated, a slow-release formulation is injected into alternate gluteal muscles every 4 weeks for long-term therapy. Adverse effects primarily involve the gastrointestinal system (eg, nausea, cramps, steatorrhea) and the heart (rate abnormalities).

Thyrotropin-Releasing Hormone

Thyrotropin-releasing hormone (TRH) is a tripeptide that stimulates the release of thyroid-stimulating hormone (TSH) from the anterior pituitary. TRH also increases prolactin production by the anterior pituitary, but has no effect on the release of GH or adrenocorticotropin (ACTH). TRH has been used in diagnostic testing of thyroid dysfunction.

Corticotropin-Releasing Hormone

Corticotropin-releasing hormone (CRH) stimulates secretion of adrenocorticotropic hormone (ACTH) from the anterior

pituitary. In response to CRH, ACTH is cleaved from a larger precursor molecule called pro-opiomelanocortin (POMC), which is cleaved into several unique biologically active peptides. CRH is used to diagnose the source of ACTH secretion abnormalities. If an ACTH-secreting tumor is located within the pituitary, exogenous CRH usually produces an increase in ACTH secretion. In contrast, if an ACTH-secreting tumor is located outside the pituitary, exogenous CRH rarely results in any change in ACTH secretion.

Gonadotropin-Releasing Hormone

Gonadotropin-releasing hormone (GnRH), a decapeptide, coordinates reproductive function in males and females by regulating release of two gonadotropins—luteinizing hormone (LH) and follicle-stimulating hormone (FSH)—from the anterior pituitary. When administered in a *pulsatile* fashion that mimics the endogenous pattern of secretion, **recombinant GnRH** (or a synthetic analog like **leuprolide**) *stimulates* gonadotropin release. Pulsatile GnRH administration is used to determine the basis of delayed puberty in adolescents. Rarely, it is used to treat infertility in both sexes that is due to hypothalamic dysfunction. In contrast, *continuous nonpulsatile* administration *inhibits* FSH and LH release by causing down-regulation of GnRH receptors in pituitary cells that normally release the gonadotropins. This type of steady dosage of GnRH agonists is used to suppress gonadotropin secretion in men with prostatic carcinoma or children with precocious puberty.

GnRH agonists are also used in women undergoing assisted reproduction technology procedures or who have a gynecologic problem that benefits from ovarian suppression such as endometriosis or uterine fibroids. In endometriosis, the presence of estrogen-sensitive endometrium outside the uterus often causes cyclical abdominal pain in premenopausal women. Pain is often reduced by preventing endometrial implants from being exposed to normal cyclical changes in the concentrations of estrogen and progesterone. Ovarian suppression induced by continuous treatment with a GnRH agonist greatly reduces estrogen and progesterone concentrations and prevents cyclical changes. Treatment with a GnRH agonist is limited to 6 months because prolonged ovarian suppression can result in decreased bone mineral density. If women experience satisfactory pain relief from GnRH agonist-induced ovarian suppression, treatment can continue with the addition of estrogen or progestins to reduce GnRH agonist-induced bone mineral loss.

GnRH antagonists (eg, **ganirelix**, **cetrorelix**, **abarelix**, **degarelix**) inhibit FSH and LH secretion in a dose-dependent manner. Ganirelix and cetrorelix can be used in controlled ovarian hyperstimulation procedures. Abarelix and degarelix are used in the treatment of advanced prostate cancer.

Prolactin-Inhibiting Hormone

Dopamine (also called prolactin-inhibiting hormone, PIH) is the primary physiologic regulator of prolactin release. Acting through D_2 dopamine receptors, dopamine inhibits prolactin release from the anterior pituitary. Prolactin deficiency is rare. Prolactin excess—hyperprolactinemia—is more common. Hyperprolactinemia can be due to impaired transport of dopamine to the pituitary (due to brain surgery, head trauma, or pituitary stalk compression from a tumor), prolactin-secreting adenomas, or an adverse drug reaction (ADR). Dopamine itself is not used to treat hyperprolactinemia. Instead, dopamine D_2 receptor agonists such as **bromocriptine** and **cabergoline** are first-line treatment.

ANTERIOR PITUITARY HORMONES

Growth Hormone (GH, or somatropin)

GH's effects are primarily mediated via insulin-like growth factor-1 (IGF-1; also known as somatomedin C), which is mainly produced in the liver. GH has anabolic effects in muscle and catabolic effects in adipose tissue; thus, shifting body composition toward increased muscle mass and decreased adiposity. GH and IGF-1 have opposite effects on insulin sensitivity. GH reduces insulin sensitivity, leading to increased blood glucose concentration; IGF-1 increases insulin sensitivity, leading to increased glucose disposal into insulin-sensitive target tissues.

Recombinant forms of human GH are **somatropin** and **somatrem**; the former is identical to endogenous GH, while the latter has an extra methionine added to the protein.

Recombinant growth hormone is used to treat GH deficiency in children and adults. Girls with Turner syndrome treated with GH frequently achieve increased final adult height. GH treatment also improves growth in children with failure to thrive secondary to chronic renal failure or HIV infection. GH is also helpful in treating adults with acquired immune deficiency syndrome (AIDS)–associated wasting. While it has typically been thought that somatopause (a decrease in GH in adults) has no pathological consequences, adults with GH deficiency often have obesity, decreased muscle mass and bone mineral density, dyslipidemia, and decreased cardiac output. When GH-deficient adults are treated with GH, many of these manifestations reverse.

Based on the fact that serum GH levels normally decrease across the lifespan, GH has been a popular component of antiaging programs, despite strong and consistent evidence from animal studies demonstrating that analogs of GH and IGF-1 actually *shorten* lifespan. Many athletes also take supraphysiological doses of GH purportedly to increase muscle mass and recover more rapidly after training despite a lack of evidence that GH enhances physical performance. The World Anti-Doping Agency, which strives to provide consistent anti-doping policies within sports organizations across the world, prohibits the use of GH and its releasing factors.

Most of the information available about adverse effects of supraphysiological doses of GH comes from individuals with endogenous excess GH (gigantism and acromegaly). GH excess in patients with acromegaly results in increased growth of the *short* bones and cartilage tissue, resulting in the classic phenotype of enlarged hands and feet and coarsened and enlarged facial features. GH excess results in insulin resistance, diabetes, excessive sweating, hypertension, congestive heart failure, carpal tunnel syndrome, neuropathy, and increased mortality. Retrospective analyses of individuals with acromegaly suggest increased frequency of benign and malignant tumors.

Thyroid-Stimulating Hormone

Thyroid-stimulating hormone (TSH) increases the uptake of iodine into cells in the thyroid gland and subsequent production of thyroid hormones. Clinically, TSH has been used as a diagnostic tool to distinguish primary hypothydroidism (when the thyroid gland does not make enough thyroid hormone) from secondary hypothyroidism (insufficient thyroid hormone production due to disorders of the pituitary gland or hypothalamus).

Adrenocorticotropin Hormone

Adrenocorticotropin hormone (ACTH) is a large peptide formed from an even larger precursor peptide, pro-opiomelanocortin. This precursor is also the source of α-melanocyte-stimulating hormone, β-endorphin, and met-enkephalin. **Cosyntropin**, a synthetic ACTH analog, is used for diagnostic purposes in patients with abnormal corticosteroid production.

Follicle-Stimulating Hormone

Follicle-stimulating hormone (FSH) stimulates gametogenesis and follicle development in women and spermatogenesis in men. Three preparations are available to be used in combination with other drugs to treat infertility in both sexes. One is called **urofollitropin**, which is a purified extract from the urine of postmenopausal women. The two recombinant forms, **follitropin-α** and **follitropin-β** differ slightly in chemical structure.

Luteinizing Hormone

In women, luteinizing hormone (LH) acts in concert with FSH to regulate gonadal steroid production, follicular development, and ovulation. In men, LH regulates testosterone production. Human chorionic gonadotropin (hCG), the placental hormone necessary during early pregnancy, is almost identical to LH in structure and mediates its actions through activation of LH receptors. Thus, hCG or its recombinant form is often used for LH action. These agents or recombinant LH (**lutropin**) are used for treatment of hypogonadism in men and women and as part of controlled ovarian hyperstimulation and assisted reproductive technology programs.

Menotropins

Menotropins are a mixture of FSH and LH purified from the urine of postmenopausal women. The product is used in combination with hCG in the treatment of hypogonadal states and as part of controlled ovarian hyperstimulation and assisted reproductive technology programs.

THYROID AND ANTITHYROID DRUGS

The thyroid gland secretes two types of hormones: calcitonin and two iodine-containing hormones, thyroxine (T_4) and triiodothyronine (T_3). Calcitonin, a peptide that is important in calcium metabolism and bone mineralization is discussed in Chapter 25. Figure 22-2 outlines the agents that are used to treat insufficient thyroid function (hypothyroidism) and excess thyroid activity (hyperthyroidism).

Thyroid function is controlled by TSH release from the anterior pituitary and by iodine availability. TSH stimulates the uptake of iodine and synthesis of thyroid hormone. In addition, TSH has growth-promoting effects on the thyroid gland. High levels of thyroid hormones inhibit TSH release, providing an effective negative feedback control mechanism.

The thyroid gland synthesizes and secretes T_3 and T_4, which are collectively known as thyroid hormone (TH). Iodine derived from food or iodine supplements (eg, iodized salt) is actively transported and highly concentrated in the thyroid gland (Figure 22-3). Tyrosine residues of the protein thyroglobulin within the gland are iodinated to form monoiodotyrosine (MIT) or diiodotyrosine (DIT). T_4 is formed from the combination of two molecules of DIT and T_3 is formed from the combination of one molecule each of MIT and DIT. In the case of inadequate iodine intake, TH cannot be synthesized and the lack of negative feedback to the anterior pituitary results in excessive TSH release. Under the persistent trophic effects of TSH, the thyroid gland enlarges, forming a goiter. However, a goiter is not always associated with a *lack* of TH production. Graves disease is an autoimmune disorder in which autoantibodies are directed against TSH receptors on the thyroid gland. Two results of this binding are excessive production of TH (hyperthyroidism) and hypertrophy of the gland, resulting in a diffuse goiter.

Most of the hormone released from the thyroid gland is T_4. Both T_3 and T_4 are transported in the blood by thyroxine-binding globulin (TBG), a protein synthesized by the liver. After dissociating from TBG and entering the target cell, T_4 is converted to T_3, which is 10 times more potent than T_4. T_3 binds to nuclear receptors that modulate the expression of genes responsible for many metabolic processes. Proteins synthesized under T_3 control differ depending on the tissue involved. These proteins include Na^+/K^+ ATPase, specific contractile proteins in smooth muscle and the heart, enzymes involved in lipid metabolism, and critical developmental components in the brain. In addition, T_3 may have a separate membrane receptor-mediated effect in some tissues. TH is essential for normal growth and

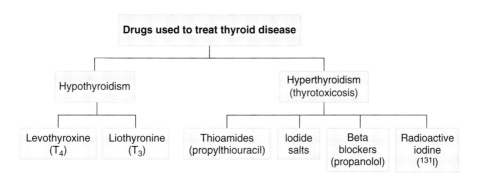

FIGURE 22-2 Drug treatment of thyroid disease is divided into supplementation with synthetic exogenous hormones when thyroid function is insufficient (hypothyroidism), or inhibition of thyroid function when thyroid hormones are in excess (hyperthyroidism).

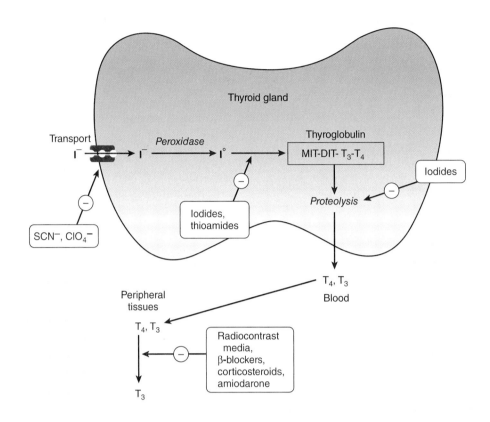

FIGURE 22-3 **Sites of action of various drugs that interfere with thyroid hormone biosynthesis.** DIT, diiodotyrosine; MIT, monoiodotyrosine; T_3, triiodothyronine; T_4, thyroxine.

development of the nervous, skeletal, and reproductive systems as well as regulation of metabolism of fats, carbohydrates, proteins, and many vitamins. Table 22-2 outlines the manifestations of hyperthyroidism and hypothyroidism.

Thyroid Drugs

Thyroid hormone therapy can be accomplished with either T_4 or T_3. Synthetic T_4 (**levothyroxine**) is usually the first choice. The long half-life of T_4 (7 days) allows once daily to weekly administration, whereas the shorter half-life of T_3 (24 hours) requires multiple daily doses. Toxicity due to excessive supplementation of TH is expressed as hyperthyroidism (Table 22-2). Older adults, individuals with cardiovascular disease, and those with long-standing hypothyroidism are highly sensitive to the stimulatory effects of T_4 on the heart. Therapists should monitor vital signs carefully and be especially cognizant of patient's perception of palpitations (arrhythmias) and angina during rehabilitation.

Antithyroid Drugs

Thyroid hormone activity can be temporarily reduced with agents that either disrupt TH synthesis (thiomides, iodide salts)

or agents that modify tissue responses to TH (β-blockers). Permanent disruption of TH activity involves destroying the gland with radiation (^{131}I) or surgical removal.

The thiomides, **propylthiouracil** (PTU) and **methimazole**, inhibit TH production by blocking iodination of the tyrosine residues of thyroglobulin and inhibiting coupling of DIT and MIT (Figure 22-3). Taken orally, thioamides are effective in most people with uncomplicated hyperthyroidism. Because synthesis (rather than release) of TH is inhibited, these agents often require 3-4 weeks for full effect. However, high-dose PTU may have faster effect because it inhibits target tissue conversion of T_4 to T_3. The most common ADR is skin rash. Rarely, severe immune reactions (vasculitis, hypoprothrombinemia, agranulocytosis) occur, but these are usually reversible. PTU is preferred in pregnancy because it is less likely than methimazole to cross the placenta and enter breast milk. However, because of the risk of fetal hypothyroidism, both thiomides are used very cautiously in pregnant and nursing women.

Iodide salts inhibit TH release and decrease the size and vascularity of the hyperplastic thyroid gland (Figure 22-3). Because iodide salts inhibit release as well as synthesis of TH, their onset of action occurs relatively rapidly—within 2-7 days. Inhibition is transient because the thyroid gland "escapes" from the iodide block after several weeks of treatment. Iodide

TABLE 22-2 Manifestations of hyperthyroidism and hypothyroidism.

System	Hyperthyroidism	Hypothyroidism
Skin and appendages	Warm, moist skin; sweating; heat intolerance; fine, thin hair; pretibial dermopathy (Graves disease)	Pale, cool, puffy; dry and brittle hair; brittle nails
Eyes, face	Retraction of upper lid with wide stare; periorbital edema; exophthalmos; diplopia (Graves disease)	Drooping of eyelids; periorbital edema, loss of temporal aspects of eyebrows; puffy, nonpitting facies; large tongue
Cardiovascular system	Decreased peripheral vascular resistance; increased heart rate, stroke volume, cardiac output, pulse pressure; high-output heart failure; increased inotropic and chronotropic effects; arrhythmias; angina	Increased peripheral vascular resistance; decreased heart rate, stroke volume, cardiac output, pulse pressure; low-output heart failure; ECG: bradycardia, prolonged PR interval, flat T wave, low voltage; pericardial effusion
Respiratory system	Dyspnea; decreased vital capacity	Pleural effusions; hypoventilation and CO_2 retention
Gastrointestinal system	Increased appetite; increased frequency of bowel movements; hypoproteinemia	Decreased appetite; decreased frequency of bowel movements; ascites
Central nervous system	Nervousness; hyperkinesia; emotional lability	Lethargy; general slowing of mental processes; neuropathies
Musculoskeletal system	Weakness and muscle fatigue; increased deep tendon reflexes; hypercalcemia; osteoporosis	Stiffness and muscle fatigue; decreased deep tendon reflexes; increased alkaline phosphatase, LDH, AST
Renal system	Mild polyuria; increased renal blood flow; increased glomerular filtration rate	Impaired water excretion; decreased renal blood flow; decreased glomerular filtration rate
Hematopoietic system	Increased erythropoiesis; anemia[a]	Decreased erythropoiesis; anemia[a]
Reproductive system	Menstrual irregularities; decreased fertility; increased gonadal steroid metabolism	Menorrhagia; infertility; decreased libido; impotence; oligospermia; decreased gonadal steroid metabolism
Metabolic system	Increased BMR; negative nitrogen balance; hyperglycemia; increased free fatty acids; decreased cholesterol and triglycerides; increased hormone degradation; increased requirements for fat- and water-soluble vitamins; increased drug metabolism	Decreased BMR; slight positive nitrogen balance; delayed degradation of insulin, with increased sensitivity; increased cholesterol and triglycerides; decreased hormone degradation; decreased requirements for fat- and water-soluble vitamins; decreased drug metabolism

AST, aspartate aminotransferase; BMR, basal metabolic rate; ECG, electrocardiogram; LDH, lactate dehydrogenase.
[a]Anemia of hyperthyroidism is usually normochromic and caused by increased red blood cell turnover. Anemia of hypothyroidism may be normochromic, hyperchromic, or hypochromic and may be due to decreased production rate, decreased iron absorption, decreased folic acid absorption, or to autoimmune pernicious anemia.

salts are used to manage a "thyroid storm" (life-threatening sudden acute exacerbation of all the symptoms of hyperthyroidism), and to prepare patients for surgical resection of a hyperactive thyroid. Usual forms are oral solutions such as Lugol solution (iodine and potassium iodide) and saturated solution of potassium iodide.

Radioactive iodine therapy using ^{131}I is the preferred treatment for most people over 21 years of age. Unlike thiomides and iodide salts, an effective dose of ^{131}I can produce a permanent nonsurgical cure for hyperthyroidism. [131]I is administered orally and rapidly taken up and concentrated in the thyroid gland. Six to twelve weeks later, the gland physically shrinks and the patient then typically becomes euthyroid or hypothyroid. When hypothyroidism develops, oral levothyroxine is given to replace TH to normal levels. Advantages of ^{131}I to treat hyperthyroidism include easy administration, effectiveness, lack of endangering other tissues, absence of pain, and low cost. [131]I should not be used in pregnant or nursing women as it crosses the placenta and enters breast milk.

β-blockers (Chapter 6) may be especially useful in controlling tachycardia and other cardiac abnormalities of severe hyperthyroidism. **Propranolol** also inhibits the conversion of T_4 to T_3 (Figure 22-3). Finally, it is helpful for the therapist to appreciate that a number of drugs that are not used in the treatment of thyroid dysfunction may affect TH levels by altering thyroid hormone synthesis, transport, or metabolism (Table 22-3). Sometimes, these changes may produce clinical signs or symptoms.

GONADAL HORMONES AND INHIBITORS

The gonadal hormones include the steroids produced by the ovaries (estrogens and progesterone) and the testes (chiefly testosterone) (Figure 22-4). Many synthetic estrogens and progestins have been produced because of their use as contraceptives. These drugs include receptor agonists, partial agonists, antagonists, and some drugs with mixed effects.

TABLE 22-3 **Effects of select drugs on thyroid function.**

Drug Effect	Drugs
Change in TH Synthesis	
Inhibition of TRH or TSH secretion without induction of hypothyroidism	Dopamine, levodopa, corticosteroids, somatostatin, metformin, heroin
Inhibition of TH synthesis or release with the induction of hypothyroidism (or occasionally hyperthyroidism)	Iodides (including amiodarone), lithium, amino-glutethimide, thioamides, ethionamide, HIV protease inhibitors
Alteration of TH Transport and Serum Total T_3 and T_4 Levels, But Usually No Modification of FT_4^a or TSH	
Increased TBG	Estrogens, tamoxifen, heroin, methadone, mitotane, fluorouracil
Decreased TBG	Androgens, anabolic steroids, glucocorticoids
Displacement of T_3 and T_4 from TBG with transient hyperthyroxinemia	Salicylates, fenclofenac, mefenamic acid, intravenous furosemide, heparin
Alteration of T_3 and T_4 Metabolism With Modified Serum T_3 and T_4 Levels, But Not FT_4 or TSH Levels	
Increased hepatic enzyme activity with enhanced degradation of TH	Phenytoin, carbamazepine, phenobarbital, rifampin, rifabutin, nicardipine, imatinib, sertraline, quetiapine
Inhibition of 5'-deiodinase with decreased T_3, and increased rT_3^b	Iopanoic acid, ipodate, amiodarone, β-blockers, corticosteroids, propylthiouracil, flavonoids
Other Interactions	
Interference with T_4 absorption from the gut	Oral bisphosphonates, cholestyramine, colestipol, aluminum hydroxide, proton pump inhibitors, sucralfate, raloxifene, ferrous sulfate, orlistat, ciprofloxacin, aluminum hydroxide, bran/fiber, soy, coffee
Induction of autoimmune thyroid disease with hypothyroidism or hyperthyroidism	Interferon-∝, interleukin-2, lithium

TBG, thyroxine-binding globulin; TH, thyroid hormone; TRH, thyroxine-releasing hormone; TSH, thyroid-stimulating hormone.
^{a}FT$_4$ is free thyroxine not bound to TBG.
^{b}rT$_3$ is an inactive deiodinated metabolite of T$_4$.

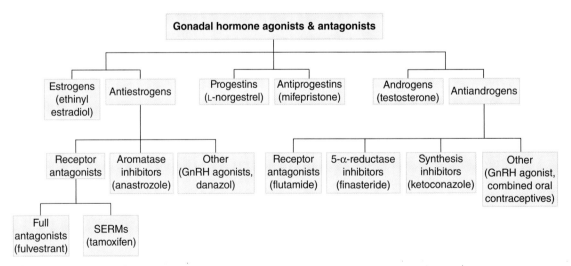

FIGURE 22-4 **Drug classes used for contraception and treatment of gonadal dysfunction.** Gonadal hormones are divided into steroids of the ovary (ie, estrogens and progesterone receptor agonists) and those of the testis (chiefly testosterone). Subsequent divisions include drugs that inhibit synthesis of steroid hormones, partial receptor agonists, receptor antagonists, and those that act as agonists in some tissues and antagonists in other tissues. This last division of mixed agonists is called selective estrogen receptor modulators (SERMs). Prototype drugs are in parentheses.

Selective estrogen receptor modulators (SERMs) are a classic example of drugs with mixed effects. In some tissues, SERMs demonstrate estrogenic effects and in other tissues SERMs have antiestrogenic effects. All synthetic androgens are derived from testosterone and have anabolic activity. A diverse group of antiandrogenic drugs is used in the treatment of prostate cancer, benign prostatic hyperplasia, and hirsutism in women.

The ovaries are the primary source of sex hormones in women during the childbearing years (ie, between puberty and menopause). During each menstrual cycle, in response to FSH and LH from the anterior pituitary, a follicle in the ovary matures, secretes increasing amounts of estrogen, releases an ovum, and finally transforms into a progesterone-secreting corpus luteum. If the ovum is not fertilized and implanted, the corpus luteum degenerates. The endometrium, which proliferated under estrogen stimulation, is shed as part of the menstrual flow, and the cycle repeats. Both estrogen and progesterone enter target cells and bind to cytosolic receptors. The receptor-hormone complex translocates into the nucleus, where it modulates gene expression.

Estrogens

Estrogen hormones (**estradiol**, **estriol**, and **estrone**) are essential for normal female sexual development. Estrogens are responsible for growth of the vagina, uterus, and uterine tubes during childhood, appearance of secondary sexual characteristics, and the growth spurt associated with puberty. Estrogen also has multiple metabolic effects. The hormone modifies serum protein levels, reduces bone resorption, enhances blood coagulability, increases plasma triglyceride and high-density lipoprotein (HDL) cholesterol, and reduces low-density lipoprotein (LDL) cholesterol. Figure 22-5 illustrates the physiologic regulation of ovarian hormone secretion and some sites of action of antiestrogens.

Pharmaceutical applications for estrogens include treatment of hypogonadism in young females, hormone replacement therapy (HRT), and as a component of contraceptives (Table 22-4). The major ovarian estrogen in nonpregnant women is estradiol. Although estradiol has low oral bioavailability, its bioavailability is increased in a micronized form. **Ethinyl estradiol** and **mestranol** are synthetic estrogens with high bioavailability that are used in hormonal contraceptives. Estradiol can also be administered via transdermal patch or vaginal cream. Long-acting esters of estradiol that are converted in the body to estradiol can be administered by intramuscular injection. Mixtures of conjugated estrogens from biologic sources (eg, **Premarin**) are used orally for HRT. HRT is used to treat estrogen deficiency resulting from premature ovarian failure, menopause, or surgical removal of the ovaries. HRT ameliorates hot flashes and atrophic changes in the urogenital tract. Estrogen is also effective in preventing bone loss and osteoporosis.

There are both short-term and long-term ADRs associated with estrogen. Dose-dependent toxicities include nausea, breast tenderness, and increased risk of migraine headache,

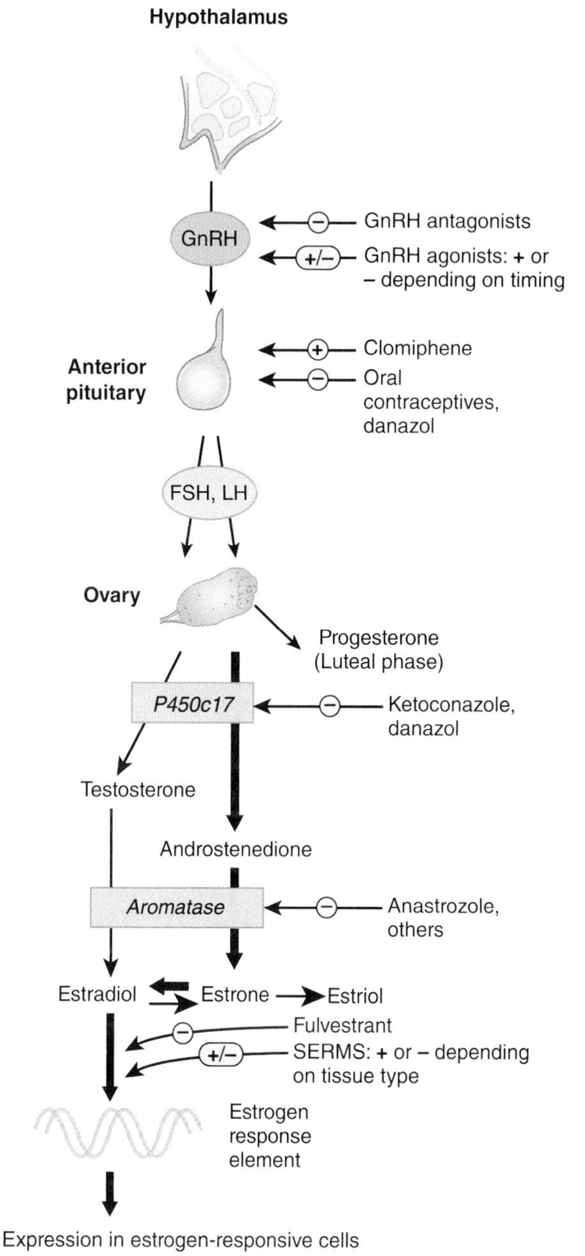

FIGURE 22-5 Control of ovarian hormone secretion, action of ovarian hormones, and select sites of action of antiestrogens. In the follicular phase, ovaries produce primarily estrogens; in the luteal phase, ovaries produce estrogens and progesterone. GnRH, gonadotropin-releasing hormone; SERMs, selective estrogen receptor modulators.

thromboembolic events (eg, deep vein thrombosis), gallbladder disease, hypertriglyceridemia, and hypertension. In hypogonadal girls, the dose of estrogen must be adjusted carefully to prevent premature closure of the epiphyses of the long bones, resulting in short stature. The relationship between long-term estrogen therapy and cancer continues to be actively investigated. When used alone for HRT in women with a uterus, estrogen increases the risk of endometrial cancer. However,

TABLE 22-4 **Common applications for gonadal hormones and hormone antagonists.**

Clinical Application	Drugs
Hypogonadism in girls, women	Conjugated estrogens ethinyl estradiol, estradiol esters
Hormone replacement therapy (HRT)	Estrogen component: conjugated estrogens, estradiol, estrone, estriol
	Progestin component: progesterone, medroxyprogesterone acetate
Oral hormonal contraceptive	Combined: ethinyl estradiol or mestranol plus a progestin
	Progestin only: norethindrone or norgestrel
Parenteral contraceptive	Medroxyprogesterone as a depot IM injection
	Ethinyl estradiol and noregestromin as a weekly patch
	Ethinyl estradiol and etonogestrel as a monthly vaginal ring
	Etonogestrel as a subcutaneous implant
	L-Norgestrel as an intrauterine device (IUD)
Postcoital (emergency) contraceptive	L-Norgestrel, combined oral contraceptives
Intractable dysmenorrhea or uterine bleeding	Conjugated estrogens, ethinyl estradiol, oral contraceptive, GnRH agonist, depot injection of medroxyprogesterone acetate
Infertility	Clomiphene; hMG and hCG; GnRH analogs; progesterone; bromocriptine
Abortifacient	Mifepristone (RU 486) and misoprostol
Endometriosis	Oral contraceptive, depot injection of medroxyprogesterone acetate, GnRH agonist, danazol
Breast cancer	Tamoxifen, aromatase inhibitors (eg, anastrozole)
Osteoporosis in postmenopausal women	Conjugated estrogens, estradiol, raloxifene
Hypogonadism in boys; men: replacement therapy	Testosterone enanthate or cypionate; methyltestosterone; fluoxymesterone, testosterone (patch)
Anabolic protein synthesis	Oxandrolone, stanozolol
Prostate hyperplasia (benign)	Finasteride
Prostate cancer	GnRH agonist or antagonist, androgen receptor antagonist (eg, flutamide)
Hirsutism	Combined oral contraceptive, spironolactone, flutamide, GnRH agonist

GnRH, gonadotropin-releasing hormone; hCG, human chorionic gonadotropin; hMG, menotropins; IM, intramuscular.

combining estrogen with a progestin can prevent this effect. Estrogen use by postmenopausal women is associated with a small increase in the risk of breast cancer, myocardial infarction, and stroke, which is not ameliorated by concurrent progestin therapy.

Progestins

Progestins are a group of chemically similar steroid hormones. Progesterone is the major progestin in humans. Progesterone induces secretory changes in the endometrium and is required to maintain pregnancy. Other progestins stabilize the endometrium, but do not support pregnancy. Unlike the estrogens, progestins do not significantly affect plasma proteins, though they do affect carbohydrate metabolism and stimulate fat deposition.

A micronized form of progestin is used orally for HRT and progesterone-containing vaginal creams are also available. Synthetic progestins (eg, **medroxyprogesterone**) have improved oral bioavailability. The 19-nortestosterone compounds differ primarily in their degree of androgenic effects. Older drugs such as **L-norgestrel** and **norethindrone** are more androgenic than the newer progestins **norgestimate** and **desogestrel**.

The major uses of progestins are as a component of HRT (see above) and as contraceptives, either alone or in combination with an estrogen. In addition, high doses of progestins are useful in preventing ovulation (and menstruation) for other purposes such as treating dysmenorrhea and endometriosis. Progesterone is also used in assisted reproductive technology programs to promote and maintain pregnancy.

The toxicity of progestins is low. In some individuals, they may increase blood pressure and decrease plasma HDL cholesterol. In premenopausal women, long-term use of high doses is associated with a reversible decrease in bone density and delayed resumption of ovulation after termination of therapy.

Hormonal Contraceptives

Hormonal contraceptives contain either a combination of an estrogen and a progestin or a progestin alone. Hormonal contraceptives are available as oral pills, long-acting injections, transdermal patches, vaginal rings, and intrauterine devices (IUDs) (Table 22-4).

Three different types of oral contraceptives for women are available in the United States. Monophasic preparations are a combination of estrogen-progestin tablets that are taken in constant dosage throughout the menstrual cycle. Biphasic and triphasic preparations are combination preparations in which the progestin or estrogen dosage, or both, changes during the month to more closely mimic hormonal changes in a menstrual cycle. The primary mechanism of action for these combination preparations is inhibition of ovulation due to inhibition of gonadotropin secretion from the anterior pituitary. Additional mechanisms include changes in the cervical mucus glands, uterine tubes, and endometrium that decrease the likelihood of fertilization and implantation. The third type of oral preparation contains only progestin. Progestin-only contraceptives do not always inhibit ovulation. Instead, they act through the other mechanisms listed.

Postcoital contraceptives are also known as "emergency" or "morning after" contraception. If administered within 72 hours after unprotected sexual intercourse, they prevent pregnancy 99% of the time by mechanisms of action that are not well understood. When administered before the LH surge, they inhibit ovulation. They also affect cervical mucus, tubal function, and endometrial lining. Several types of oral preparations are effective: estrogens alone, L-norgestrel (progestin alone), combination pills containing an estrogen and a progestin, and mifepristone (RU 486), a progesterone antagonist. Since nausea and vomiting are common, most preparations are administered with antiemetics. Other ADRs include headache, dizziness, breast tenderness, and abdominal and leg cramps.

Combination hormonal contraceptives have additional clinical uses, including prevention of estrogen deficiency in young women with primary hypogonadism after their growth has been achieved (Table 22-4). Combinations of hormonal contraceptives and progestins alone are used to treat acne, hirsutism, dysmenorrhea, and endometriosis. Users of combination hormonal contraceptives have reduced risks of ovarian cysts, ovarian and endometrial cancer, benign breast disease, and pelvic inflammatory disease as well as a lower incidence of ectopic pregnancy, iron deficiency anemia, and rheumatoid arthritis.

The incidence of dose-dependent toxicity has fallen since low-dose combined oral contraceptives were introduced. The two most notable adverse effects include thromboembolism and the potential for increased risk of developing breast cancer at a younger age (though not an elevated lifetime risk). Increased risk of thromboembolism is due to the action of the estrogenic component on liver synthesis of blood coagulation factors. There is a well-documented increase in the risk of thromboembolic events (myocardial infarction, stroke, deep vein thrombosis, pulmonary embolism) in smokers, older women, women with a personal or family history of such problems, and women with genetic defects that affect the production or function of clotting factors. However, risk of thromboembolism incurred by the use of combined hormonal contraceptives is usually less than that imposed by pregnancy.

Other toxicities of hormonal contraceptives include nausea, breast tenderness, headache, increased skin pigmentation, and depression. The low-dose combined oral and progestin-only contraceptives cause significant breakthrough bleeding, especially during the first few months of therapy. Preparations containing older, more androgenic progestins can cause weight gain, acne, and hirsutism.

Antiestrogens

Antiestrogens include therapeutic agents that have been designed to inhibit the synthesis of estrogen (aromatase inhibitors), antagonize all estrogen receptors (**fulvestrant**), or act as selective estrogen receptor modulators (SERMs) that act as agonists in some tissues and as partial agonists or antagonists in other tissues.

Aromatase inhibitors such as **anastrozole** and **letrozole** are nonsteroidal inhibitors of aromatase, the enzyme required for estrogen synthesis. These drugs are used in the treatment of breast cancer (Chapter 31).

Fulvestrant is a pure estrogen receptor antagonist, meaning that it blocks the effects of endogenous estrogen at estrogen receptors in *all* tissues. It is used in treatment of breast cancer in those who have become resistant to tamoxifen.

The first and one of the most widely prescribed SERMs is **tamoxifen**. Tamoxifen is effective in the treatment of hormone-responsive breast cancer because it acts as an *antagonist* to prevent receptor activation by endogenous estrogens (Figure 22-5). Tamoxifen is also used prophylactically to reduce the incidence of breast cancer in women who are at very high risk. However, tamoxifen acts as an *agonist* at endometrial estrogen receptors, which promotes hyperplasia and increases the risk of endometrial cancer. Tamoxifen frequently causes hot flashes (antagonist effect) and increases risk of venous thrombosis (agonist effect). In bone, tamoxifen has more agonist than antagonist estrogenic actions, thus preventing osteoporosis in women who are taking the drug for breast cancer. **Toremifene**, a SERM structurally related to tamoxifen, has similar properties, indications, and toxicities. **Raloxifene** is a SERM with partial agonist action on bone. It is approved for prevention of osteoporosis in postmenopausal women and the prevention of breast cancer in high-risk women. Like tamoxifen, raloxifene has antagonist effects in breast tissue and reduces the incidence of breast cancer in women who are at very high risk. Unlike tamoxifen, the drug has no estrogenic effects on endometrial tissue. Adverse effects also include hot flashes and increased risk of venous thrombosis. **Clomiphene** selectively blocks estrogen receptors in the anterior pituitary, thus reducing the negative feedback from endogenous estrogen, which results in increased FSH and LH secretion. This SERM-induced increase in gonadotropins stimulates ovulation in anovulatory women who wish to become pregnant. A newer SERM called **bazedoxifene** is approved for treatment of menopausal symptoms and prevention of postmenopausal osteoporosis when used in combination with conjugated estrogens.

Antiprogestins

Mifepristone (RU 486) is an orally active steroid antagonist of progesterone and glucocorticoid receptors. Mifepristone is primarily used to terminate early pregnancies (during the first 7 weeks after conception). It can be given orally as a single dose or over 2-4 days. The combination of mifepristone and a prostaglandin E analog (**misoprostol**) effectively terminates pregnancy in over 95% of women treated in early pregnancy. Adverse effects includes the cramping and bleeding associated with passing the pregnancy, nausea, vomiting, and diarrhea, which are primarily due to misoprostol.

Danazol is a weak partial agonist that binds to progestin, androgen, and glucocorticoid receptors. Danazol also inhibits several cytochrome P450 (CYP) enzymes involved in gonadal steroid synthesis. The drug is sometimes used in the treatment of endometriosis and fibrocystic breast disease. Major adverse effects include weight gain, acne, increased hair growth, hot flashes, and muscle cramps. Its use is contraindicated in pregnancy and breast-feeding.

Androgens

The hypothalamic-pituitary control of the secretion of testosterone and related androgens is presented in Figure 22-6. Testosterone and related androgens are produced in the testes, adrenal glands, and, to a small extent, the ovaries. Testosterone is synthesized from progesterone and dehydroepiandrosterone (DHEA). The latter also has a sulfated form (DHEAS). In the plasma, testosterone is partly bound to a transport protein, sex hormone–binding globulin (SHBG). Testosterone itself is active in some tissues, but the enzyme 5α-reductase converts it to dihydrotestosterone (DHT), which is the active hormone in many tissues. After unbinding from its transport protein, the hormone can enter an androgen-responsive cell and bind to cytosolic receptors (Figure 22-6). The hormone-receptor complex enters the nucleus and modulates the expression of target genes.

Testosterone and its derivatives have androgenic actions (increased male characteristics) and anabolic actions (increased muscle mass and red blood cell production). Testosterone is necessary for normal development of the male fetus and infant and is responsible for major changes in the male at puberty. These changes include growth of the penis, larynx, and skeleton; development of facial, pubic, and axillary hair; darkening of skin; and, enlargement of muscle mass. After puberty, testosterone maintains secondary sex characteristics, fertility, and libido. Testosterone also helps maintain normal bone density. Finally, testosterone (as dihydrotestosterone) acts on hair cells to cause male-pattern baldness.

Because of rapid hepatic metabolism, orally administered testosterone has little effect, but orally active variants are available. Testosterone may also be given by injection of long-acting esters or as a transdermal patch. Many androgens have been synthesized in an effort to increase their anabolic effects (primarily to increase muscle mass) without increasing their androgenic actions. For example, **oxandrolone** and

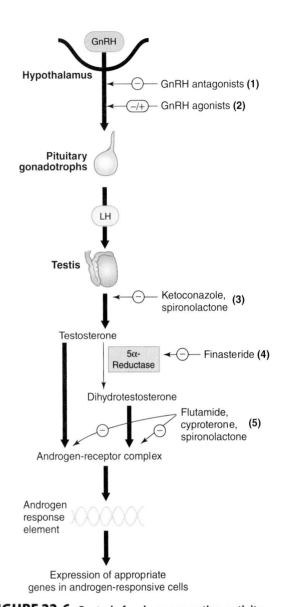

FIGURE 22-6 **Control of androgen secretion, activity of androgens, and some sites of action of antiandrogens:** **(1)** competitive inhibition of gonadotropin-releasing hormone (GnRH) receptors; **(2)** stimulation (+) or inhibition (−) by GnRH agonists; **(3)** inhibition of testosterone synthesis by ketoconazole and possibly spironolactone; **(4)** inhibition of dihydrotestosterone production by finasteride; and **(5)** inhibition of androgen binding at its receptor by flutamide and other drugs.

stanozolol are drugs that have an increased ratio of anabolic: androgenic action in animal testing. However, in humans, all of the so-called anabolic steroids have androgenic effects.

The primary clinical use of androgens is for replacement therapy in hypogonadism (Table 22-4). They have also been used to stimulate red blood cell production in certain anemias and to promote weight gain in patients with wasting syndromes (eg, AIDS-associated wasting). The anabolic effects have been exploited illicitly by athletes in attempts to increase muscle mass and strength and enhance athletic performance. Doses taken for these purposes are often many times higher than those prescribed to treat medical conditions. Many amateur and professional athletic organizations ban the use of androgens in their respective sports. The World Anti-Doping Agency includes *all* anabolic androgenic steroids on the Prohibited List.

Most of the toxicities associated with androgens are predictable based on their physiologic actions. Use of androgens by females results in menstrual irregularity and virilization, which includes hirsutism, enlarged clitoris, and deepening of the voice. In women who are pregnant with a female fetus, exogenous androgens can cause virilization of the fetus' external genitalia. In men, high doses of androgens cause feedback inhibition at the anterior pituitary and conversion of exogenous androgens to estrogens. This results in feminization characterized by gynecomastia, testicular shrinkage, and infertility. High doses also cause behavioral changes including hostility and aggression ("roid rage") (Chapter 21). In both sexes, high doses of anabolic steroids can cause cholestatic jaundice, elevation of liver enzyme levels, possibly hepatocellular carcinoma, increased lipid levels (resulting in atherosclerosis), and sodium retention (resulting in hypertension).

Antiandrogens

Decreasing the effects of androgens is an important mode of therapy for both benign and malignant prostate disease, precocious puberty, hair loss, and hirsutism. Figure 22-6 outlines sites in which drugs inhibit the androgen pathway.

Starting at the top of the hypothalamic-pituitary axis, a reduction in gonadotropin secretion, especially LH secretion, lowers the production of testosterone. As described earlier, this can be effectively accomplished with long-acting depot preparations of leuprolide or similar GnRH agonists. This continuous nonpulsatile administration of GnRH agonists is used in prostatic carcinoma. During the first week of therapy, an androgen receptor antagonist such as flutamide is added to prevent the tumor flare that can result from the surge in testosterone synthesis caused by the agonist, before receptor downregulation. Within several weeks, testosterone production falls to low levels.

Another way to decrease the action of androgens is to inhibit steroid hormone synthesis. All steroid hormones are derivatives of cholesterol. **Ketoconazole**, an antifungal agent (Chapter 29), inhibits CYP enzymes necessary for synthesis of gonadal and adrenal steroids. Ketoconazole has been used to suppress adrenal steroid synthesis in individuals with steroid-responsive metastatic tumors. **Spironolactone**, a drug used principally as a potassium-sparing diuretic (Chapter 7), is also used in the treatment of hirsutism in women. Its antiandrogenic action comes from two distinct actions. First, it inhibits 17α-reductase, an enzyme involved in androgen synthesis. Second, spironolactone competes with DHT for androgen receptors.

As discussed earlier, 5α-reductase converts testosterone to DHT. Some tissues, notably the prostate and hair follicles, depend on DHT rather than testosterone for androgenic stimulation. Drugs such as **finasteride** and **dutasteride** (which has a longer half-life) are 5α-reductase inhibitors used to treat benign prostatic hyperplasia. At lower dose, finasteride is used for the treatment of male pattern baldness. Because 5α-reductase inhibitors do not interfere with the action of testosterone, they are less likely than other antiandrogens to cause impotence, infertility, and loss of libido.

At the target tissues, androgen receptor antagonists can be used to inhibit androgenic action. Flutamide and related drugs are nonsteroidal compounds that act as competitive antagonists at androgen receptors. These drugs are used to decrease the action of endogenous androgens in men with prostate cancer.

Finally, combined hormonal contraceptives can be used in women with hirsutism, which is caused by excessive production of androgenic steroids. The estrogen in the contraceptive causes the liver to increase production of sex hormone–binding globulin, which in turn acts to reduce the concentration of free androgen in the blood that is responsible for promoting the male-pattern hair growth.

REHABILITATION RELEVANCE

Many drugs are available that either mimic or inhibit endogenous hormones. Summarized below are adverse effects of drugs or drug classes mostly likely to affect rehabilitation.

- **Hypertension** is a potential dose-dependent adverse effect associated with estrogens, progestins, and levothyroxine. Levothyroxine and octreotide (somatostatin analog) may induce **heart rate abnormalities** in some individuals. Therapists should be aware that older adults and those with cardiovascular disease are more likely to experience the cardiac stimulatory effects of levothyroxine.

- Estrogens, hormonal contraceptives, and the SERMs tamoxifen and raloxifene are associated with an **increased risk of thromboembolic events**. Patients should be educated about signs/symptoms of deep vein thrombosis (DVT). If a DVT is suspected based on signs/symptoms and modified Wells clinical prediction rule, a definitive diagnostic test (eg, Doppler or D-dimer test) should be requested and therapy held until appropriate anticoagulation therapy has been instituted.

- A **negative impact on plasma lipid profile** may occur with the estrogens and in some individuals taking progestins. While some dyslipidemias may respond positively to exercise alone (eg, decreased plasma HDL cholesterol), a comprehensive diet, exercise, and medication program may be indicated to achieve an ideal plasma lipid profile.

- **Hot flashes** are associated with the SERMs tamoxifen and raloxifene and the antiprogestin danazol. Individuals may have a decreased capacity to consistently thermoregulate during aerobic activities. Since higher levels of physical activity in general may reduce the likelihood of moderate to severe hot flash symptoms in mid-life women, promotion of exercise in a cool, well-ventilated area may allow women to participate.

- In individuals taking GH or androgens as performance-enhancing drugs, therapists should encourage honest discussion regarding the broad constellation of adverse effects associated with taking these hormones in supraphysiological doses. If possible, communication should include the physician.

CASE CONCLUSION

The exogenous thyroid medication the patient recently started has likely resulted in hyperthyroidism. The adverse effects of levothyroxine did not manifest until she was exercising. Hyperthyroidism decreased the patient's exercise tolerance directly through an effect on skeletal muscles (weakness, muscle fatigue) and indirectly through altered cardiac (increased heart rate, arrhythmias) and pulmonary (dyspnea, decreased vital capacity) function. The therapist recommended that the patient discontinue her exercise program until her physician is able to reevaluate her and perform the appropriate thyroid function tests. Because cardiac arrhythmias are common with hyperthyroidism, the therapist immediately informed the physician of the patient's vital signs and her current clinical presentation.

CHAPTER 22 QUESTIONS

1. Growth hormone does *not* play a key role in which of the following physiologic actions?

   a. Regulation of protein, fat, and carbohydrate metabolism
   b. Regulation of normal adult height
   c. Regulation of lean body mass
   d. Regulation of secondary sexual characteristics

2. Which of the following would stimulate gonadotropin (FSH and LH) secretion?

   a. Continuous nonpulsatile administration of gonadotropin-releasing hormone
   b. Pulsatile administration of gonadotropin-releasing hormone
   c. Gonadotropin-releasing hormone antagonists
   d. Levothyroxine

3. Which of the following drugs is *not* associated with an increased risk of thromboembolic events?

   a. Testosterone
   b. Estrogens
   c. Hormonal contraceptives
   d. Tamoxifen

4. Which of the following is true regarding treatment of hypothyroidism?

   a. Synthetic T_4 (levothyroxine) is usually the first choice.
   b. Synthetic T_3 (liothyronine) is usually the first choice.
   c. Thyroid-stimulating hormone (TSH) is usually the first choice.
   d. Thyrotropin-releasing hormone (TRH) is usually the first choice.

5. Which of the following would be anticipated in an individual taking growth hormone in supraphysiological doses as a performance-enhancing drug?

   a. Hypotension
   b. Bradycardia
   c. Testicular shrinkage
   d. Diabetes mellitus

6. Potential treatments for an individual with hyperthyroidism does *not* include which of the following?

   a. Radioactive iodine therapy using ^{131}I
   b. Iodide salts
   c. Radioactive synthetic T_4
   d. Surgical removal of the thyroid gland

7. Which of the following conditions is likely to be treated with recombinant forms of human growth hormone?

   a. Endometriosis
   b. Prostate cancer
   c. Osteoporosis
   d. Acquired immune deficiency syndrome-associated wasting

8. Which of the following is an anticipated manifestation of hypothyroidism?

   a. Emotional lability
   b. Tachycardia
   c. Carbon dioxide retention
   d. Heat intolerance

9. Which of the following is true regarding treatment of endometriosis with a gonadotropin-releasing hormone agonist?

   a. Treatment beyond 6 months can result in decreased bone mineral density.
   b. Hirsutism is a common adverse drug reaction.
   c. Testosterone production increases.
   d. Plasma growth hormone increases.

10. Which of the following conditions is *not* an indication for the used of selective estrogen receptor modulators (SERMs)?

    a. Hormone-responsive breast cancer
    b. Prophylaxis of breast cancer in women at very high risk
    c. Uterine fibroids
    d. Prophylaxis of osteoporosis in postmenopausal women

Corticosteroids and Corticosteroid Antagonists

CASE STUDY

The patient is a 20-year-old cross-country runner in her junior year of college with complaints of right heel pain for the past few months. The team physician diagnosed her with plantar fasciitis. He prescribed meloxicam, a nonsteroidal anti-inflammatory drug (NSAID), to take on an "as needed" basis to decrease pain and inflammation and referred her to physical therapy. The patient has no other significant medical problems. Upon examination, the physical therapist noted that the patient had pain with palpation of the right calcaneal plantar fascia insertion, decreased active and passive talocrural joint dorsiflexion, and decreased passive ankle dorsiflexion with the knee extended (indicating decreased flexibility of the gastrocnemius-soleus complex). Finally, the therapist noted that the patient's running shoes provided little pronation support and were worn beyond their functional life span.

REHABILITATION FOCUS

The cortical region of the adrenal gland produces and releases many corticosteroids into the blood. Corticosteroids comprise two major physiologic and pharmacologic groups: glucocorticoids and mineralocorticoids (Figure 23-1). A common mistake is for clinicians to use the term "corticosteroid" when their intent is to specifically discuss only the *glucocorticoid* subclass of corticosteroids, the steroids that have significant anti-inflammatory and immunosuppressive effects. In this text, the appropriate term "glucocorticoid" will be used, but the reader should be aware that in literature and in verbal communication, the broader term corticosteroid is frequently used instead.

The glucocorticoid class of pharmacologic agents significantly influences the clinical practice of physical therapists for several reasons. First, many patients referred for rehabilitation have previously taken or are currently taking glucocorticoids. Local glucocorticoid injections are commonly used in the treatment of a wide variety of musculoskeletal conditions such as shoulder impingement syndrome, adhesive capsulitis, De Quervain's tenosynovitis, trochanteric bursitis, as well as osteoarthritis of the knee, hand, hip, and spine. While these agents decrease pain and inflammation at the site of tissue injury, repeated injections may weaken connective tissue. Physical therapy interventions are often necessary adjuncts to pharmacotherapy if optimal outcome with minimal recurrence is to be achieved. Second, long-term use of glucocorticoids, especially when administered systemically, often results in adverse effects that may require the physical therapist to modify the plan of care. For example, prolonged systemic glucocorticoid use increases the incidence of type 2 diabetes mellitus, hypertension, muscle wasting, thinning of the skin, poor wound healing, and increased risk of infection. In an attempt to mitigate these adverse drug reactions (ADRs), the therapist may prescribe exercise programs to improve glycemic control, decrease blood pressure, and promote muscle hypertrophy (or at least ameliorate drug-induced muscle wasting). The prudent therapist may decrease the intensity of soft tissue mobilization and avoid taping to decrease the risk of delayed wound healing and skin tears, respectively. All therapists should be aware that aseptic necrosis of the hip is a well-documented toxicity of long-term systemic glucocorticoid use. This condition occurs when blood supply to the head and neck of the femur diminishes, causing tiny breaks in the bone that can eventually result in fractures and bone collapse. Clinical presentation is typically increasing pain with weightbearing, but with minimal loss of range of motion. Suspicion of this condition with confirmation of the patient's history of prolonged systemic glucocorticoid use should prompt urgent medical referral for appropriate imaging. Last, physical therapists often use glucocorticoids as one intervention within a multicomponent plan of care to treat inflammatory connective tissue conditions. Therapists deliver glucocorticoids transcutaneously by iontophoresis or phonophoresis. For drug delivery, iontophoresis uses electromotive charge-charge repulsion, whereas phonophoresis uses the mechanical energy of ultrasound. These modalities increase glucocorticoid transcutaneous flux and can improve clinical outcomes in conditions ranging from plantar fasciitis to temporomandibular disorders. Some therapists may mistakenly assume that when dexamethasone sodium phosphate, the drug most commonly used in iontophoresis, fails to decrease a patient's pain or inflammation that

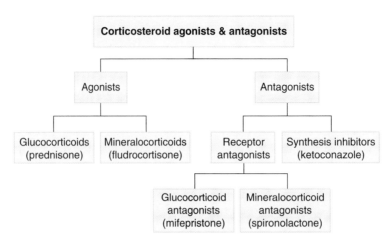

FIGURE 23-1 **Classification of drugs that mimic or block the effects of endogenous corticosteroids.** Prototype drugs are in parentheses.

this drug is not an effective anti-inflammatory agent. In fact, dexamethasone is approximately 30 times more potent with respect to its anti-inflammatory actions than endogenous cortisol; thus, the issue the therapist must consider is whether the drug has effectively penetrated the skin to *reach* the target area. Two critical issues consistently debated in the literature for these drug delivery modalities include the depth of tissue penetration and parameters that optimize transcutaneous drug delivery. The therapist should also note that localized drug delivery does not prevent systemic absorption. Because phonophoretic or iontophoretic administration of glucocorticoids may require a prescription, therapists should consult appropriate state authorities prior to administering these drugs.

BACKGROUND

The endogenous corticosteroids are essential for life. All corticosteroids are synthesized from cholesterol. Glucocorticoids have important effects on intermediary metabolism, catabolism, immune responses, and inflammation. Mineralocorticoids regulate sodium and potassium transport in the collecting tubules of the kidney. A third group of corticosteroids is the adrenal androgens (dehydroepiandrosterone [DHEA] and androstenedione). These constitute the major endogenous precursors of estrogen in females in whom ovarian function is deficient or absent (eg, postmenopausal) and in preadolescent males. Drugs that modulate the physiologic effects of endogenous corticosteroids either mimic the corticosteroids or inhibit corticosteroid synthesis or receptor interactions.

Like other hormones under the control of the hypothalamic and pituitary endocrine system, glucocorticoids provide feedback inhibition of their own production by acting in the hypothalamus and pituitary. Glucocorticoids inhibit the production of corticotropin-releasing factor (CRF) within the hypothalamus and adrenocorticotropic hormone (ACTH) within the pituitary. CRF controls the release of ACTH, which in turn regulates corticosteroid production within the adrenal

cortex. A key action of taking an exogenous glucocorticoid is activation of this feedback inhibition system. As a result, endogenous adrenal steroid production is suppressed. After prolonged systemic treatment, it takes weeks to months (depending on the potency and duration of the exogenous glucocorticoid) for the patient's own adrenal gland to make and release sufficient levels of cortisol. A large number of synthetic glucocorticoids are available. They can be delivered by almost any route, including oral, inhalation, injection, and topical.

GLUCOCORTICOIDS

Mechanism of Action

In the blood, lipophilic steroid hormones bind to carrier proteins. At the target cell, the steroid hormone unbinds from the carrier molecule, enters the cell, and binds to an intracellular receptor. The hormone-receptor complex translocates to the nucleus where it alters gene expression by binding to glucocorticoid response elements (GREs) (Figure 23-2). Tissue-specific responses to steroids are made possible by the presence of different protein regulators in each tissue that control the interaction between the hormone-receptor complex, other transcription factors, and particular response elements.

Organ and Tissue Effects

Glucocorticoids have such widespread and diverse effects because almost every cell in the body expresses glucocorticoid receptors. Glucocorticoids are important regulators of intermediary metabolism of carbohydrates, lipids, and proteins. They cause a general catabolic effect. Glucocorticoids increase breakdown of fat and protein and decrease the uptake of glucose by muscle and adipose tissue. Glucocorticoids also stimulate gluconeogenesis. As a result, blood glucose level rises, and insulin secretion is stimulated. The net result of

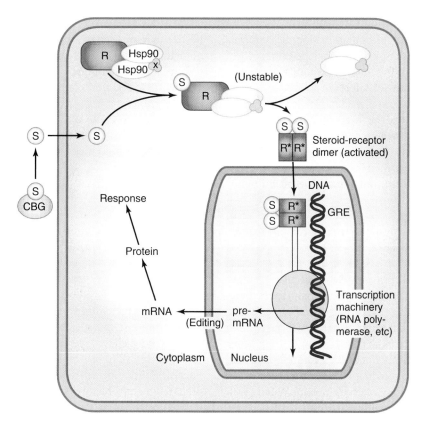

FIGURE 23-2 Mechanism of glucocorticoid action. This figure models the interaction of a steroid (S), with its receptor (R) and the subsequent events in a target cell. The steroid is present in the blood—bound to the corticosteroid-binding globulin (CBG)—but enters the cell as the free form (S). The intracellular receptor (R) is bound to stabilizing proteins, including heat shock protein 90 (Hsp90) and several others. When the complex binds a molecule of steroid, the Hsp90 and associated molecules are released. The steroid-receptor complex enters the nucleus as a dimer, binds to the glucocorticoid response element (GRE) of the DNA, and regulates gene transcription. The resulting mRNA is edited and exported to the cytoplasm for the production of the protein that produces the final hormone response.

glucocorticoids' actions is increased plasma concentration of free fatty acids, amino acids, and glucose. Cortisol, the endogenous glucocorticoid released from the adrenal gland, is often called the body's "stress hormone" because of its ability to increase fuel in the blood in times of fasting or other physiological or psychological stressors.

Chronic systemic use of high doses of glucocorticoids results in a characteristic "cushingoid" appearance, named after the hypercortisolism associated with either excessive pituitary production of ACTH (Cushing's disease) or with excessive adrenal production of cortisol (Cushing's syndrome). Both lipolysis and lipogenesis are stimulated, but there is a net increase of fat deposition in certain areas, particularly the face, shoulders, and back. The cushingoid appearance includes a "moon face" and "buffalo hump" on the posterior base of the neck. Because the drugs stimulate muscle protein breakdown and amino acid release, chronic glucocorticoid use results in skeletal muscle wasting. In addition, lymphoid and connective tissue, fat, and skin undergo atrophy under the influence of high concentrations of these steroids. Catabolic effects on bone can lead to osteoporosis, with the highest rate of bone loss occurring within the first 3-6 months of glucocorticoid treatment, and a slower decline continuing with persistent use.

Vertebral fractures are most common because glucocorticoids have greater effects on trabecular bone than on cortical bone. In children, glucocorticoids inhibit growth.

Glucocorticoids have very important anti-inflammatory and immunosuppressive effects (Chapters 32 and 34), which make these drugs extremely useful therapeutically, but chronic use is also responsible for many serious adverse effects. Regardless of the inciting cause, inflammation involves the extravasation of leukocytes from the blood into the affected tissue. Glucocorticoids dramatically alter the distribution and function of leukocytes—increasing the number of neutrophils and decreasing the number of lymphocytes, eosinophils, basophils, and monocytes in circulation—while inhibiting the migration of *all* white blood cells from the blood to the affected tissue. These drugs also inhibit the ability of macrophages and other antigen-presenting cells to respond to antigens. Fundamental mechanisms underlying these anti-inflammatory effects include decreases in the production of cytokines that participate in inflammatory reactions (eg, interleukin-1, tumor necrosis factor-α) as well as decreases in eicosanoid metabolism. In the latter process, glucocorticoids inhibit the enzyme responsible for the synthesis of arachidonic acid, resulting in decreased expression of prostaglandins and leukotrienes, the key products that induce and perpetuate the diverse effects involved in acute inflammation. The immunosuppressive effects of glucocorticoids include inhibition of mechanisms involved in cell-mediated immunity, especially those dependent on lymphocytes. Glucocorticoids are actively lymphotoxic and, for this reason, are important in the treatment of hematologic cancers. The drugs do not interfere with the development of normal acquired immunity, but can delay rejection reactions in patients with organ transplants.

Endogenous cortisol has many other effects besides those on macronutrient metabolism, inflammation, and immunosuppression. Cortisol has permissive effects on actions of other hormones. For example, if cortisol is low or absent in the circulation, the expected vasoconstriction response of vascular smooth muscle to catecholamines like epinephrine and norepinephrine will not be as robust. In contrast, high levels of circulating glucocorticoids increase the vascular sensitivity to catecholamines, which is one reason that hypertension is a characteristic of Cushing's syndrome. Another reason for hypertension in Cushing's syndrome is that cortisol is required for normal renal excretion of water loads. Thus, in conditions of excess cortisol or exogenous glucocorticoids, there is a salt-retaining (and thus, water-retaining) effect. Glucocorticoids also have effects on the central nervous system. When given in large doses, especially for long periods of time, these drugs can cause profound behavioral changes. Large doses of glucocorticoids also stimulate gastric acid secretion and decrease resistance to ulcer formation.

Clinical Uses

Glucocorticoids play an important role in the treatment of both adrenal and nonadrenal disorders. Examples of common therapeutic uses are presented in Table 23-1. Glucocorticoids are essential to preserve life in patients with chronic adrenal cortical insufficiency (Addison's disease); high doses are necessary in acute adrenal insufficiency (addisonian crisis), which can be precipitated in individuals with Addison's disease by infection, surgery, or trauma. Glucocorticoids are also used in certain types of congenital adrenal hyperplasia, in which synthesis of abnormal forms of cortisol are stimulated by ACTH. In these conditions, administration of a potent synthetic glucocorticoid suppresses ACTH secretion sufficiently to reduce synthesis of the abnormal steroids.

Glucocorticoid therapy is used far more frequently in *nonadrenal* disorders. These drugs play an important role in the treatment of conditions that physical therapists encounter frequently in their practice: inflammatory conditions (eg, arthritis, bursitis, cerebral edema, asthma), autoimmune disorders (eg, systemic lupus erythematosus, rheumatoid arthritis), and the prevention and treatment of organ transplant rejection. Other applications include the treatment of hematopoietic cancers, chemotherapy-induced vomiting, hypercalcemia, and high-altitude sickness. **Betamethasone,** a synthetic glucocorticoid with a low degree of protein binding, is given to women in premature labor to hasten maturation of the fetal lungs. Glucocorticoids are typically not curative. Rather, they are used to suppress the inflammatory and immunological processes that cause many of the clinical manifestations of many conditions. The degree of benefit conferred by glucocorticoids differs considerably in various disorders, and long-term therapy with these drugs is undertaken with great consideration because of their toxicity. They are used only when the seriousness of the disorder warrants their use and when less hazardous measures have been exhausted.

Important Glucocorticoids

The major endogenous glucocorticoid is cortisol and its synthetic equivalent is called **hydrocortisone**. Endogenous cortisol secretion is regulated by ACTH and varies with the circadian rhythm. The peak plasma cortisol level occurs in the morning and the trough occurs about midnight. In the plasma, cortisol is 95% bound to corticosteroid-binding globulin. Exogenously administered cortisol is well absorbed from the gastrointestinal tract and is cleared by the liver. Compared with its synthetic congeners, cortisol has a short duration of action (half-life of ~60-90 minutes). Although it diffuses poorly across normal intact skin, topical hydrocortisone preparations are readily absorbed across inflamed skin and mucous membranes. Cortisol also has a small, but significant, salt-retaining mineralocorticoid effect.

The mechanism of action of synthetic glucocorticoids is identical to that of endogenous cortisol. However, these drugs have been chemically modified to have longer half-lives and durations of action, reduced salt-retaining effects, and better penetration of lipid barriers for topical activity. A large number of glucocorticoid preparations are available for use (Table 23-2). Special glucocorticoids have been developed for use in asthma and other conditions in which activity on mucous membranes or skin is required, but systemic effects need to be avoided. For example, **beclomethasone** and **budesonide** (drugs for chronic obstructive pulmonary disease or asthma) readily penetrate airway mucosa, but have very short half-lives after they enter the blood, so that systemic effects and toxicity are greatly reduced.

Adverse Effects

Nearly 1% of the population in the United States is receiving prolonged glucocorticoid therapy. Thus, physical therapists must be aware of their adverse effects, which may require modification of interventions and/or medical referral. The major adverse effects are those resulting from the hormonal actions that manifest as iatrogenic Cushing's syndrome and have been described earlier. Drugs such as **cortisone** and hydrocortisone have some mineralocorticoid effects that promote chronic salt and water retention, which can lead to hypertension. In recognition of the profound immunosuppressive effects of glucocorticoids, therapists need to vigilantly adhere to standard precautions and be aware of the potential for hidden infections that do not present with expected signs and symptoms

TABLE 23-1 Some therapeutic indications for the use of glucocorticoids in nonadrenal disorders.

Disorder	Examples
Allergic reactions	Angioneurotic edema, asthma, bee stings, contact dermatitis, drug reactions, allergic rhinitis, serum sickness, urticaria
Collagen-vascular disorders	Giant cell arteritis, systemic lupus erythematosus, mixed connective tissue syndromes, polymyositis, polymyalgia rheumatica, rheumatoid arthritis, temporal arteritis
Eye diseases	Acute uveitis, allergic conjunctivitis, choroiditis, optic neuritis
Gastrointestinal diseases	Inflammatory bowel disease, nontropical sprue, subacute hepatic necrosis
Hematologic disorders	Acquired hemolytic anemia, acute allergic purpura, leukemia, lymphoma, autoimmune hemolytic anemia, idiopathic thrombocytopenic purpura, multiple myeloma
Systemic inflammation	Acute respiratory distress syndrome (sustained therapy with moderate dosage accelerates recovery and decreases mortality)
Infections	Acute respiratory distress syndrome, sepsis
Inflammatory conditions of bones and joints	Arthritis, bursitis, tenosynovitis
Nausea and vomiting	Large dose of dexamethasone reduces emetic effects of chemotherapy and general anesthesia
Neurologic disorders	Cerebral edema (large doses of dexamethasone are given to patients following brain surgery to minimize cerebral edema in postoperative period), multiple sclerosis
Organ transplants	Prevention and treatment of rejection (immunosuppression)
Pulmonary diseases	Aspiration pneumonia, bronchial asthma, prevention of infant respiratory distress syndrome, sarcoidosis
Renal disorders	Nephrotic syndrome, glomerulonephritis
Skin diseases	Atopic dermatitis, dermatoses, lichen simplex chronicus (localized neurodermatitis), mycosis fungoides, pemphigus, seborrheic dermatitis, xerosis
Thyroid diseases	Malignant exophthalmos, subacute thyroiditis
Miscellaneous	Hypercalcemia, mountain sickness

of inflammation. When systemic glucocorticoids are used for short durations (< 2 weeks), serious adverse effects are not common. However, behavioral changes such as insomnia, euphoria ("steroid high"), depression, and occasionally acute psychosis often occur earlier. Acute peptic ulcers may also occur, even after short duration treatment.

An important consequence of chronic glucocorticoid therapy is adrenal suppression secondary to inhibition of ACTH

TABLE 23-2 Properties of representative corticosteroids.

Agent	Duration of Action (hr)	Anti-Inflammatory Activity[a]	Salt-Retaining Activity[a]	Topical Activity
Primarily Glucocorticoid				
Cortisol (hydrocortisone)	8-12	1	1	0
Prednisone	12-24	4	0.3	(+)
Triamcinolone	15-24	5	0	+++
Dexamethasone	24-36	30	0	+++++
Primarily Mineralocorticoid				
Aldosterone	1-2	0.3	3000	0
Fludrocortisone	8-12	10	125-250	0

[a]Potency relative to cortisol.

secretion by the pituitary. The inability of the adrenal glands to produce and secrete adequate cortisol can occur when glucocorticoids are systemically administered for more than 2 weeks. Abrupt discontinuation of glucocorticoid therapy can result in a potentially life-threatening addisonian crisis. To avoid adrenal insufficiency in patients who have had long-term therapy, additional "stress doses" may need to be given during serious illness or before major surgery. It may take many months for endogenous cortisol levels to return to normal. Therefore, individuals who are being withdrawn from glucocorticoids after protracted use should have their doses tapered slowly over the course of several months to allow adequate recovery of adrenal function. Occasionally, some patients may remain hypoadrenal.

Methods for minimizing glucocorticoid toxicity include alternate-day therapy to reduce pituitary suppression, dose tapering soon after achieving a therapeutic response, and local administration (eg, aerosols for asthma, injections for soft tissue and joint inflammation). Injectable glucocorticoid agents have different potency and solubility, and solubility is inversely correlated with the duration of action. **Triamcinolone** and **methylprednisolone** are two agents commonly injected into soft tissue and synovial joints to treat the decreased mobility and pain in arthritis, bursitis, trigger finger, De Quervain's tenosynovitis, and carpal tunnel syndrome. There is strong evidence that glucocorticoid injections worsen long-term outcomes for individuals with lateral epicondylalgia. In addition, glucocorticoids are usually not injected into tendons because these structures are particularly prone to injury post-injection and other interventions (eg, eccentric training) are more effective. For these reasons, physicians avoid glucocorticoid injections for Achilles and patellar tendinopathies.

Glucocorticoid injections are typically adjuvant therapy for appropriate musculoskeletal conditions that are given with or after initiation of physical therapy. Therapeutic responses to injections are variable. If a therapeutic effect is achieved, a maximum of four injections per year is recommended due to concern that repeated use may accelerate normal aging-related articular cartilage atrophy or may weaken tendons or ligaments. Because of the possibility of local tissue tears due to temporarily high concentrations of glucocorticoids, strenuous physical activity of the injected region should be avoided for approximately 2 weeks following injection. In addition, a minimum of 4-6 weeks should pass between glucocorticoid injections.

Extra-articular glucocorticoid injections seem to be relatively safe. A low incidence of adverse reactions has been reported that include skin depigmentation and atrophy, cellulitis, and plantar fat atrophy. Systemic effects are possible; the most commonly reported is hyperglycemia in individuals who have diabetes.

MINERALOCORTICOIDS

The major endogenous mineralocorticoid in humans is aldosterone, which has previously been discussed in connection with control of its secretion by angiotensin II and with

hypertension (Chapters 4 and 7). Secretion of aldosterone is regulated by both ACTH and the renin-angiotensin system and is important in the regulation of blood volume and blood pressure (Figure 4-5). Aldosterone has a short half-life and little glucocorticoid activity (Table 23-2). The mechanism of aldosterone action is similar to that of glucocorticoids. The mineralocorticoid receptor shares similar homology with the glucocorticoid receptor. Other mineralocorticoids include **deoxycorticosterone** (the naturally occurring precursor of aldosterone) and a synthetic analog, **fludrocortisone**. Fludrocortisone is the most widely used mineralocorticoid and it also has significant glucocorticoid activity (Table 23-2). Because of its long duration of action, fludrocortisone is used for replacement therapy after surgical removal of the adrenal gland and for chronic, stable Addison's disease.

CORTICOSTEROID ANTAGONISTS

To antagonize the effects of endogenous corticosteroids, either corticosteroid receptor antagonists or inhibitors of corticosteroid synthesis are used. The mineralocorticoid receptor antagonists, **spironolactone** and **eplerenone**, were discussed in connection with diuretics (Chapter 7) and heart failure (Chapter 9). **Mifepristone** (RU 486) is an antagonist of glucocorticoid and progesterone receptors. Its use to terminate early pregnancies was discussed in Chapter 22. Mifepristone has also been used in the treatment of Cushing's syndrome due to ectopic ACTH production or adrenal carcinoma, but is only recommended when other therapeutic interventions have failed.

Ketoconazole is an antifungal drug that is used (at higher doses than necessary for treating fungal infections) to nonselectively inhibit the synthesis of adrenal corticosteroids and gonadal steroids (Figures 22-5 and 22-6). It has been used in several conditions in which reduced steroid levels are desirable: adrenal carcinoma, hirsutism, breast cancer, and prostate cancer. **Aminoglutethimide** is a potent inhibitor of adrenal steroids. This drug blocks the conversion of cholesterol to pregnenolone, an early step in the steroid biosynthesis pathway. Thus, aminoglutethimide inhibits the production of cortisol, aldosterone, and the adrenal androgens. Aminoglutethimide may be used in conjunction with other drugs to decrease steroid secretion in individuals with adrenocortical cancer, but its use is limited by its broad actions.

REHABILITATION RELEVANCE

Systemic glucocorticoids, especially when taken over long periods of time, have *predictable adverse effects* based on their hormonal actions. The rate of development of iatrogenic Cushing's syndrome depends on dosage and duration of glucocorticoid use, as well as the genetic background of the individual.

- **Type 2 diabetes mellitus** is typically treated with diet and insulin. Therapists should incorporate an exercise program to improve glycemic control. Exacerbation of exercise-induced hyperglycemia should be monitored with capillary blood glucose checks.

- **Muscle wasting** due to excess glucocorticoids predominantly affects fast-twitch glycolytic (type IIb) fibers. Weakness and myopathy are especially notable in proximal muscles, with pelvic girdle muscles more severely affected than the arms. Adequate protein intake is helpful in preventing acceleration of muscle loss. Resistance exercise can help mitigate muscle atrophy.
- **Hypertension** increases the risk for cardiovascular dysfunction such as angina pectoris or dysrhythmias. Therapists need to monitor blood pressure and heart rate in patients before and after therapy interventions.
- **Behavioral changes** are common, even after only a few days of treatment. Emotional lability, even within a single therapy session, is not uncommon. Therapists should educate patients that these changes are a predictable ADR and not to place too much emphasis on analysis of these emotions.

- **Immunosuppression** increases the patient's risk of infection. Patients, families, and caregivers should be educated about the importance of handwashing and maintaining a clean patient environment to decrease the risk of infection. Physical therapists should be more aware of the likelihood of an occult infection due to the suppression of cardinal signs and symptoms of inflammation.
- **Gastrointestinal distress** can present as nausea, vomiting, or abdominal discomfort. Because of the increased risk of peptic ulcers, therapists should inform the medical team of signs and symptoms to determine if further work-up is indicated.
- **Edema** varies, depending on the particular glucocorticoid agent used. Because drugs such as cortisone and hydrocortisone have glucocorticoid and mineralocorticoid activity, these drugs will cause more water retention than agents such as methylprednisone and prednisone, which have less water-retaining properties. If edema is negatively affecting functional mobility and rehabilitation goals, therapists should alert the medical team.

CASE CONCLUSION

Multiple factors contribute to plantar fasciitis, which is a common cause of heel pain in both athletes and nonathletes. For the current patient, contributing causes were likely limited ankle dorsiflexion range of motion and worn-out running shoes that were unable to protect against excessive pronation that increases stress on the plantar fascia. The plan of care for plantar fasciitis typically includes some combination of the following interventions: oral NSAIDs, glucocorticoid injections into the fascia, iontophoresis of a glucocorticoid directed into the fascia, stretching of the gastrocnemius-soleus complex and the plantar fascia itself, taping, orthotics aimed at supporting the longitudinal arch, and night splints. The physical therapist instructed the patient

how to effectively stretch the plantar fascia and gastrocnemius-soleus muscle complex and advised her to consider different running shoes or to replace her current shoes more frequently to help prevent recurrent bouts of plantar fasciitis. Over 2-3 weeks (across 6 treatment sessions), the therapist iontophoresed a solution of 0.4% dexamethasone sodium phosphate into the plantar region. Iontophoresis of dexamethasone sodium phosphate provides short-term pain relief and functional improvement for individuals with plantar fasciitis. For those with symptoms that do not improve with conservative rehabilitation, cortisone injections into the plantar fascia, extracorporeal shockwave therapy, or - as a last resort - surgical procedures may be utilized.

CHAPTER 23 QUESTIONS

1. Which of the following is *not* an adverse effect of prolonged systemic glucocorticoid use?

   a. Vertebral fractures
   b. Hypoglycemia
   c. Proximal muscle wasting
   d. Immunosuppression

2. Which mechanism is partly responsible for the anti-inflammatory actions of glucocorticoids?

   a. Increased production of arachidonic acid
   b. Increased production of interleukin-1
   c. Increased release of lymphocytes in circulation
   d. Inhibition of white blood cell migration from circulation to affected tissue

3. Individuals with chronic adrenal cortical insufficiency (Addison's disease) must receive exogenous glucocorticoids to survive.

   a. True
   b. False

4. Which of the following is *not* true regarding adrenal suppression that occurs as a result of chronic systemic glucocorticoid use?

   a. Exogenous glucocorticoids must be discontinued when patients have a serious illness.
   b. Adrenal suppression can occur when exogenous glucocorticoids are given for less than a month.
   c. Higher doses of exogenous glucocorticoids are given when patients have a major surgery.
   d. Individuals who have taken glucocorticoids for a long time have their doses tapered gradually to allow recovery of adrenal function.

5. Which of the following adverse drug reactions might be expected even after short-duration systemic glucocorticoid use?

   a. Moon face
   b. Behavioral changes
   c. Buffalo hump
   d. Muscle wasting

6. Which strategy is *not* used to decrease the toxicity of glucocorticoids?

   a. Alternate-day therapy
   b. Dose tapering soon after therapeutic response
   c. High oral doses for long durations
   d. Local administration

7. Which of the following conditions is likely to worsen with glucocorticoid injections?

   a. Bursitis
   b. Arthritis
   c. Tenosynovitis
   d. Lateral epicondylalgia

8. What is the recommended maximum number of glucocorticoid injections into the same soft tissue or joint per year?

   a. 1
   b. 2
   c. 4
   d. 8

9. Which of the following is true regarding glucocorticoid-induced muscle wasting?

   a. It affects primarily fast-twitch type IIb muscle fibers.
   b. It affects primarily large aerobically adapted muscles.
   c. It affects primarily distal lower extremity muscles.
   d. It affects primarily distal upper extremity muscles.

10. Which of the following drugs is *not* a corticosteroid antagonist?

    a. Mifepristone
    b. Ketoconazole
    c. Hydrocortisone
    d. Aminoglutethimide

Pancreatic Hormones and Antidiabetic Drugs

S.L. is a 50-year-old woman with a body mass index of 30 kg/m² and a 4-year history of type 2 diabetes. Her only medication is metformin, which she takes twice per day. She is a lawyer with a sedentary lifestyle. She admits that she also struggles to adequately monitor her diet. Her recent fingerstick blood glucose levels have ranged from 95 to 280 mg/dL, with the higher values taken after meals. At her recent medical checkup, her A1C was 8.7%, elevated from her previous measurement at 7.5%. Because current metformin monotherapy has failed to control her hyperglycemia, the physician discussed the risks of chronic hyperglycemia as well as options for achieving glycemic control. Following this discussion, S.L. expressed a renewed interest in making a stronger attempt at lifestyle management. The physician encouraged this new commitment. She recommended an outpatient rehabilitation clinic for development of an appropriate exercise program as well as consultation with a dietitican for dietary control. She also prescribed another antidiabetic agent, repaglinide, to decrease postprandial blood glucose elevations. For the past month, S.L. has been participating in an aerobic and resistance exercise program 5 times per week, as initially prescribed by a physical therapist. Today, she arrived at the clinic for a reevaluation and advancement of her exercise program. After assessment of baseline vital signs, the physical therapist started S.L. on the treadmill for an aerobic warm-up. Within 10 minutes, S.L. became diaphoretic and shaky. The therapist assisted her off the treadmill and into a chair. S.L. performed a fingerstick blood glucose reading, which was 53 mg/dL. The therapist brought her some fruit juice and hard candy. Within 30 minutes, S.L. felt well and a second fingerstick blood glucose reading was 92 mg/dL.

REHABILITATION FOCUS

Across the world, 8.5% of adults have diabetes mellitus. In the United States, more than 30 million people have diabetes and approximately 84 million adults have prediabetes. Thus, over one-third of Americans are directly affected by this chronic disease or are on its path. Because the risk of developing type 2 diabetes increases with age, obesity, and lack of physical activity, its prevalence is expected to grow.

Physical therapists commonly treat individuals burdened by diabetic complications such as heart disease, end-stage renal disease, amputation, and blindness. Lifestyle management—diabetes self-management education, medical nutrition therapy, physical activity, smoking cessation counseling, and psychosocial care—is a fundamental cornerstone of diabetes prevention and diabetes care. The importance of *regular* exercise in glycemic control has been increasingly appreciated as the molecular mechanisms of glucose disposal have been elucidated. Muscle contractions move glucose transporters to the surface of muscle fibers, increasing glucose disposal within trained muscle fibers. In a simple analogy, trained muscles can be viewed like sponges that "soak up" glucose from the blood. If larger muscle groups are exercised, larger "sponges" are available to "soak up" excess blood glucose. Exercise not only improves blood glucose control, but also reduces cardiovascular risk factors, contributes to weight loss, and improves well-being. Clinical trials have provided strong evidence for the ability of aerobic and resistance exercise to decrease hemoglobin A1C (a long-term measure of glycemic control) in adults with type 2 diabetes.

Lifestyle management forms the foundation for both type 1 and type 2 diabetic care. For most individuals with type 2 diabetes, antidiabetic medications are required to control chronic hyperglycemia and some may additionally require insulin. For those with type 1 diabetes, insulin is required to control chronic hyperglycemia. Figure 24-1 shows the drug classes used in the treatment of diabetes.

BACKGROUND

The islets of Langerhans in the pancreas contain at least five hormone-producing types of endocrine cells (Table 24-1). These include glucagon-producing alpha cells, insulin- and amylin-producing beta cells, somatostatin-producing delta cells, ghrelin-producing epsilon cells, and pancreatic polypeptide-producing F cells. The most common disease related to pancreatic function is diabetes mellitus. Diabetes mellitus is

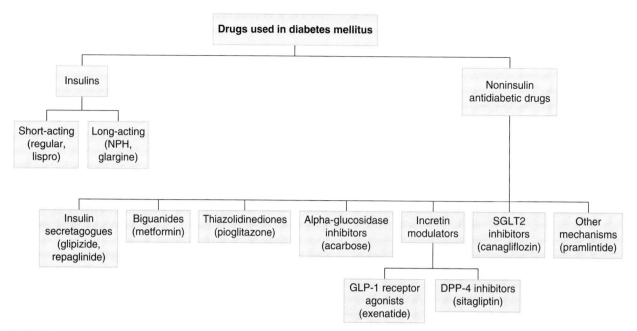

FIGURE 24-1 **Drug classes used in the treatment of diabetes mellitus may be initially divided into insulin and noninsulin antidiabetic drugs.** The noninsulin antidiabetic agents are subsequently divided into seven classes based on mechanism of action. Prototype or example drugs are in parentheses.

defined as elevated blood glucose due to a deficiency of insulin secretion by beta cells, with or without concurrent impairment of insulin action (ie, insulin resistance).

Insulin is a small protein hormone synthesized from a larger prohormone called proinsulin. Proinsulin is arranged in two chains (A and B) that are connected to each other by a connecting peptide (C-peptide). Within the Golgi apparatus of beta cells, proinsulin is cleaved into two peptide chains that are cross-linked by disulfide bridges and the 31-amino acid C-peptide. In response to triggers for insulin release (eg, increase in blood glucose), beta cells release vesicles containing insulin and C-peptide in equimolar amounts. C-peptide does not appear to have any significant physiologic action.

TABLE 24-1 **Pancreatic islet cells and their secretory products.**

Cell Types[a]	Approximate Percentage of Islet Mass	Secretory Products
Alpha (A) cell	20	Glucagon, proglucagon
Beta (B) cell	75	Insulin, C peptide, proinsulin, amylin
Delta (D) cell	3-5	Somatostatin
Epsilon cell	< 1	Ghrelin
F cell (PP cell)	1	Pancreatic polypeptide (PP)

[a]Within pancreatic polypeptide-rich lobules of adult islets, located only in the posterior portion of the head of the human pancreas, glucagon cells are scarce (< 0.5%) and F cells make up as much as 80% of the cells.

Pancreatic beta cells release insulin at a low basal rate, and at a much higher rate in response to a variety of stimuli, especially glucose. Additional physiologic triggers for insulin release include increased plasma levels of certain amino acids, hormones such as glucagon-like polypeptide 1 (GLP-1), glucose-dependent insulinotropic polypeptide (GIP), high concentrations of free fatty acids, and parasympathetic stimulation to beta cells.

Figure 24-2 illustrates a well-defined mechanism by which glucose triggers insulin release. In beta cells, increased extracellular glucose increases intracellular adenosine triphosphate (ATP) concentration, which closes ATP-dependent potassium channels. Closure of potassium channels results in fewer positive ions leaving the cell, which causes membrane depolarization. This depolarization opens voltage-gated calcium channels. The resulting increase in intracellular free calcium triggers exocytosis of vesicles containing insulin.

Insulin circulates freely in the blood and exerts its effects by activating insulin receptors located on almost *all* cells. The insulin receptor is a transmembrane tyrosine kinase receptor. When activated by insulin binding, the insulin receptor phosphorylates itself as well as a set of intracellular proteins that comprise signaling pathways. Within the cell, this series of phosphorylations results in multiple effects including translocation of glucose transporters (GLUTs) to the plasma membrane, changes in activity of enzymes involved in carbohydrate, protein, and lipid metabolism, and complex effects on cell growth and division. Thus, insulin's actions can be grouped into two broad categories: metabolic effects on macronutrient synthesis and growth-promoting effects on DNA synthesis, cell division, and differentiation.

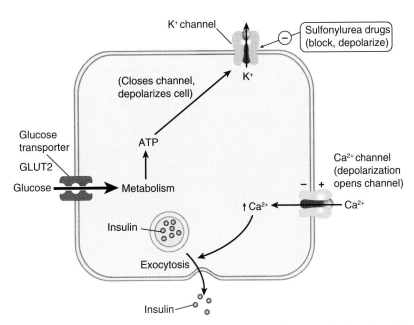

FIGURE 24-2 **Model of how insulin is released from a pancreatic beta cell by glucose and sulfonylurea drugs.** In the resting cell with normal (low) ATP levels, potassium moves out of the cell (down its concentration gradient) through ATP-gated potassium channels. This conductance maintains a relatively negative membrane potential. In this state, insulin release is minimal. If extracellular (blood) glucose concentration rises, glucose enters the cell (via a glucose transporter, GLUT2), intracellular ATP production increases, ATP binds to and closes potassium channels, and the cell depolarizes. Voltage-gated calcium channels open in response to depolarization, allowing calcium to enter the cell. Increased intracellular calcium results in increased insulin secretion. Sulfonylurea drugs bind to and close ATP-dependent potassium channels, thereby depolarizing the membrane and increasing insulin release.

By facilitating glucose uptake into cells and affecting many enzymes, insulin has important effects in almost every tissue of the body, but its principal targets are liver, muscle, and adipose tissue. Table 24-2 outlines insulin's physiologic effects in these target tissues. In the liver, insulin increases glycogen synthesis by both increasing the activity of enzymes that convert glucose to glycogen and inhibiting the enzymes involved in glycogenolysis and gluconeogenesis. Insulin also decreases protein breakdown and increases synthesis and storage of triglycerides and formation of very low-density lipoproteins (VLDLs). In muscle, insulin stimulates glucose uptake by recruiting GLUT4 transporters to the plasma membrane. Through its effects on enzymes in metabolic pathways, insulin promotes glycogen synthesis, glycolysis, and carbohydrate oxidation. Insulin promotes protein synthesis (by increasing net amino acid uptake) and inhibits protein breakdown. In adipose tissue, insulin also promotes glucose uptake through GLUT4 transporters. This insulin-facilitated glucose uptake is used to fuel the synthesis of triglycerides. Simultaneously, insulin inhibits the breakdown of triglycerides to glycerol and free fatty acids. In addition, insulin stimulates synthesis of lipoprotein lipase, which liberates fatty acids from circulating chylomicrons and VLDLs. This effect allows free fatty acids to enter adipocytes and be converted into triglycerides. Ultimately, insulin-facilitated glucose uptake into liver, muscle, and fat boosts supplies of glycogen and lipids that can be used later to supply the energy that will be needed during fasting (when insulin concentration is at its lowest).

DIABETES MELLITUS

Diabetes mellitus may be diagnosed based on plasma glucose criteria (either fasting plasma glucose ≥ 126 mg/dL or 2-hour plasma glucose ≥ 200 mg/dL during an oral glucose tolerance test), or hemoglobin A1C criteria. When plasma glucose levels are in the normal range, approximately 4-6% of hemoglobin A is irreversibly glycated by glucose; this glycosylated hemoglobin is called hemoglobin A1C. In individuals with *chronic* hyperglycemia, the percentage of hemoglobin that is glycosylated—the A1C fraction—is elevated. Thus, the A1C serves as an index of plasma glucose levels over the previous 8-12 weeks, whereas blood or urine glucose concentration reflects glucose control near the time of sample collection. In nondiabetic individuals, A1C levels are less than 5.7%. In individuals with prediabetes (impaired glucose tolerance) who are at high risk for developing the disease, A1C levels are 5.7-6.4%. The A1C diagnostic criterion for diabetes is ≥ 6.5%.

Diabetes can be classified into three major categories: type 1, type 2, and gestational. Other forms due to causes such as diseases of the exocrine pancreas (eg, cystic fibrosis and pancreatitis) or drug-induced are not as common.

Type 1 Diabetes Mellitus

Type 1 diabetes is the result of selective autoimmune beta-cell destruction, usually leading to absolute insulin deficiency. Individuals are typically diagnosed in childhood with the hallmark symptoms of polyuria and polydipsia, and roughly

TABLE 24-2 Endocrine effects of insulin.

Effects on liver
Reversal of catabolic features of insulin deficiency
  Inhibits glycogenolysis
  Inhibits conversion of fatty acids and amino acids to keto acids
  Inhibits conversion of amino acids to glucose
Anabolic actions
  Promotes glucose storage as glycogen (induces glucokinase and glycogen synthase; inhibits phosphorylase)
  Increases triglyceride synthesis and very low-density lipoprotein (VLDL) formation

Effects on muscle
Increased protein synthesis
  Increases amino acid transport
  Increases ribosomal protein synthesis
Increased glycogen synthesis
  Increases glucose transport
  Induces glycogen synthase and inhibits phosphorylase

Effects on adipose tissue
Increased triglyceride storage
  Induces lipoprotein lipase to hydrolyze triglycerides from lipoproteins
  Promotes glucose transport into adipocytes, providing glycerol phosphate to permit esterification of fatty acids supplied by lipoprotein transport
  Inhibits intracellular lipase

one-third present with diabetic ketoacidosis (DKA). DKA is a dangerous condition resulting from excessive adipose tissue breakdown (due to lack of insulin) and accumulation of ketones. Type 1 diabetes can occur in adulthood, though onset and clinical presentation may be more variable. Type 1 DM is found in all ethnic groups, with the highest incidence in people from northern Europe and Sardinia. Susceptibility appears to involve a multifactorial genetic linkage, but only 10-15% of patients have a positive family history. Most individuals with type 1 diabetes present with significant beta cell loss and insulin administration is *required* to control hyperglycemia and prevent ketosis.

Type 2 Diabetes Mellitus

Type 2 diabetes accounts for 90-95% of all diabetes. Type 2 diabetes is characterized by relative (rather than absolute) insulin deficiency in the setting of peripheral insulin resistance. Insulin resistance is a state in which insulin's primary target tissues are not as *responsive* to insulin. Although insulin is produced by beta cells, the amount secreted (which may be quite high) is inadequate to overcome the resistance of the tissues. Circulating endogenous insulin is typically sufficient to prevent ketoacidosis, but inadequate to prevent hyperglycemia. The impaired insulin action also affects fat metabolism, resulting in increased free fatty acid flux and triglyceride levels, and a low serum concentration of high-density lipoprotein (HDL), the lipoprotein that has a protective effect against

atherosclerosis. Over time, a given individual may have more insulin resistance or more beta-cell deficiency, and the abnormalities may be mild or severe.

Most, but not all, individuals with type 2 diabetes are overweight or obese. Excess weight in itself causes some degree of insulin resistance. Thus, the onset of type 2 diabetes often occurs in adulthood. However, incidence in children and adolescents is rising due to the increased prevalence of obesity in young people. Although insulin resistance may improve with weight reduction and/or pharmacologic treatment of hyperglycemia, it is seldom restored to normal. Type 2 diabetes can initially be controlled with diet, exercise, and oral glucose-lowering agents or noninsulin injectable medications. Some individuals may have progressive beta-cell failure and eventually require the addition of insulin to their drug therapy.

Dehydration in untreated and poorly controlled individuals with type 2 diabetes can lead to a life-threatening condition called nonketotic hyperosmolar coma. In this condition, blood glucose may rise 6-20 times the normal range, and an altered mental state develops that may progress to loss of consciousness. Urgent medical care and rehydration is required. Although people with type 2 diabetes ordinarily do not develop ketosis, ketoacidosis may occur as the result of a stressor such as infection or use of a medication that enhances insulin resistance such as a glucocorticoid (Chapter 23).

Gestational Diabetes Mellitus

Gestational diabetes is defined as any abnormality in glucose levels noted for the first time during pregnancy. Gestational diabetes is diagnosed in approximately 7% of pregnancies in the United States. During pregnancy, placental hormones produce insulin resistance, particularly in the last trimester. Because gestational diabetes carries risks for maternal and fetal outcomes, it is recommended that pregnant women be tested either at the first prenatal visit (in women with diabetes risk factors) or at 24-28 weeks of gestation (in women with lower diabetes risk). The preferred therapy for gestational diabetes is insulin because it does not cross the placenta to a great extent. **Metformin** and **glyburide** may be used, but both cross the placenta. All oral antidiabetic drugs lack long-term safety data.

INSULIN

All individuals with type 1 diabetes require exogenous insulin therapy to control hyperglycemia and avoid DKA. In addition, approximately 30% of people with type 2 diabetes require insulin therapy, either alone or in conjunction with oral antidiabetic drugs. Insulin is also the first-line agent recommended for treatment of gestational diabetes.

Although insulins derived from animals (pig or cow) are still available in other parts of the world, these are no longer available in the United States. Human insulin is manufactured by recombinant DNA technology and dispensed as regular

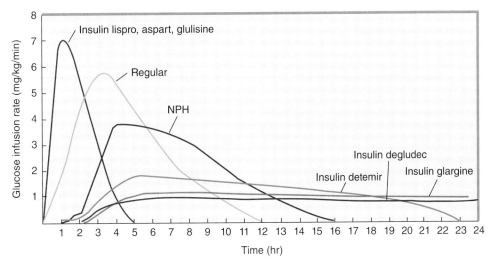

FIGURE 24-3 **Extent and duration of action of various types of insulin as indicated by the glucose infusion rates (mg/kg/min) required to maintain a constant plasma glucose concentration.** Durations of action shown are typical of an average dose of 0.2-0.3 units/kg; except for insulin lispro and insulin aspart, duration increases when dosage is increased.

(R) and neutral protamine Hagedorn (NPH). Because endogenous insulin has a half-life of only a few minutes in the circulation, many insulin preparations are formulated to release the hormone slowly into the circulation. There are also six analogs of human insulin: three rapidly acting formulations and three long-acting formulations. The ratio of zinc and other substances to insulin influences the rate of release of active hormone from the site of administration and the duration of action (Figure 24-3). Table 24-3 shows the bioavailability characteristics for the available insulins. Since insulin is a peptide hormone, it cannot be taken orally because it will be degraded by endogenous peptidases. Instead, insulin is typically administered via subcutaneous injection (using disposable needles and syringes, pen-sized injectors, or a continuous insulin infusion device). Inhaled insulin is also available. The goals of insulin therapy are to control both basal and postprandial (after a meal) plasma glucose levels, while minimizing the risk of hypoglycemia.

Short-Acting Insulin Preparations

Short-acting insulins include **regular insulin**, the three rapidly acting insulins (**insulin lispro**, **insulin aspart**, and **insulin glulisine**), and **inhaled insulin** (technosphere insulin). Regular crystalline-zinc insulin is a rapid-onset and short-action formulation. Regular insulin is used in maintenance regimens, alone or mixed with long-acting preparations. Before the development of the other short-acting insulins, regular insulin was the primary rapid-onset agent. Intravenous infusions of regular insulin are used to treat DKA and during perioperative management of diabetics that require insulin.

Insulin lispro, insulin aspart, and insulin glulisine are rapidly acting insulins that contain transpositions of two amino acids or replacement of one or more native amino acids. These changes alter physical properties of the peptides so that they dissolve more rapidly at the site of administration and enter the circulation faster than regular insulin (Table 24-3). Thus,

TABLE 24-3 **Bioavailability characteristics of the insulins.**

Insulin Preparations	Onset of Action	Peak Action	Effective Duration
Insulins lispro, aspart, glulisine	5-15 min	1-1.5 hr	3-4 hr
Human regular	30-60 min	2 hr	6-8 hr
Technosphere inhaled insulin	5-15 min	1 hr	3 hr
Human NPH	2-4 hr	6-8 hr	10-20 hr
Insulin glargine	0.5-1 hr	Flat	~ 24 hr
Insulin detemir	0.5-1 hr	Flat	17 hr
Insulin degludec	0.5-1 hr	Flat	More than 42 hr

while regular insulin has an onset of action 30-60 minutes after subcutaneous injection, these formulations have a very rapid onset of action of 5-15 minutes. Rapidly acting insulins should be taken 15 minutes before a meal (compared with 45 minutes for regular insulin). Patients should be taught to eat a readily absorbable carbohydrate early in the meal to avoid hypoglycemia. For most commonly used dosages of insulin lispro, insulin aspart, and insulin glulisine, increasing the dose only increases the maximum effect, not the duration of effect, which remains at about 4 hours.

In 2006, the Food and Drug Administration (FDA) approved a special inhalation formulation of regular insulin. This was the first insulin formulation that did not require injection. Interest was too low to support continued production and the drug was discontinued. However, the second rapidly acting inhaled insulin was approved by the FDA for use in adults in 2014. This recombinant regular insulin is called technosphere insulin. After inhalation from the single-use device, peak plasma insulin level occurs within 12-15 minutes and median time to maximal effect is approximately 1 hour. Cartridges containing 4, 8, or 12 units should be inhaled immediately before a meal. The most common adverse effect is cough, affecting almost one-third of trial patients. Inhaled insulin is contraindicated in individuals who smoke or have chronic pulmonary disease. Prior to using inhaled insulin, spirometry should be performed to determine potential lung disease, and then again at 6 months and annually after initiation.

Long-Acting Insulin Preparations

Neutral protamine Hagedorn (NPH) is an intermediate-acting insulin whose absorption and onset of action are delayed by combining regular insulin with protamine, a highly basic protein. Its onset of action is approximately 2-4 hours with an effective duration of 10-20 hours (Table 24-3). NPH insulin is usually mixed (in the syringe or purchased premixed) with regular, lispro, aspart, or glulisine insulins and administered 2-4 times daily.

"Peakless" insulins with very slow onset and prolonged action include **insulin glargine**, **insulin detemir**, and **insulin degludec** (Table 24-3). Insulins glargine and detemir achieve a peakless plateau within 3-6 hours and maintain a relatively constant plasma insulin level for up to 24 hours. These formulations are usually given either in the morning only or in the morning and evening to help control basal plasma glucose levels. This stable basal insulin level may be supplemented with injections of insulin lispro or regular insulin during the day to meet requirements of carbohydrate intake. Because insulin glargine is very acidic, it should not be mixed with other insulins to avoid loss of efficacy. Insulin degludec is the newest long-acting insulin and has the longest duration of action (exceeding 42 hours).

Insulin Delivery Systems

The standard mode of insulin therapy is subcutaneous injection with disposable plastic syringes with attached needles.

Common syringe sizes include 1 mL (100 units), 0.5 mL (50 units), and 0.3 mL (30 units). The smallest syringe is popular because many individuals with diabetes do not take more than 30 units of insulin in a single injection. Rotation of injection sites is recommended to avoid lipodystrophy of subcutaneous adipose tissue that can occur if the same site is repeatedly injected.

Portable pen-sized injectors eliminate the need for carrying insulin vials and syringes. Some insulin pens contain replaceable cartridges, whereas others are disposable.

Continuous subcutaneous insulin infusion (CSII) pumps avoid the need for multiple daily injections. The pump contains a reservoir (for rapid-acting insulins only), program chip, keypad, and display screen. The pager-sized pump is placed on a belt or in a pocket. An infusion set is inserted subcutaneously, usually in the abdomen. Insulin is infused through thin plastic tubing connecting the reservoir to the infusion set. Every 2-3 days, the insulin reservoir, tubing, and infusion set must be changed using sterile techniques. The programmable pump delivers basal and bolus insulin doses, based on blood glucose self-monitoring results. Basal 24-hour insulin rates are typically preprogrammed, but patients still have the ability to make basal adjustments. For example, the individual can decrease basal insulin rates for many hours after intense exercise to decrease the risk of hypoglycemia. The patient still uses bolus amounts of insulin to decrease high blood glucose levels and to cover mealtime insulin requirements. Bolus amounts are either dynamically programmed or use preprogrammed algorithms. In the latter case, the patient enters both the carbohydrate content ingested and current plasma glucose level and the pump calculates the appropriate dose of insulin. While CSII pumps have flexibility advantages over multiple daily subcutaneous injections, their use requires involvement and commitment by the patient.

Adverse Effects of Insulin

The most common complication is hypoglycemia, which results from excessive insulin action. Hypoglycemia can be very dangerous because brain damage may result. People with advanced renal disease, older adults, and children younger than 7 years are most susceptible to hypoglycemia and its detrimental effects. In individuals with *intact* hypoglycemic awareness, rapid development of hypoglycemia causes autonomic hyperactivity. Sympathetic manifestations include tachycardia, palpitations, sweating, and tremulousness. Parasympathetic manifestations include nausea and hunger. If untreated, hypoglycemia may progress to convulsions and coma. In diabetics who experience frequent hypoglycemic episodes, these autonomic warning signs can be less frequent or even absent. These individuals can develop severe manifestations of hypoglycemia, including confusion, weakness, bizarre behavior, coma, or seizures without warning. Every person with diabetes who is receiving hypoglycemic drug therapy should have an identification bracelet, necklace, or card in the wallet or purse, as well as some form of rapidly absorbed

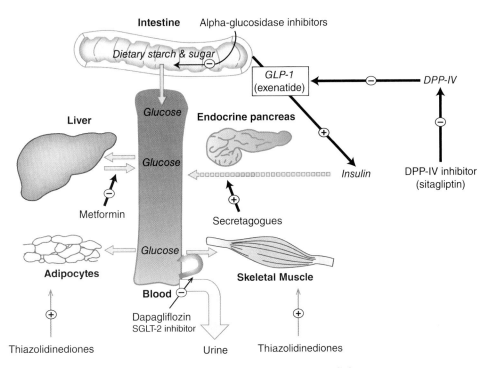

FIGURE 24-4 Major actions of the primary antidiabetic drugs used to treat type 2 diabetes.

glucose. To reverse hypoglycemia, prompt administration of glucose or simple sugars is essential. The glucose may be given either as sugar or candy by mouth or as intravenous glucose. When unconsciousness prevents oral glucose administration, an intramuscular injection of glucagon can be used to raise serum glucose concentrations.

Insulin-induced immunologic complications occur when antibodies to insulin or noninsulin protein contaminants are formed. This can result in resistance to insulin's action or allergic reactions. With the current use of highly purified human insulins, immunologic complications are very uncommon. Insulin may also cause weight gain, which is particularly undesirable in patients with type 2 diabetes, who frequently have excess weight.

NONINSULIN ANTIDIABETIC DRUGS

Figure 24-1 shows the seven categories of blood glucose-lowering agents available to treat type 2 diabetes: (1) insulin secretagogues that stimulate endogenous insulin secretion (sulfonylureas, meglitinides, D-phenylalanine derivatives); (2) drugs that primarily act to decrease hepatic gluconeogenesis (biguanides); (3) drugs that act on liver, muscle, and fat to increase glucose uptake and decrease hepatic gluconeogenesis (thiazolidinediones); (4) drugs that slow intestinal glucose absorption (α-glucosidase inhibitors); (5) agents that modulate incretins (GLP-1 receptor agonists, dipeptidyl peptidase 4 [DPP-4] inhibitors); (6) drugs that inhibit glucose reabsorption in the

kidney (sodium-glucose co-transporter 2 [SGLT2] inhibitors), and (7) agents that act by other mechanisms (pramlintide). With the exception of pramlintide, which can be used for treating both type 1 and type 2 diabetes, these agents are only used in the treatment of type 2 diabetes. All are taken orally, except the GLP-1 agonists and pramlintide, which are injected subcutaneously. Figure 24-4 illustrates the major sites of action for noninsulin drugs used to treat type 2 diabetes and Table 24-4 outlines their physiologic effects and duration of action.

Insulin Secretagogues

Insulin secretagogues stimulate the release of endogenous insulin. Most of the insulin secretagogues are in the chemical class known as **sulfonylureas**. The sulfonylureas close the ATP-regulated potassium channels in pancreatic beta cell membranes; channel closure depolarizes the cells, which triggers insulin release (Figure 24-2). Insulin secretagogues are not effective in diabetics who lack functional beta cells. The second-generation sulfonylureas **glyburide**, **glipizide**, **gliclazide**, and **glimepiride** are considerably more potent and used more commonly than the older agents such as **tolbutamide** or **chlorpropamide**.

Repaglinide and **nateglinide** are newer insulin secretagogues. Repaglinide is from a chemical class called meglitinides, whereas nateglinide is a D-phenylalanine derivative. Both of these drugs also promote insulin release by closing ATP-regulated potassium channels in pancreatic beta cell membranes. The most notable difference between these newer drugs and the sulfonylureas is their more rapid onset and shorter duration of

TABLE 24-4 Representative drugs used to treat type 2 diabetes mellitus.

Drug	Physiological Effect	Duration of Action (hours)	Adverse drug reactions
Insulin secretagogues	Reduce plasma glucose in people with functioning beta cells		
Sulfonylureas Glipizide Glyburide Glimepiride Gliclazide (not available in United States)		10-24	Hypoglycemia Weight gain
Meglitinides Repaglinide		1-3 (with rapid onset of action)	
D-Phenylalanine derivative Nateglinide		< 4 (with rapid onset of action)	
Biguanides Metformin	Decreases endogenous glucose production	12-24	GI symptoms, lactic acidosis (rare); decreased vitamin B_{12} absorption
Thiazolidinediones Pioglitazone Rosiglitazone	Decrease insulin resistance	> 24	Fluid retention, edema, anemia, weight gain, bones fractures in women, may worsen heart disease and increase risk of myocardial infarction
α-Glucosidase inhibitors Acarbose Miglitol	Reduce conversion of starch and disaccharides to monosaccharides; reduce postprandial hyperglycemia	3-4 (with rapid onset of action)	GI symptoms (flatulence, diarrhea, abdominal pain)
Incretin modulators	Reduce postprandial hyperglycemia, increase glucose-mediated insulin release, lower plasma glucagon, delay gastric emptying, decrease appetite		
GLP-1 receptor agonists[a] Exenatide Liraglutide Albiglutide Dulaglutide		5-10	GI symptoms (nausea, vomiting), pancreatitis
DPP-4 inhibitors Sitagliptin Saxagliptin Linagliptin Alogliptin		~ 24	Upper respiratory infections, headache, pancreatitis, rare allergic reactions
SGLT2 Inhibitors Canagliflozin Dapagliflozin Empagliflozin	Increase glucosuria, lower plasma glucose level	Half-life ~ 10-14	Genital and urinary tract infections, osmotic diuresis, hypotension
Amylinomimetic[a,b] Pramlintide		3	GI symptoms, hypoglycemia, headache

DPP-4, dipeptidyl peptidase 4; GI, gastrointestinal; GLP-1, glucagon-like polypeptide-1; SGLT2, sodium-glucose cotransporter 2.
[a]Parenteral (subcutaneous) administration.
[b]Pramlintide is also used to treat type 1 diabetes.

action. These drugs are taken just before meals to reduce the postprandial rise in blood glucose concentration.

Hypoglycemia is the most common adverse effect of the secretagogues. Occasionally, rash and allergy are reported. The older sulfonylureas (tolbutamide and chlorpropamide) are extensively bound to serum proteins. Thus, drugs that compete for protein binding may enhance their hypoglycemic effects. Because of chlorpropamide's long duration of action, prolonged hypoglycemic reactions can occur. These are more common in older adults and the drug is contraindicated in this group. Like insulin, the insulin secretagogues also cause weight gain.

Biguanides

Metformin is the only biguanide available in the United States. Biguanides act by a poorly understood mechanism to reduce both postprandial and fasting glucose levels in people with type 2 diabetes. Proposed mechanisms of action include reduced hepatic gluconeogenesis, stimulation of glycolysis in peripheral tissues, reduction of glucose absorption from the gastrointestinal tract, and reduction of plasma glucagon. Metformin's duration of action is intermediate compared to most other oral antidiabetic drugs (Table 24-4).

Metformin is recommended as first-line therapy for type 2 diabetes. The drug does not increase body weight (as do other oral antidiabetic drugs and insulin) or provoke hypoglycemia. Metformin has been shown to decrease the risk of macrovascular and microvascular complications associated with diabetes. This contrasts with other therapies that have only been shown to modify microvascular morbidity. The landmark Diabetes Prevention Program also demonstrated that metformin is useful in *preventing* the onset of type 2 diabetes in middle-aged obese individuals with prediabetes, though it did not prevent diabetes in older, leaner prediabetics.

The most common adverse drug reactions associated with metformin are gastrointestinal (nausea and diarrhea), occurring in up to 20% of patients. The most serious toxicity is lactic acidosis. Increased risk of lactic acidosis presumably arises because metformin inhibits gluconeogenesis, so the drug may also impair conversion of lactic acid to glucose, an important reaction normally performed in the liver. Patients at greatest risk for lactic acidosis are those with renal or liver disease, alcoholism, or conditions that predispose them to tissue anoxia and excess lactic acid production, such as chronic cardiopulmonary dysfunction. Metformin also inhibits vitamin B_{12} absorption, which may result in vitamin B_{12} deficiency after many years of use. Screening for vitamin B_{12} deficiency is recommended because this condition may present as a peripheral neuropathy and be misdiagnosed as diabetic neuropathy.

Thiazolidinediones

Thiazolidinediones decrease insulin resistance by increasing target tissue sensitivity to insulin. The two drugs in this class are **rosiglitazone** and **pioglitazone**. Thiazolidinediones bind to and activate the nuclear receptors called peroxisome proliferator-activated receptor-gamma (PPAR-γ). Activation of PPAR-γ receptors regulates the transcription of genes encoding proteins involved in carbohydrate and lipid metabolism, insulin signal transduction, and adipose tissue differentiation. The thiazolidinediones increase glucose uptake in muscle and adipose tissue (via increased glucose transporter expression), inhibit hepatic gluconeogenesis, decrease free fatty acid levels, modify the plasma lipid profile, and alter levels of adipose tissue hormones (adipokines).

Thiazolidinediones reduce both fasting and postprandial hyperglycemia. They are used as monotherapy or in combination with insulin or other anitdiabetic agents. Adverse effects have limited more widespread use of thiazolidinediones.

Troglitazone, the first thiazolidinedione introduced, was removed from the market because of hepatotoxicity. Although rosiglitazone and pioglitazone appear to carry less risk of serious liver dysfunction, liver function should be monitored and these drugs are not recommended for use in people with active liver disease. Thiazolidinediones can cause volume expansion, which presents as edema and mild anemia, especially when combined with exogenous insulin. Due to concerns of increased risk of cardiovascular events, rosiglitazone's use is restricted in some countries. Heart failure and other cardiovascular complications may occur and use is contraindicated in individuals with moderate or severe heart failure. Weight gain occurs, especially when thiazolidinediones are combined with insulin or sulfonylureas. Some evidence suggests loss of bone mineral density and increased risk of fractures in women. Because pioglitazone and troglitazone induce cytochrome P450 enzymes, these drugs can reduce plasma concentrations of drugs also metabolized by these enzymes (eg, oral contraceptives, cyclosporine) and thus potentially their effectiveness.

Alpha-glucosidase Inhibitors

Acarbose and **miglitol** inhibit α-glucosidase, an enzyme necessary for converting complex starches and disaccharides to monosaccharides that can be transported from the intestinal lumen into the blood. By delaying digestion and absorption of starch and disaccharides, α-glucosidase inhibitors reduce postprandial hyperglycemia. These drugs have no effect on fasting blood sugar. Both drugs are taken before meals, can be used as monotherapy, or in combination with other antidiabetic drugs.

Gastrointestinal adverse effects including flatulence, diarrhea, and abdominal pain have limited the use of α-glucosidase inhibitors. These unpleasant effects are caused by increased fermentation of unabsorbed carbohydrate by bacteria in the colon and resulting gas production. The adverse effects lessen with ongoing use because distal segments of the small intestine begin expressing α-glucosidase, which increases glucose absorption and decreases movement of carbohydrate into the colon. Patients taking α-glucosidase inhibitors who experience hypoglycemia should be treated with oral glucose (dextrose) and not sucrose because the absorption of sucrose will be delayed.

Incretin Modulators (GLP-1 Receptor Agonists and Dipeptidyl Peptidase 4 [DPP-4] Inhibitors)

When glucose is consumed *orally*, it stimulates a higher insulin response compared to an equivalent glucose dose administered *intravenously*. This finding suggested the existence of a gastrointestinal tract-derived substance that stimulates insulin release. Further research led to discovery of two hormones released from endocrine cells in the intestines in response to food. These gut hormones—incretins—were identified as GLP-1 and glucose-dependent insulinotropic peptide (GIP). GLP-1 also delays gastric emptying, inhibits glucagon secretion, and produces a sense of satiety. Because GLP-1 is quickly broken down by dipeptidyl peptidase 4 (DPP-4), native GLP-1 cannot be used therapeutically to enhance endogenous insulin release. Instead, four metabolically stable GLP-1 receptor agonists have been designed: **exenatide**, **liraglutide**, **albiglutide**, and **dulaglutide**.

All of the GLP-1 receptor agonists are administered via subcutaneous injections. These drugs are administered before breakfast and dinner (exenatide), once daily (liraglutide), or once weekly (albiglutide, dulaglutide, exenatide LAR). GLP-1 receptor agonists are adjunctive therapy for people with type 2 diabetes. Weight loss occurs, which is more prominent with exenatide and liraglutide; this effect contributes to glycemic control as weight loss in itself reduces insulin resistance.

The most frequent adverse effects are nausea and vomiting as well as hypoglycemia when used in conjunction with sulfonylurea drugs. GLP-1 receptor agonists may increase the risk of pancreatitis; patients are advised to get immediate medical care if they experience persistent and severe abdominal pain. GLP-1 agonists are not used in people with personal or family history of medullary thyroid cancer or multiple endocrine neoplasia syndrome type 2 because animal studies showed these agents stimulated thyroidal C-cell tumors.

An alternative approach to increasing the activity of incretins is the use of DPP-4 inhibitors to prolong the action of endogenously released GLP-1 and GIP. In the United States, there are four oral DPP-4 inhibitors, often referred to as the "gliptins": **sitagliptin**, **saxagliptin**, **linagliptin**, and **alogliptin**. The gliptins are taken daily either as monotherapy or in combination with other oral antidiabetic agents. Therapy results in A1C reductions ranging from 0.4% to 1.0%. With the exception of linagliptin, elimination is via the kidney, so dosages must be reduced in people with renal impairment. Adverse effects of the gliptins include headache, nasopharyngitis, increased risk of infections (upper respiratory tract and urinary tract), and hypersensitivity reactions ranging from urticaria to anaphylaxis. Hypoglycemia may occur when the gliptins are combined with insulin or insulin secretagogues. Last, the risk of pancreatitis may be increased.

Sodium-Glucose Cotransporter 2 (SGLT2) Inhibitors

Glucose is freely filtered by the renal glomeruli and is entirely reabsorbed by sodium-glucose cotransporters (SGLTs) located in the proximal tubules. Sodium-glucose transporter 2 (SGLT2) is the cotransporter responsible for approximately 90% of glucose reabsorption (Figure 7-7). Inhibition of SGLT2 decreases the blood glucose level in diabetics by allowing glucose to be lost in the urine (glucosuria). Three SGLT2 inhibitors—**canagliflozin**, **dapagliflozin**, and **empagliflozin**—are approved for use alone or in combination with other oral antidiabetic agents or insulin in people with type 2 diabetes. Therapy results in A1C reductions comparable to the gliptins. Treatment also results in modest weight loss ranging from 2 to 5 kg. Based on their mechanism of action, SGLT2 inhibitors are not as effective in chronic kidney disease; their use is contraindicated in individuals with low glomerular filtration rates. Osmotic diuresis can deplete intravascular volume and cause hypotension. Main adverse effects include increased incidence of genital and urinary tract infections. Dapagliflozin may increase the risk of breast and bladder cancers. Last, canagliflozin (and possibly the other SGLT2 inhibitors) may decrease bone mineral density. Canagliflozin also carries a black box warning for increased risk of leg and foot amputation.

Pramlintide

Amylin is a 37-amino acid protein that is co-secreted with insulin from the pancreatic beta cells. **Pramlintide** is a synthetic analog of amylin. Administration of pramlintide has multiple effects. The drug reduces postprandial glucose elevation (by prolonging gastric emptying), reduces glucagon secretion, and suppresses appetite. Pramlintide is injected subcutaneously immediately before eating; levels peak within 20 minutes. The drug is approved for treating individuals with type 1 and 2 diabetes who have not been able to decrease postprandial blood glucose to target levels. However, pramlintide is not very useful in type 2 diabetics who can use the GLP-1 receptor agonists instead. Concurrent rapid-acting mealtime insulin dosages should be decreased to avoid hypoglycemia. Severe hypoglycemia is more common in patients with type 1 diabetes. In addition to hypoglycemia, headaches, nausea, vomiting, and loss of appetite are the major adverse effects.

GLUCAGON

Glucagon is a hormone secreted by alpha cells of the endocrine pancreas. Glucagon acts through G protein-coupled receptors to stimulate adenylate cyclase and increase intracellular cyclic adenosine monophosphate (cAMP). Activation of glucagon receptors increases hepatic glycogenolysis and gluconeogenesis, increases heart rate and contractility, and relaxes smooth muscle, particularly smooth muscle in the gastrointestinal tract.

Glucagon is used to treat severe hypoglycemia in patients with diabetes or insulin-secreting tumors, but its hyperglycemic action requires intact hepatic glycogen stores. The drug is administered intramuscularly or intravenously. In the management of severe adrenergic β-blocker overdose, glucagon may be the most effective method for stimulating the depressed heart because it increases cardiac cAMP without accessing β receptors. Glucagon is also valuable for radiographic studies of the bowel or abdomen when temporary reduction of motility is necessary for optimal visualization.

TREATMENT OF DIABETES MELLITUS

Management of the individual with diabetes includes education, diet (eg, limiting carbohydrate intake, caloric restriction), weight loss (especially in type 2 diabetes) and exercise, as well as insulin and/or other antidiabetic drugs. Education of both patient and family is a fundamental and ongoing component of care. Topics must include type of diabetes, blood glucose measurement, rationale for controlling hyperglycemia, and benefits of optimal glycemic control. For people taking insulin, users must understand the relationship between the action profiles of different insulins, timing and carbohydrate content of meals, and necessary insulin adjustments for exercise and infections. Last, the patient and family should recognize signs and symptoms of hypoglycemia, understand methods to decrease its incidence, and have rapidly absorbed carbohydrates always available.

Based on the frequency of cardiovascular and other diabetes-related complications, the American Diabetes Association (ADA) regularly revises glycemic targets. Acceptable glycemic control includes an A1C less than 7%, premeal blood glucose levels of 90-130 mg/dL, and less than 180 mg/dL 1 hour and less than 150 mg/dL 2 hours after meals. Many studies have shown that tight glycemic control benefits individuals with both type 1 and type 2 diabetes by decreasing the risk of microvascular complications (eg, renal and retinal damage), myocardial infarction, and death related to diabetic complications. Less stringent A1C targets are sometimes used for individuals treated with insulin or insulin secretagogues (due to the increased risk of hypoglycemia), children, those with limited life expectancy, and those with significant microvascular and macrovascular disease.

Type 1 Diabetes Mellitus

Treatment for type 1 diabetes involves dietary instruction and insulin therapy. Most people with type 1 diabetes require at least 3 or 4 insulin injections per day to effectively control hyperglycemia. Roughly 40% of the total insulin dosage is the longer-acting insulins used to cover basal insulin requirements. The rapidly acting insulins are used for meals, snacks, and corrections of high blood glucose levels. Pramlintide may be added for improved control of postprandial glucose levels. The individual must also pay careful attention to factors that change insulin requirements such as deviations from the regular diet, exercise, infection, and other forms of stress. While the risk of hypoglycemic reactions is increased in tight control regimens, it is not enough to obviate the benefits of better control for most individuals.

Type 2 Diabetes Mellitus

Type 2 diabetes is usually a progressive disease, and treatment for an individual generally escalates over time. The cornerstone of initial treatment is intensive lifestyle interventions (diet and exercise) to lose weight and decrease insulin resistance. If lifestyle interventions are not sufficient to normalize blood glucose levels, initial drug therapy is usually monotherapy with metformin. Although the initial response to metformin is usually good, erosion of glycemic control within 5-10 years is common. If metformin alone is not successful, a second drug is added. Choice of the second drug is individualized, depending on agent efficacy, hypoglycemic risk, effect on weight, adverse effects, and cost. If two agents are not sufficient for glycemic control, a third agent may be added.

Type 2 diabetes involves insulin resistance and often, eventual inadequate insulin production due to beta-cell failure. Thus, pharmacotherapy often combines an agent that augments insulin's action with one that increases insulin blood levels. The former includes metformin, thiazolidinediones, or α-glucosidase inhibitors; the latter includes insulin secretagogues, exenatide, or insulin itself. If the combination of oral drugs and injectable GLP-1 receptor agonists fails to achieve glycemic control, insulin therapy is typically initiated. Sulfonylureas, metformin, thiazolidinediones, and some insulin formulations are long-acting drugs that help control both fasting and postprandial blood glucose levels. In contrast, repaglinide, α-glucosidase inhibitors, exenatide, regular insulin and the rapidly acting insulins are short-acting drugs that primarily target postprandial glucose levels.

REHABILITATION RELEVANCE

Exercise is a key component of lifestyle management of diabetes. Exercise improves insulin sensitivity and can facilitate weight loss, which can delay pharmacotherapy in some individuals with type 2 diabetes. People with type 1 diabetes can also improve glycemic control with a regular exercise program. Aerobic exercise may assist in weight control and improve cardiovascular fitness, which can decrease the risk of macrovascular complications.

In 2018, the ADA recommended that most adults with diabetes should engage in ≥ 150 minutes of moderate to vigorous intensity aerobic activity per week. To decrease insulin resistance, daily exercise—or, at least not allowing more than 2 days to elapse between exercise sessions—is recommended. Aerobic activity bouts should ideally be at least 10 minutes, with the goal of approximately 30 minutes per day or more. Resistance training should be performed at least twice per week. Children and adolescents with prediabetes or diabetes should engage in ≥ 60 minutes per day of moderate- to vigorous-intensity aerobic activity, with vigorous muscle-strengthening and bone-strengthening activities at least 3 days per week.

While preexercise evaluation has not been routinely recommended, the ADA states that providers should assess individuals with diabetes for conditions that might contraindicate certain types of exercise or predispose them to injury. Physical therapists may be ideal healthcare providers to prescribe and appropriately monitor and adjust exercise programs for individuals with complications such as hypertension, autonomic neuropathy, peripheral neuropathy, and history of foot ulcers or Charcot foot. If there is high risk for or presence of cardiovascular pathophysiology, stress testing should precede the design of an exercise program. In people with long-standing diabetes, autonomic neuropathy can affect heart rate. Ratings of perceived exertion (RPE) may be better indicators of exercise intensity than percentage of estimated maximal heart rate. Moderate intensity exercise corresponds to an RPE approximately 12-13 on the Borg RPE. Diabetic foot screens should be performed prior to exercise to determine degree of protective sensation and any necessary modifications of exercise mode and footwear.

For individuals taking insulin and/or insulin secretagogues, exercise may cause hypoglycemia if medication dose or carbohydrate consumption is not altered. If preexercise glucose levels are less than 100 mg/dL, patients may need to ingest added carbohydrates, lower preexercise insulin dose (or *during* exercise with an insulin pump), modify time of day exercise is performed, and/or change the intensity and duration of exercise. Therapists should remember that hypoglycemic symptoms may not be present, or they may mimic increased exertion. Due to increased insulin sensitivity, some patients experience hypoglycemia after exercise that may last for hours. Hypoglycemia is less common with noninsulin antidiabetic medications and preventive measures for hypoglycemia are typically not needed. Exercise is contraindicated when ketosis is present because exercise may exacerbate ketoacidosis. People should also not exercise when fingerstick blood glucose values exceed 300 mg/dL.

Below are adverse effects of antidiabetic drugs or drug classes mostly likely to affect rehabilitation.

- **Hypoglycemia** is most common with insulin and insulin secretagogues. Hypoglycemia may also occur with GLP-1 receptor agonists, DPP-4 inhibitors, pramlintide, and α-glucosidase inhibitors, especially when these medications are combined with insulin or the secretagogues. Patients should be advised to have readily absorbable carbohydrates

available. Clinic gyms should stock glucose or candy, juice, or (nondiet) soda. Patients taking α-glucosidase inhibitors who experience hypoglycemia should be given glucose and not sucrose. Glucose levels should be checked prior to aerobic activities and patients should be informed that hypoglycemia may occur during exercise or up to 24 hours after exercise.

- **Weight gain** is most common with insulin and insulin secretagogues, but also occurs with the thiazolidinediones. Encourage intensive lifestyle management with emphasis on caloric restriction and exercise for weight control.

- **Gastrointestinal disturbances** ranging from nausea and vomiting to flatulence and diarrhea may limit participation in rehabilitation. These effects are most common with metformin, α-glucosidase inhibitors, GLP-1 receptors agonists, and pramlintide.

- **Lactic acidosis** with metformin is rare, but more likely to occur in people with cardiorespiratory insufficiency and alcoholism. Symptoms of lactic acidosis include rapid onset of abdominal pain, muscle pain, diarrhea, and unusual sleepiness. If lactic acidosis is suspected, immediate medical care should be sought.

- **Cardiovascular complications** may occur with thiazolidinediones. Monitor vital signs and be alert for signs or symptoms of exercise intolerance.

- **Decreased bone mineral density** has been reported with the use of thiazolidinediones and SGLT2 inhibitors. Emphasize weightbearing and resistance exercises and be especially alert for increased risk of fractures.

- **Pancreatitis** has been reported in people taking GLP-1 receptor agonists. Immediate medical care is indicated if patients experience persistent and severe abdominal pain.

- **Decreased vitamin B$_{12}$ absorption** may occur in long-term users of metformin. Patients with suspected diabetic neuropathy symptoms should be screened for vitamin B$_{12}$ deficiency.

- **Hypotension** may occur with use of SGLT2 inhibitors. To prevent syncope, assist patients with positional changes and provide a cool-down period following exercise.

CASE CONCLUSION

S.L. recalled that she took her regular dose of repaglinide before a small protein-dominant lunch and then walked the ½ mile to the PT clinic. S.L.'s symptomatic hypoglycemia noted during today's session was likely the result of a combination of factors. First, her diligent participation in almost daily exercise for the past month improved insulin sensitivity. Second, repaglinide is a short-acting insulin secretagogue. She took this medication before a small meal with

low carbohydrate content. The combination of taking a drug that increased insulin secretion from the beta cells with little carbohydrate, walking to the clinic, and then walking on the treadmill, on the background of improved insulin sensitivity likely resulted in today's hypoglycemic event. The physical therapist advised S.L. to return to her physician for a reevaluation of her medications in the face of her current changing glycemic control.

CHAPTER 24 QUESTIONS

1. Which of the following does *not* decrease insulin resistance?

   a. Exercise
   b. Insulin secretagogues
   c. Pioglitazone
   d. Rosiglitazone

2. Which of the following drugs is considered first-line therapy for type 2 diabetes?

   a. Glyburide
   b. Insulin
   c. Metformin
   d. Pioglitazone

3. Which of the following drugs increases the risk of hypoglycemia?

   a. Glucagon
   b. Glyburide
   c. Metformin
   d. Pioglitazone

4. Which of the following drugs, or drug classes, does *not* have weight gain as an adverse effect?

   a. Metformin
   b. Insulin
   c. Insulin secretagogues
   d. Thiazolidinediones

5. Which of the following formulations of insulin would most likely be given to control the postprandial rise in blood glucose level?

   a. Insulin detemir
   b. Insulin glargine
   c. Insulin lispro
   d. NPH insulin

6. Which of the following drugs is *not* used in the treatment of type 1 diabetes?

   a. Insulin lispro
   b. Inhaled insulin
   c. Glyburide
   d. Pramlintide

7. Which of the following drugs, or class of drugs, for type 2 diabetes must be injected subcutaneously?

   a. Insulin secretagogues
   b. Metformin
   c. Sodium-glucose transporter 2 (SGLT2) inhibitors
   d. Pramlintide

8. Which of the following drugs, or drug classes, has as an adverse effect of vitamin B_{12} deficiency that may lead to peripheral neuropathy and be misdiagnosed as diabetic neuropathy?

   a. GLP-1 receptors agonists
   b. Insulin
   c. Metformin
   d. Thiazolidinediones

9. Which of the following statements is true regarding the inhalation formulation of insulin?

   a. This formulation is a rapidly acting insulin.
   b. This formulation is a long-acting insulin.
   c. The formulation is ideal for individuals with diabetes who also have chronic pulmonary disease.
   d. This drug formulation is reserved only for individuals with type 2 diabetes.

10. Which of the following statements is true regarding continuous subcutaneous insulin infusion (CSII) pumps?

    a. These pumps only deliver basal (background) insulin doses.
    b. These pumps deliver basal (background) and bolus insulin doses.
    c. These pumps are only used to deliver long-acting insulins.
    d. These pumps are used to deliver preprogrammed doses of insulin and do not allow the user to make changes.

CHAPTER

Drugs that Affect Bone Mineral Homeostasis

25

CASE STUDY

L.T. is a 55-year-old man with a 20-year history of rheumatoid arthritis (RA) and body mass index of 28 kg/m². He has had bilateral knee joint replacements, the most recent performed 2 years ago. L.T. ambulates with two single-point canes to increase mobility and decrease knee pain. Three weeks ago, he was diagnosed with locally invasive prostate cancer. Prior to starting pharmacotherapy for prostate cancer, he received a bone mineral density study that revealed osteoporosis. The oncologist referred L.T. to rehabilitation for development of a conditioning program as part of an osteoporosis management strategy. L.T.'s current pharmacotherapy for RA includes nonsteroidal anti-inflammatory drugs and disease-modifying antirheumatic drugs (Chapter 34) as well as long-term intermittent use of glucocorticoids (Chapter 23) during acute RA flare-ups. The pharmacotherapy for prostate cancer is designed to suppress testosterone production and destroy in situ cancer cells. Suppression of endogenous testosterone production will be accomplished by continuous dosing with goserelin plus flutamide for the first several weeks (Chapter 22). Radiation therapy will be initiated to destroy in situ cancer cells in the prostate. To help prevent further bone loss, L.T. also began taking over-the-counter vitamin D and calcium carbonate and the prescription drug alendronate. These agents are to be continued as long as goserelin is administered.

REHABILITATION FOCUS

Physical therapists are well aware that bones provide support for the body and serve as attachment sites for muscles to enable mobility. Every day, therapists evaluate and provide interventions for the most common dysfunctions of the skeletal system—fractures and osteoporosis. While clinicians know that calcium and vitamin D are required for "strong bones," the dynamic regulation of bone mineral homeostasis is extremely complex with old theories being revised and intricate interplays among hormones and other endogenous substances still being discovered.

Calcium and phosphate are the major mineral constituents of bone and are also two of the most important minerals for general cellular function. Accordingly, the body has evolved a complex set of mechanisms by which calcium and phosphate homeostasis is carefully maintained. Approximately 98% of the 1-2 kg of calcium and 85% of the 1 kg of phosphorus in the human adult are found in bone, the primary reservoir for these minerals. Bone is constantly remodeling, with ready exchange of minerals with free ions in the extracellular fluid. Bones not only serve as the principal structural support for the body, but also provide space within the bone marrow for hematopoiesis. Dysfunction in bone mineral homeostasis can have many clinical consequences. Obviously, disruptions of its rigid structural support can result in osteoporosis and fractures.

Abnormalities in bone mineral homeostasis can also result in electrolyte disturbances, with manifestations of muscle weakness, tetany, and coma. Finally, hematopoietic capacity may be reduced in conditions such as infantile osteopetrosis.

The average American diet provides 600-1000 mg of calcium per day, of which a net amount of approximately 100-250 mg is absorbed. Absorption principally occurs in the duodenum and upper jejunum, whereas secretion principally occurs in the ileum. The amount of phosphorus in the American diet is about the same as that of calcium. However, the efficiency of phosphate absorption (mostly in the jejunum) is greater, ranging from 70% to 90%, depending on intake. The movement of calcium and phosphate across the intestinal and renal epithelia is closely regulated. In the steady state, renal excretion of calcium and phosphate balances intestinal absorption. Most of the time, more than 98% of filtered calcium and 85% of filtered phosphate are reabsorbed by the kidneys.

There are likely more than a dozen endogenous hormones and growth factors that regulate calcium and phosphate homeostasis. However, the three primary regulators are vitamin D, parathyroid hormone (PTH), and fibroblast growth factor 23 (FGF23). Secondary regulators such as calcitonin, estrogens, and glucocorticoids modulate bone mineral homeostasis under certain physiologic conditions. Endogenous agents (or drugs that mimic or inhibit their actions) and exogenous agents are used in the treatment of bone mineral disorders (Figure 25-1).

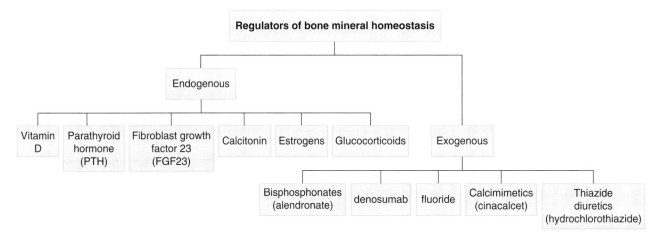

FIGURE 25-1 **Regulators of bone mineral homeostasis may be divided into endogenous regulators and exogenous agents.** Vitamin D, parathyroid hormone, and fibroblast growth factor 23 are primary regulators, whereas calcitonin, estrogens, and glucocorticoids play modulatory roles. Exogenous agents such as bisphosphonates, denosumab, calcimimetics, and thiazide diuretics are used to prevent or treat disorders of bone. Fluoride is primarily used as an additive in toothpaste to reduce dental cavities. Under exogenous agents, prototype drugs are in parentheses.

ENDOGENOUS REGULATORS

Primary Regulators

Vitamin D

The term *vitamin D*, when used without a subscript, refers to a group of fat-soluble steroids, the most important of which are vitamin D_2 (ergocalciferol) and vitamin D_3 (cholecalciferol). Both are prohormones, meaning that they are biologically inactive; metabolic conversion in the liver and kidney is required to gain biologic activity. The precursor to vitamin D_2 is found in plants and fungi, whereas the precursor to vitamin D_3 is found in the skin. Vitamin D_3 is produced under the influence of ultraviolet B (UVB) radiation from the precursor 7-dehydrocholesterol in the skin. The precursor of vitamin D_2 also undergoes transformation with UVB radiation. Few foods naturally contain vitamin D, but vitamins D_2 and D_3 can be ingested in fortified foods such as milk and in supplements.

Of the natural metabolites of vitamin D, 25-hydroxyvitamin D (**calcifediol**) formed in the liver and 1,25-dihydroxyvitamin D (1,25[OH]$_2$D) or **calcitriol**, formed in the kidney are available for clinical use. Several synthetic analogs of 1,25(OH)$_2$D are also used to extend the utility of this natural metabolite to treat a variety of conditions. Because it is fat-soluble, vitamin D and its metabolites circulate bound to vitamin D-binding protein (DBP). However, it is the free, unbound forms of the metabolites that have biologic activity. This has clinical relevance given that levels of DBP can increase (estrogen therapy, late pregnancy) and decrease (liver disease, nephrotic syndrome). When evaluating an individual's vitamin D status, measurement of a single marker of the total 25(OH)D level may not accurately measure the bioavailable metabolites. In addition, some metabolites bind less well to DBP and consequently have shorter half-lives, which influences treatment strategies. Excess vitamin D is stored in adipose tissue.

The primary effect of vitamin D metabolites (especially 1,25[OH]$_2$D) is a net increase in serum levels of calcium and phosphate by increasing both the intestinal absorption and bone resorption of these minerals as well as decreasing their renal excretion (Table 25-1). Since their effects in the gastrointestinal tract are greater than those in the kidney, vitamin D also increases urinary calcium. Active vitamin D metabolites are required for normal bone mineralization. Vitamin D deficiency results in the softening of bones, presenting as rickets in growing children and osteomalacia in adults. Specific receptors for 1,25(OH)$_2$D have been identified in almost all tissues, not just bone, intestine, and kidney. More recent efforts to create analogs of 1,25(OH)$_2$D that do not increase blood calcium concentration are being made. The goal is to target nonclassic tissues to modulate the newly appreciated roles of vitamin D in the regulation of endocrine function, immunity, and muscle function. The diverse actions of vitamin D are initiated by changes in gene expression that are mediated by activation of the intracellular vitamin D receptor.

Clinically, vitamin D supplements and synthetic derivatives are used in the treatment of deficiency states (eg, nutritional deficiency, intestinal osteodystrophy), chronic kidney or liver disease, hypoparathyroidism, and nephrotic syndrome. For individuals with chronic kidney or liver disease or hypoparathyroidism, the active form of vitamin D (calcitriol) is required. To treat secondary hyperparathyroidism associated with renal failure, calcitriol reduces PTH (which corrects the hypocalcemia) and improves bone disease, but calcitriol can cause hypercalcemia and hypercalciuria. To address the latter concern, **doxercalciferol**, **paricalcitol**, and **calcipotriene** (**calcipotriol**) were developed. These agents are active vitamin D analogs that cause less hypercalcemia in all individuals as well as less hypercalciuria, if renal function is normal. In combination with calcium supplementation and other drugs, vitamin D is used in the prevention and treatment of osteoporosis in older adults. Moreover, a number of calcitriol analogs

TABLE 25-1 Actions of parathyroid hormone (PTH), vitamin D, and fibroblast growth factor 23 (FGF23) on intestine, bone, and kidney.

	PTH	Vitamin D	FGF23
Intestine	Increased calcium and phosphate absorption by increased 1,25(OH)$_2$D	Increased calcium and phosphate absorption by 1,25(OH)$_2$D	Decreased calcium and phosphate absorption by decreased 1,25(OH)$_2$D production
Kidney	Decreased calcium excretion, increased phosphate excretion, stimulation of 1,25(OH)$_2$D production	Calcium and phosphate excretion may be decreased by 25(OH)D and 1,25(OH)$_2$D^a	Increased phosphate excretion Decreased 1,25(OH)$_2$D production
Bone	High doses increase calcium and phosphate resorption Low doses increase bone formation	Increased calcium and phosphate resorption by 1,25(OH)$_2$D Bone formation may be increased by 1,25(OH)$_2$D	Decreased mineralization due to hypophosphatemia and low 1,25(OH)$_2$D levels
Net effect on serum levels	Calcium increased Phosphate decreased	Calcium and phosphate increased	Phosphate decreased

^{a}Direct effect. Vitamin D also indirectly increases urine calcium because of increased intestinal calcium absorption and decreased PTH.

are being synthesized in an effort to examine their potential usefulness in a variety of inflammatory and malignancy conditions. For example, topical calcipotriene (calcipotriol) is currently used to treat psoriasis, a hyperproliferative skin disorder. The main hazard associated with chronic overdose of vitamin D and/or its metabolites is hypercalcemia, hyperphosphatemia, and hypercalciuria.

Parathyroid Hormone

Parathyroid hormone (PTH) is an 84-amino acid peptide hormone released from the parathyroid glands primarily in response to changes in serum calcium levels. If the free (ionized) calcium serum level falls, PTH is released. The net effect of PTH is to *increase* serum calcium and *decrease* serum phosphate (Table 25-1). In the kidney, PTH increases calcium (and magnesium) reabsorption while reducing reabsorption of phosphate (and amino acids, bicarbonate, sodium, chloride, and sulfate). Another important action of PTH in the kidney is its stimulation of calcitriol production, which will increase serum calcium by increasing intestinal absorption. In a feedback manner, active vitamin D metabolites directly inhibit PTH synthesis. In bone, PTH promotes bone remodeling (Figure 25-2). PTH increases the activity and number of osteoclasts, the cells responsible for bone resorption, but it does so indirectly. First, PTH activates G protein-coupled receptors on bone-forming osteoblasts, inducing a membrane-bound protein called RANK ligand (RANKL). RANKL then acts on osteoclast precursors and osteoclasts to increase both their number and activity. Thus, bone remodeling is actually initiated by osteoclastic bone resorption and followed by osteoblastic bone formation. Although PTH enhances both bone resorption and bone formation, the net effect of *excess* PTH is increased bone resorption. However, when administered in low, intermittent doses, PTH produces a net increase in bone

formation. Based on this effect, a shortened recombinant form of PTH called PTH 1-34 (**teriparatide**) and the synthetic analog **abaloparatide** are used in the treatment of osteoporosis. The full-length recombinant form of PTH (**Natpara**) is used to treat hypoparathyroidism.

Fibroblast Growth Factor 23

Fibroblast growth factor 23 (FGF23) is a protein made by osteoblasts and osteocytes and released in response to elevated levels of serum 1,25(OH)$_2$D (calcitriol) and phosphate. Its main function appears to be regulation of serum phosphate. In the kidney, FGF23 decreases reabsorption and increases excretion of phosphate, thus lowering serum phosphate. As the most recently discovered primary regulator of bone mineral homeostasis, FGF23 is not currently used as a drug.

Interaction of Vitamin D, PTH, and FGF23

Table 25-1 summarizes the principal actions of vitamin D, PTH, and FGF23 on intestine, kidney, and bone. The net effect of vitamin D is to raise serum levels of calcium and phosphate; the net effect of PTH is to raise serum calcium and lower serum phosphate; the net effect of FGF23 is to lower serum phosphate.

Figure 25-3 illustrates the interactions and feedback mechanisms that regulate calcium and phosphate homeostasis. The two primary regulators of PTH secretion are calcium and phosphate. In the parathyroid gland, specialized G protein-coupled receptors sense extracellular ionized calcium concentration and couple this with intracellular calcium concentration. When extracellular calcium falls, intracellular calcium falls in parallel and parathyroid cells secrete more PTH. Conversely, a rise in intracellular calcium concentration in parathyroid cells inhibits PTH secretion. Phosphate ion also affects PTH secretion, albeit indirectly. Phosphate binds with calcium and decreases the concentration of ionized calcium. Thus, an increase in

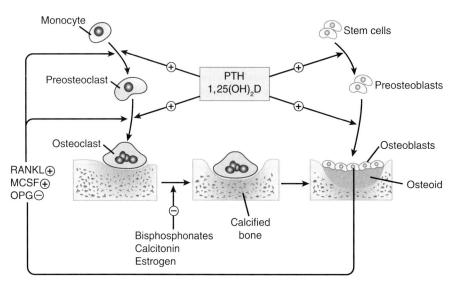

FIGURE 25-2 **Parathyroid hormone (PTH) and 1,25(OH)₂D regulate bone formation and resorption (ie, bone turnover).** This is done by activating precursor differentiation and stimulating osteoblast production of signaling factors such as RANK ligand (RANKL), macrophage-colony-stimulating factor (MCSF), and osteoprotegerin (OPG).

serum phosphate reduces the ionized calcium concentration, which enhances PTH secretion. In the kidney, high levels of calcium and phosphate reduce production of 1,25(OH)₂D (calcitriol) and increase production of 24,25(OH)₂D, another vitamin D metabolite. Since calcitriol is far more potent than 24,25(OH)₂D at increasing serum calcium and phosphate, the net effect of calcitriol's action is feedback inhibition of vitamin D's main action. Calcitriol inhibits PTH secretion through a direct action on PTH gene transcription. This provides yet another negative feedback loop because PTH is a major stimulus for calcitriol production. The ability of calcitriol to inhibit PTH secretion directly can be exploited by administering calcitriol analogs that have less effect on serum calcium. Such drugs are proving useful in the management of the secondary

hyperparathyroidism that accompanies renal failure, and may be useful in selected cases of primary hyperparathyroidism. In the last feedback loop, calcitriol stimulates FGF23 production, which inhibits calcitriol production while promoting hypophosphatemia. Resulting hypophosphatemia inhibits FGF23 production and stimulates calcitriol production.

Secondary Regulators

Compared to the role of the three primary regulators discussed above, the physiological role of the secondary regulators on bone mineral homeostasis is minor. However, in pharmacological doses, these may be used therapeutically to treat bone mineral disorders.

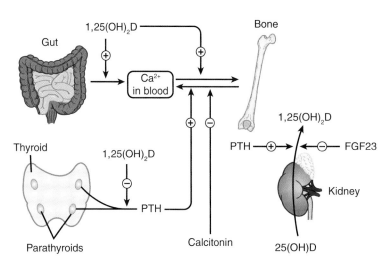

FIGURE 25-3 **Hormonal interactions controlling bone mineral homeostasis.** 1,25(OH)₂D is produced in the kidney. Parathyroid hormone (PTH) promotes its production and fibroblast growth factor 23 (FGF23) inhibits its production. Once formed, 1,25(OH)₂D increases intestinal calcium and phosphate absorption; in those with vitamin D deficiency, 1,25(OH)₂D promotes bone formation. PTH stimulates bone resorption, while calcitonin inhibits bone resorption. Extracellular Ca²⁺ and 1,25(OH)₂D inhibit PTH synthesis.

Calcitonin

Calcitonin is a peptide hormone secreted by the parafollicular cells of the thyroid gland. The principal effect of calcitonin is to lower serum calcium and phosphate by inhibiting bone resorption and inhibiting renal reabsorption of both minerals. Calcitonin not only reduces renal reabsorption of calcium and phosphate, but also of sodium, potassium, and magnesium.

In cases of calcitonin excess (thyroid tumor) or deficiency (thyroidectomy), no obvious disturbances have been identified. Therapeutic administration of calcitonin is useful to acutely lower serum calcium in Paget's disease and hypercalcemia. During initial stages of exogenous calcitonin administration, bone formation is not impaired. With continued use, both formation and resorption of bone are reduced. Calcitonin can be used in the treatment of osteoporosis and has been shown to increase bone mass and reduce the incidence of spine fractures. However, other drugs (eg, bisphosphonates) are more effective.

Calcitonin is administered by injection or nasal spray. Because human calcitonin has a short half-life, salmon calcitonin is used more frequently. In pharmacologic dosages, calcitonin reduces gastric acid output by inhibiting gastrin secretion, and increases secretion of sodium, potassium, chloride, and water into the gut, which may cause abdominal pain and diarrhea.

Estrogens

These compounds were previously discussed (Chapter 22) in relation to their regulation of sexual development, metabolism, and reproduction. Estrogens and selective estrogen receptor modulators (SERMs) such as **raloxifene** prevent or delay bone loss in postmenopausal women. This effect may be the result of more than one mechanism. First, estrogens increase the concentration of 1,25(OH)$_2$D in the blood, which inhibits PTH-stimulated bone resorption. Estrogens also increase the liver's production of DBP so that the total concentration of vitamin D metabolites in the circulation increases. Last, estrogen has direct effects on bone remodeling (Figure 25-2). Long-term estrogen treatment to treat postmenopausal osteoporosis fell out of favor due to well-documented cardiovascular and cancer risks.

Glucocorticoids

Glucocorticoids (Chapter 23) inhibit bone mineral homeostasis by antagonizing vitamin D-stimulated intestinal calcium transport, stimulating renal calcium excretion, and blocking bone formation. As a result, chronic systemic use of glucocorticoids is a common cause of osteoporosis in adults and stunted skeletal development in children. However, glucocorticoids are useful in the intermediate-term treatment of hypercalcemia associated with lymphomas and granulomatous diseases such as sarcoidosis.

EXOGENOUS AGENTS

A variety of other types of drugs are used to regulate bone mineral homeostasis. Some, like the bisphosphonates and **denosumab**, were developed especially for this purpose, while others like the thiazide diuretics have found clinical value in treating certain disorders of bone mineral homeostasis.

Bisphosphonates

The bisphosphonates (**alendronate**, **etidronate**, **ibandronate**, **pamidronate**, **risedronate**, **tiludronate**, **zoledronate**) are short-chain organic polyphosphate compounds that are used to treat osteoporosis, Paget's disease, and hypercalcemia associated with some cancers. Bisphosphonates reduce bone resorption and turnover by inhibiting osteoclast activity (Figure 25-2). The ability of these drugs to increase bone mineral density (BMD) likely extends beyond slowing down the formation and breakdown of the hydroxyapatite crystals that comprise bone. Bisphosphonates have other complex cellular effects including inhibition of vitamin D production, calcium transport, and glycolysis in bone cells.

Bisphosphonate therapy is one of the most common strategies to prevent and treat all forms of osteoporosis (eg, postmenopausal, glucocorticoid-induced). Chronic bisphosphonate therapy with the newer agents slows osteoporosis progression, increases BMD, and reduces spine and hip fractures over 5 years. Pamidronate, zoledronate, or etidronate are the preferred agents for treatment of the hypercalcemia associated with Paget's disease and malignancy.

Oral bioavailability of bisphosphonates is low (< 10%), and food impairs absorption even further. Thus, patients are advised to take these drugs on an empty stomach. Roughly one half of the absorbed drug accumulates in bone, which is retained for months to years, while the rest is excreted unchanged in the urine. To minimize the major adverse effect of esophageal and gastric irritation (rarely, ulceration), patients are advised to take these drugs with large quantities of water, remain upright for 30 minutes, and avoid situations that permit esophageal reflux (ie, activities that increase intra-abdominal pressure). For the prevention or treatment of osteoporosis, once-weekly or once-monthly oral administration of large doses of a bisphosphonate is as efficacious as daily administration of smaller doses and does not result in more toxicity. Intravenous bisphosphonate infusions circumvent the adverse effect of esophageal irritation. Quarterly (ibandronate) or annual (zoledronate) intravenous infusions have been found to be effective. This route of administration is relatively free of adverse reactions (except for a short flu-like syndrome that typically only occurs after the first infusion). Although osteonecrosis of the jaw has been reported, it is very rare in the usual doses used for osteoporosis. Oversuppression of bone turnover may explain the incidence of subtrochanteric femur fractures during long-term bisphosphonate treatment.

Denosumab

Denosumab is a monoclonal antibody that binds to and prevents the action of RANKL (Figure 25-2). Thus, denosumab inhibits osteoclast formation, maintenance, and survival. Denosumab is as effective as the potent bisphosphonates in decreasing bone resorption and is used in the treatment of osteoporosis. Denosumab can also be used to limit growth of bone metastases or bone loss due to drugs that suppress gonadal function. Denosumab is given subcutaneously every month or 6 months (depending on the indication). Because many immune cells also produce RANKL, there may be an increased risk of infection. Like with the bisphosphonates, denosumab carries the potential risk of osteonecrosis of the jaw and subtrochanteric fracture due to the suppression of bone turnover.

Fluoride

Fluoride accumulates in bone and teeth, where it may stabilize their hydroxyapatite crystal structures. Appropriate concentrations of fluoride ion in drinking water (0.5-1.0 ppm) or as an additive in toothpaste have a well-documented ability to reduce dental caries. Although epidemiological observations have demonstrated fewer vertebral compression fractures in areas with fluoridated water, clinical trials of fluoride have not consistently demonstrated a reduction in fractures. The Food and Drug Administration (FDA) has not approved fluoride for the prevention or treatment of osteoporosis. Acute fluoride toxicity (usually caused by ingestion of rat poison) causes gastrointestinal and neurologic symptoms. Chronic toxicity (fluorosis) includes ectopic bone formation (exostoses) and calcified bumps on bones.

Calcimimetics

Cinacalcet is the first approved agent in this new class of drugs that lowers PTH by activating the calcium-sensing receptor in the parathyroid gland. Cinacelcet has been approved to treat hyperparathyroidism secondary to chronic kidney disease and to treat the hypercalcemia associated with parathyroid carcinoma. Adverse effects include hypocalcemia and adynamic bone disease (profoundly decreased bone cell activity).

Thiazide Diuretics

This drug class was previously discussed in relation to treatment of hypertension (Chapter 7). In bone mineral disorders, thiazide diuretics can facilitate renal excretion of calcium. Thiazides are useful in reducing hypercalciuria and nephrolithiasis in people with idiopathic hypercalciuria. They are not used to treat osteoporosis.

PHARMACOTHERAPY FOR SELECT BONE MINERAL DISORDERS

Osteoporosis

Osteoporosis is an abnormal loss of bone that predisposes an individual to fractures. Clinically, the condition is defined as a bone density of 2.5 standard deviations below that of the healthy average young adult (30 years of age), typically measured by dual-energy x-ray absorptiometry at certain sites. The most common forms of osteoporosis are postmenopausal and age related. However, osteoporosis can result from chronic systemic administration of glucocorticoids or other drugs, endocrine diseases such as thyrotoxicosis or hyperparathyroidism, malabsorption syndromes, alcohol abuse, and cigarette smoking.

Both endogenous hormones and exogenous agents are used individually or in combination to treat osteoporosis. Figure 25-4 compares the effects of several agents on BMD over time. The postmenopausal form of osteoporosis is secondary to the reduced estrogen production that accompanies menopause; it can be treated with estrogen (with progestin to prevent endometrial cancer in women with a uterus). However, concerns about increases in breast cancer risk and cardiovascular adverse events have reduced enthusiasm for this form of therapy. The selective estrogen receptor modulator (SERM) raloxifene (Chapter 22) avoids the increased risk of

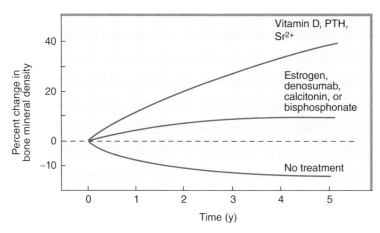

FIGURE 25-4 Typical changes in bone mineral density (BMD) with time after the onset of menopause, with and without treatment. Without treatment, men and women lose bone during aging. Vitamin D, parathyroid hormone (PTH), and strontium (Sr^{2+}) promote new bone formation and can increase BMD throughout the period of treatment. However, high doses of PTH and vitamin D also cause bone resorption. In contrast, estrogen, denosumab, calcitonin, and bisphosphonates block bone resorption, leading to a transient increase in BMD because bone formation is not initially decreased. Over time, both bone formation and bone resorption are decreased and BMD reaches a new plateau.

breast and uterine cancer associated with estrogen supplementation while maintaining the benefit to bone. Although not as effective as estrogen at increasing bone density, raloxifene reduces the risk of breast cancer and decreases the risk of spinal (but not hip) fractures. In contrast, bisphosphonates and teriparatide protect against both fracture types. Raloxifene does not prevent hot flushes and imposes the same increased risk of venous thrombosis as estrogen.

To counter the reduced intestinal calcium transport associated with osteoporosis, vitamin D therapy is sometimes employed along with dietary calcium supplementation. Although several large studies have shown that vitamin D supplementation (800 IU/day) with calcium increases BMD and reduces falls and fractures, the dual supplement regimen is usually given in conjunction with other drugs used to treat osteoporosis. Calcitriol and other vitamin D metabolites are used in other countries to increase BMD and decrease fractures, but the FDA has not approved these agents for osteoporosis.

Bisphosphonates are the most popular drugs used to treat osteoporosis of various causes because they increase BMD and reduce the risk of fractures in the hip, spine, and other locations. Since bisphosphonates are such potent inhibitors of bone turnover, this effect may account for the noted increase in subtrochanteric femur fractures in patients taking bisphosphonates for years. This is the basis for some clinicians recommending a drug "holiday" after ≥ 5 years of bisphosphonate therapy to help promote normal bone growth, if the fracture risk of discontinuing drug treatment is not high. Currently, there is no consensus regarding how long it is best to take a bisphosphonate.

Teriparatide (recombinant form of PTH 1-34) is given subcutaneously once daily. This drug stimulates new bone formation and is associated with a substantial reduction in the incidence of fractures, but is currently approved for only 2 years of use. Denosumab, the RANKL inhibitor, is also injected subcutaneously. This monoclonal antibody has comparable efficacy to bisphosphonates with regards to reducing risk of spinal and nonspinal fractures in the treatment of postmenopausal osteoporosis. Calcitonin is also approved for the treatment of postmenopausal osteoporosis. While calcitonin increases bone mass, this drug is not as effective as bisphosphonates or teriparatide; calcitonin reduces the incidence of fractures, but only in the spine. Though not yet approved by the FDA, **strontium ranelate** is used in Europe to treat osteoporosis. This drug increases BMD by inhibiting bone resorption (by blocking osteoclast differentiation and promoting osteoclast apoptosis) and increasing bone formation.

Nutritional Vitamin D Insufficiency or Deficiency

Because of vitamin D's newly discovered roles in many systems besides the skeletal system, the "optimal" level of vitamin D has been reexamined. As a result, several expert panels have produced guidelines. Serum levels of vitamin D are measured in nanograms/mL of 25(OH)D. A level of 25(OH)D above 10 ng/mL is necessary to prevent rickets or osteomalacia.

However, 20-30 ng/mL may be necessary to optimize intestinal uptake of calcium, build and maintain BMD, reduce falls and fractures, and decrease the incidence of several diseases (eg, diabetes mellitus, autoimmune diseases, cancer). The Institute of Medicine (IOM) recommends a serum level of 20-30 ng/mL, but states that up to 50 ng/mL is safe. The IOM based their recommendations on stronger data (from randomized controlled trials) supporting vitamin D's skeletal effects and not on weaker data supporting vitamin D's purported nonskeletal effects. The Endocrine Society states that the appropriate lower limit should be 30 ng/mL. For individuals between 1 and 70 years of age, 600 IU/day is thought to be sufficient to meet these goals; up to 4000 IU/day is considered safe. Factors that contribute to lower serum vitamin D levels include: older age, obesity, limited sun exposure (or use of sunscreens), dark complexion, and malabsorption issues (eg, Crohn's disease, gastric bypass surgery, cystic fibrosis). Vitamin D *insufficiency* (25[OH]D concentration of 20-30 ng/mL) or vitamin D *deficiency* (25[OH]D concentration < 20 ng/mL) can be treated by higher dosages of vitamin D (1000-4000 IU/day or 50,000 IU/wk for several weeks).

Chronic Kidney Disease

The major problems of chronic kidney disease (CKD) that impact bone mineral homeostasis are deficient calcitriol production and retention of phosphate, which reduces ionized serum calcium. As a result of low serum calcium, individuals present with secondary hyperparathyroidism. With reduced calcitriol production, less calcium is absorbed from the intestine and less bone is resorbed. FGF23 levels increase early in CKD, which can further reduce calcitriol production in the kidney. The most common clinical presentation in CKD is hypocalcemia and hyperphosphatemia. The skeletal manifestation of renal osteodystrophy includes a mixture of osteomalacia (abnormal bone formation due to inadequate mineralization) and osteitis fibrosa (excessive bone resorption with fibrotic replacement of calcified matrix). Some individuals with CKD may become hypercalcemic, most often as a result of severe secondary hyperparathyroidism. Vitamin D supplementation is often prescribed for dialysis patients in chronic renal failure. The choice of vitamin D metabolite depends upon the type and extent of bone disease and hyperparathyroidism. In the United States, doxercalciferol and paricalcitol are approved for treating secondary hyperparathyroidism of CKD. Regardless of the drug employed, careful attention to serum calcium and phosphate levels is required. Calcium supplements and phosphate restriction are used in combination with vitamin D metabolites. Serum PTH levels are monitored to determine whether therapy is correcting or preventing secondary hyperparathyroidism. Vitamin D metabolites are monitored to assess compliance, absorption, and metabolism.

Other Clinical Disorders

A number of gastrointestinal and hepatic conditions (eg, biliary cirrhosis, bariatric surgery) may result in abnormal calcium and phosphate homeostasis that ultimately leads to bone disease. This intestinal osteodystrophy likely results from abnormal calcium or vitamin D intestinal absorption. Clinically, the bone disease secondary to gastrointestinal dysfunction manifests as osteoporosis and osteomalacia, but without osteitis fibrosa that characterizes renal osteodystrophy. Treatment includes high doses of vitamin D (25,000-50,000 IU one to three times per week) or its analogs in conjunction with dietary calcium supplementation.

Nephrotic syndrome is a condition characterized by malfunctioning or damaged glomeruli. The syndrome includes loss of protein in the urine (with accompanying low serum albumin levels), high plasma lipids, and significant edema. Individuals with nephrotic syndrome lose vitamin D metabolites in the urine, likely due to loss of DBP. Subsequently, some individuals may develop bone disease. Though no trials with vitamin D have been carried out in this population, treatment includes vitamin D supplementation.

Paget's disease is a localized bone disease characterized by uncontrolled osteoclastic bone resorption with secondary increases in disorganized new bone formation. Although the disease is fairly common, symptomatic bone disease is less common. The definitive cause of the condition is unknown. The goal of treatment is to reduce bone pain and stabilize or prevent other problems such as progressive deformity, hearing loss, high-output cardiac failure, and immobilization hypercalcemia. Calcitonin and bisphosphonates are first-line agents for treatment of Paget's disease.

REHABILITATION RELEVANCE

Physical therapists develop exercise programs, which when combined with pharmacotherapy and diet, may delay the onset and extent of osteoporosis. Therapists also treat individuals with pain and dysfunction resulting from osteoporosis-induced fractures. Multiple exercise formats including weightbearing (eg, walking, stair climbing), resistance (eg, weight lifting, swimming), and aerobic have been shown to delay osteoporosis.

Of these, resistance training may provide the strongest stimulus for bone remodeling and reduced bone loss. In contrast to pharmacotherapy and diet modification, exercise can maintain and improve cardiovascular and respiratory status. Exercise can also increase strength and improve balance, which have the added benefit of reducing the likelihood of falls and associated fractures. Finally, exercise may enhance pharmacologically stimulated bone formation, suggesting that the combination of exercise and drug therapy may optimize building and maintaining bone mass. Risks of drug therapy relevant to rehabilitation are highlighted below.

- **Esophageal irritation or ulceration** can occur with bisphosphonates. Patients taking bisphosphonates within 30 minutes prior to a therapy session may experience esophageal pain if they are horizontal during the session. Have patients take bisphosphonates after or at least 1 hour prior to therapy sessions.
- **Gastrointestinal distress** may occur with calcitonin, teriparatide, or SERMs such as raloxifene. Therapy sessions may exacerbate symptoms. If possible, schedule therapy sessions for days when these drugs are not administered.
- SERMs such as raloxifene may cause **hot flushes and nausea**. Therapy sessions may exacerbate hot flushes. Cooler temperatures in treatment rooms may help.
- **Chest pain, dyspnea, and dizziness** can occur with teriparatide. Therapists should be alert to these symptoms, assess potential causal factors, and recognize that exercise may exacerbate these adverse effects.
- **Osteonecrosis of the jaw and subtrochanteric fractures** are rare but significant potential adverse effects associated with bisphosphonates and denosumab. When working with individuals taking these drugs, therapists should spend additional time providing education about the increased risk of fracture after a fall and performing careful differential diagnosis when evaluating temporomandibular joint dysfunction.

CASE CONCLUSION

L.T. ambulates independently into the outpatient therapy clinic with both canes. He states that recurring painful RA flare-ups prevent him from participating in aerobic activities. The near constant knee pain limits him to household or limited community ambulation. Typically, his upper body function does not limit his activities, except in acute RA flare-ups. After evaluation, the physical therapist recommended upper extremity resistance exercises (as pain and acute RA flare-ups allow) and an aquatherapy program that included ambulation on the clinic's underwater treadmill at a water level that the patient found comfortable. L.T. initially participated in the program at the clinic under therapist supervision, then continued at a local recreation center where he could walk at a comfortable speed in the shallow end of the pool. The therapist asked L.T. to return once every other week for reevaluation and treatment modification. The therapist also encouraged

L.T. to attempt swimming when he feels more comfortable in the water. The oncologist referred L.T. for development of a conditioning program in recognition of his low BMD, which probably stems from intermittent (though long-term) glucocorticoid use and minimal physical activity. In addition, the antiandrogen pharmacotherapy for prostate cancer will suppress bone mineralization, progressing the osteoporosis. The purpose of vitamin D, calcium, and alendronate is to limit further bone mineralization loss. An appropriate conditioning program in conjunction with anti-osteoporosis drugs will help minimize further bone loss and *may* increase bone mineralization. Although aquatic exercise is not as effective as resistance exercise in preventing bone demineralization in the lower extremities, L.T.'s current limitations preclude consistent resistance training. Aquatic therapy has the added benefits of maintaining cardiovascular and respiratory functions.

CHAPTER 25 QUESTIONS

1. Which of the following is *not* a primary regulator of bone mineral homeostasis?

   a. Estrogen
   b. Parathyroid hormone
   c. Vitamin D
   d. Fibroblast growth factor 23

2. Which drug increases the risk of esophageal irritation?

   a. Vitamin D
   b. Calcitonin
   c. Alendronate
   d. Raloxifene

3. Which of the following drugs for osteoporosis decreases the risk of spinal, but not hip fractures?

   a. Raloxifene
   b. Zoledronate
   c. Teriparatide
   d. Denosumab

4. Which of the following agents is *least* likely to cause gastrointestinal distress?

   a. Calcitonin
   b. Teriparatide
   c. Vitamin D
   d. Raloxifene

5. Which of the following conditions may thiazide diuretics be used to treat?

   a. Hypercalciuria
   b. Hyperthyroidism
   c. Osteoporosis
   d. Osteomalacia

6. At what serum concentration range of 25(OH)D is an individual considered vitamin D deficient?

   a. < 20 ng/mL
   b. 20-30 ng/mL
   c. 30-40 ng/mL
   d. 40-50 ng/mL

7. Which of the following is a monoclonal antibody that inhibits the action of RANK ligand?

   a. Strontium ranelate
   b. Denosumab
   c. Calcipotriol
   d. Cinacelcet

8. Which of the following drugs is used to treat the secondary hyperparathyroidism of chronic kidney disease?

   a. Teriparatide
   b. Fluoride
   c. Calcitonin
   d. Doxercalciferol

9. Which of the following is the main adverse effect associated with chronic vitamin D overdose?

   a. Anemia
   b. Hypophosphatemia
   c. Hypocalcemia
   d. Hypercalcemia

10. Which of the following conditions is *not* an indication for the use of bisphosphonates?

    a. Osteoporosis
    b. Paget's disease
    c. Hypocalcemia
    d. Hypercalcemia

Antihyperlipidemic Drugs

P.E. is a 43-year-old Hispanic man employed on an assembly line at an automotive plant. Four weeks ago, he was involved in an industrial accident in which he experienced muscular strains to his lower extremities and low back. He was evaluated at the onsite clinic, placed on light duty, and referred to an outpatient physical therapy clinic. P.E. has a body mass index of 27 kg/m^2, hypertriglyceridemia, and high plasma low-density lipoprotein (LDL) cholesterol. He is taking gemfibrozil and niacin to improve his lipid profile. During his first visit to the outpatient physical therapist 3 weeks ago, he complained of diffuse muscle and joint pain in both legs and his back. He also stated that his legs felt weak. During the first week of rehabilitation, supportive therapy for pain relief only slightly improved his ability to function in light duty work. Last week, he began a work-hardening program to enable him to return to full-time regular work. During the program, he complained that his previous pain and muscle weakness increased. The physical therapist initially assumed that his pain might be related to initiating exercises included in the work-hardening program and noted this in the chart as suspected delayed onset muscle soreness (DOMS). P.E. continued performing the work-hardening program and the therapist reevaluated his functional status the following week. Upon questioning, P.E. denied any changes in his medications since his initial evaluation. He also denied taking over-the-counter medications or dietary supplements. However, he added that he started taking "red yeast rice" approximately 5 weeks ago because he heard that it lowers "bad cholesterol." When asked why he did not include this on the initial evaluation form, he stated: "the form only asked for medications, and red yeast rice is just a naturally occurring cholesterol-lowering supplement."

REHABILITATION FOCUS

Hyperlipidemia increases the risk of atherosclerosis, stroke, and heart disease. Optimal improvement in blood lipid profiles occurs when individuals make lifestyle changes (exercise, weight reduction, and decreased consumption of saturated and *trans* fat) along with antihyperlipidemic drug therapy. Several drug classes used to treat hyperlipidemia may have adverse effects that clinically manifest as myalgia, arthralgia, and muscle weakness. Although the precise mechanism of these symptoms and signs is uncertain, hypotheses range from mitochondrial dysfunction due to inhibition of ubiquinone (a coenzyme involved in the electron transport chain) to dysfunctional fatty acid metabolism. The most commonly prescribed class of antihyperlipidemic drugs is the HMG-CoA reductase inhibitors, known more commonly as statins. Observational studies indicate that there are particular concerns in rehabilitating patients taking statins. Resistance training and aerobic exercise—especially with increasing intensity—increase the risk of myalgias and skeletal muscle symptoms in individuals taking statins. Investigation into the presence of risk factors for statin-induced myopathy can help the physical therapist determine whether the patient's clinical presentation is more consistent with musculoskeletal dysfunction, drug-related adverse effects, or the combination of both.

BACKGROUND

Atherosclerosis—the abnormal accumulation of lipids and products resulting from an inflammatory response in the walls of arteries—is the leading cause of death in the Western world. Heart attacks, angina pectoris, peripheral arterial disease, and strokes are common sequelae of atherosclerosis. Improving plasma lipid profiles has been shown to prevent the sequelae of atherosclerosis and decrease mortality in people with a history of cardiovascular disease and hyperlipidemia. Figure 26-1 outlines the six drug classes used to decrease plasma lipid concentration (hyperlipidemia) and to prevent or reverse associated atherosclerosis. Although the drugs are generally safe and effective, adverse effects include drug-drug interactions and toxic reactions in skeletal muscle and the liver.

Because lipids—mainly cholesterol and triglycerides—are hydrophobic, they are transported in the blood by macromolecular complexes termed lipoproteins. Lipoproteins are

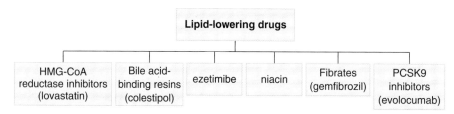

FIGURE 26-1 **The six classes of lipid-lowering drugs based on mechanisms of action.** Example drugs are in parentheses. PCSK9, proprotein convertase subtilisin/kexin type 9.

composed of a lipid core surrounded by apolipoproteins that regulate both the uptake and off-loading of lipids and interactions with cell membrane receptors. The lipoproteins that are primarily responsible for delivering cholesterol to peripheral tissues are called the low-density lipoproteins (LDLs). Those primarily responsible for delivering triglycerides to peripheral tissues are called the very-low-density lipoproteins (VLDLs). LDLs and VLDLs are produced in the liver and contain a key apolipoprotein called B-100. Lipoproteins that contain apolipoprotein (apo) B-100 convey lipids into arterial walls. Catabolism of chylomicrons that are synthesized in the intestinal wall from dietary fat results in the formation of apolipoprotein B-48, which can also enter the artery wall. Lipoproteins that contain apo B-100, and potentially those that contain apo B-48, may be involved in the atherosclerotic process.

Cells that need cholesterol or triglycerides can uptake these lipids from B-100-containing lipoproteins by receptor-mediated endocytosis or by scavenger receptors. Receptor-mediated uptake is a carefully regulated process that protects cells from being overloaded with lipids. In contrast, uptake by scavenger receptors is an unregulated process that can overwhelm the ability of a cell to safely sequester potentially toxic lipids. Macrophages in arterial walls use scavenger receptors to take up circulating lipoproteins, especially particles with apolipoproteins that have been modified by free radicals (ie, oxidized). When these macrophages become overloaded with lipids, they transform into distressed foam cells that initiate a local inflammatory response. Engorged foam cells, foam cells that have burst, and many products of the inflammatory response form the core of an atherosclerotic plaque. Whereas plaques can slowly occlude coronary and cerebral vessels,

clinical symptoms are more frequently precipitated by rupture of unstable plaques, leading to occlusive thrombi.

High-density lipoproteins (HDLs) also originate in the liver. However, these lipoproteins exert several *anti*atherogenic effects. HDLs participate in the reverse pathway: they remove cholesterol from the artery wall and inhibit the oxidation of *pro*-atherogenic lipoproteins. Low plasma HDL is an independent risk factor for coronary artery disease (CAD), whereas high plasma HDL is associated with decreased risk for CAD.

Plasma lipids are often measured after a 10-hour fast. Desirable and elevated levels are presented in Table 26-1. The risk of atherosclerotic heart disease increases with high concentrations of atherogenic lipoproteins such as LDL ("bad cholesterol"), and low concentrations of HDL ("good cholesterol"). Additional risk factors include personal and family history of atherosclerosis, obesity, cigarette smoking, and excessive alcohol intake.

Premature or accelerated development of atherosclerosis is strongly associated with elevated levels of total cholesterol and LDL cholesterol. In contrast, the link between hypertriglyceridemia (elevated plasma triglycerides while fasting) and atherosclerosis is less well defined. However, it is clear that severe hypertriglyceridemia such as that associated with chylomicronemia, a recessive genetic disorder that prevents the normal uptake or metabolism of chylomicrons, is correlated with a high incidence of lipid-filled foam cells in the bone marrow, spleen, and liver. Regulation of plasma lipoprotein levels involves a balance among dietary fat intake, hepatic processing, and utilization by peripheral tissues. *Primary* disturbances in regulation occur in various familial diseases that reflect a variety of genetic determinants. *Secondary*

TABLE 26-1 Lipid Guidelines from the National Cholesterol Education Program (2001).

	Optimal	Near Optimal/ Above Optimal	Borderline High	High	Very High
Total Cholesterol	< 200		200-239	≥ 240	
LDL cholesterol	< 100	100-129	130-159[a]	160-189	≥ 190
Triglycerides	< 150		150-199	200-499	≥ 500

LDL, low-density lipoprotein.

[a]Considered as high if coronary disease or more than 2 risk factors are present.

All values given in mg/dL. High-density lipoprotein (HDL) risk profile is opposite of the other lipoproteins. Ideally, triglyceride concentration should be below 120 mg/dL. HDL ≥ 60 is high and reduces cardiovascular risk. HDL ≤ 40 is low and considered to increase cardiovascular risk. Additional information may be found from the ATPIII Guidelines At-A-Glance Quick Desk Reference at https://www.nhlbi.nih.gov/files/docs/guidelines/atglance.pdf.

TABLE 26-2 Primary hyperlipoproteinemias and their treatment.

Disorder	Manifestations	Diet + Single Drug[a]	Drug Combination
Primary chylomicronemia (familial lipoprotein lipase, cofactor deficiency; others)	Chylomicrons and VLDL increased	Omega-3 fatty acids Fibrate or niacin	Fibrate plus niacin
Familial hypertriglyceridemia	VLDL increased; chylomicrons may be increased	Omega-3 fatty acids Fibrate or niacin	Fibrate plus niacin
Familial combined hyperlipoproteinemia	VLDL predominantly increased	Omega-3 fatty acids Statin, fibrate, or niacin	Two or three of the single agents[b]
	LDL predominantly increased	Statin, ezetimibe, or niacin	Two or three of the single agents
	VLDL, LDL increased	Omega-3 fatty acids Statin or niacin	Niacin or fibrate plus statin[b]
Familial dysbetalipoproteinemia	VLDL remnants, chylomicron remnants increased	Omega-3 fatty acids Fibrate, statin, or niacin	Statin plus fibrate or niacin
Familial Hypercholesterolemia			
Heterozygous	LDL increased	Statin, resin, niacin, or ezetimibe	Two or three of the individual drugs
Homozygous	LDL increased	Atorvastatin, rosuvastatin, ezetimibe, or PCSK9 MAB	Combinations of some of the single agents
Familial ligand-defective apo B-100	LDL increased	Statin, niacin, or ezetimibe	Two or three of the single agents
Lp(a) hyperlipoproteinemia	Lp(a) increased	Niacin	

HDL, high density lipoprotein; LDL, low density lipoprotein; Lp(a), lipoprotein a; VLDL, very low density lipoprotein.
[a]Single-drug therapy with omega-3 dietary supplement should be evaluated before drug combinations are used.
[b]Therapeutic discussion of specific agents not included in text.

disturbances are associated with a Western diet (ie, high in red meat, dairy products, refined sugars, and saturated and *trans* fats and low in fruits, vegetables, whole grains, fish, and legumes), many endocrine conditions, and diseases of the liver or kidneys. Table 26-2 presents the treatment for primary hyperlipoproteinemias.

TREATMENT STRATEGIES

Dietary measures are the first method of management and may be sufficient to reduce lipoprotein levels to a desirable range. Cholesterol, saturated fats, and *trans* fats are the primary dietary factors that contribute to elevated LDL levels, whereas total fat and caloric restriction is important in management of triglycerides. Therapeutic diets are designed to reduce the total intake of these substances. In some individuals, omega-3 fatty acids found in fish oils (but not those found in plants) can profoundly lower plasma triglycerides. In contrast, omega-6 fatty acids found in high proportion in some vegetable oils (eg, sunflower, corn, soybean) may increase triglycerides. Finally, a high blood level of homocysteine, a homologue of the amino acid cysteine, initiates pro-atherogenic changes in vascular endothelium. Individuals with hyperhomocysteinemia can reduce the plasma level by restricting total protein intake to the amount required for amino acid replacement.

The decision to add drugs to the treatment strategy for hyperlipidemia depends on the specific metabolic defect and its potential for causing atherosclerosis or pancreatitis. For the particular patient, the specific choice of drug depends on the lipid abnormality. Antihyperlipidemic drug therapy can reduce hepatic cholesterol synthesis (statins), reduce cholesterol (ezetimibe) and bile acid (resins) absorption from the intestine, decrease secretion of lipoproteins (niacin), reduce LDL concentration (PCSK9 inhibitors), or increase peripheral clearance of lipoproteins (fibrates). Figure 26-2 illustrates the sites of action for four of the antihyperlipidemic drug classes. Drug therapy for hyperlipidemia can cause slow physical *regression* of plaques. The well-documented reduction in acute coronary events following vigorous drug treatment is attributable chiefly to reduction of inflammatory activity, which is evident within 2-3 months after starting therapy. With the exception of PCSK inhibitors that are injected subcutaneously, these agents are administered orally.

HMG-COA REDUCTASE INHIBITORS (STATINS)

The hepatic hydroxymethylglutaryl-coenzyme A [HMG-CoA] reductase inhibitors reduce *total* plasma cholesterol by competitively inhibiting the rate-limiting enzyme (HMG-CoA reductase)

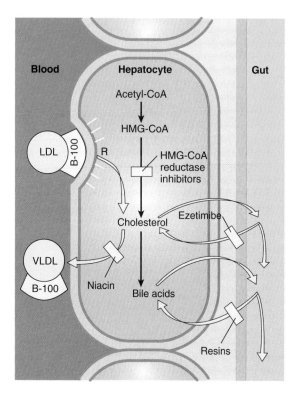

FIGURE 26-2 **Sites of action of HMG-CoA reductase inhibitors (statins), niacin, ezetimibe, and resins.** Inhibition by a drug class is shown by a "rectangle" across the arrow representing the normal metabolic pathway. Low-density lipoprotein (LDL) receptors are increased by treatment with resins and HMG-CoA reductase inhibitors. R, LDL receptor; VLDL, very-low-density lipoproteins.

for cholesterol synthesis in the liver (Figure 26-2). As a result, the liver compensates by increasing the number of high-affinity LDL receptors, which clear LDL from the blood. Statins are the most

effective agents at reducing LDL plasma levels (Table 26-3), especially when used in combination with other drug classes (Table 26-2). Statins also produce modest decreases in plasma triglycerides and small increases in HDL cholesterol.

Lovastatin and **simvastatin** are prodrugs. The other HMG-CoA reductase inhibitors (**atorvastatin, fluvastatin, pravastatin, rosuvastatin**) are active as given. The plasma half-lives of statins vary widely, from atorvastatin with a half-life of 1-3 hours to rosuvastatin with a half-life of 19 hours.

Statins also have direct antiatherosclerotic effects. The impaired synthesis of isoprenoids and decreased prenylation of Rab and Rho proteins reduce atherosclerotic inflammation and may play a role in decreasing subsequent coronary and atherosclerotic stroke events.

The statins are commonly used because they are effective and well tolerated. Large clinical trials have shown that they reduce the risk of coronary events and mortality in individuals with and without heart disease. (Fluvastatin has less maximal efficacy than the other drugs in this group.) Due to evidence that this class of drugs is teratogenic, statins should be avoided in pregnancy.

There are several common adverse effects of statins. Mild elevations of liver enzymes (aminotransferases) may occur, but these are not often associated with significant hepatic damage. Individuals with pre-existing liver disease or a history of alcohol abuse may have higher risk for hepatic toxicity. Statins may increase blood glucose levels, which can lead to development of type 2 diabetes. Some statin users have also reported mild cognitive impairment (forgetfulness, confusion).

Perhaps the most well-known adverse effect of statins is myopathy. Its true incidence is unknown, likely due in part to the fact that there is little consensus on its definition. Signs and symptoms of statin-induced myopathy can include myalgia, myopathy, and rhabdomyolysis. Myalgia includes muscle pain or weakness *without* elevated plasma creatine kinase

TABLE 26-3 Lipid-modifying effects of antihyperlipidemic drugs.

Drug	LDL Cholesterol	HDL Cholesterol	Triglyceride
Statins			
Atorvastatin[a]	−25% to −50%	+5% to +15%	↓↓
Fluvastatin	−20% to −30%	+5% to +10%	↓
Lovastatin[b]	−25% to −40%	+5% to +10%	↓
Resins	−15% to −25%	+5% to +10%	±[c]
Ezetimibe	−20%	+5%	±
Fibrates	−10% to −15%[d]	+15% to +20%	↓↓
Niacin	−15% to −25%	+25% to +35%	↓↓

HDL, high-density lipoprotein; LDL, low-density lipoprotein; ±, variable, if any.
[a]Rosuvastatin has similar effect.
[b]Pravastatin has similar effect.
[c]Resins can increase serum triglyceride concentrations in some patients with combined hyperlipidemia.
[d]Fibrates can increase LDL cholesterol in some patients with combined hyperlipidemia.

(CK). Creatine kinase is an intracellular enzyme found in various cell types, especially muscle, that is released when such cells are damaged. Myopathy refers to symptoms of myalgia, weakness or cramps, plus an otherwise unexplained elevation in CK ≥ 10 times the upper limit of normal. An increase in creatine kinase release from skeletal muscle (subtype CK-MM) is noted in about 10% of statin-users; in a few patients, severe muscle pain, joint pain (arthralgia), and even rhabdomyolysis may occur. Rhabdomyolysis is the rarest and most severe adverse effect. This condition results from acute necrosis of skeletal muscle fibers with subsequent leakage of cellular contents into the circulation and urine. Rhabdomyolysis can produce asymptomatic illness with elevated plasma CK or a life-threatening condition associated with extreme elevations in plasma CK, electrolyte imbalances, acute renal failure, and disseminated intravascular coagulation. Rhabdomyolysis usually resolves when statin use is discontinued, unless it is unrecognized and severe enough to cause death.

Statin-induced myopathy may occur with monotherapy, however the incidence increases when combined with certain other drugs. Because statins are metabolized by the cytochrome P450 (CYP) system, drugs or foods (eg, grapefruit juice) that inhibit CYP activity increase the risk of hepatotoxicity and myopathy. Red yeast rice is a fermentation product that contains variable amounts of naturally occurring lovastatin. Thus, combined use of statins and this dietary supplement should be avoided. Other risk factors for statin-induced myopathy include (but are not limited to): high-statin dosage, polypharmacy, impaired hepatic and renal function, diabetes mellitus, untreated hypothyroidism, advanced age (>65 years) and frailty, small body frame, infection, female sex, recent surgery, and excessive alcohol intake. Last, physical exercise appears to increase the likelihood for developing statin-induced myopathy.

RESINS

Bile acid-binding resins (**cholestyramine**, **colestipol**, and **colesevelam**) are large nonabsorbable polymers that bind bile acids in the intestine (Figure 26-2). By preventing the reabsorption of bile acids secreted by the liver, these agents divert hepatic cholesterol to the synthesis of new bile acids, thereby reducing the amount of cholesterol in the tightly regulated intracellular pool. A compensatory increase in the synthesis of hepatic high-affinity LDL receptors increases the removal of circulating LDL lipoproteins. The resins modestly reduce plasma LDL cholesterol, but have little effect on HDL cholesterol or triglycerides (Table 26-3). In some people with familial combined hyperlipidemia, resins increase plasma VLDL.

The resins are used in patients with hypercholesterolemia (Table 26-2). They may help reduce pruritus in patients with cholestasis and bile salt accumulation.

Adverse effects include bloating, constipation, and an unpleasant gritty taste. Resins may impair the absorption of vitamins (eg, vitamin K, dietary folates) and drugs (eg,

digitalis, thiazides, warfarin, pravastatin, fluvastatin). Heartburn and diarrhea are occasionally reported.

EZETIMIBE

Ezetimibe is used either alone or in combination with other antihyperlipidemic drugs to treat hypercholesterolemia (Table 26-2). As monotherapy, ezetimibe reduces LDL cholesterol by about 20% (Table 26-3). When combined with a statin, it is even more effective.

Ezetimibe is a prodrug converted in the liver to its active glucuronide form, undergoes enterohepatic recirculation, and has a 22-hour half-life. Ezetimibe inhibits the enzyme NPC1L1, which is involved in the gastrointestinal uptake of cholesterol and phytosterols. Phytosterols are naturally occurring compounds found in plant cell membranes that normally enter gastrointestinal epithelial cells, but then are immediately transported back into the intestinal lumen (Figure 26-2). By inhibiting NPC1L1 and thus preventing absorption of *dietary* cholesterol and cholesterol that is excreted in bile, ezetimibe reduces the cholesterol in the tightly regulated hepatic pool. Again, the liver compensates by increasing synthesis of high-affinity LDL, which increases the removal of LDL lipoproteins from the blood. Because of ezetimibe's direct role in inhibiting phytosterol transport, the drug is also used to treat phytosterolemia, a rare genetic disorder that results from impaired export of phytosterols.

Ezetimibe does not appear to be metabolized by the CYP system. The drug is well tolerated, though when combined with statins, may increase the risk of hepatic toxicity. Serum concentrations of its active form are increased by fibrates and reduced by cholestyramine.

NIACIN (NICOTINIC ACID)

Niacin (vitamin B_3), but not nicotinamide (another form of vitamin B_3) has multiple antihyperlipidemic actions. This water-soluble vitamin lowers plasma LDL cholesterol and triglyceride concentrations and increases HDL cholesterol concentrations, but only at dosages multifold *higher* than that found within a multivitamin supplement (Table 26-2).

In adipose tissue, niacin decreases release of fatty acids and triglycerides into the blood, which would be converted to VLDL by the liver. Niacin also directly reduces VLDL secretion from the liver (Figure 26-2). Consequently, LDL formation and plasma concentration is reduced (Table 26-3). In the capillaries, niacin increases triglyceride removal from VLDL, which accounts for the reduction in serum triglyceride concentrations. Niacin is the most effective antihyperlipidemic agent in increasing plasma HDL. By decreasing the catabolic rate of HDL, the plasma level of HDL cholesterol rises.

Niacin also decreases circulating fibrinogen and increases tissue plasminogen activator (tPA), the enzyme involved in breaking down blood clots. Combined, these effects decrease the risk of thrombus formation and increase the dissolution of thrombi. Last, niacin is also the only antihyperlipidemic drug to decrease lipoprotein a, or—"Lp(a)"—in most patients. Lp(a) is formed from LDL and (a) protein. The (a) protein is homologous with plasminogen (Chapter 11), but is not activated by tPA. Instead, (a) protein acts as an inhibitory substrate for tPA. Lp(a) is found in atherosclerotic plaques and contributes to coronary artery disease by inhibiting thrombolysis.

Cutaneous flushing is a common adverse effect of niacin. Pretreatment with aspirin or other nonsteroidal anti-inflammatory drugs reduces flushing intensity, suggesting that this effect is mediated by prostaglandin release. Tolerance to the flushing reaction usually develops within a few days. Dose-dependent nausea and abdominal discomfort often occur. Pruritus and other skin conditions have been reported. Moderate elevations of liver enzymes and even severe hepatotoxicity may occur. Hyperuricemia occurs in about 20% of patients. Niacin has been shown to induce minor insulin resistance in diabetic and nondiabetic individuals. Finally, niacin may potentiate the action of some antihypertensive drugs.

FIBRIC ACID DERIVATIVES (FIBRATES)

Fibric acid derivatives (eg, **gemfibrozil**, **fenofibrate**) are used to treat hypertriglyceridemia (Table 26-2). Because these drugs have only small effects on LDL cholesterol, they are often combined with other antihyperlipidemic agents to treat individuals with elevated plasma LDL and VLDL. The fibrates also produce a modest increase in HDL cholesterol (Table 26-3).

The fibrates are ligands for the peroxisome proliferator-activated receptor-alpha (PPAR-α) protein, a receptor that regulates the transcription of genes involved in lipid metabolism. In adipose tissue, this interaction with PPAR-α increases the activity of lipoprotein lipase, which enhances clearance of triglyceride-rich lipoproteins. In striated muscle and liver, fibrates increase fatty acid oxidation. In the liver, this effect limits the supply of triglycerides necessary for VLDL synthesis.

Nausea is the most common adverse effect of gemfibrozil. Skin rashes also frequently occur. A few patients show decreases in white blood counts or hematocrit, and these drugs can potentiate the action of anticoagulants. Because there is an increased risk of cholesterol gallstones, fibrates should be used with caution in those with a history of cholelithiasis. When used in combination with statins, the fibrates significantly increase the risk of myopathy.

PCSK9 INHIBITORS

Proprotein convertase subtilisin/kexin type 9 (PCSK9) is an enzyme expressed primarily in the liver, but is also found in nonhepatic sites including atherosclerotic plaques. Multiple regulators of PCSK9 exist, and PCSK9 may have a role in lipid and glucose regulation. The role of PCSK9 in lipid regulation is related to its binding at hepatic LDL receptors, which results in LDL receptor internalization and lysosomal degradation.

As a result of fewer hepatic cellular surface LDL receptors, the ability of the liver to bind and internalize extracellular LDL decreases, thus increasing circulating LDL. A decrease in circulating PCSK9 results in increased expression of hepatic LDL receptors and decreased circulating LDL.

Available therapeutic PCSK9 inhibitors are humanized monoclonal antibodies called **evolocumab** and **alirocumab**. At the highest doses, treatment results in a 70% reduction in plasma LDL concentration. Additional reductions in triglycerides, apo B-100, and Lp(a) also occur. Use of PCSK9 inhibitors added to a baseline statin regimen results in additional lowering of plasma LDL and reduced cardiovascular events. PCSK9 inhibitors are only used in individuals who have familial hypercholesterolemia or clinical atherosclerotic cardiovascular disease that require additional lowering of plasma LDL level. They are given with the maximal tolerated statin dosage and/or ezetimibe. The major adverse effect is injection site reactions. Infrequent adverse effects include respiratory infections and flu-like symptoms.

COMBINATION THERAPY

Initially, each individual with hyperlipidemia is treated with dietary modification. To achieve the desired effect on triglycerides and various lipoproteins (VLDL, LDL, and HDL), a drug or drug combination is often added to dietary control to achieve *maximal* improvement in lipid profile with *minimal* toxicity. The most common combinations are listed in Table 26-2. Certain drug combinations present challenges. For example, resins interfere with the absorption of certain statins (pravastatin, cerivastatin, atorvastatin, and fluvastatin), so statins must be taken at least 1 hour before or 4 hours after the resins. Combining statins with either fibrates or niacin increases the risk of myopathy. The benefit of combinations is continuously being evaluated in clinical trials. For example, in a patient with both elevated triglycerides and LDL cholesterol, only a high intensity stain is recommended.

REHABILITATION RELEVANCE

Lipid-lowering drugs are a component of a multidimensional regimen that includes exercise (which can increase plasma HDL concentration) and dietary changes (to lower LDL and total plasma cholesterol levels). At the same time, many of these drugs may interfere with health and exercise programs in some individuals.

- **Arthralgia**, **myalgia**, **myopathy**, **and rhabdomyolysis** are potential adverse effects of several lipid-lowering drug classes. Incidence is higher with statins and when combinations of different drug classes are taken. The physical therapist should attempt to differentiate pain associated with exercise from that associated with adverse effects of these drugs. Statin-induced muscle symptoms often involve large, proximal, and symmetrical muscle groups, with lower extremity or calf muscles affected more often than upper extremities. If the patient presents with any of these manifestations, the therapist should contact the referring healthcare provider. After review and clearance by the prescribing healthcare provider, the therapist may consider decreasing the intensity of aerobic and resistance exercises until symptoms resolve.

- **Flushing** is a significant adverse effect with niacin. Although not directly related to rehabilitation outcomes, this adverse effect may decrease attendance or participation in rehabilitation sessions. If the patient complains of significant flushing, the therapist should contact the referring provider, as the resolution is simple and effective.

- Several anithyperlipidemic drug classes may cause **hepatic dysfunction** and careful monitoring may be required.

CASE CONCLUSION

If P.E.'s lower extremity muscle and joint pain and weakness and low back pain were the result of his accident, these symptoms would be expected to decrease after three weeks. In addition, if his symptoms were the result of DOMS, they would not be expected to occur *immediately* after exercise. Instead, DOMS presents more often as progressive muscle pain with restricted range of motion of affected muscle groups that develops 12-48 hours after exercise, but subsides within 96 hours. To facilitate the differential diagnosis, the physical therapist asked additional questions related to the onset, pattern, and duration of muscle weakness and pain and the patient's current medication regimen. After learning that the patient was taking red yeast rice, the therapist referred P.E. back to the original healthcare provider for further evaluation with this additional information. Blood analyses revealed elevated creatine kinase (subtype CK-MM) and mildly elevated myoglobin. P.E. was diagnosed with myopathy, likely associated with the combination of red yeast rice and antihyperlidemic medications. *Some* dietary supplements of red yeast rice contain lovastatin and other naturally occurring statins. When P.E. combined a statin-containing supplement with niacin and gemfibrozil, this resulted in medication-induced myopathy and associated clinical manifestations.

CHAPTER 26 QUESTIONS

1. Hypertriglyceridemia is most commonly associated with which of the following disorders?

   a. Acute kidney failure
   b. Atherosclerosis
   c. Acute pancreatitis
   d. Acute liver failure

2. Which of the following drugs is a monoclonal antibody?

   a. Niacin
   b. Lovastatin
   c. Colestipol
   d. Evolocumab

3. Which of the following drugs inhibits the enzyme proprotein convertase subtilisin/kexin type 9 (PCSK9)?

   a. Alirocumab
   b. Atorvastatin
   c. Cholestyramine
   d. Ezetimibe

4. Which of the following is responsible for removing cholesterol from the atherosclerotic plaques and returning it to the liver?

   a. Low-density lipoproteins
   b. Intermediate density lipoproteins
   c. High-density lipoproteins
   d. Chylomicrons

5. Which of the following drugs decreases plasma concentration of low-density lipoproteins (LDLs) and total cholesterol by inhibiting hepatic synthesis of cholesterol?

   a. Evolocumab
   b. Colestipol
   c. Lovastatin
   d. Niacin

6. Which of the following drugs decreases plasma cholesterol by binding cholesterol in the intestinal lumen and inhibiting its uptake into the body?

   a. Cholestyramine
   b. Ezetimibe
   c. Lovastatin
   d. Niacin

7. Which of the following drugs would be most effective at reducing hypertriglyceridemia?

   a. Cholestyramine
   b. Clofibrate
   c. Ezetimibe
   d. Fluvastatin

8. Which of the following drugs is associated with the highest potential incidence for myopathy and rhabdomyolysis?

   a. Colesevelam
   b. Evolocumab
   c. Ezetimibe
   d. Pravastatin

9. Which of the following drugs is also a vitamin?
    a. Colesevelam
    b. Ezetimibe
    c. Niacin
    d. Rosuvastatin

10. Which of the following drug classes is most efficacious in lowering LDL cholesterol?
    a. Fibrates
    b. Niacin
    c. Resins
    d. Statins

Antibacterial Agents

CASE STUDY

C.J. is a 56-year-old white woman with a 40-year history of type 1 diabetes mellitus. Two weeks ago, she suffered a myocardial infarction (MI) for which she was hospitalized for several days. Prior to her MI, C.J. had been evaluated at an outpatient wound clinic for neuropathic ulcers on both feet. Three weeks after her MI, C.J. returns to the wound clinic for her first treatment. The physical therapist notes increased erythema around the right foot ulcer since the evaluation. The therapist contacts the primary healthcare provider to report the patient's change in status. The wound is cultured and is positive for *Staphylococcus aureus*. The patient is given oral clindamycin to treat the wound infection and returns to the wound clinic the following week. The physical therapist notes that the erythema on the right foot has receded. As the therapist is taking wound measurements, C.J. mentions that she has been experiencing abdominal cramping and frequent bouts of watery diarrhea for the past several days. She has not reported this to her physician because she felt that this was a minor problem and did not want to "bother her doctor." The physical therapist discusses with C.J. that her diarrhea may be related to the antibiotic therapy and encourages her to relay the signs and symptoms to her physician as soon as possible.

INTRODUCTION TO ANTIMICROBIAL DRUGS

Infectious diseases are among the most common forms of illness. Thus, many patients undergoing physical rehabilitation may be taking one or more antimicrobial drugs. While many of these drugs may have little direct impact on functional rehabilitation outcomes, they certainly have an impact on the overall health status of the patient.

The next four chapters address agents used to treat infections caused by bacteria, viruses, fungi, protozoa, and helminths (worms). After gaining access into the human body, these pathogens can cause illnesses ranging from minor infections to life-threatening illnesses. Antimicrobial drugs are among the most dramatic examples of advances of modern medicine.

Many infectious diseases once considered incurable and lethal are now amenable to treatment, although the development of resistant organisms threatens the continued success of antimicrobial drugs. Antimicrobial drugs are classified and identified according to the primary type of infectious organism they are used to treat (eg, antibacterial, antiviral, antifungal).

The remarkably powerful and specific activity of antimicrobial drugs is due to their *selective toxicity*—that is, drugs are designed to selectively target structures that are either unique to microorganisms or much more important in them than in humans. Therefore, a general understanding of microbial structure and function is necessary to understand the mechanisms of action of antimicrobial agents. Notably, selective toxicity is *not* perfect, and antimicrobials may exert some adverse effects in humans.

BACTERIAL PATHOGENICITY

Bacterial infections harm humans in several ways. Bacteria can directly damage or destroy human cells by releasing toxins, and they can compete with human cells for vital nutrients. In addition, bacteria trigger the immunocompetent host to mount an immune response that may damage not only pathogenic bacteria, but also the host's cells and tissues.

It is noteworthy to mention that not all bacteria living *on* and *in* the human body are harmful. Recent attention and investigation have focused on understanding the role of a variety of microorganisms that live in association with the human body—the so-called *human microbiome*. In the average human, bacteria in particular outnumber human cells by a factor of 10. Bacteria that are part of our normal flora are generally not pathogenic and in fact may be essential for maintaining health. For example, *Escherichia coli* that normally inhabit the gastrointestinal (GI) tract assist in digestion of food, synthesize essential nutrients such as vitamin K, and inhibit the growth of other potentially pathogenic organisms. Antibiotic therapy—the use of antibacterial agents—often results in the eradication of normal gut flora. The result can be an intestinal environment conducive to the proliferation of pathogenic microbes (eg, yeasts, *Clostridium difficile*).

BACTERIAL STRUCTURE AND NOMENCLATURE

Target sites for antibiotics include the cell wall or membranes surrounding the bacterium, the bacterial deoxyribonucleic acid (DNA) or ribonucleic acid (RNA), or structures involved in bacterial reproduction (the ribosome and associated proteins). To understand the mechanisms of action for various antibiotics, the general structure of bacteria must be appreciated.

Fungi, protozoa, and multicellular organisms are eukaryotes that have membrane-bound nuclei containing their genetic material. In contrast, bacteria are single-celled prokaryotes that lack membrane-bound organelles, but still have a characteristic organization. All or most of the bacterial DNA forms a long circular molecule in a region called the nucleoid. In an area physically separate from the nucleoid, small circular DNA in the form of plasmids may also be present. Plasmids replicate independently of chromosomal DNA and often carry critical genes that benefit the bacterium's survival in certain conditions. Genes that confer resistance to antibiotics are often contained in plasmid DNA (ie, plasmid-mediated resistance). Both chromosomal nucleoid DNA and plasmid DNA are subject to mutations that can be passed on to daughter cells. Bacteria can also exchange genetic material by a process called conjugation, thus allowing passage of drug resistance genes without mutation. An RNA polymerase transcribes nucleoid and plasmid DNA into messenger RNA.

Ribosomal function is the same in prokaryotic and eukaryotic cells—ribosomes translate messenger RNA into a new protein chain, the final product of the gene. Ribosomal structure is characterized as 70S in prokaryotes and as 80S in eukaryotes. (The "S" unit refers to how a molecule sediments under centrifugal force in an ultracentrifuge.) The bacterial 70S ribosome is comprised of two major subunits: 30S and 50S. Certain antibiotic classes (eg, the aminoglycosides) specifically target the 70S ribosome.

All bacterial cells (except mycoplasmas) have a cell wall that lies external to the cytoplasmic membrane. The cell wall is a structure not found in eukaryotes. The cell wall's rigidity maintains the cell's integrity, preventing lysis due to high internal osmotic pressure. Bacteria are classified as *gram positive* or *gram negative* according to their cell wall structure. The primary structural component of the cell wall is a peptidoglycan, a polymer of sugars and charged amino acids, which makes the peptidoglycan highly polar. In gram-positive bacteria, the peptidoglycan forms a very thick hydrophilic layer external to the cell membrane. The thick hydrophilic surface of gram-positive bacteria can be digested by lysozyme (an enzyme present in body secretions and intracellular organelles), but it provides protection against most other enzymes and bile in the intestine. **Penicillin** and cephalosporin antibiotics inhibit synthesis of the bacterial cell wall by disrupting peptidoglycan formation. In gram-negative bacteria, the peptidoglycan layer is thinner and anchored to an overlying outer membrane (Figure 27-1). The outer membrane is relatively hydrophobic. To allow hydrophilic nutrients to enter the cell, gram-negative bacteria have special pores formed by proteins called porins.

The cell wall is a primary determinant of the ultimate shape of the bacterium, which is an important characteristic for bacterial identification. In general, the shape of bacteria can be categorized as spherical (cocci), rod (bacilli), or helical (spirilla). Although each bacterium is named according to its genus and species (eg, *Staphylococcus aureus*), bacteria are often categorized by common characteristics such as shape and histologic staining properties. For example, gram-positive cocci include bacteria that stain in a certain manner (determined by the gram-positive cell wall) and are spherical in shape (cocci). This group includes *S aureus* and *Streptococcus pneumoniae*.

A common way to classify antibiotics is on the basis of their site of action: (1) inhibitors of bacterial cell wall synthesis, (2) inhibitors of bacterial protein synthesis, and (3) inhibitors of bacterial DNA synthesis. Antimycobacterial drugs are discussed separately.

PRINCIPLES OF ANTIBIOTIC THERAPY

Some antibiotics are *bactericidal* (ie, kill bacteria), while others are *bacteriostatic* (ie, inhibit bacterial growth). Certain antibiotics may be bacteriostatic at lower concentrations and bactericidal at higher concentrations. Bacteriostatic antibiotics can successfully treat infections in individuals with intact

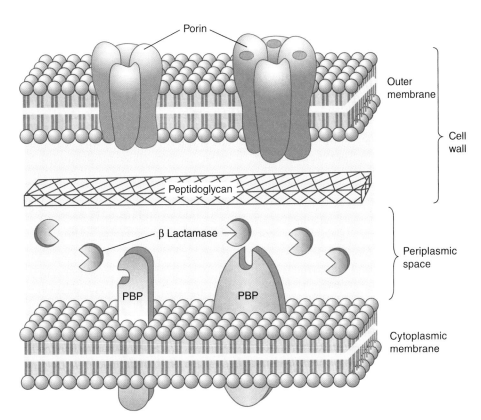

FIGURE 27-1 **A simplified diagram of the cell envelope of a gram-negative bacterium.** The outer membrane is a lipid bilayer present in gram-negative, but not gram-positive bacteria. Porins penetrate the outer membrane; these proteins form channels that provide hydrophilic access to the cytoplasmic membrane. The peptidoglycan layer, unique to bacteria, is much thicker in gram-positive bacteria than in gram-negative bacteria. The outer membrane (only in gram-negative bacteria) and the peptidoglycan layer constitute the cell wall. Penicillin-binding proteins (PBPs) are membrane proteins that cross-link peptidoglycan. If present, β-lactamases reside in the periplasmic space or on the outer surface of the cytoplasmic membrane. These enzymes may destroy β-lactam antibiotics that penetrate the outer membrane.

immune systems because they prevent the bacterial population from increasing, and allow host defense mechanisms to eradicate the remaining population. For bacteriostatic drugs (eg, tetracyclines), the concentrations that inhibit growth are much lower than those that kill bacteria. Bactericidal antibiotics are preferred for treating infections in immunocompromised individuals because they are able to eradicate an infection even in the absence of normal host defense mechanisms. For bactericidal drugs (eg, aminoglycosides), there is little difference between concentrations that inhibit growth of bacteria and those that kill bacteria.

Dosage regimens with antibiotics have traditionally used multiple daily doses to maintain plasma concentrations above the minimal inhibitory concentration (MIC) for as long as possible. However, the in vivo effectiveness of some antibiotics (eg, aminoglycosides) results from a *concentration-dependent* killing action. As the plasma level is increased above the MIC, these agents kill an increasing proportion of bacteria and do so at a more rapid rate. Many other antibiotics (eg, penicillins and cephalosporins) cause *time-dependent* killing of bacteria, wherein their in vivo efficacy is directly related to time above the MIC and becomes independent of concentration once the MIC has been reached.

Some drugs exert a *postantibiotic effect* in which inhibition of bacterial growth continues after plasma levels have fallen to low levels. The mechanisms of the postantibiotic effect are unclear, but may reflect the time required by bacteria to synthesize new enzymes and cellular components, persistence of the antibiotic at target binding sites, or enhanced susceptibility of bacteria to host defense mechanisms. The postantibiotic effect contributes to the efficacy of once-daily administration of aminoglycosides, and may also contribute to the efficacy of the fluoroquinolones.

ANTIBIOTIC RESISTANCE

The major problem threatening the continued success of *all* antimicrobial drugs—not just antibiotics—is the development of resistant organisms. The mechanisms underlying microbial resistance to drugs existed long before the clinical use of such drugs. Since these mechanisms are already present in nature, an inevitable consequence of antimicrobial use is the *selection* of resistant microorganisms. For example, to escape the effects of antibiotics, bacteria may produce drug-inactivating enzymes, change the structure of target receptors, increase antibiotic efflux via drug transporters, and decrease cell wall permeability to antibiotics. Many strategies have been employed to mitigate microbial resistance. These include the use of additional agents that protect against enzymatic inactivation, the use of antibiotic combinations, the introduction of new (and often expensive) chemical derivatives of established antibiotics, and efforts to avoid indiscriminate use or misuse of antibiotics. One must always consider that use of an antibiotic *now* can increase the opportunity for bacteria to develop resistance to that antibiotic in the future.

Antibiotic resistance is a worldwide public health challenge. The increasing prevalence of resistant organisms requires the use of more broad-spectrum, less effective, or more toxic antibiotics. Infections caused by antimicrobial-resistant pathogens are associated with higher costs, morbidity, and mortality. In the United States, the Centers for Disease Control and Prevention (CDC) estimates that at least 2 million people contract an antibiotic-resistant infection, and roughly 23,000 people die annually.

To address antibiotic resistance, attention has focused on eliminating misuse of antibiotics. Antibiotic misuse can occur in many ways. Clinically, misuse includes antibiotic use in people who are unlikely to have bacterial infections, use of antibiotics for unnecessarily long periods, and use of multiple drugs or broad-spectrum antibiotics when not needed. Agriculturally, large quantities of antibiotics have been used to stimulate animal growth and prevent infection, especially for animals raised in crowded conditions. This antibiotic use has added to selection pressure, eliminating only the most susceptible organisms and leaving the more resistant ones to proliferate. In 2013, the Food and Drug Administration (FDA) in the United States announced a program to phase out the nontherapeutic use of antibiotics in livestock.

Penicillins are among the most misused antibiotics, having been used irrationally for nonsusceptible infections and in agriculture for many decades. As a result, the prevalence of methicillin-resistant strains of *Staphylococcus aureus* (MRSA) continues to increase. Broad-spectrum penicillins also eradicate normal flora, thereby predisposing the patient to colonization and superinfection with opportunistic, drug-resistant species present within the hospital environment.

Addressing increasing antimicrobial resistance around the world is difficult because patients, prescribers, inpatient facilities, pharmaceutical companies, as well as agricultural users do not have adequate and recognizable incentives to act in ways that would help conserve antibiotic effectiveness. Collaborative global approaches that extend across multiple health and agricultural sectors will be needed to slow the tide of antimicrobial resistance.

INHIBITORS OF BACTERIAL CELL WALL SYNTHESIS

The major antibiotics that inhibit bacterial cell wall synthesis are penicillins and cephalosporins. These agents only kill bacterial cells that are actively growing and creating new cell walls. They are called β-lactam antibiotics because they share an unusual four-member ring structure called a β-lactam ring. The β-lactam antibiotics include some of the most effective, widely used, and well-tolerated antimicrobial agents.

The selective toxicity of the β-lactams and other cell wall synthesis inhibitors is due to specific actions on the synthesis of cell walls—structures that are unique to bacteria. More than 50 antibiotics that act as cell wall synthesis inhibitors are currently available, with individual spectra of activity that afford a wide range of clinical applications. Figure 27-2 outlines the cell wall synthesis inhibitors.

Penicillins

All penicillins are derivatives of 6-aminopenicillanic acid and contain a β-lactam ring structure that is essential for antibacterial activity. Penicillin subclasses have additional chemical modifications that confer differences in antimicrobial activity, susceptibility to acid and enzymatic hydrolysis, and biodisposition. Penicillins vary in their resistance to gastric acid and, therefore, vary in their oral bioavailability. Except for

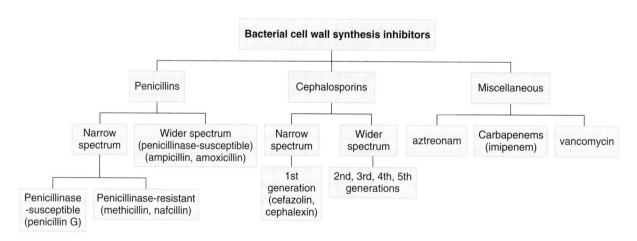

FIGURE 27-2 Classification of drugs that inhibit bacterial cell wall synthesis. Prototype agents are in parentheses.

amoxicillin, oral penicillins should generally *not* be given with food to minimize binding to food proteins and acid inactivation. Thus, patients are typically advised to take penicillins 1-2 hours before or after meals. Penicillins are not metabolized extensively; they are usually excreted unchanged in the urine via glomerular filtration and tubular secretion. **Ampicillin** and **nafcillin** are excreted partly in the bile. The plasma half-lives of most penicillins vary from 30 to 60 minutes. Two forms of **penicillin G**, the prototype of a subclass of penicillins with a limited antibacterial spectrum, are administered intramuscularly and have long plasma half-lives because the active drug is released very slowly into the blood. Most penicillins cross the blood-brain barrier only when the meninges are inflamed (eg, in meningitis).

Mechanisms of Action and Resistance

The β-lactam antibiotics inhibit cell wall synthesis by binding to specific receptor proteins called penicillin-binding proteins (PBPs) located in the bacterial cytoplasmic membrane. This binding inhibits the transpeptidation reaction that cross-links the peptidoglycan chain components of the cell wall, and activates autolytic enzymes that cause lesions in the bacterial cell wall (Figure 27-1).

The most common method of bacterial resistance to β-lactam antibiotics is the production of enzymes called β-lactamases (penicillinases) that hydrolyze the β-lactam ring of these drugs, resulting in the loss of antibacterial activity. Many bacteria (especially *Staphylococcus* species and many gram-negative organisms) produce β-lactamases. About 90% of all staphylococcal strains both in the hospital and in the community are β-lactamase producers. To prevent inactivation of the β-lactam ring, penicillins are sometimes administered in combination with inhibitors of bacterial β-lactamases (eg, clavulanic acid, sulbactam, tazobactam).

A second mechanism of resistance that bacteria exploit is structurally modifying their target PBPs. Modifications in target PBPs are responsible for methicillin resistance (in staphylococci) and penicillin resistance (in pneumococci and enterococci). In some gram-negative bacteria, resistance may be due to impaired penetration of antibiotics to their target PBPs. To cross the outer membrane that distinguishes gram-negative from gram-positive bacteria, β-lactams must enter the cell via porins (Figure 27-1). By altering porin structures, some bacteria may impede β-lactam access to their target PBPs. Finally, some gram-negative bacteria may produce efflux pumps that effectively expel some β-lactam agents that get past the outer membrane.

Clinical Uses

Figure 27-2 outlines penicillins into narrow and wider spectrum agents, with "spectrum" referring to the number of organisms against which they provide antibacterial activity. These antibiotics may also be classified by whether they are susceptible to bacterial penicillinase (β-lactamase).

Among the narrow-spectrum *penicillinase-susceptible agents,* penicillin G is the prototype. Clinical uses include treatment for infections caused by common streptococci, meningococci, gram-positive bacilli, and spirochetes. Many strains of pneumococci are now resistant to penicillins. Most strains of *Staphylococcus aureus* and a significant number of strains of *Neisseria gonorrhoeae* are resistant via production of β-lactamases. However, penicillin G is still the first-line drug for syphilis. **Penicillin V**, the oral equivalent of penicillin G, is only used in minor oropharyngeal infections due to its poor bioavailability, narrow spectrum, and need for multiple daily dosing. Instead, amoxicillin is often used.

The narrow-spectrum *penicillinase-resistant* subclass includes **methicillin**, nafcillin, and **oxacillin**. Methicillin, the prototype of this class, is no longer used clinically because of the high incidence of adverse effects, especially nephritis. The primary use of nafcillin and oxacillin is in the treatment of suspected or known methicillin-susceptible and penicillin-resistant staphylococcal infections. However, use of these drugs has decreased dramatically due to increasing rates of methicillin resistance in staphylococci (methicillin-resistant *S aureus* [MRSA] and methicillin-resistant *S epidermidis* [MRSE]). Notably, these two strains—important in many hospital-acquired infections—are resistant to all penicillins and are often resistant to multiple antimicrobial drugs. Vancomycin (see below) may be used in some of these cases.

Ampicillin and amoxicillin have a wider spectrum than penicillin G. Because these drugs are penicillinase susceptible, their antibacterial effect is enhanced when administered in combination with penicillinase inhibitors (eg, clavulanic acid). Ampicillin and amoxicillin (better oral absorption than ampicillin) are often used to treat urinary tract infections (UTIs), otitis media, pneumonia, and bacteremias resulting from infections with susceptible bacterial species. **Piperacillin** and **ticarcillin**, available as coformulations with penicillinase inhibitors, have activity against several gram-negative bacteria, including *Pseudomonas*, *Enterobacter*, and some *Klebsiella* species. Most drugs in this subclass have synergistic actions when used with aminoglycosides (inhibitors of protein synthesis discussed later in chapter).

Adverse Effects

The penicillins are remarkably nontoxic, which unfortunately may encourage inappropriate use. Most serious adverse drug effects (ADRs) are due to nephrotoxicity and hypersensitivity reactions. All penicillins are cross-sensitizing and cross-reacting, so cross-allergenicity among the different penicillins should be assumed. About 5-10% of individuals with a history of penicillin reaction have an allergic response when given a penicillin again. Allergic reactions include urticaria, severe pruritus, fever, joint swelling, hemolytic anemia, nephritis, and in rare cases anaphylaxis. Nafcillin is associated with neutropenia. Ampicillin frequently causes maculopapular skin rash that does not appear to be an allergic reaction.

Large oral doses of penicillins, especially ampicillin, may cause nausea, vomiting, and diarrhea. Gastrointestinal upset may be caused by direct irritation or by overgrowth of gram-positive organisms or yeasts. Ampicillin has been implicated in pseudomembranous colitis.

Cephalosporins

The cephalosporins are also β-lactam antibiotics. They vary in their antibacterial activity and are designated first-, second-, third-, fourth-, or fifth-generation drugs according to the order of their introduction into clinical use (Figure 27-2). Several cephalosporins are available for oral use, but most are administered parenterally. Cephalosporins with side chains may undergo hepatic metabolism, but the major elimination mechanism is renal excretion via active tubular secretion. **Cefoperazone** and **ceftriaxone** are excreted mainly in the bile. Most first- and second-generation cephalosporins do not enter the cerebrospinal fluid even when the meninges are inflamed.

Mechanisms of Action

Cephalosporins' bactericidal activity results from binding to PBPs in bacterial cell membranes and interfering with bacterial cell wall synthesis. Cephalosporins have a broader spectrum of activity than the penicillins because they are less susceptible to many penicillinases produced by staphylococci. However, bacterial resistance to cephalosporins can result from production of other β-lactamases, decreases in membrane permeability to cephalosporins, and altered PBP structures. Methicillin-resistant staphylococci are also resistant to cephalosporins.

Clinical Uses

Cefazolin (parenteral) and **cephalexin** (oral) are examples of first-generation cephalosporins. Clinical uses include treatment of infections caused by many strains of *E Coli, Klebsiella pneumoniae*, and gram-positive cocci. Cefazolin is the drug of choice for surgical prophylaxis and for many streptococcal and staphylococcal infections that require intravenous therapy. These agents are *not* active against MRSA, most gram-negative cocci, enterococci, and most gram-negative rods.

Second-generation agents include **cefaclor**, **cefamandole**, **cefuroxime**, **cefprozil**, **cefotetan**, and **cefoxitin**. Members of this subclass usually have less activity against gram-positive organisms than first-generation drugs, but have extended gram-negative coverage. Marked differences in activity, pharmacokinetics, and toxicity occur among second-generation agents. Examples of clinical uses include infections caused by *Bacteroides fragilis* (eg, peritonitis, diverticulitis) and *Haemophilus influenzae* or *Moraxella catarrhalis* (eg, sinusitis, otitis, lower respiratory infections).

Characteristic features of third-generation drugs (eg, **ceftazidime**, **cefoperazone**, **cefotaxime**, **ceftizoxime**, **ceftriaxone**, **cefixime**) include increased activity against gram-negative organisms resistant to other β-lactam drugs and

ability to penetrate the blood-brain barrier (except cefoperazone and cefixime). Individual drugs have activity against *Pseudomonas* (cefoperazone, ceftazidime) and *B fragilis* (ceftizoxime). Drugs in this subclass are usually reserved for treatment of serious infections (eg, bacterial meningitis) that are resistant to most other drugs. The exceptions are ceftriaxone (parenteral) and cefixime (oral), which are currently drugs of choice to treat gonorrhea. Likewise, in acute otitis media, a single injection of ceftriaxone is usually as effective as a 10-day treatment course with amoxicillin.

Cefepime is the only fourth-generation cephalosporin. The drug has the widest antibacterial spectrum of the cephalosporins, combining the gram-positive activity of the first-generation drugs and the broader gram-negative spectrum of the third-generation drugs. Cefepime is more resistant to β-lactamases produced by gram-negative organisms, including *Enterobacter, Haemophilus, Neisseria,* and some penicillin-resistant pneumococci.

Ceftaroline fosamil is the first fifth-generation cephalosporin. It is a prodrug of the active metabolite ceftaroline and is the first β-lactam antibiotic with activity against MRSA to be approved for clinical use in the United States. Though ceftaroline fosamil was approved to treat community-acquired pneumonia and skin and soft tissue infections, it has been used to treat complicated infections including bacteremia, endocarditis, and osteomyelitis.

Adverse Effects

Cephalosporins may elicit a variety of hypersensitivity reactions identical to those of penicillins, including fever, skin rashes, nephritis, granulocytopenia, hemolytic anemia, and anaphylaxis. However, the chemical nucleus of cephalosporins is sufficiently different from that of penicillins so that some individuals with a history of penicillin allergy may sometimes be treated successfully with a cephalosporin. However, individuals with a history of *anaphylaxis* to penicillins should not receive cephalosporins. Complete cross-hypersensitivity among different cephalosporins should be assumed.

Cephalosporins may cause pain at intramuscular injection sites and phlebitis after intravenous administration. They may increase the nephrotoxicity of aminoglycosides when the two are administered together. Drugs containing a methylthiotetrazole group (eg, cefamandole, cefoperazone, cefotetan) may cause hypoprothrombinemia and disulfiram-like reactions with ethanol.

Other β-Lactam Drugs

Several other β-lactam drugs are of clinical importance. **Aztreonam** is neither a penicillin nor a cephalosporin. It is a monobactam, named for its chemical structure that contains one β-lactam ring. Aztreonam is resistant to β-lactamases produced by certain gram-negative rods, but has no activity against gram-positive bacteria or anaerobes. The drug inhibits cell wall synthesis by preferentially binding to a specific penicillin-binding protein. It is synergistic with aminoglycosides. Aztreonam is administered intravenously, and is eliminated via renal tubular secretion. There is no cross-allergenicity with penicillins; penicillin-allergic patients tolerate aztreonam without reaction. Major toxicity is uncommon. Adverse effects include GI upset with possible superinfection, vertigo, and headache.

Imipenem, **doripenem**, **meropenem**, and **ertapenem** are carbapenems. While they contain the β-lactam ring structure, they have low susceptibility to β-lactamases. Carbapenems have wide activity against gram-positive cocci (including some penicillin-resistant pneumococci), gram-negative rods, and anaerobes. The carbapenems are administered parenterally, and are especially useful for infections caused by organisms resistant to other antibiotics. However, MRSA strains of staphylococci are resistant.

Because a renal enzyme inactivates imipenem, this drug is administered with **cilastatin**, an inhibitor of this enzyme. The ADRs of imipenem-cilastatin include GI distress, skin rash, and, at very high plasma levels, central nervous system (CNS) toxicity (confusion, encephalopathy, seizures). Meropenem, doripenem, and ertapenem are much less likely to cause seizures than imipenem. Individuals with penicillin allergy may be allergic to carbapenems, but the incidence is very low (< 1%). Ertapenem has a long half-life, and its intramuscular injection causes pain and irritation.

β-Lactamase Inhibitors

An obvious problem with using β-lactam antibiotics such as penicillins and cephalosporins is that many bacteria produce β-lactamases that inactivate these agents. **Clavulanic acid**, **sulbactam**, and **tazobactam** are β-lactamase inhibitors that have no antibacterial action themselves, but are potent inhibitors of many (not all) bacterial β-lactamases. These agents are only available in fixed combinations with certain penicillins and cephalosporins to treat infections caused by bacteria that produce β-lactamases.

Other Inhibitors of Cell Wall Synthesis

Vancomycin is a glycopeptide antibiotic produced by a strain of *Streptococcus*. The drug binds to a unique set of amino acids used in cross-linking the peptidoglycan cell wall. As a result, chains of the peptidoglycan cannot be cross-linked and the cell wall is disrupted, making the bacterial cell susceptible to lysis. Vancomycin is not absorbed from the GI tract, so the drug is only given orally to treat bacterial infections *within* the small intestine or colon. Given parenterally, vancomycin penetrates most tissues and is eliminated unchanged in the urine. Thus, dosage modification is mandatory in individuals with renal impairment.

Vancomycin has a narrow spectrum of activity, but this drug is important in the treatment of serious bloodstream infections and endocarditis caused by MRSA. In combination with other drugs, vancomycin is also recommended for treating meningitis caused by penicillin-resistant pneumococci. Oral vancomycin is a first-choice drug to treat moderate to severe colitis caused by *C difficile*. **Teicoplanin** and

telavancin, other glycopeptide antibiotics, have similar characteristics. Telavancin has a boxed warning due to nephrotoxicity. In addition, the drug is contraindicated in pregnant women because it is a potential teratogen.

Some strains of enterococci and staphylococci have become resistant to vancomycin (ie, vancomycin-resistant enterococci [VRE] and vancomycin-resistant *S aureus* [VRSA]). Resistance to vancomycin is due to a single amino acid change in the bacterial binding site for vancomycin, which significantly decreases its binding affinity. The prevalence of VRE is increasing and poses a serious clinical problem because such organisms usually exhibit multiple-drug resistance. Likewise, strains of MRSA have been reported with intermediate resistance to vancomycin, leading to treatment failures.

Frequent toxic effects of parenteral vancomycin include phlebitis at the site of administration, chills, fever, and nephrotoxicity. Rapid intravenous infusion may cause diffuse flushing ("red man syndrome") caused by histamine release. This reaction can be minimized using a slow infusion (preferred method) or pretreatment with an antihistamine. Ototoxicity is less common.

Daptomycin is a newer lipopeptide agent that is chemically different from vancomycin, but has a similar spectrum of activity and indications. Its advantage is that it may be active against several strains of VRE and VRSA. Daptomycin is not indicated for pneumonia because pulmonary surfactant antagonizes daptomycin. The ADRs include myopathies (generalized muscle pain, cramps, or weakness) associated with elevations in creatine kinase. Thus, patients given daptomycin should be monitored for skeletal muscle dysfunction and creatine kinase elevation. In addition, transitory peripheral neuropathies have been reported.

Other inhibitors of cell wall synthesis include **bacitracin**, **fosfomycin**, and **cycloserine**. Bacitracin is a peptide antibiotic that interferes with a late stage in cell wall synthesis in gram-positive organisms. Because of its marked nephrotoxicity, this antibiotic is limited to topical use. Typically, bacitracin is combined with polymyxin and neomycin in an ointment base for treating skin or mucous membrane infections due to mixed bacterial flora. Bacitracin solutions in saline can also be used for irrigation of joints, wounds, or the pleural cavity. Fosfomycin inhibits an early stage of bacterial cell wall synthesis. Oral fosfomycin may be used to treat uncomplicated UTIs and prostatitis. With multiple dosing, resistance emerges quickly and diarrhea is common. Cycloserine prevents formation of a functional bacterial peptidoglycan. Because of its potential neurotoxicity (tremors, seizures, psychosis), cycloserine is only used to treat strains of *Mycobacterium tuberculosis* (the causative agent of tuberculosis) that are resistant to first-line antituberculous drugs.

INHIBITORS OF BACTERIAL PROTEIN SYNTHESIS

The basic process by which mammalian and bacterial cells make proteins is similar. In both mammalian and bacterial cells, the specific genetic information contained within DNA

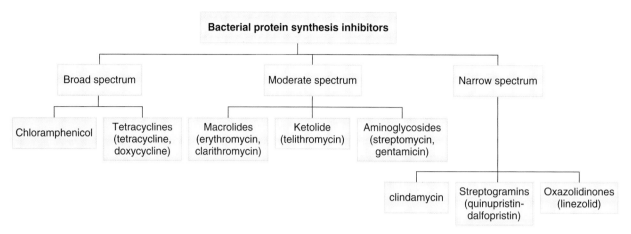

FIGURE 27-3 **Classification of drugs that inhibit bacterial protein synthesis based on spectrum of antibacterial activity.** Prototype agents are shown in parentheses.

is transcribed into messenger RNA (mRNA). Next, mRNA is translated into a new polypeptide or protein chain. The role of ribosomes in this process is to move along the mRNA chain, recruit transfer RNA (tRNA) molecules that carry different amino acids, and join the incoming amino acids to the growing polypeptide chain. There are critical differences between mammalian and bacterial ribosomal subunits and in the chemical composition and functional specificities of component nucleic acids and proteins. These differences form the basis of selective toxicity of certain antibiotics against bacteria without causing major effects on protein synthesis in mammalian cells.

Although drugs in this class vary dramatically in their chemical structure and spectrum of antimicrobial efficacy (Figure 27-3), each agent inhibits bacterial protein synthesis by acting at the level of the bacterial ribosome. **Chloramphenicol**, tetracyclines, and aminoglycosides were the first inhibitors of bacterial protein synthesis to be discovered. Due to their broad spectrum of antibacterial activity and low toxicities, these drugs were overused. As a result, many once highly susceptible bacterial species have become resistant, and these drugs are now used for more selected targets.

Mechanisms of Action

Most antibiotics in this subclass are *bacteriostatic* inhibitors of protein synthesis that act at the ribosomal level. Bacteria have 70S ribosomal complexes with 50S and 30S subunits. With the exception of tetracyclines and aminoglycosides, the binding sites for these antibiotics are on the 50S ribosomal subunit. Chloramphenicol, **clindamycin**, and the macrolides prevent a step called transpeptidation, in which the next new amino acid is added to the nascent peptide chain. Tetracyclines bind to the 30S ribosomal subunit at a site that blocks the binding of amino acid-carrying tRNA (charged tRNA) to the acceptor site of the ribosome-mRNA complex. **Linezolid** binds to a unique site on the 50S ribosome and blocks formation of the tRNA-ribosome-mRNA complex. The streptogramins are *bactericidal* for most susceptible organisms. They bind

to the 50S ribosomal subunit, and prevent extrusion of the nascent polypeptide chain. In addition, streptogramins inhibit enzymes that synthesize tRNA, leading to a decrease in free tRNA within the cell.

Chloramphenicol

Chloramphenicol is effective orally as well as parenterally, though the oral formulation in no longer available in the United States. Chloramphenicol is distributed throughout all tissues, readily crossing the placental and blood-brain barriers. The drug undergoes enterohepatic cycling, and is mostly inactivated by the liver. Because chloramphenicol inhibits hepatic drug-metabolizing enzymes, the half-lives of certain drugs (eg, phenytoin, tolbutamide, warfarin) is increased.

Clinical Uses

Chloramphenicol is a broad-spectrum antibiotic that is active against both aerobic and anaerobic gram-positive and gram-negative organisms. The drug is not active against *Chlamydia*. Clinically significant resistance occurs through the formation of plasmid-encoded enzymes that inactivate chloramphenicol. Because of its bacterial resistance and toxicity as well as the availability of many other effective agents, chloramphenicol has very few uses as a systemic drug and is rarely used in the United States. Chloramphenicol may be considered for treating serious typhus and Rocky Mountain spotted fever infections, or as an alternative to β-lactam antibiotics for treating bacterial meningitis in individuals with significant hypersensitivity reactions to penicillin. In many parts of the world, topical chloramphenicol (eye drops) is still commonly used in the treatment of conjunctivitis.

Adverse Effects

Adults (though not children) taking chloramphenicol occasionally develop nausea, vomiting, and diarrhea. Oral or vaginal candidiasis may occur due to alteration of normal microbial flora. A common ADR is a dose-related reversible suppression of red blood cell production. A rare adverse effect that is unrelated to dose is aplastic anemia, which involves suppressed production of *all* blood cells. Unfortunately, aplastic anemia occurs more frequently with prolonged use and is usually irreversible. If newborns are given high dosages, chloramphenicol may accumulate because infants lack effective metabolic mechanisms for the drug. The resulting gray baby syndrome is characterized by decreased red blood cells (cyanosis), vomiting, flaccidity, hypothermia, and cardiovascular collapse.

Tetracyclines

Tetracyclines (**tetracycline, doxycycline, minocycline, demeclocycline, tigecycline**) are broad-spectrum bacteriostatic antibiotics that inhibit protein synthesis in gram-positive and gram-negative bacteria, *Rickettsia* (the cause of Rocky Mountain spotted fever and some other difficult-to-treat infections)*, Chlamydia, Mycoplasma, Borrelia* (the cause of Lyme disease), and some protozoa. For the most part, the tetracyclines have only minor differences in their activities against specific organisms, with the exception of tigecycline that retains activity against organisms resistant to other tetracyclines. Susceptible microorganisms accumulate tetracyclines intracellularly via passive diffusion and energy-dependent transport systems in their cell membranes. Tetracyclines have little effect on mammalian protein synthesis because an active efflux mechanism prevents their intracellular accumulation.

Pharmacokinetics and Mechanisms of Resistance

Oral absorption for each of the drugs in this class is variable and may be impaired by foods and multivalent cations (calcium, iron, aluminum). For example, tetracycline and demeclocyline should be taken on an empty stomach, while oral absorption of doxycycline and minocycline is not impaired by food. Because tigecycline has very poor oral absorption, this tetracycline is formulated only for intravenous use. Tetracyclines are distributed widely and cross the placental barrier. All of the tetracyclines undergo enterohepatic cycling. Doxycycline is excreted mainly in feces; the other tetracyclines are eliminated primarily in the urine. Tetracyclines are classified as short-acting (tetracycline), intermediate-acting (demeclocyline), and long-acting (doxycycline and minocycline) based on their half-lives. Tigecycline has the longest half-life of the tetracyclines.

Plasmid-mediated resistance to tetracyclines is widespread. The most important resistance mechanisms are the development of efflux pumps for active extrusion of tetracyclines and ribosomal protein modification. Plasmids that include genes involved in producing efflux pumps for tetracyclines commonly include resistance genes for multiple antibiotics. Many tetracycline-resistant organisms are still susceptible to tigecycline because this drug is not a substrate of the efflux pumps.

Clinical Uses

A tetracycline is the drug of choice in infections caused by *Mycoplasma pneumoniae* (in adults), *Chlamydia, Rickettsia,* and *Vibrio* (eg, cholera). Specific tetracyclines are used in the treatment of GI ulcers caused by *Helicobacter pylori* (tetracycline), in Lyme disease (doxycycline), and sometimes in the meningococcal carrier state (minocycline), if the strain is not resistant. Doxycycline is sometimes used in the prevention of malaria and in the treatment of amebiasis (Chapter 29). Doxycycline is also an alternative drug in the treatment of syphilis in people with penicillin allergy. In combinations with other drugs, the tetracyclines can be used for treating plague, tularemia, and brucellosis. Other uses include the treatment of respiratory infections caused by susceptible organisms, leptospirosis, some nontuberculous mycobacterial infections, and acne. Demeclocycline was rarely used as an antibacterial. Rather, this drug is used more in the treatment of inappropriate antidiuretic hormone (ADH) secretion because it inhibits the renal actions of ADH.

Tigecycline has a broader spectrum than the other tetracyclines because it is not affected by the common resistance mechanisms. Tigecycline's antimicrobial activity includes gram-positive cocci resistant to methicillin (MRSA strains) and vancomycin (VRE strains), β-lactamase-producing gram-negative bacterial strains, anaerobes, chlamydiae, and mycobacteria.

Adverse Effects

Hypersensitivity reactions to tetracyclines are uncommon. Most of the ADRs are due to direct toxicity of the tetracycline agent or due to alterations in microbial flora. Effects on the GI system range from mild nausea and diarrhea to severe, possibly life-threatening colitis. Disturbances in the normal flora are due to suppression of tetracycline-susceptible organisms and overgrowth of resistant organisms, especially pseudomonas, staphylococci, and candida. This can result in intestinal disturbances, anal pruritus, vaginal or oral candidiasis, or enterocolitis. However, the risk of *C difficile* colitis may be lower with the tetracyclines than with other antibiotics.

Tetracyclines bind to calcium deposited in newly formed bone or teeth in young children. Fetal exposure to tetracyclines may lead to tooth enamel dysplasia and discoloration and irregularities in bone growth. Although usually contraindicated in pregnancy, there may be situations in which the benefit of administering tetracyclines outweighs the risk. If taken for long periods of time in children under 8 years of age, tetracyclines may cause similar changes in teeth and bone. High doses of tetracyclines, especially in pregnant women and those with preexisting hepatic disease, may impair liver function and lead to hepatic necrosis. Likewise, in individuals with kidney disease, tetracyclines may exacerbate renal dysfunction. Systemic tetracyclines may enhance skin photosensitivity, particularly in fair-skinned individuals. Dose-dependent reversible dizziness, vertigo, and tinnitus have been reported with doxycycline and minocycline.

Macrolides

The macrolide antibiotics **erythromycin**, **azithromycin**, and **clarithromycin** are large cyclic lactone ring structures with attached sugars. The macrolides have good oral bioavailability, but azithromycin absorption is impeded by food. Macrolides distribute to most body tissues, but azithromycin is unique in that the levels achieved in tissues and in phagocytes are considerably higher than those in the plasma. The elimination of erythromycin (via biliary excretion) and clarithromycin (via hepatic metabolism and urinary excretion of intact drug) is fairly rapid (half-lives 2-6 hours). In contrast, azithromycin is eliminated slowly (half-life 2-4 days), mainly in urine as unchanged drug. Oral **fidaxomicin**, a narrow-spectrum macrolide with negligible systemic absorption used to treat *C difficile* infection, is discussed in Chapter 30.

Resistance to macrolide antibiotics typically involves efflux pump mechanisms and the production of an enzyme (methylase) that alters the drugs' ribosomal binding site. Cross-resistance among the macrolides is complete; that is, if an organism is resistant to one macrolide agent, it will be resistant to all other macrolides. In the case of methylase-producing bacterial strains, there is partial cross-resistance with other drugs that bind to the same ribosomal site as macrolides, including clindamycin and streptogramins. Resistance in *Enterobacteriaceae* is due to formation of drug-metabolizing esterases.

Clinical Uses

Erythromycin, the prototype in this class, has a narrower spectrum of action but continues to be active against several important pathogens: many species of *Campylobacter, Chlamydia, Mycoplasma, Legionella,* gram-positive cocci (including β-lactamase-producing staphylococci), and some gram-negative organisms. Erythromycin does *not* have activity against MRSA or penicillin-resistant *Streptococcus pneumoniae.*

The spectra of activity of azithromycin and clarithromycin are similar to erythromycin, but include greater activity against *Chlamydia, Mycobacterium avium* complex, and *Toxoplasma* species. Clarithromycin is approved for prophylaxis against and treatment of *M avium* complex and as a component of drug regimens for ulcers caused by *H pylori.* Because of its long half-life, the use of azithromycin may permit one-daily dosing and shortening of the duration of antibiotic treatment in many cases.

Adverse Effects

Oral administration of macrolide antibiotics often causes anorexia, nausea, vomiting, and diarrhea. Stimulation of gut motility is the most common reason for discontinuing erythromycin and choosing another antibiotic. This action is sometimes exploited therapeutically to treat patients with gastroparesis. A hypersensitivity-based acute cholestatic hepatitis (fever, jaundice, impaired liver function) may occur with **erythromycin estolate**, an older formulation of the drug. This condition usually resolves. Because erythromycin and clarithromycin inhibit several hepatic cytochrome P450 (CYP) enzymes, these drugs increase plasma levels of anticoagulants, carbamazepine, cisapride, digoxin, and theophylline. Drug interactions are uncommon with azithromycin because this agent does not inhibit CYPs.

Ketolide: Telithromycin

Ketolides are structurally related to macrolides. At the time of this writing, **telithromycin** is the only ketolide available. Telithromycin has limited clinical availability because its use can result in hepatitis and liver failure. Many macrolide-resistant microbial strains are susceptible to telithromycin because the drug binds more tightly to bacterial ribosomes and is a poor substrate for bacterial efflux pumps that mediate resistance. Telithromycin is currently only indicated for treatment of mild to moderately severe community-acquired bacterial pneumonia. Anyone receiving this drug must be given an FDA-approved patient medication guide detailing the drug's risks.

Clindamycin

Clindamycin inhibits bacterial protein synthesis via a mechanism similar to that of the macrolides, although it is not chemically related. Mechanisms of resistance include alteration of the drug's ribosomal binding site and enzymatic inactivation of the drug. Cross-resistance between clindamycin and the macrolides is common. Gram-negative aerobes are intrinsically resistant because the cell wall is impermeable to clindamycin. The drug is available by oral, intravenous, and topical administration methods. Good tissue penetration occurs after oral absorption. Clindamycin is eliminated partly by metabolism and partly by biliary and renal excretion.

Clindamycin is indicated for treating skin and soft tissue infections caused by streptococci and staphylococci. The drug may be active against community-acquired strains of MRSA, though resistance is increasing. Clindamycin is used in the treatment of severe infections caused by anaerobes such as *Bacteroides* (most common bacteria in the colon) that often participate in mixed infections. Clindamycin (sometimes in combination with an aminoglycoside or cephalosporin) is used to treat: penetrating wounds of the abdomen and the gut; infections originating in the female genital tract (eg, septic abortion and pelvic abscesses); and lung and periodontal abscesses. Clindamycin has been used as a back-up drug against gram-positive cocci, and is currently recommended for prophylaxis of endocarditis in individuals with cardiac valve disease who are allergic to penicillin. In people with AIDS, clindamycin plus primaquine is an effective alternative to trimethoprim-sulfamethoxazole for moderate to moderately severe *Pneumocystis jirovecii* pneumonia. For AIDS-related toxoplasmosis of the brain, clindamycin is used in combination with pyrimethamine. Adverse effects of clindamycin include GI irritation, skin rashes, neutropenia, and hepatic dysfunction. Use of clindamycin is also a risk factor for diarrhea and colitis due to *C difficile.*

Streptogramins

Quinupristin-dalfopristin is a combination of two streptogramins. The combination has rapid bactericidal activity that lasts longer than the half-lives of the individual compounds. Antibacterial activity includes penicillin-resistant pneumococci, methicillin-resistant and vancomycin-resistant staphylococci (MRSA and VRSA, respectively), and vancomycin-resistant *Enterococcus faecium*. Administered intravenously, the combination product may cause pain at the infusion site and an arthralgia-myalgia syndrome. Streptogramins are potent inhibitors of CYP3A4 and thus increase plasma levels of many drugs, including cisapride, cyclosporine, diazepam, nonnucleoside reverse transcriptase inhibitors, and warfarin.

Oxazolidinones

Linezolid was the first drug in the class of antibiotics called the oxazolidinones. Linezolid binds to a unique site on one of the bacterial ribosomal subunits. Resistance can occur with decreased affinity of linezolid for this binding site. There is currently no cross-resistance with other protein synthesis inhibitors. Linezolid is used in the treatment of vancomycin-resistant *E faecium* infections, healthcare-associated and community-acquired pneumonia, and complicated or uncomplicated skin and soft tissue infections caused by susceptible gram-positive bacteria. The drug is also used in the treatment of multidrug-resistant tuberculosis and *Nocardia* infections. Linezolid is available in both oral and parenteral formulations. The primary adverse effect is hematologic; thrombocytopenia and neutropenia occur, most commonly in immunosuppressed patients. When administered with serotonergic drugs, linezolid has been associated with cases of serotonin syndrome.

Tedizolid is the active metabolite of the prodrug tedizolid phosphate. This new oxazolidinone is highly active against gram-positive bacteria, including MRSA. Orally or intravenously, the drug can be used to treat acute skin and soft tissue infections. Potential advantages over linezolid include increased potency against staphylococci and once-daily dosing (due to longer half-life). Tedizolid may have lower risk of serotonergic toxicity.

Aminoglycosides

Important aminoglycosides include **gentamicin**, **tobramycin**, **amikacin**, **streptomycin**, **neomycin**, and **spectinomycin**. Aminoglycosides are useful mainly against aerobic gram-negative rods. A primary advantage of aminoglycosides is that they can often be used in once-daily dosing protocols, which lends itself to outpatient therapy and can be more effective and less toxic than traditional dosing regimens. Aminoglycosides have greater efficacy when administered as a single large dose because their bactericidal effectiveness is concentration dependent. That is, as the plasma level is increased above the MIC, aminoglycosides kill an increasing proportion of bacteria and do so more rapidly. Aminoglycosides can also exert

a postantibiotic effect, in which their killing action continues when plasma levels have declined below measurable levels. A single large daily dose of an aminoglycoside generally results in fewer adverse effects because toxicity depends both on a critical plasma concentration and on the time that such a level is exceeded. With single large doses, the time above such a threshold is shorter than with administration of multiple smaller doses.

The aminoglycosides are structurally related amino sugars attached by glycosidic linkages. All of the aminoglycosides are polar compounds, so they are not absorbed after oral administration. Therefore, they must be given intramuscularly or intravenously for systemic effect. They have limited tissue penetration and do not readily cross the blood-brain barrier. The major mode of excretion is via the kidney, and plasma levels of these drugs are greatly affected by changes in renal function. With normal renal function, the elimination half-life of aminoglycosides is 2-3 hours. For traditional dosing regimens of 2 or 3 times daily, peak serum levels are measured 30-60 minutes after administration and trough level just before the next dose. With once-daily dosing, peak plasma levels are less important since they will be expectedly high (though maximal doses are established).

Mechanism of Action and Resistance

To kill bacteria, aminoglycosides must penetrate the bacterial cell envelope. This process is partly dependent on oxygen-dependent active transport; therefore, these agents have minimal activity against strict anaerobes. To assist entry of aminoglycosides into bacterial cells, aminoglycosides are almost always coadministered with a cell wall synthesis inhibitor such as a β-lactam antibiotic.

Once inside the bacterial cell, aminoglycosides bind to the 30S ribosomal subunit and interfere with protein synthesis in at least three ways: (1) blocking formation of the initiation complex, (2) causing misreading of mRNA, and (3) inhibition of translocation (Figure 27-4).

Bacterial resistance to the aminoglycosides can be due to failure of the drugs to penetrate the bacterial cell or due to plasmid-mediated formation of inactivating enzymes. The latter effect is the primary mechanism of resistance, though individual aminoglycosides have varying susceptibilities to such enzymes.

Clinical Uses

Aminoglycosides are mostly used against gram-negative enteric (ie, intestinal) bacteria. The main differences among the individual aminoglycosides lie in their activities against specific organisms, particularly gram-negative rods. Gentamicin, tobramycin, and amikacin are important drugs for the treatment of serious infections caused by aerobic gram-negative bacteria, including *E coli* and *Enterobacter, Klebsiella* (especially important in respiratory infections and urinary tract infections), *Proteus, Providencia, Pseudomonas,* and *Serratia* (important in septicemia and pulmonary infections) species. These aminoglycosides also have activity against other species (eg, *H influenzae, Moraxella*

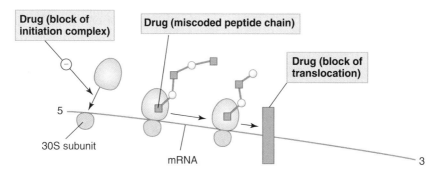

Normal bacterial cell

Initiation codon

50S subunit

Nascent peptide chain

5

30S subunit

mRNA

3

Aminoglycoside-treated bacterial cell

Drug (block of initiation complex)

Drug (miscoded peptide chain)

Drug (block of translocation)

5

30S subunit

mRNA

3

FIGURE 27-4 **Mechanisms of action of the aminoglycosides.** Normal bacterial protein synthesis is shown in the top panel. In the bottom panel, three unique aminoglycoside effects have been described: block of formation of the initiation complex; miscoding of amino acids in the nascent peptide chain due to misreading of the mRNA; and block of translocation on the mRNA. Block of movement of the ribosome may occur after the formation of a single initiation complex, resulting in an mRNA chain with only a single ribosome on it, a so-called monosome.

catarrhalis, Shigella), although they are not drugs of choice for infections caused by these organisms. When used alone, aminoglycosides are not reliably effective for treating infections caused by gram-positive cocci. Antibacterial synergy may occur when aminoglycosides are used in combination with cell wall synthesis inhibitors. For example, aminoglycosides may be combined with penicillins to treat pseudomonal, listerial (important in some cases of meningitis), and enterococcal infections. However, due to toxicity, these combinations are used less often when alternative regimens are available.

Resistance to streptomycin has occurred for most previously susceptible bacterial species. Now, streptomycin is mainly used as a second-line agent in the treatment of tuberculosis, but the drug is only used in combination with other agents to prevent emergence of resistance. For nontuberculous infections, intramuscularly administered streptomycin can be given in combination with an oral tetracycline in the treatment of plague, tularemia (rabbit fever), and sometimes brucellosis. Streptomycin may be useful to treat some enterococcal infections that are resistant to several other aminoglycosides. Because of the risk of irreversible vestibular dysfunction, streptomycin should not be used when other drugs will serve.

Owing to its toxic potential and higher resistance rates than other aminoglycosides, neomycin is only used topically or locally (eg, in the GI tract to eliminate aerobic bowel flora). Chapter 29 discusses the use of **paromomycin** as an

alternative drug for treating visceral leishmaniasis and intestinal infections with other parasites. Spectinomycin is structurally related to the aminoglycosides. Although this drug is no longer available in the United States, it is an important backup drug that is administered as a single intramuscular dose for treating gonorrhea, most commonly in individuals with allergic reactions to β-lactam antibiotics.

Adverse Effects

All aminoglycosides are ototoxic and nephrotoxic. Auditory or vestibular damage (or both) may occur and may be irreversible. Auditory impairment, which may manifest as tinnitus and hearing loss (initially high frequency), is more likely with amikacin. Vestibular dysfunction that may manifest as vertigo, ataxia, and loss of balance is more likely with gentamicin and tobramycin. These toxic risks are proportionate to the plasma levels of the aminoglycoside. Precautions taken to reduce these risks include once-daily dosing (versus traditional dosing regimens), monitoring plasma drug levels with appropriate dose modification, and avoiding any additive ototoxicity during dosing (eg, avoiding use of loop diuretics). Because ototoxicity has been reported after fetal exposure, aminoglycosides are contraindicated in pregnancy unless their potential benefits are judged to outweigh risk.

Renal toxicity usually takes the form of acute tubular necrosis, which is often reversible. This ADR is more common

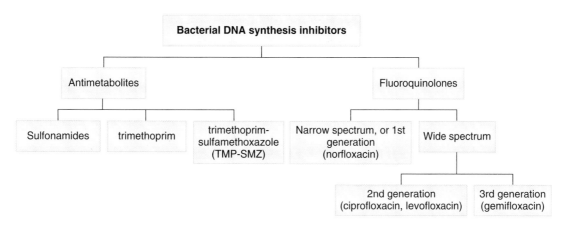

FIGURE 27-5 **Drugs that inhibit bacterial DNA synthesis: sulfonamides, trimethoprim, and fluoroquinolones.** Prototype agents are shown in parentheses.

in older adults and in those concurrently receiving amphotericin B, cephalosporins, or vancomycin. Gentamicin and tobramycin are the most nephrotoxic aminoglycosides. Allergic skin reactions may occur in patients and contact dermatitis may occur in healthcare personnel handling these drugs. Neomycin is most likely to cause this effect.

INHIBITORS OF BACTERIAL DNA SYNTHESIS

The sulfonamides, **trimethoprim**, and the fluoroquinolones comprise the group of drugs that exert antibacterial effects by interfering with bacterial DNA synthesis (Figure 27-5).

Sulfonamides and Trimethoprim

Mechanism of Action and Pharmacokinetics

Sulfonamides and trimethoprim are called antifolate drugs because they interfere with folic acid synthesis. Folic acid and folate are forms of vitamin B_9. Folic acid is the synthetic form found in fortified foods and supplements, and folate is the anionic form found naturally in foods. Folic acid is necessary for DNA replication; thus, it is necessary for production and maintenance of new cells (Chapter 11). While mammals rely on exogenous (ie, dietary) folate, many bacteria cannot and therefore must rely on enzymes to synthesize folate from its precursor, para-aminobenzoic acid (PABA). Antifolate drugs inhibit folic acid synthesis at different stages (Figure 27-6). Their selective toxicity results from the fact that mammalian cells utilize dietary folic acid, so inhibition of folic acid synthesis will primarily affect bacteria.

Sulfonamides competitively inhibit dihydropteroate synthase and can also act as substrates for this enzyme, resulting in the formation of nonfunctional forms of folic acid. Trimethoprim selectively inhibits bacterial dihydrofolate reductase, which prevents formation of the active form of folic acid. Bacterial dihydrofolate reductase is 4-5 orders of magnitude

more sensitive to trimethoprim inhibition than the mammalian form of dihydrofolate reductase. Sulfonamides are infrequently used as monotherapy because microbial resistance is common. The combination of **trimethoprim and sulfamethoxazole** (**TMP-SMZ**) causes a *sequential blockade* of folic acid synthesis, resulting in a synergistic and often bactericidal action against a wide spectrum of microorganisms (Figure 27-6). Resistance to this drug combination occurs but has been relatively slow in development.

The sulfonamides are weakly acidic compounds that have a chemical nucleus resembling PABA, the substrate with which they compete. Individual sulfonamide drugs differ mainly in their pharmacokinetic properties and clinical uses. Shared pharmacokinetic features include modest tissue penetration, hepatic metabolism, and excretion of both intact drug and acetylated metabolites in the urine. Sulfonamides

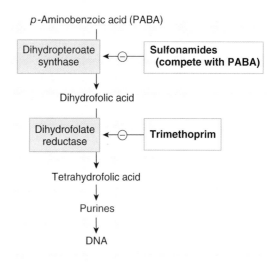

FIGURE 27-6 **Inhibitory effects of sulfonamides and trimethoprim on folic acid synthesis.** Inhibition of two successive steps in the formation of tetrahydrofolic acid constitutes sequential blockade and results in antibacterial synergy.

can be divided into three major groups: (1) oral absorbable, (2) oral nonabsorbable, and (3) topical. The oral absorbable agents have a wide distribution, including the CNS, placenta, and fetus.

Trimethoprim is a weak base and is trapped in acidic environments, reaching high concentrations in prostatic and vaginal fluids. A large fraction of trimethoprim is excreted unchanged in the urine.

Clinical Uses

Among the oral absorbable sulfonamides, sulfamethoxazole is only used as a fixed-dose combination with trimethoprim (TMP-SMZ) in the United States. The drug combination is active against a wide variety of bacteria, including both methicillin-sensitive and methicillin-resistant *S aureus*. TMP-SMZ is effective for treating UTIs, prostatitis, uncomplicated skin and soft tissue infections, and bone and joint infections. This drug combination is also effective for infections such as *P jiroveci* pneumonia, toxoplasmosis, and nocardiosis (Chapter 29). Oral **sulfadiazine plus pyrimethamine** (a dihydrofolate reductase inhibitor) works synergistically as a first-line treatment for toxoplasmosis. **Sulfasalazine** is the oral nonabsorbable agent commonly used in inflammatory bowel disease (eg, ulcerative colitis, enteritis). Several sulfonamides are used topically to treat bacterial ophthalmic and wound infections. **Sodium sulfacetamide** ophthalmic solution or ointment is effective for treating bacterial conjunctivitis. **Silver sulfadiazine** cream is used to help prevent infection of burn wounds.

Adverse Effects

Adverse effects of the sulfonamides include allergic reactions, hepatotoxicity, nephrotoxicity, and GI discomfort such as nausea, vomiting, and diarrhea. Allergic reactions, including skin rashes and fever, are common. Historically, cross-allergenicity among the individual sulfonamides was assumed. However, recent evidence suggests that this is not the case and many individuals that are allergic to nonantibiotic sulfonamides (eg, oral hypoglycemics, thiazides) can tolerate the sulfonamide antibiotics. Common drug interactions include competition with warfarin and methotrexate for plasma protein binding, which transiently increases the plasma levels of these drugs. Sulfonamides can displace bilirubin from plasma proteins, with the risk of severe newborn jaundice and kernicterus if used in the third trimester of pregnancy. Persons with glucose-6-phosphate dehydrogenase (G6PD) deficiency may suffer hemolysis if sulfonamides are given.

Trimethoprim may cause the predictable adverse effects of an antifolate drug, including megaloblastic anemia, leukopenia, and granulocytopenia. These effects are usually ameliorated by supplementary folinic acid. The combination of TMP-SMX may also cause any of the ADRs associated with sulfonamides. Individuals with AIDS given TMP-SMX have a high incidence of adverse effects, including fever, rashes, leukopenia, and diarrhea.

Fluoroquinolones

Mechanism of Action and Pharmacokinetics

Fluoroquinolones are usually bactericidal against a variety of gram-positive and gram-negative organisms. Fluoroquinolones selectively inhibit two enzymes critical for bacterial DNA synthesis: topoisomerase II (DNA gyrase) and topoisomerase IV. Inhibition of DNA gyrase prevents relaxation of positively supercoiled DNA, a step that is required for normal transcription. Inhibition of topoisomerase IV interferes with the separation of replicated chromosomal DNA during cell division. Like aminoglycosides, the fluoroquinolones also exhibit postantibiotic effects. Resistance has emerged rapidly to the older fluoroquinolones. Resistance to one fluoroquinolone—particularly if it is of a high level—generally indicates cross-resistance to all other fluoroquinolones.

All of the fluoroquinolones have good oral bioavailability, although some antacids that contain multivalent cations may interfere. All except **norfloxacin** penetrate most tissues and achieve adequate plasma levels for use in systemic infections. Elimination of most fluoroquinolones is through the kidneys; dosage reductions are usually needed in renal dysfunction. The exception is **moxifloxacin**, which is eliminated by hepatic metabolism and biliary excretion. Half-lives of fluoroquinolones are usually 3-8 hours, but the agents eliminated by nonrenal routes have half-lives from 10 to 20 hours.

Fluoroquinolones are classified by "generation" based on their antimicrobial spectrum of activity (Figure 27-5). Norfloxacin, a first-generation agent that is no longer available in the United States, has the least activity against both gram-negative and gram-positive organisms. Second-generation fluoroquinolones include **ciprofloxacin, levofloxacin, enoxacin, lomefloxacin, ofloxacin,** and **pefloxacin**. These agents have excellent activity against gram-negative bacteria and moderate to good activity against gram-positive cocci. In the United States, ciprofloxacin and levofloxacin are the two most frequently systemically administered fluoroquinolones. Ciprofloxacin is the most active against gram-negative bacteria, especially *P aeruginosa*. Methicillin-susceptible *S aureus* strains are usually susceptible to this group, but methicillin-resistant strains of staphylococcus are usually resistant. To help prevent emergence of resistance, fluoroquinolones are typically given with a second drug (eg, rifampin) when treating staphylococcal strains. The third-generation fluoroquinolones (**gatifloxacin, gemifloxacin,** and **moxifloxacin**) are not as active as the second-generation agents against gram-negative organisms, but have improved activity against gram-positive organisms, including *S pneumoniae* and some strains of staphylococci.

Clinical Uses

All of the fluoroquinolones (except for moxifloxacin) are effective in the treatment of UTIs caused by many bacterial strains. Fluoroquinolones (except norfloxacin) have been used widely for respiratory tract, skin, bone, intra-abdominal, joint, and soft tissue infections caused by many drug-resistant organisms including *Pseudomonas* and *Enterobacter*. Ciprofloxacin is the first-line drug for prophylaxis and treatment of anthrax, whereas levofloxacin is only approved for prophylaxis of anthrax. Fluoroquinolones have also been used in the meningococcal carrier state, for prophylaxis of bacterial infections in neutropenic patients, and as part of the multidrug regimen in the treatment of tuberculosis.

Adverse Effects

Overall, fluoroquinolones are very well tolerated. Gastrointestinal distress is the most common ADR. In addition, these drugs may cause skin rashes, headache, dizziness, insomnia, abnormal liver function tests, and photosensitivity. Some fluoroquinolones prolong the QT_c interval. Their use should therefore be avoided in individuals with known prolongation of the QT_c interval and those on certain antiarrhythmic or other drugs that increase the QT_c interval.

Fluoroquinolones are not recommended for use in children or in pregnancy because they have caused cartilage problems in animal models. Tendonitis is a complication that may be serious because of the risk of tendon rupture. Risk factors for tendonitis include older age, renal insufficiency, and concurrent glucocorticoid use. Peripheral neuropathy may develop any time during treatment with fluoroquinolones. Neuropathy may persist for months to years after drug administration has ceased. In some cases, the neuropathy may be permanent. Last, because of the effect of systemic gatifloxacin on plasma glucose levels in people with diabetes, gatifloxacin is now only available as an ophthalmic preparation in the United States. Although many of these potential ADRs are not common, the FDA has required a boxed warning on all fluoroquinolones that these drugs be reserved for those individuals who do not have alternative treatment options.

ANTIMYCOBACTERIAL DRUGS

Mycobacteria are slow-growing aerobic gram-positive bacteria that are widespread in the environment and in animals. The peptidoglycan layer has a different chemical basis than gram-positive or gram-negative bacteria. The outer envelope contains a variety of complex lipids called mycolic acids, which create a waxy layer that provides resistance to drying and other environmental factors. As a result, mycobacteria can survive for prolonged periods in the environment and are effectively transmitted by airborne droplets. After entering host cells, mycobacteria survive as intracellular parasites in macrophages.

Mycobacterial infections are generally slowly developing chronic conditions. Because mycobacterial cell wall components promote immunologic reactions, a significant portion of the clinical pathology is attributable to the host immune response rather than to direct bacterial toxicity. For all mycobacterial infections, social and environmental factors as well as genetic predisposition play a role. Major human pathogens include *M tuberculosis* and *M leprae*, the causative agents of tuberculosis and leprosy, respectively. Mycobacteria other than tuberculosis are associated with several other conditions, usually in immunocompromised individuals. In the United States, *M avium* complex is an increasingly important pathogen in people with AIDS.

Figure 27-7 outlines the drugs used against major mycobacterial infections. Chemotherapy for tuberculosis, leprosy, and other nontuberculous mycobacteria is complicated by numerous factors, including: (1) limited information about the mechanisms of antimycobacterial drug actions; (2) the rapid development of resistance; (3) the intracellular location of mycobacteria; (4) the chronic nature of mycobacterial disease that requires protracted drug treatment (months to years, depending on which drugs are used) that is associated with drug toxicities; and (5) patient compliance with the regimen. Chemotherapy of mycobacterial infections almost always involves prolonged use of drug combinations of two or more drugs to delay the emergence of resistance and to enhance antimycobacterial efficacy.

Drugs Used in Tuberculosis

The major drugs used in tuberculosis are **isoniazid (INH)**, **rifampin**, **ethambutol**, and **pyrazinamide**. Actions of these agents on *M tuberculosis* are bactericidal or bacteriostatic, depending on drug concentration and strain susceptibility. Treatment of pulmonary tuberculosis usually begins with a three- or four-drug combination regimen depending on the known or anticipated rate of resistance to INH. Table 27-1 outlines recommended treatment regimens for drug-susceptible tuberculosis. Therapy is typically initiated with INH, rifampin,

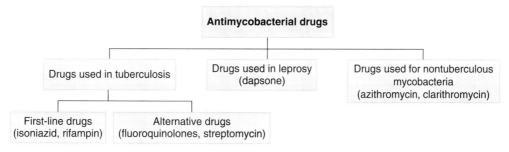

FIGURE 27-7 **Drugs that inhibit mycobacteria can be classified according to their use in tuberculosis, leprosy, and nontuberculous mycobacterial infections.** Prototype agents are shown in parentheses.

TABLE 27-1 Recommended treatment for drug-susceptible tuberculosis.

Regimen (in order of preference)	Intensive Phase (min duration = 8 wks)		Continuation Phase (min duration = 18 wks)[a]		
	Drugs	Dosing Interval	Drugs	Dosing Interval	Comments
1	INH RIF PZA EMB	7 day/wk[b]	INH RIF	7 day/wk[b]	Preferred regimen
2	INH RIF PZA EMB	7 day/wk[b]	INH RIF	3 day/wk	Preferred alternative if less frequent DOT is needed.
3	INH RIF PZA EMB	3 day/wk	INH RIF	3 day/wk	Caution in individuals with HIV and/or cavitary disease due to concerns for treatment failure, relapse, drug resistance
4	INH RIF PZA EMB	7 day/wk × 2 wk, then 2 day/wk × 6 wk	INH RIF	2 day/wk	Avoid in individuals with HIV or those with smear-positive and/or cavitary disease

DOT, directly observed therapy; EMB, ethambutol; HIV, human immunodeficiency virus; INH, isoniazid; PZA, pyrazinamide; RIF, rifampin.
[a]Experts recommend prolonged continuation phase (31 weeks) for patients with cavitation on initial chest radiograph and positive cultures at the end of the intensive treatment phase.
[b]May consider 5 days per week if needed for DOT. No studies compare 5 versus 7 doses per week, but extensive experience suggests efficacy of this regimen.

ethambutol, and pyrazinamide until the susceptibility of the strain is known. In susceptible isolates, ongoing therapy with INH and rifampin (the most active drugs) is continued for an additional 4 months. When this combination is administered for 9 months, 95-98% of tuberculosis cases are cured (if the strain is susceptible). Directly observed therapy (DOT) regimens, in which a healthcare provider witnesses ingestion of the antituberculosis agents, are recommended in noncompliant patients and in drug-resistant tuberculosis.

Isoniazid

Isoniazid is structurally similar to pyridoxine (vitamin B_6). The drug is well absorbed orally and is able to penetrate cells to act on intracellular mycobacteria. Isoniazid is metabolized in the liver and its rate of metabolism varies among ethnic groups. Fast metabolizers (half-life ~60-90 minutes) may require higher dosage than slow metabolizers (half-live ~3-4 hours) for equivalent therapeutic effects.

Isoniazid inhibits synthesis of mycolic acids that form an essential component of mycobacterial cell walls. Isoniazid is the single most important drug used in tuberculosis and is a component of most drug combination regimens (Table 27-1). Because resistance emerges rapidly if used alone, INH is always used together with other antituberculosis drugs in treatment of *active* infection. Isoniazid is only given as the sole drug for treatment of *latent* infection, including purified protein derivative (PPD) skin test converters, and individuals who have close contact with patients with active disease.

Neurotoxic effects are common and include peripheral neuropathy, restlessness, muscle twitching, and insomnia. Neuropathy is more likely to occur in slow INH metabolizers and those with predisposing conditions such as malnutrition, alcoholism, diabetes, AIDS, and uremia. Pyridoxine can be given to reduce this toxicity without impairing the antibacterial action. Isoniazid is hepatotoxic and may cause abnormal liver function tests, jaundice, and hepatitis. Risk of hepatotoxicity increases with age; fortunately, hepatotoxicity is rare in children. Isoniazid may inhibit hepatic metabolism of drugs (eg, phenytoin). Hemolysis and a lupus-like syndrome have been reported.

Rifampin

Rifampin is bactericidal against susceptible *M tuberculosis* organisms. When given orally, it is well absorbed and distributed to most body tissues, including the CNS. The drug undergoes enterohepatic cycling and is partially metabolized in the liver. Both free drug and metabolites are eliminated mainly in the feces. Rifampin inhibits DNA-dependent RNA polymerase in *M tuberculosis* and many other microorganisms. If rifampin is used alone, changes in drug sensitivity of the polymerase emerges rapidly, leading to resistance.

Like INH, rifampin is always used in combination with other drugs to treat active tuberculosis infections because resistance develops rapidly if the drug is used alone. However, rifampin can be used as the single drug in treatment of latent tuberculosis in INH-intolerant individuals or in those who have close contact with patients carrying INH-resistant strains. Rifampin has other uses in bacterial infections. Alone, rifampin can be used to eliminate meningococcal carriage; in combination therapy, rifampin can be used to eliminate staphylococcal carriage. Rifampin combination therapy is also used in the treatment of serious staphylococcal infections (eg, osteomyelitis, prosthetic joint infections).

Rifampin imparts a harmless orange color to urine, sweat, tears, and contact lenses (soft lenses may be permanently stained). Occasional ADRs include rashes, thrombocytopenia, nephritis, and liver dysfunction. Rifampin commonly causes light-chain proteinuria and may impair antibody responses. If given less often than twice weekly, rifampin may cause a flu-like syndrome (chills, fever, myalgias) and anemia.

Rifampin strongly induces liver drug-metabolizing enzymes and enhances the elimination rate of many drugs, including some anticonvulsants, anticoagulants, contraceptive steroids, cyclosporine, ketoconazole, and methadone. **Rifabutin** is less likely to cause drug interactions than rifampin and is equally effective as an antimycobacterial agent. Rifabutin is usually preferred over rifampin in treating tuberculosis in people with AIDS because rifampin affects the metabolism of many HIV medications through induction of the cytochrome P450 system.

Ethambutol

Ethambutol is well absorbed orally and distributed to most tissues, including the CNS when the meninges are inflamed. A large fraction is eliminated unchanged in the urine. Dose reduction is necessary in renal failure. Ethambutol interferes with mycobacterial cell wall synthesis by inhibiting arabinosyl transferases involved in the synthesis of arabinogalactan, a component of mycobacterial cell walls. Resistance occurs rapidly via if the drug is used alone. Ethambutol is a component of combination drug treatment of active tuberculosis. The drug can also be used in combination with other drugs to treat nontuberculous mycobacterial infections such as *Mycobacterium avium complex* (MAC).

The most common ADRs are dose-dependent visual disturbances, including loss of visual acuity, red-green color blindness, and possible retinal damage (from prolonged use at high doses). Most of these effects regress if the drug is stopped promptly. Baseline and monthly visual acuity and color discrimination testing is recommended, with particular attention to individuals on higher doses or with renal dysfunction. Ethambutol is relatively contraindicated in children too young to allow assessment of visual acuity and red-green color discrimination. Other neurotoxic effects include headache, confusion, and peripheral neuropathy.

Pyrazinamide

Pyrazinamide is well absorbed orally and penetrates most body tissues, including inflamed meninges. The drug is partly metabolized to pyrazinoic acid, and both parent molecule and metabolite are excreted in the urine. Plasma half-life of pyrazinamide is increased in hepatic or renal failure.

Pyrazinamide is taken up by macrophages and exerts its action against mycobacteria contained within lysosomes. Pyrazinamide is an important front-line drug used in combination with INH and rifampin in short-course (6-month) regimens as a "sterilizing" agent active against any residual intracellular mycobacteria that could cause relapse (Table 27-1). Resistance develops rapidly if the drug is used alone, but there is minimal cross-resistance with other antimycobacterial drugs.

Approximately 40% of patients develop nongouty polyarthralgia (ie, pain at multiple joints). Hyperuricemia commonly occurs, though is usually asymptomatic. Other ADRs include myalgia, GI irritation, maculopapular rash, hepatic dysfunction, and photosensitivity.

Alternative Drugs

Alternative drugs are typically only used in certain cases, including: (1) resistance to first-line agents, (2) failure of clinical response to first-line agents, (3) serious treatment-limiting adverse reactions to first-line agents. These drugs are considered second-line drugs because they are no more effective, and their toxicities are often more serious than those of the major drugs used to treat tuberculosis. Second-line agents include streptomycin, amikacin, fluoroquinolones, linezolid, rifabutin (for patients without HIV), **rifapentine**, **ethionamide**, **aminosalicylic acid (PAS)**, **capreomycin**, cycloserine, and **bedaquiline**. As with first-line agents, these drugs are always used in combinations.

Drugs Used in Leprosy

Mycobacterium leprae is the causative agent of leprosy (Hansen's disease). *M leprae* grows intracellularly, typically within skin and endothelial cells and Schwann cells of peripheral nerves. Onset of leprosy is very gradual (mean incubation period ~5 years) and the spectrum of disease is broad, depending on the host's immune response. Leprosy requires close and prolonged contact for transmission. Transmission is directly related to overcrowding and poor hygiene, and likely occurs via droplets from nose and mouth. The annual incidence of leprosy in the United States is only 150 cases, while worldwide there are roughly 250,000 cases.

Several drugs closely related to the sulfonamides have been used effectively in long-term treatment of leprosy. **Dapsone** (diaminodiphenyl sulfone) remains the most active drug against *M leprae*. Like the sulfonamides, its mechanism of action involves inhibition of folic acid synthesis. Dapsone can be given orally, penetrates tissues well, undergoes enterohepatic cycling, and is eliminated in the urine, partly as acetylated metabolites. Dapsone is rarely used alone in leprosy, but rather in combination with rifampin and with or without **clofazimine**. In addition to its use in leprosy, dapsone is an alternative drug for the prevention and treatment of *P jiroveci* pneumonia in people with AIDS.

Clofazimine causes GI irritation and pinkish brown discoloration of the skin. Dapsone is usually well tolerated. Common adverse effects of dapsone include GI irritation, fever, skin rashes, and methemoglobinemia. Hemolysis may occur, especially in individuals with glucose-6-phosphate dehydrogenase deficiency.

Drugs for Nontuberculous Mycobacterial Infections

In the United States, many infections resulting from mycobacteria are caused by "atypical mycobacteria." These pathogens are now referred to as *nontuberculous mycobacteria*. In general, these nontuberculous species are less susceptible to the antituberculous drugs, but may be susceptible to drugs such as the macrolides (eg, azithromycin, clarithromycin), sulfonamides, and tetracyclines.

An important pathogen in this group is *M avium* complex (MAC), which includes both *M avium* and *M intracellulare*. MAC is a main cause of disseminated infections in late stages of AIDS. In patients with CD4 counts less than 50/microliter, clarithromycin or azithromycin is recommended as prophylaxis for disseminated MAC. Treatment of MAC infections requires a combination of drugs, typically azithromycin or clarithromycin with ethambutol and possibly the addition of rifabutin.

REHABILITATION RELEVANCE

Physical therapists routinely treat patients receiving antibacterial drugs. Therapists often treat patients with infections directly related to their need for rehabilitation, such as after significant burns, open wounds, or surgery. More often, therapists are working with patients whose infections such as pneumonia or UTIs may not be directly related to their rehabilitation needs. These infections are common in both hospitalized patients and those receiving outpatient or home healthcare.

A large number of antibacterial agents are currently in clinical use. Many factors are considered in the choice of a particular drug. These include the species of bacterium (if known), the bacterium's drug susceptibility (if known), the location of the infection (which often points to the most likely organism), the severity of infection, the adverse effect profile of the antibiotic under consideration, as well as any impairment in the elimination mechanisms (eg, renal or liver dysfunction).

A serious problem of antibacterial therapy is the increasing prevalence of resistant strains. As healthcare professionals, physical therapists should educate patients about the role *each* individual plays in limiting the development of drug-resistant bacteria. Specifically, patients can be reminded that:

(1) antibacterial drugs should be used cautiously and not overused, and (2) once a drug regimen has been initiated, it should be completed as directed. Physical therapists also have a responsibility in preventing the spread of infections (Chapter 30). Handwashing between patients, appropriately disinfecting or sterilizing rehabilitation equipment (eg, assistive devices, gait belts) between patients, and maintaining sterile techniques when necessary (ie, wound care) can limit infection transfer.

Physical therapists should be able to recognize classes of antibacterial agents and their adverse effect profiles. The most common adverse effects associated with many antibacterial drugs are hypersensitivity (ie, allergic) reactions and GI disturbances. Listed below are the adverse effects of drugs covered in this chapter that are most likely to affect rehabilitation, as well as potential ways to mitigate their influence.

- The antibiotics with the highest potential to cause **hypersensitivity or allergic reactions** are the penicillins, cephalosporins, and sulfonamides. Most penicillins have generic names that end with "*-illin*." The generic names of most agents in the cephalosporin class begin with "*cef-*" and those in the sulfonamide class begin with "*sulfa-*." Allergic reactions can include rash or urticaria, severe itching, wheezing, ultraviolet sensitivity, fever, joint swelling, and in rare cases anaphylaxis. If an allergic reaction is suspected, this should be reported to the medical team or primary care provider (PCP) immediately.

- Perhaps the majority of antibacterial drugs are associated with **gastrointestinal problems**. Symptoms range from nausea, vomiting, and diarrhea to superinfection with resistant organisms and colitis. If signs and symptoms routinely interfere with therapy, altering therapy times around GI problems may improve patient participation. Certain antibiotics (eg, clindamycin, fluoroquinolones) pose more significant risk for *C difficile* infection. If patients demonstrate or report frequent watery stools, the PCP or medical team should be informed immediately to determine the necessity of testing for infection with *C difficile*.

- Many antibiotics (especially chloramphenicol, erythromycin, clarithromycin, fluoroquinolones, and rifampin) cause **significant drug-drug interactions**. If plasma levels of other drugs increase, patients may experience increased adverse effects. If plasma levels of other drugs decrease, their efficacy may be decreased.

- Intravenous infusions of cephalosporins and vancomycin may cause **phlebitis** at the injection site. Pain and edema may limit mobility in the affected extremity. Weightbearing on the affected extremity should be as tolerated, following any restrictions set by the PCP.

- Certain antibiotics **inhibit production of red blood cells** (eg, chloramphenicol), **white blood cells** (eg, clindamycin, linezolid, trimethoprim) **or platelets** (eg, linezolid). Anemia limits exercise tolerance. Therapists should closely monitor symptoms of exercise intolerance because pulse oximetry may not adequately represent oxygenation. Leukocytopenia increases patients' susceptibility to infection. Physical therapists should be vigilant with infection control precautions and consider treating the patient in his/her own room in preference to areas with larger pathogenic exposures (eg, therapy gym). Thrombocytopenia increases patients' susceptibility to bleeding and bruising. Conservative sharp wound debridement, deep tissue massage, or resistance exercise that places significant pressure on bony or small surface areas should be avoided (eg, resistive tubing around the ankle).

- The fluoroquinolones (individual generic drug names tend to end in "-*oxacin*") may cause **tendonitis** that can limit range of motion and strength of involved joints. To mitigate the risk of tendon rupture, strengthening exercises around symptomatic joints should be avoided.

- **Dizziness or vertigo** has been reported with the tetracyclines doxycycline and minocycline, the aminoglycosides, and the fluoroquinolones. Because these symptoms increase the risk of falling, therapists should employ fall risk reduction strategies including patient and caregiver education, increased guarding, and provision of assistive devices, as indicated.

- The aminoglycosides and vancomycin are nephrotoxic and **ototoxic**. If the patient reports (or the therapist observes) decreased hearing acuity or vestibular function, these symptoms should be reported immediately to the PCP. **High-frequency hearing loss**, more common with amikacin and kanamycin, may limit patients' ability to follow the therapist's instructions. **Vertigo, ataxia, and loss of balance** (more common with gentamicin and tobramycin) may limit mobility and increase risk of falling.

- Drugs used to treat tuberculosis commonly cause **neurotoxic effects** (isoniazid, ethambutol), **visual changes** (ethambutol, pyrazinamide), and **nongouty polyarthralgia** (pyrazinamide) that may hinder participation in rehabilitation programs. Neurotoxic and visual changes associated with antimycobacterial drugs should be reported to the PCP. In the absence of serious toxicity, the patient should be strongly encouraged to continue with the drug regimen because compliance is required for eradication of the infectious organism. If symptoms are limiting activity, rehabilitation goals may need to be postponed until the drug regimen has been completed.

CASE CONCLUSION

The therapist recognized that C.J.'s report of diarrhea might indicate more than a straightforward adverse effect of antibiotic therapy. While gastrointestinal distress is common with many antibiotics, use of clindamycin in particular is a significant risk factor for *Clostridium difficile* infection. C.J.'s report of frequent watery diarrhea along with abdominal cramping for more than a couple days increased the therapist's concern that the patient may be presenting with symptoms of *C difficile* infection. Because of the potential for *C difficile* infection to cause life-threatening complications such as dehydration, pseudomembranous colitis, and even death, the physical therapist alerted the primary care physician of C.J.'s status to facilitate urgent follow-up, if deemed necessary.

CHAPTER 27 QUESTIONS

1. Which of the following drugs may be used to treat infections caused by methicillin-resistant staphylococcus (MRSA)?

    a. Cefazolin
    b. Vancomycin
    c. Penicillin G
    d. Nafcillin

2. Which of the following is *not* a recognized mechanism of bacterial resistance to antibiotics?

    a. Production of β-lactam rings
    b. Production of β-lactamases
    c. Modifications in target penicillin binding proteins
    d. Decreased cell wall permeability to antibiotics

3. Which of the following statements is true regarding the cephalosporins?

    a. The bactericidal effects of cephalosporins result from inhibition of bacterial protein synthesis.
    b. Cephalosporins are classified by generation according to their spectrum of activity.
    c. The cephalosporins can only be administered parenterally.
    d. Some individuals with a history of penicillin allergy may be treated successfully with a cephalosporin.

4. Which of the following drug classes does *not* have its antibacterial effect by inhibiting the synthesis of bacterial cell walls?

    a. Cephalosporins
    b. Penicillins
    c. Aminoglycosides
    d. Carbapenems

5. Which of the following antibiotic classes is associated with significant ototoxicity?

   a. Penicillins
   b. Aminoglycosides
   c. Tetracyclines
   d. Cephalosporins

6. Tendonitis and neuropathy are potential adverse reactions for which of the following drug classes?

   a. Tetracyclines
   b. Cephalosporins
   c. Carbapenems
   d. Fluoroquinolones

7. Which of the following statements is true?

   a. Chemotherapy for mycobacterial infections requires multidrug regimens over long periods (ie, months).
   b. Leprosy is the most common mycobacterial infection in the United States.
   c. Mycobacteria rarely develop resistance to treatment when an individual drug is used as monotherapy.
   d. Drugs that target mycobacteria have few adverse effects.

8. Which of the following drugs used in the treatment of tuberculosis is associated with loss of visual acuity?

   a. Isoniazid
   b. Ethambutol
   c. Pyrazinamide
   d. Rifampin

9. Which of the following is the primary drug used to treat leprosy?

   a. Dapsone
   b. Doxycycline
   c. Dalfopristin
   d. Tetracycline

10. Which of the following has been associated with the development of antibiotic resistance?

    a. Use of a single antibiotic for a selective bacterium
    b. Use of antibiotics over short periods of time
    c. Use of broad-spectrum antibiotics
    d. Use of narrow-spectrum antibiotics

Antiviral Agents

F.M. is a 44-year-old man who has been human immunodeficiency virus (HIV) positive for 10 years. On his most recent physician visit, he was hyperglycemic and dyslipidemic. Although his weight has been stable over the past several years, he noted that his legs appear thinner and his waist is definitely larger. The patient's antiretroviral therapy regimen includes two nucleoside reverse transcriptase inhibitors, a nonnucleoside reverse transcriptase inhibitor, a protease inhibitor, and a pharmacokinetic booster. Since his HIV infection has responded very well to this drug regimen, F.M.'s physician is currently reluctant to switch to a protease inhibitor-sparing regimen. Instead, she has referred him to a physical therapist to assess the efficacy of a nonpharmacological approach to treating the hyperglycemia, dyslipidemia, and lipodystrophy.

REHABILITATION FOCUS

Viral infections such as HIV or hepatitis B virus (HBV) are chronic. Once acquired, the individual rarely eliminates the virus. Such chronic viral infections pose a unique problem in healthcare. These diseases may accelerate aging, resulting in physical decline beyond that based on the person's chronologic age. Pharmacotherapy for such infections is lifelong. Although many antiviral agents limit the extent of systemic damage, especially when initiated early during infection, very few can completely cure viral infections. Patients taking antiviral agents also face challenges in adhering to complicated drug regimens. For example, antiretroviral therapy (ART) regimens generally require persons infected with HIV that demonstrate acquired immunodeficiency syndrome (AIDS) to take multiple drugs—antiviral drugs and drugs for comorbidities—*every day* on a chronic basis. Antihepatitis B drug regimens are also complex and chronic, as are some antiherpetic drug regimens. In addition, the adverse effects of systemic antiviral agents may cause some patients to abandon treatment.

Most research on debilitation associated with viral infections has focused on the HIV/AIDS population. These individuals demonstrate higher rates of pain disorders, physical deconditioning, psychiatric disorders, and cardiovascular and metabolic diseases. These dysfunctions likely result from both the disease process and the pharmacotherapy. Individuals with chronic HIV infection often seek additional nonpharmacological therapies to improve health and fitness, body image, reduce metabolic and cardiovascular comorbidities, and decrease chronic pain and depression. Adherence

to exercise programs has demonstrated beneficial effects in *all* these areas. A systematic review found that 41-50 minutes of aerobic exercise 3-4 times per week was associated with higher CD4 cell counts, but not reduced viral load. Resistance programs have demonstrated higher adherence rates than aerobic programs. However, individuals with HIV/AIDS demonstrate higher dropout rates from physical intervention programs compared to other populations with similar comorbidities.

Therapists must be sensitive to the profound impact chronic infectious diseases and the antiviral drugs used to treat them have on patients' abilities to participate in therapy sessions and to achieve some therapy goals. Adverse drug reactions (ADRs) may delay treatment sessions. In the inpatient setting, frequent brief sessions may be more effective and tolerable than a single longer session. Pain due to peripheral neuropathies or myalgia may shift the treatment plan toward pain alleviation using more passive interventions such as heat modalities or transcutaneous electrical nerve stimulation. Flexibly managing therapy sessions around the patients' best time optimizes their ability to reach rehabilitation goals.

Because HIV directly targets the immune system, people with AIDS are among the most immunocompromised individuals. In addition to ART, those with AIDS are often taking prophylactic medications to prevent opportunistic infections from other viruses, bacteria, fungi, and miscellaneous pathogens. Therapists should be alert to new signs and symptoms of acute infections and report these immediately to the referring healthcare provider to facilitate aggressive treatment in early infectious stages. Therapists must be especially vigilant in practicing standard precautions, which includes staying home or avoiding patient care when illness strikes the therapist.

BACKGROUND

Viral infections range from those that cause minor illnesses, such as the common cold and cold sores, to life-threatening diseases, such as viral hepatitis, AIDS, Ebola, and severe acute respiratory syndrome (SARS). In addition, some viruses are associated with the development of certain types of cancer. For example, chronic HBV infection is associated with hepatic cancer, certain strains of human papillomavirus are the primary causative agent of cervical cancer, and HIV is associated with increased cancer risk due to decreased immunosurveillance.

Virus transmission can occur in many ways. The most common ways that virions enter the body are via inhaled droplets (eg, rhinovirus, the causative agent of the common cold), contaminated food or water (eg, hepatitis A), direct contact from an infected host's body fluids (eg, HIV, HBV, hepatitis C; HCV), or direct inoculation by bites of infected vectors (eg, dengue fever).

A virion (infective form of the virus) consists only of nucleic acids (deoxyribonucleic acid [DNA] or ribonucleic acid [RNA]) surrounded by a protein shell, or capsid. Some viruses have an additional glycoprotein coat called an envelope. Viruses are obligate intracellular parasites. That is, unlike bacteria, viruses depend on living host cells to replicate and function. Viruses must enter the host cell through its plasma membrane and take command of the host cell's synthetic processes in order to replicate itself and spread. Antiviral drugs can potentially exert their actions by interfering at several stages of viral replication, including: (1) viral attachment and entry into the host cell; (2) uncoating of the viral nucleic acid; (3) synthesis of early viral regulatory proteins; (4) synthesis of viral RNA or DNA; (5) late protein synthesis and processing; (6) viral packaging and assembly; and (7) virion release. Figure 28-1 presents an overview of viral infection and potential sites for inhibition of viral replication.

ANTIVIRAL AGENTS

Viruses are complicated chemotherapy targets for several reasons. Since viruses rely entirely on host cells' machinery to function, selective pharmacologic destruction of a virus without destroying human cells is difficult. Early treatment is critical, but frequently not possible because viral replication often peaks *before* clinical symptoms develop. Many antiviral agents also rely on a normal immune system to destroy the virus. Thus, immune suppression often lengthens viral illnesses. Antiviral drugs are virustatic—meaning that they are only active against the replicating virus and do not affect the latent virus. Figure 28-2 outlines the antiviral drugs against herpes, HIV, influenza, HBV, and HCV covered in this chapter.

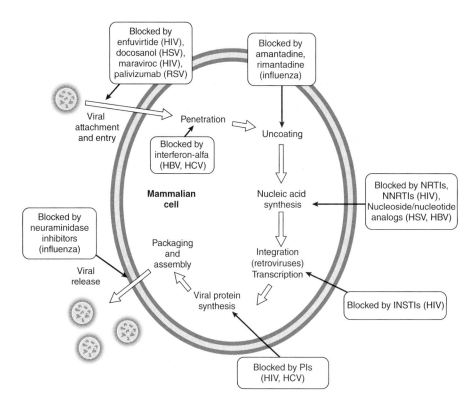

FIGURE 28-1 **Major steps for viral infection of a host cell include viral attachment and entry, penetration, uncoating, nucleic acid synthesis, integration (for retroviruses), transcription, protein synthesis, and packaging and assembly of new virions to be subsequently released.** Antiviral drugs target specific sites to inhibit viral replication. Abbreviations are defined in the text.

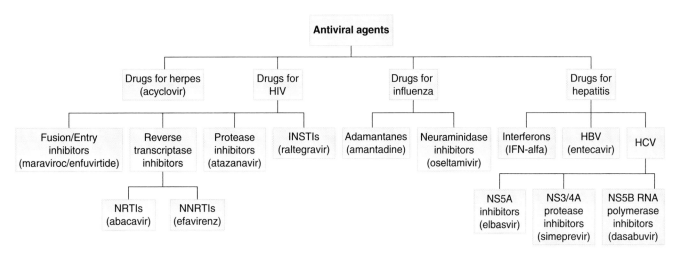

FIGURE 28-2 **Antiviral drugs used to treat herpes, HIV, influenza, and hepatitis B and C.** Prototypical drugs are listed in parentheses. HBV, hepatitis B; HCV, hepatitis C; HIV, human immunodeficiency virus; IFN, interferon; INSTIs, integrase strand transfer inhibitors; NNRTIs, nonnucleoside reverse transcriptase inhibitors; NRTIs, nucleoside/nucleotide reverse transcriptase inhibitors; NS, nonstructural.

Vaccines can effectively prevent infection from certain viruses such as influenza A and B, or HBV. Active and passive immunizations are discussed briefly at the end of the chapter.

GENERAL MECHANISMS OF ACTION AND RESISTANCE

Mechanisms of Action

Many antiviral drugs have similar chemical structures and mechanisms of action. Many are nucleoside or nucleotide analogs; that is, these drugs consist of complete or modified ribose/deoxyribose rings or modified purine (adenine or guanine) or pyrimidine (cytosine, uracil, thymidine) bases. Some antiviral drugs require phosphorylation in order to be active. The nucleoside analogs require triphosphorylation, whereas the nucleotide analogs only require biphosphorylation. The nucleotides require the transfer of only two high-energy phosphate groups to be active because they already have a covalently bound phosphate group in their original structure. These ribose ring or base modifications inhibit viral RNA or DNA replication by either blocking the enzymatic site of the viral protein and/or by terminating the viral nucleic acid chain elongation. For some drugs, the inhibition is irreversible, while for others it is reversible. This description is true for the antiretroviral nucleoside/nucleotide reverse transcriptase inhibitors used in treating HIV infection, several of the drugs used to treat HBV infection, and NS5B RNA polymerase inhibitors working at the enzymatic site of NS5B to treat HCV infection. The selective toxicity of these drugs is due to their preferred binding by *viral* proteins (rather than by host cell proteins) and termination of viral nucleic chain replication.

Pharmacokinetics

Concomitant food intake may enhance, inhibit, or have no effect on the oral bioavailability of antiviral drugs. For example, the bioavailability of saquinavir (an anti-HIV drug) is increased if consumed with a high-fat meal because its absorption is enhanced. There is no antiviral drug *class* effect to account for these differences. Rather, differences are related to the medicinal chemistry of each specific drug. Metabolism and elimination of antiviral drugs is also influenced by both hepatic and renal function. **Ritonavir** is a unique example of a drug that can be used to manipulate oral bioavailability of other drugs. Ritonavir is an HIV protease inhibitor, but this drug is also an inhibitor of hepatic enzymatic pathways responsible for first-pass metabolism of multiple antiviral drugs. As such, ritonavir is formulated with multiple antiretroviral and anti-HCV drugs to decrease first-pass metabolism of these drugs and thus improve their oral bioavailability. **Cobicistat** is another drug formulated with antiretroviral drugs to increase their bioavailability by inhibiting their first-pass hepatic metabolism. These agents reduce the required dosage of other antiviral drugs and diminish their ADRs. For this reason, ritonavir and cobicistat are referred to as pharmacokinetic "boosters" or "enhancers." The pharmacokinetics for antiviral drugs is complex; the interested reader should refer to additional resources related to the specific drug.

The elimination half-life of antiviral drugs varies with both drug class and individual drug. Many of the nucleoside/nucleotide analogs have a *plasma* elimination half-life and an *intracellular* half-life. For example, ganciclovir (an antiherpes drug) has a plasma elimination half-life of 4 hours, but an intracellular half-life of 16-24 hours. The longer intracellular half-life is due to the phosphorylation and subsequent intracellular entrapment of the drug.

Viral Drug Resistance

Mutations that cause changes in viral structure and/or viral enzymes often lead to the emergence of drug-resistant viral strains. Therefore, antiviral drugs that have similar chemical structures and mechanisms of action demonstrate crossover viral resistance in which resistance to a particular antiviral drug often results in resistance to other antiviral drugs. One of the most important trends in viral chemotherapy, especially in the management of HIV infection, has been the introduction of combination drug therapy, in which more than one stage of viral replication is inhibited. The benefits of combined antiviral therapy include greater clinical effectiveness and prevention, or at least delay of, viral drug resistance.

ANTIHERPES DRUGS

Second to the common cold and flu (influenza) viruses, herpes viruses are one of the leading causes of human viral disease. The most common herpes viruses are herpes simplex virus type 1 (HSV-1), herpes simplex virus type 2 (HSV-2), varicella-zoster virus (VZV), Epstein-Barr virus (EBV), and cytomegalovirus (CMV). For the majority of individuals infected by *any* herpes virus, the virus remains in the body for the life of the individual. Herpes infections are well known for remaining latent for months or even years. Then, in response to some trigger, the virus is reactivated, and the patient once again becomes symptomatic. Examples of triggers that reactivate the virus include sun exposure, concurrent viral illness, or immunosuppression.

The HSV-1 strain is the primary culprit responsible for orofacial (eg, cold sores) and ocular infections. The HSV-2 strain generally causes genital infections. Notably, HSV-1 and HSV-2 can cause outbreaks at either body site by direct contact with infectious secretions or mucous membranes. During the primary infection, HSV spreads from infected epithelial and mucosal cells to nearby sensory nerve endings and is transported along axons to the cell bodies. The precise cell(s) harboring the virus in the chronic disease state may be either germinal epithelial cells at the site of infection or the neurons. The virus enters the cell nucleus, where it persists indefinitely in a latent state. Recurrent HSV symptoms occur due to reactivation of the virus, producing vesicular lesions as well as intermittent asymptomatic viral shedding. Lesions usually heal within 2 weeks. Relapsing episodes are often physically and psychologically distressing. Pregnant women who are shedding may transmit the virus during delivery, with severe and potentially fatal consequences to the neonate.

In its primary infection, VZV causes chickenpox (herpes varicella) in children and is rapidly spread via airborne droplets and contact with lesions. Herpes zoster, also known as shingles, is a *reactivation* of a previous infection with VZV. Roughly 2-3 days before vesicular skin lesions appear, the patient often experiences pain along affected dermatomes (ie, those dermatomes innervated by neurons that harbor the reactivated HSV). The area generally remains painful until lesions heal in 3-4 weeks. Shingles cannot be contracted from someone who has shingles, because the infection always comes from reactivation of the latent VZV infection in the patient's own spinal cord ganglia. However, the primary infection,

chickenpox, *can* be transmitted from a person with herpes zoster to someone who has not already had chickenpox, or the chickenpox vaccine.

CMV infections occur primarily in the setting of advanced immunosuppression and are typically due to reactivation of latent infection. Dissemination of infection results in end-organ disease, including retinitis, colitis, esophagitis, central nervous system (CNS) disease, and pneumonitis. The incidence of CMV infections has markedly decreased in persons infected with HIV due to the advent of potent antiretroviral therapy. However, reactivation of CMV infection after organ transplantation is still prevalent.

Most drugs used to treat herpes viruses are nucleoside/nucleotide analogs that inhibit viral DNA polymerases, the enzymes that assist in viral replication. As stated previously, most antiviral drugs are bioactivated via phosphorylation through virus-specific and/or host enzymes to active drug forms. When the bioactivation of these drugs is selective, they are trapped inside the virally infected cells. These drugs are incorporated into the viral DNA as the virus replicates. Therefore, these agents are not effective against the latent, nonreplicating virus. As a class, the nucleoside/nucleotide analogs of these drugs have longer intracellular half-lives compared to their plasma elimination half-lives due to phosphorylation and intracellular trapping. In general, plasma elimination half-lives are less than 8 hours, while intracellular half-lives are substantially longer, ranging up to 24 hours for ganciclovir and several months for foscarnet, which is incorporated into bone. Acyclovir, famciclovir, and penciclovir may be used during pregnancy.

Acyclovir and Congeners

Acyclovir, **ganciclovir**, and **penciclovir** share similar chemical structures and mechanisms of action and also demonstrate cross-resistance. Acyclovir is a guanosine nucleoside analog that is activated first by virus-specific enzymes and then by host enzymes to form acyclovir triphosphate (Figure 28-3). The triphosphorylated drug competes with deoxyguanosine triphosphate for the viral DNA polymerase enzymatic site. Acyclovir then becomes incorporated into the viral DNA, but because the drug lacks the necessary position for nucleotide attachment, the DNA chain elongation terminates. In addition, acyclovir is irreversibly bound to the DNA template. Ganciclovir and penciclovir are similar guanosine nucleoside analogs, with similar mechanisms of activation by triphosphorylation. Ganciclovir terminates elongation of the viral DNA chain and competitively inhibits the DNA polymerase, whereas penciclovir only competitively inhibits the DNA polymerase. Acyclovir may be administered topically, orally or intravenously. Ganciclovir is usually administered intravenously. Due to poor oral absorption, penciclovir is only used topically.

Following oral administration, the prodrugs **valacyclovir** and **famciclovir** are converted to acyclovir and penciclovir, respectively, by first-pass metabolism. When valacyclovir and famciclovir are taken orally, blood levels of acyclovir and

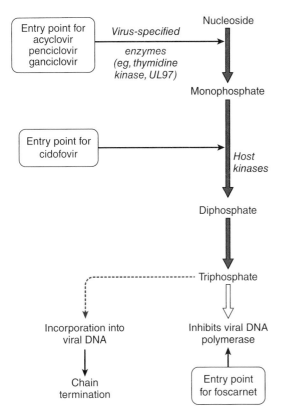

FIGURE 28-3 **Mechanism of action of antiherpetic drugs.** Drugs listed within the boxes denote their specific entry point into the viral synthesis pathway. Their integration at these points results in inhibition of the DNA polymerase and/or nucleic acid chain elongation termination. Acyclovir, penciclovir, and ganciclovir require triphosphorylation to act as a substrate for the DNA polymerase; the first phosphorylation is mediated by a viral enzyme, which causes the active metabolite to accumulate only in infected cells. Cidofovir requires only two phosphorylations to be active. Foscarnet does not require phosphorylation to be active.

penciclovir may be 3-5 times higher than when acyclovir and penciclovir are taken orally. Viral resistance to these drugs results from either modification of the enzymatic site of the DNA polymerase, or modification of viral-specific enzymes responsible for the initial phosphorylation of these drugs.

Clinically, antiherpes drugs may decrease the duration of symptoms by 2 days and time to lesion healing by 4 days. These drugs are also administered prophylactically to prevent viral reactivation. Viral outbreak may resume upon termination of treatment with increased risk of viral resistance to one or more of these drugs. Systemic drug delivery results in headache, nausea, and diarrhea. Tremors, delirium, and seizures have also been reported for acyclovir, but not the others. Nondefined peripheral neuropathies, myelosuppression, confusion, and psychiatric disorders have been reported for ganciclovir.

Cidofovir is a cytosine nucleotide analog that is bioactivated exclusively by host cell enzymes (Figure 28-3). The drug is active against HSV, CMV, adenovirus, poxviruses, and polyomaviruses, including many acyclovir-resistant strains. Cidofovir is

generally administered topically or intravenously. Intravenous cidofovir is used to treat CMV retinitis and mucocutaneous HSV infections. As a nucleotide, the drug is diphosphorylated to the active form by host kinases. The phosphorylated drug inhibits the DNA polymerase and is incorporated into the DNA chain. Cidofovir is dose-dependently nephrotoxic and may cause metabolic acidosis.

Foscarnet inhibits viral DNA polymerase, RNA polymerase, and HIV reverse transcriptase without requiring phosphorylation or other type of activation (Figure 28-3). Foscarnet blocks the pyrophosphate binding site of these enzymes and inhibits cleavage of pyrophosphate from deoxynucleotide triphosphates. The drug is only available intravenously, and penetrates well into tissues, including the CNS. Foscarnet is an alternative drug for the prophylaxis and treatment of CMV infections, and has minimal cross-resistance. The ADRs may be severe, including nephrotoxicity, hypo- or hypercalcemia, hyperphosphatemia, and genitourinary ulcerations. The CNS effects include headache, hallucinations, and seizures.

Docosanol is a saturated 22-carbon aliphatic alcohol that inhibits fusion between the host cell plasma membrane and the HSV envelope, thereby preventing viral entry into host cells and subsequent viral replication. Topical docosanol cream is available without a prescription. If applied within 12 hours of onset of prodromal symptoms, docosanol shortens healing time in recurrent orofacial herpes. Minimal ADRs are reported with topical application.

ANTI-HIV DRUGS

Human immunodeficiency virus strikes the immune system, specifically targeting CD4+ T lymphocytes. Depletion of infected CD4 cells ultimately leads to profound immunosuppression. Acquired immune deficiency syndrome is symptomatic disease, characterized by the development of a wide spectrum of opportunistic infections and malignancies either acquired or reactivated due to the immunosuppression caused by HIV. HIV/AIDS is a global health problem. Routes of infection include sexual intercourse, intravenous drug use, and vertical transmission from mother to fetus.

To understand the drugs used in the treatment of HIV, the life cycle of HIV must be briefly examined (Figure 28-4). HIV is a retrovirus, meaning that it is an enveloped virus with a single-stranded RNA (not DNA) genome. To enter host CD4+ cells, the viral envelope glycoprotein (gp) 160, a combination of gp120/gp41, binds to the host cell surface, resulting in a conformational change to the gp120/gp41. This change allows access to the chemokine receptors (CCR5 or CXCR4) on the surface of the white blood cells. The virus then fuses with the host cell membrane and uncoats as it enters the host cell. After uncoating, viral replication depends on the viral reverse transcriptase, which transcribes the viral genome from single-stranded RNA into double-stranded DNA. This newly formed double-stranded DNA is integrated into the human host's genome by a viral integrase. Integrated viral DNA is then transcribed by a

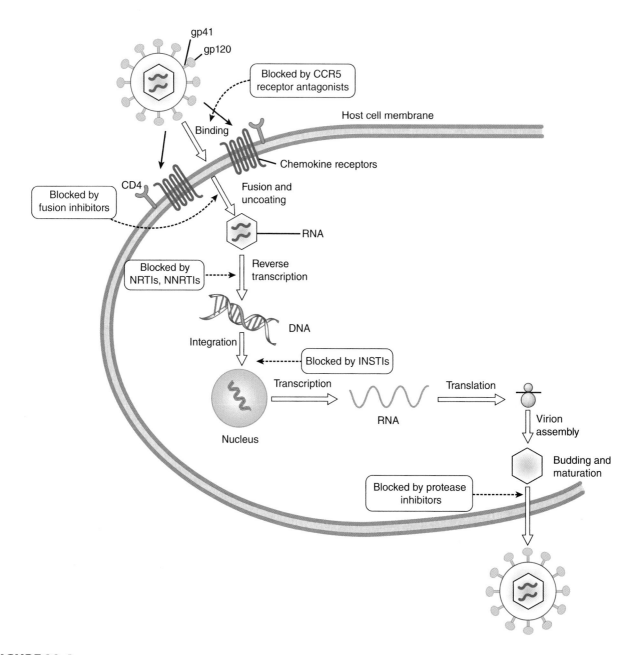

FIGURE 28-4 Life cycle of HIV. Binding of viral glycoproteins to host cell CD4 and chemokine receptors leads to fusion of the viral and host cell membranes via gp41 and entry of the virion into the cell. After uncoating, reverse transcription copies the single-stranded HIV RNA genome into double-stranded DNA, which is integrated into the host cell genome. Gene transcription by host cell enzymes produces messenger RNA, which is translated into proteins that assemble into immature noninfectious virions that bud from the host cell membrane. Maturation into fully infectious virions is through proteolytic cleavage. INSTIs, integrase strand transfer inhibitors; NNRTIs, nonnucleoside reverse transcriptase inhibitors; NRTIs, nucleoside/nucleotide reverse transcriptase inhibitors.

host polymerase enzyme into messenger RNA, which is translated into proteins that assemble into immature noninfectious virions that bud from the host cell membrane. Subsequent proteolytic cleavage allows maturation into fully infectious virions.

There are two major types of HIV. HIV-1 is the most widespread worldwide, whereas HIV-2, a less pathogenic variant, is found primarily in western Africa. Discussion of antiretroviral agents in this chapter is specific to HIV-1. Patterns of susceptibility of HIV-2 to these agents may vary; however, there is innate resistance of HIV-2 to the non-nucleoside/nucleotide reverse transcriptase inhibitors and enfuvirtide as well as a lower barrier of resistance to nucleoside/nucleotide reverse transcriptase inhibitors and protease inhibitors.

At this time, there is no cure for HIV infection or AIDS. However, pharmacotherapy has dramatically improved both the length and quality of life for HIV-infected individuals, and can delay the onset of AIDS. Without pharmacological treatment, most infected individuals die within a few years after the onset

TABLE 28-1 Major antiretroviral drugs used against HIV.

Class	Prototype	Other Significant Agents
Nucleoside reverse transcriptase inhibitors	Abacavir	Emtricitabine, lamivudine
Nucleotide reverse transcriptase inhibitors	Tenofovir disoproxil fumarate	Tenofovir alafenamide
Nonnucleoside reverse transcriptase inhibitors	Delavirdine	Efavirenz, etravirine, nevirapine, rilpivirine
Integrase strand transfer inhibitors	Dolutegravir	Elvitegravir, raltegravir
Protease inhibitors	Indinavir	Atazanavir, darunavir, fosamprenavir, lopinavir, nelfinavir, ritonavir, saquinavir, tipranavir
CCR-5 antagonist	Maraviroc	
Fusion inhibitor	Enfuvirtide	

Tenofovir alafenamide and tenofovir disoproxil fumarate are both prodrugs of the active compound, tenofovir. Both prodrugs require metabolism prior to activation, although the site of activation for each prodrug differs. Maraviroc and enfuvirtide are the only drugs in their respective classes.

of symptoms. Currently, the standard of care in treating HIV infection involves initiating antiretroviral therapy (ART) that requires 3-4 antiretroviral drugs. If possible, ART is initiated *before* symptoms appear. The goal of combination regimens is to inhibit or stop viral replication at a number of distinct steps (Figure 28-4). Compared with the administration of a single antiretroviral agent, combination therapy increases the efficacy of drug therapy, decreases the risk of developing drug resistance, and reduces viral load (amount of virus in the blood).

Table 28-1 outlines the five classes of antiretroviral agents currently available: fusion/penetration inhibitors, nucleoside/nucleotide reverse transcriptase inhibitors (NRTIS), nonnucleoside reverse transcriptase inhibitors (NNRTIs), integrase strand transfer inhibitors (INSTIs), and protease inhibitors (PIs). Drug combinations are tailored to each patient depending on many variables, including potency, viral resistance, patient tolerance, convenience, and adherence to drug regimen. With the exception of the fusion inhibitor enfuvirtide, the anti-HIV agents are all available as oral formulations. Drug management of HIV/AIDS is subject to change as newer agents become available. New pharmacotherapies are being sought that offer the advantages of once-daily dosing, smaller pill size, lower incidence of ADRs, new viral targets, and antiviral activity against strains that are resistant to other agents.

Fusion/Entry Inhibitors

Enfuvirtide and **maraviroc** are the newest classes of antiretroviral agents. These drugs do not require phosphorylation for activation, and there is only a plasma elimination half-life. There is no stated contraindication for the use of these drugs during pregnancy.

Enfuvirtide is a synthetic 36-amino-acid peptide that binds to the gp41 portion of the viral envelope, preventing the conformational change and viral entry (Figure 28-4). The drug is metabolized by proteolysis and must be administered subcutaneously. Enfuvirtide lacks cross-resistance with other currently approved antiretroviral drug classes. The most common ADRs are local injection site reactions (painful erythematous nodules) that rarely lead to drug discontinuation. Other potential adverse effects include insomnia, headache, dizziness, and nausea. Hypersensitivity reactions rarely occur.

Maraviroc binds specifically and selectively to the host cell surface chemokine receptor CCR5. Maraviroc is approved for use in combination with other antiretroviral agents in adults infected only with CCR5-tropic HIV-1. Potential ADRs include upper respiratory tract infection, cough, fever, rash, dizziness, myalgia and arthralgia, diarrhea, and sleep disturbance. Hepatotoxicity and increased risk of myocardial ischemia and infarction have been reported with this drug. Maraviroc is contraindicated in persons with severe or end-stage renal impairment. Caution is advised when used in individuals with preexisting hepatic impairment and in those coinfected with HBV or HCV.

Nucleoside/Nucleotide Reverse Transcriptase Inhibitors

The NRTIs were the first group of drugs used to treat HIV infection. NRTIs selectively inhibit the HIV reverse transcriptase at the enzymatic site after phosphorylation by host cell kinases (Figure 28-4). The reverse transcriptase incorporates the phosphorylated NRTI into the growing viral DNA chain, which stops chain elongation. If NRTIs are used as single agents to treat HIV, resistance emerges rapidly. However, resistance is rare in combination regimens. As newer agents have become available, several older NRTIs have been used less frequently because of either suboptimal safety or inferior efficacy. **Zalcitabine** is no longer marketed, and regimens containing **zidovudine**, **didanosine**, or **stavudine** are infrequently recommended as first-line regimens and are not subsequently discussed.

Abacavir is a guanosine nucleoside analog. **Lamivudine** is a cytosine nucleoside analog with inhibitor activity against the reverse transcriptase in HIV as well as the DNA polymerase in HBV. **Tenofovir disoproxil fumarate** is a nucleotide analog of adenosine. In the blood, tenofovir disoproxil fumarate is converted to the active drug tenofovir. Like lamivudine, tenofovir has inhibitory activity against reverse transcriptase in HIV and the DNA polymerase in HBV. **Tenofovir alafenamide** is another prodrug that is converted to tenofovir in hepatocytes and lymphoid cells, which improves the target bioavailability and reduces systemic toxicity. To illustrate this point, tenofovir blood levels are up to 90% lower with the alafenamide prodrug compared to the disoproxil fumarate prodrug. Because NRTIs require phosphorylation prior to antiviral activity, they have both plasma half-lives and longer intracellular half-lives. The plasma elimination half-lives may be as short as 1.5 hours for abacavir and up to 12-17 hours for tenofovir disoproxil fumarate. **Emtricitabine** is a fluorinated analog of lamivudine with an intracellular half-life greater than 24 hours, which allows for once-daily dosing.

Common ADRs of the NRTIs include nausea, diarrhea, and headache. Severe adverse effects are associated with most NRTIs, with the exception of lamivudine. All NRTIs may be associated with mitochondrial toxicity, which manifests as peripheral neuropathy, pancreatitis, and lipodystrophy. Lipodystrophy is the redistribution and accumulation of body fat that results in central obesity, dorsocervical fat enlargement (buffalo hump), peripheral and facial wasting, breast enlargement, and a cushingoid appearance. Lipodystrophy and insulin resistance occur least frequently with use of tenofovir, lamivudine, emtricitabine, and abacavir. The NRTIs have the potential to cause a rare, but serious lactic acidosis and severe hepatic steatosis, both of which are likely due to mitochondrial damage in liver cells. Symptoms include severe nausea, vomiting, and persistent abdominal pain. NRTI administration will likely be suspended in these cases. Liver toxicity is less common with lamivudine and abacavir. Risk factors include obesity, prolonged treatment with NRTIs, and preexisting liver dysfunction.

Each NRTI agent has unique adverse effects. For example, in a small percentage of patients taking abacavir, potentially fatal hypersensitivity reactions can occur. Symptoms usually occur in the first 6 weeks of therapy and include fever, malaise, vomiting, diarrhea, and anorexia. Alcohol is contraindicated with abacavir because consumption increases drug plasma concentration and increases the risk of ADRs. Abacavir has also been reported to increase the risk of myocardial infarction. Lamivudine may increase insomnia. Last, because tenofovir disoproxil fumarate is formulated with lactose, this may increase gastrointestinal (GI) manifestations in patients who are lactose intolerant.

Nonnucleoside/Nucleotide Reverse Transcriptase Inhibitors

The NNRTIs bind directly to HIV-1 reverse transcriptase. The binding site of NNRTIs is near—but distinct—from that of the NRTIs (Figure 28-4). The binding of these drugs leads to a conformational structural change to the viral transcriptase that results in allosteric inhibition of RNA- and DNA-dependent DNA polymerase activity. Unlike the NRTI agents, NNRTIs neither compete with nucleoside triphosphates nor require phosphorylation to be active. The second-generation NNRTIs (**etravirine, rilpivirine**) have higher potencies, longer half-lives, and reduced adverse-effect profiles compared with the older NNRTIs (**delavirdine, efavirenz, nevirapine**). The plasma elimination half-lives for these drugs vary from 6 hours for delavirdine to 50 hours for rilpivirine. Like the NRTIs, resistance can occur rapidly if these drugs are used as monotherapy. There is no cross-resistance between NRTI and NNRTI drugs. As a class, ADRs associated with NNRTIs include varying levels of GI distress and skin rashes, including Stevens-Johnson syndrome. For some drugs such as delavirdine, the onset of skin rash occurs within the initial 3 weeks of therapy. There are additional unique adverse effects associated with NNRTIs. Efavirenz and rilpivirine both increase total serum cholesterol levels, while etravirine increases serum cholesterol, triglyceride, and glucose levels. Along with these metabolic changes, there is increased risk of lipodystrophy and accompanying cardiovascular risks. Nevirapine increases the risk of fulminant hepatitis, and rilpivirine is associated with prolongation of the QT interval. Of the drugs in this class, efavirenz and rilpivirine are recommended for use during pregnancy. NNRTI agents are metabolized by the cytochrome P450 (CYP) system, which increases the likelihood of drug-drug adverse interactions.

Integrase Strand Transfer Inhibitors

The integrase function is essential to replication in both HIV-1 and HIV-2 strains (Figure 28-4). **Raltegravir, elvitegravir**, and **dolutegravir** are prescribed in the United States. These drugs competitively inhibit the integrase and thus prevent the insertion of the double-stranded viral DNA into the host cell's genome. Without this integration, the viral DNA cannot be transcribed and the viral replication process is terminated. None of these drugs require phosphorylation prior to antiviral activity. Plasma elimination half-lives range from 9 to 14 hours. All integrase strand transfer inhibitors have similar concomitant food intake restrictions. The pharmacokinetic "boosters" cobicistat or ritonavir previously discussed have both been used to increase oral bioavailability of dolutegravir. As a class, these drugs are well tolerated. Most common ADRs include headaches and GI dysfunction. Hepatotoxicity is clinically observed and patients are monitored. Rare severe events include rhabdomyolysis and systemic hypersensitivity. Insomnia has been reported with dolutegravir. Raltegravir has been documented to cause severe skin reactions such as Stevens-Johnson syndrome.

Protease Inhibitors

During the later stages of the HIV growth cycle, the *gag* and *gag-pol* gene products are translated into polyproteins, and these become immature budding particles. The HIV protease is responsible for cleaving these precursor molecules to produce the final structural proteins of the mature virion core. Protease inhibitors prevent post-translational cleavage of the Gag-Pol polyprotein that is required for functional viral protein conformations. Thus, PIs result in the production of immature, noninfectious HIV particles (Figure 28-4). Unlike the NRTIs, PIs do not require phosphorylation prior to antiviral activity. The plasma elimination half-lives for this class vary from 2.8 hours for **indinavir** to as long as 11 hours with **atazanavir** and **fosamprenavir**. Fosamprenavir is a prodrug converted to **amprenavir**. Fosamprenavir oral suspension contains propylene glycol and is contraindicated for young children and pregnant women. The fosamprenavir oral solution also contains several times the daily dosage of vitamin E, so supplemental vitamin E is contraindicated.

As a class, PIs are associated with GI intolerance that may be dose-limiting. The comorbidities of hyperglycemia, hyperlipidemia, and lipodystrophy often occur with these drugs with a median onset time of about 1 year after treatment initiation. Atazanavir has the lowest incidence of these effects. Insulin resistance is more common with **lopinavir**. Due to these ADRs, individuals with AIDS that are receiving PIs within an ART regimen often receive counseling about heart disease as a new complication. The PIs, notably lopinavir, may also be associated with PR and QT interval prolongation. In contrast, **saquinavir** has a lower incidence of QT interval prolongation. Drug-induced hepatitis has been reported to varying degrees with all PIs. Whether the PIs are associated with bone loss and osteoporosis after long-term use is under investigation. An increased risk of intracranial hemorrhage has been reported in individuals receiving **tipranavir/ritonavir**. **Darunavir**, fosamprenavir, and tipranavir are sulfonamides; caution should be used in patients with a history of sulfonamide allergy. PIs are metabolized by the CYP system, increasing the likelihood of drug-drug adverse interactions.

Preexposure Prophylaxis

There is no vaccine for HIV. However, the Centers for Disease Control and Prevention (CDC) recommend an oral combination of tenofovir disoproxil and emtricitabine as preexposure prophylaxis (PrEP) to reduce the likelihood of HIV infection in high-risk individuals (eg, those in an ongoing sexual relationship with an HIV-positive partner, those who have injected drugs and shared needles in the past 6 months). According to the CDC, daily PrEP can lower risk of getting HIV from sex by more than 90% and from injection drug use by more than 70%.

ANTI-INFLUENZA DRUGS

Influenza virus strains are classified by their core proteins (ie, A, B, or C), species of origin (eg, avian, swine), and geographic site of isolation. Influenza A, the only strain that causes pandemics, is classified into 16 H (hemagglutinin) and 9 N (neuraminidase) known subtypes based on surface proteins. Although influenza B viruses usually only infect people, influenza A viruses can infect a variety of animal hosts, providing an extensive reservoir. There are two major classes of anti-influenza drugs, adamantanes and neuraminidase inhibitors. Treatment is recommended for individuals with severe infection or those at high risk for complications. The neuraminidase inhibitors have activity against both influenza A and influenza B, whereas the adamantanes only have activity against influenza A viruses. None of these drugs require phosphorylation prior to antiviral activity. Thus, these drugs have only plasma elimination half-lives. Birth defects have been reported for the adamantanes following exposure during pregnancy.

Adamantanes

Amantadine and its derivative, **rimantadine**, block the M2 proton ion channel of the virus particle and inhibit uncoating of the viral RNA within infected host pulmonary epithelial cells, thus preventing viral replication. They have plasma elimination half-lives of 12-18 and 24-36 hours, respectively. They are active against influenza A only. In the absence of resistance, both amantadine and rimantadine are 70-90% protective in the prevention of clinical illness when initiated before exposure and shorten the duration of clinical illness by 1-2 days when administered as treatment. However, due to high rates of resistance, these agents are no longer recommended for the prevention or treatment of influenza. The most common GI adverse effects are nausea and anorexia. Nervousness, concentration difficulties, insomnia, and lightheadedness are common. More serious CNS adverse effects include marked behavioral changes, delirium, hallucinations, agitation, and seizures possibly due to altered dopaminergic neurotransmission. These CNS effects are less frequent with rimantadine. (See Chapter 18 for role of dopamine neurotransmission and psychiatric dysfunctions.) Both amantadine and rimantadine are teratogenic and embryotoxic in rodents, and birth defects have been reported after exposure during pregnancy.

Neuraminidase Inhibitors

The neuraminidase inhibitors **oseltamivir**, **peramivir**, and **zanamivir** halt the spread of influenza infection within the respiratory tract by interfering with release of progeny influenza A and B virus from infected host pulmonary epithelial cells. These agents competitively and reversibly inhibit the viral neuraminidase enzymatic site, resulting in clumping of newly released influenza virions to each other and to the membrane of the infected cell.

Initiation of therapy within 48 hours after the onset of illness modestly decreases the duration of symptoms. Once-daily prophylaxis is 70-90% effective in preventing disease after exposure. Oseltamivir is an orally administered prodrug that is activated by hepatic esterases and widely distributed throughout the body. ADRs include nausea, vomiting, and headache. Taking oseltamivir with food does not interfere with absorption and may decrease nausea and vomiting. Fatigue and diarrhea have also been reported and appear to be more common with prophylactic use. Neuropsychiatric events of self-injury or delirium have been reported, particularly in adolescents and adults living in Japan. Zanamivir is administered directly to the respiratory tract via inhalation. Only 10-20% of the active compound reaches the lungs; the remainder is deposited in the oropharynx. Because ADRs associated with zanamivir include cough and bronchospasm (occasionally severe), reversible decrease in pulmonary function, and transient nasal and throat discomfort, zanamivir is not recommended for patients with underlying airway disease. Peramivir is a newer, intravenously administered neuraminidase inhibitor for the treatment of acute uncomplicated influenza in adults. As with the other neuraminidase inhibitors, starting treatment within 48 hours of symptoms is optimal. The main ADR is diarrhea. As with oseltamivir, an increased risk of hallucinations, delirium, and abnormal behavior has been reported in individuals with influenza receiving peramivir. The half-lives for peramivir and oseltamivir are 6-10 and 20 hours, respectively. Zanamivir (administered by inhalation) has a pulmonary half-life of 2.8 hours.

ANTIHEPATITIS AGENTS

Viral hepatitis is an inflammation of the liver. Of the various viruses that cause hepatitis, HBV and HCV infections are most commonly treated pharmacologically. Chronic inflammation of the liver due to viral infections results in cirrhosis and increased risk for hepatic cancer. HBV is a DNA virus with a DNA polymerase containing reverse transcriptase activity, and a potential to develop a latent intracellular covalently closed circular DNA that may act as a reservoir for future replication. Thus, HBV is a chronic infection. In contrast, HCV is a single-stranded RNA virus, with an RNA polymerase for replication. With HCV infection, spontaneous remission (disappearance of the signs and symptoms) occurs within 6 months in 20-35% of individuals. As a result, treatment for HCV is usually delayed until that time to determine if the viral infection will spontaneously resolve. Several drugs are currently licensed in the treatment of HBV or HCV.

Interferons

Interferons (IFNs) are signaling proteins released by host cells in response to many pathogens, including viruses. Clinically, IFNs are injected subcutaneously or intramuscularly in the treatment of HBV and HCV. Interferons work through plasma membrane receptors on multiple cell types in the body. These drugs increase the proliferation and longevity of cytotoxic T cells, increase macrophage phagocytosis, and inhibit multiple steps in the viral penetration and replication process. HBV may be treated with **IFN alfa-2b**,

whereas HCV may be treated with **IFN alfa-2a**, IFN alfa-2b, or **IFN alfacon-1**. Attachment of polyethylene glycol (PEG) to the interferons dramatically increases their half-lives from around 2.5 hours, up to 160 hours. Pegylated IFNs decrease the frequency of injections as well as the immunogenicity. Pegylated IFN derivatives include IFN alfa-2a for treatment of HBV, and IFN alfa-2b in the treatment of HCV. The ADRs of these drugs include myelosuppression, myalgia and arthralgia, weight loss, profound psychiatric disorders, cardiotoxicities, and unmasking of autoimmune diseases. Due to response rates lower than 50% and a number of absolute contraindications for IFNs, a newer class of direct-acting antiviral drugs (discussed below) has largely replaced the use of IFNs to treat viral hepatitis.

Treatment of HBV Infection

There is no specific treatment for *acute* HBV infection, which frequently resolves spontaneously. Cure is rare for *chronic* HBV. However, currently licensed drugs suppress HBV DNA to undetectable levels, which is one of the main goals of chronic HBV therapy. Several nucleoside/nucleotide analogs are used to inhibit the DNA polymerase, and some drugs also cause chain termination after incorporation into the viral DNA. These drugs are all phosphorylated by cellular kinases. In contrast to other antiviral drug classes, the intracellular half-life for these drugs is not always longer than the plasma elimination half-life. For example, entecavir has an intracellular half-life of 15 hours and a plasma elimination half-life of 128-149 hours, allowing for once-a-day dosing. There are no specific guidelines contraindicating these drugs during pregnancy.

Adefovir dipivoxil is the prodrug of adefovir, an adenine nucleotide analog, which both inhibits the DNA polymerase and causes chain termination. **Entecavir** is a guanosine nucleotide analog that inhibits the DNA polymerase, and is unique in its ability to inhibit the reverse transcription of the negative DNA strand and synthesis of the positive DNA strand. As previously discussed, tenofovir disoproxil fumarate, an adenosine analog, is a prodrug of tenofovir and another nucleotide for the treatment of HBV (as well as HIV). Tenofovir disoproxil fumarate is unique in that resistance has not been documented in clinical trials even after 8 years of therapy. Tenofovir alafenamide is also used in the treatment of HBV infections. Lamivudine, previously discussed in the HIV section, also inhibits the DNA polymerase in HBV. Lamivudine is distinctly advantageous because this drug is safe to administer to patients with decompensated liver disease. Unfortunately, clinical use of lamivudine is limited by the development of resistance within 1 year of drug initiation in 15-30% of patients.

Nausea, diarrhea, fatigue and headache are common ADRs of these drugs. Myalgia and arthralgia are also common to many, but not all, of these drugs. Adefovir has the potential to cause lactic acidosis and hepatic steatosis, whereas entecavir is documented to cause only the lactic acidosis. Tenofovir is noted to decrease bone density with chronic therapy.

TABLE 28-2 Drug combinations used to treat hepatitis C virus (HCV).

First Drug	Viral Site of Inhibition	Required Additional Drug/s Used in Conjunction with First Drug	Viral Site/s of Inhibition
Daclatasvir	NS5A	Sofosbuvir	NS5B polymerase
Dasabuvir	NS5B polymerase	Ombitasvir, paritaprevir and ritonavir[a]	NS5A NS3/4A protease
Elbasvir	NS5A	Grazoprevir	NS3/4A protease
Ledipasvir	NS5A	Sofosbuvir	NS5B polymerase
Ombitasvir[b]	NS5A	Paritaprevir ritonavir[a]	NS3/4A protease
Simeprevir[c]	NS3/4A protease	Sofosbuvir	NS5B polymerase
Velpatasvir	NS5A	Sofosbuvir	NS5B polymerase

NS, nonstructural protein.

These drugs may be used with or without ribavirin included in the drug regimen.

[a]Ritonavir is pharmacokinetic booster included to increase the oral bioavailability of the other drugs by reducing first-pass metabolism.

[b]Ombitasvir may be administered with paritaprevir and ritonavir with or without dasabuvir.

[c]Simeprevir/sofosbuvir drug formulation may or may not include ribavirin.

Treatment of HCV Infection

For decades, the mainstay of therapy for chronic HCV infection was a combination of pegylated interferon and ribavirin, which demonstrated a cure rate of only 40-60%. **Ribavirin** is a guanosine nucleoside analog that requires phosphorylation prior to inhibiting HCV replication at multiple steps including capping of viral mRNA and RNA-dependent polymerase activity. Significant ADRs associated with ribavirin include a dose-dependent hemolytic anemia, depression, fatigue, nausea, and pruritus.

In 2011, the development of oral direct-acting antivirals (DAAs) dramatically altered the treatment of chronic HCV. Treatment with standard DAA regimens can permanently eradicate HCV infection, resulting in cure rates of 90-97%. Following completion of treatment, the remission of HCV infection has increased for up to 2 years with only a 5% relapse. Other advantages of DAA regimens include shorter treatment duration (12 weeks compared with 48 weeks), less frequent dosing, elimination of the need for injectable agents, and fewer serious ADRs. The downside of DAAs is that the regimens are very expensive.

Of the DAAs, only **sofosbuvir** is a nucleotide analog requiring phosphorylation prior to antiviral activity. The plasma elimination half-lives of DAAs range from 12 to 15 hours for **daclatasvir** to 31 hours for **grazoprevir**. The mechanism of action of DAAs is inhibition of a variety of nonstructural (NS) proteins involved in the replication and enzymatic processing of the HCV nucleic material and proteins. Daclatasvir, **elbasvir**, **ledipasvir**, **ombitasvir**, and **velpatasvir** inhibit the viral NS5A protein that is involved in HCV replication and assembly. The NS5B is an RNA-dependent RNA polymerase involved in post-translational processing necessary for HCV replication. Antiviral drugs directed at this protein have inhibitory activity following binding at the enzymatic site and allosteric sites. Thus, there are both nucleoside/nucleotide drugs that inhibit the enzymatic site and nonnucleoside/nucleotide drugs that inhibit the allosteric site. Sofosbuvir is a uridine nucleotide analog that inhibits the enzymatic site of the RNA polymerase, resulting in chain termination. **Dasabuvir** inhibits the polymerase following binding at the allosteric site, and does not have a nucleoside/nucleotide structure. The last viral target for DAAs is the NS3/4A protease that is involved in post-translational processing and replication of HCV. NS3/4A protease inhibitors include grazoprevir, **paritaprevir**, and **simeprevir**. Although simeprevir is one of the earliest protease inhibitors available, it is considered a second-generation drug due to its high binding affinity and specificity for NS3/4A.

Common ADRs of DAAs include nausea, headache and fatigue. Pruritus and insomnia are associated with dasabuvir, ombitasvir and paritaprevir. Asthenia is associated with ledipasvir and dasabuvir. Simeprevir may also result in photosensitivity, hyperbilirubinemia, and pruritus. To improve remission rates and decrease viral resistance, new therapy regimens have these drugs being used in combination (Table 28-2). These drugs are not recommended for treatment of HCV during pregnancy.

VACCINES AND IMMUNE GLOBULINS: ACTIVE AND PASSIVE IMMUNIZATIONS

Vaccines consist of whole virions or viral fragments that are completely inactivated (dead) or partially inactivated (live attenuated). Active immunization involves inoculation with a vaccine that triggers the host immune system to produce antibodies and cell-mediated immunity against the antigen. Thus, active immunization provides immunity to subsequent exposure to that particular virus. The ideal vaccine produces complete prevention of the viral disease, prevention of carrying the virus (carrier state), production of long-lasting immunity with a minimum number of immunizations, absence of toxicity, and convenience for mass immunizations (eg, inexpensive and easy to administer). Although inoculation with live attenuated products imparts longer-lasting immunity than inoculation with dead antigens, the risk of contracting the viral disease is greater. Examples of live attenuated vaccines include those for measles, mumps, and rubella (MMR), poliovirus (the oral vaccine), and herpes varicella zoster virus. Vaccines containing dead viral antigens include those for rabies and both hepatitis A and B viruses. Currently, vaccines are available for many viral infections. Whereas some vaccinations are required by state laws (eg, measles and polio for children attending public school), others are only administered to high-risk populations (eg, influenza for older adults).

Unlike active immunization, which requires the individual's immune system to produce its *own* antibodies after inoculation with an antigen, passive immunization is the transfer of *preformed* antibodies (immunoglobulins) to an individual. Passive immunization allows an individual to gain immediate immunity. However, since the individual does not produce his/her own antibodies, immunity is only temporary. Passive immunization products generally contain high titers of antibodies directed against a specific antigen or the products may simply contain antibodies found in most of the population. Passive immunization is used for: (1) individuals who are unable to form antibodies (eg, congenital agammaglobulinemia); (2) prevention of disease when time does not permit active immunization (eg, postexposure); (3) treatment of certain diseases normally prevented by immunization (eg, tetanus); and (4) treatment of conditions for which active immunization is unavailable or impractical (eg, snakebite). Antibodies can be derived from animal or human sources. Immunizations derived from human antibodies have the advantages of avoiding the risk of hypersensitivity reactions and having a longer half-life than those from animal sources.

REHABILITATION RELEVANCE

The development and clinical application of new antiviral drugs have significantly improved the quality of life and longevity in patients with chronic viral infections. As a result, many patients with chronic infections are dying *with* these infections rather than *from* these infections. Due to the chronic nature of viral pharmacotherapy and the broad spectrum of adverse effects, not a single organ system is unaffected by these drugs. The ADRs of these drugs vary from minor to life-threatening. As a general rule, appointment times may need to be adjusted and therapy goals revised to account for some adverse effects. As an example, if a patient demonstrates increased severity or incidence of ADRs, patients could be instructed to schedule appointments just prior to dosing when

plasma levels are at their lowest and associated ADRs should be diminished. Below is a summary of ADRs associated with antiviral drugs that have a direct impact on physical therapy treatment and outcomes as well as potential solutions.

- **Nausea**, **vomiting**, and **diarrhea** are common GI manifestations resulting from all drug classes. Patients may be unable to attend scheduled appointments and achieve therapy goals. Adjust therapy appointments for times when the GI manifestations are diminished.
- **Skin rash** is an adverse effect for individual antiviral drugs in different drug classes. Although minor, a rash may be a prelude to Stevens-Johnson syndrome or epidermal necrolysis. Several antiviral drugs are sulfonamides that carry an increased risk of skin hypersensitivity reactions. Regardless of the underlying cause, if the therapist observes a rash, the patient should be instructed to contact the prescribing healthcare professional at the earliest opportunity.
- The incidence of **angina pectoris**, **myocardial infarction**, and **cardiac arrhythmias** may increase in individuals taking antiviral drugs. These adverse effects may be the direct result of certain drugs on cardiac function. Alternatively, some drugs—including the entire class of antiretroviral PIs—cause metabolic dysfunction, resulting in hyperglycemia, hypercholesterolemia, hypertriglyceridemia, and lipodystrophy. Careful monitoring of casual plasma glucose levels and monitoring of cardiac function should be conducted during therapy sessions. Development of a long-term conditioning program may improve lipid and glucose profiles and reduce morbidity and mortality associated with these adverse effects.
- **Hyperglycemia** due to peripheral insulin resistance may occur with some antiviral drugs. Patients should monitor blood glucose levels. Therapists should prescribe an appropriate regular exercise program since exercise improves insulin sensitivity (see Chapter 24).
- **Myalgia**, **arthralgia**, and **asthenia** might limit participation in therapy. Goals and treatment interventions should be adjusted when these adverse effects are present.
- **Depression**, **psychosis**, and **hallucinations** may alter patient attendance and compliance with therapy. If therapy goals cannot be altered to accommodate, therapy sessions may need to be discontinued until these ADRs are resolved. Consultation with the referring healthcare professional may be appropriate.
- Central nervous system adverse effects of **tremors**, **seizures**, **confusion**, **delirium**, and **insomnia** associated with individual antiviral drugs negatively affect the ability to participate in physical therapy. Consultation with the referring healthcare professional may be indicated.
- **Increased risk of infection** may be the direct result of the viral infection (eg, HIV) or myelosuppression resulting from specific antiviral drugs. If the infection is severe, therapy sessions may have to be significantly altered or discontinued until the infection is resolved. The therapist

should consult with the referring healthcare professional to determine the appropriate action.

- **Peripheral neuropathy** in the hands and feet may be the direct effect of individual antiviral drugs, or a consequence of chronic hyperglycemia or lipodystrophy associated with certain antiviral drugs. The physical therapist should provide appropriate guidelines for insensate foot care to patients who have peripheral sensory neuropathies. If peripheral muscle weakness is also present, the patient may require appropriate orthotics or other ambulatory aids.

If the peripheral neuropathy is new or progressing, this assessment should be reported to the referring healthcare professional.

- Zanamivir may cause **bronchial irritation** that exacerbates pulmonary dysfunction in patients with asthma or obstructive airway disease. Therapy sessions and goals need to be altered to account for breathing difficulties.
- **Increased fall risk** may result from one or more of the previously discussed adverse effects. The patient and therapist should discuss and begin appropriate fall-risk prevention guidelines.

CASE CONCLUSION

At the rehabilitation clinic, the physical therapist prescribed an aerobic and progressive resistance exercise program for F.M. His exercise program included 40 minutes of moderate intensity aerobic activity and 20 minutes of resistance training 3-4 times per week. Resistance training focused primarily on large muscle groups of the lower extremities. At subsequent visits, the therapist advanced the exercises appropriately while monitoring vital signs to ensure the progression was within his tolerance. F.M. has been stringently following his exercise program for 6 months. He is quite pleased with the results, noting that his belt fits better now and he has more strength and mass in his legs. At his physician's reassessment, F.M.'s metabolic profile also improved significantly: decreased total cholesterol and increased HDL cholesterol, decreased fasting blood glucose, and decreased resting blood pressure.

Without question, antiretroviral therapy has increased the lifespan and improved quality of life for individuals with HIV infection. As individuals with HIV/AIDS live longer, other comorbidities have emerged, either as a result of the pharmacotherapy, the chronic nature of the infection, or the emergence of cardiovascular and metabolic diseases that are common in the general population. Protease inhibitors traditionally included in ART regimens are often associated with development of dyslipidemia, insulin resistance, and lipodystrophy. For adults infected with HIV, an exercise regimen including aerobic and resistance training for at least 20 minutes, performed 3 times per week for at least 5 weeks appears to be safe and improve fitness and body composition. Specifically, resistance and aerobic exercise has been shown to help HIV-infected individuals gain lean body mass, decrease truncal adiposity, and decrease total cholesterol and triglyceride concentrations. Such changes may help prevent or mitigate potential cardiovascular and metabolic complications. Other recommendations include smoking cessation and reduction in dietary fat.

CHAPTER 28 QUESTIONS

1. Which of the following drugs does *not* require phosphorylation to inhibit herpetic DNA polymerase activity?

   a. Foscarnet
   b. Cidofovir
   c. Acyclovir
   d. Docosanol

2. Which of the following is a prodrug of penciclovir?

   a. Valacyclovir
   b. Famciclovir
   c. Fosamprenavir
   d. Tenofovir disoproxil fumarate

3. Which of the following is the allosteric inhibitor of the NS5B RNA-dependent RNA polymerase in the hepatitis C virus?

   a. Delavirdine
   b. Sofosbuvir
   c. Dasabuvir
   d. Simeprevir

4. Which of the following antiretroviral drugs has minimal cross-resistance with the other drugs listed below?

   a. Tenofovir
   b. Abacavir
   c. Lamivudine
   d. Efavirenz

5. Which of the following drugs is a pharmacokinetic "booster" that decreases the first-pass hepatic metabolism of other antiretroviral drugs?

    a. Ritonavir
    b. Fosamprenavir
    c. Indinavir
    d. Amprenavir

6. Taking vitamin E supplements may be contraindicated with which of the following drugs?

    a. Foscarnet
    b. Fosamprenavir
    c. Atazanavir
    d. Lopinavir

7. Which of the following drug classes has the highest risk for insulin resistance as an adverse effect?

    a. Antiherpetic drugs
    b. Nucleoside/nucleotide reverse transcriptase inhibitors
    c. Protease inhibitors
    d. Neuraminidase inhibitors

8. Which of the following drugs may increase the risk of psychiatric disorders due to increased dopaminergic activity in the central nervous system?

    a. Zanamivir
    b. Peramivir
    c. Ribavirin
    d. Amantadine

9. Which of the following drugs is *not* clinically used in the treatment of both HIV and HBV infections?

    a. Lamivudine
    b. Adefovir dipivoxil
    c. Tenofovir disoproxil fumarate
    d. Tenofovir alafenamide

10. Which of the following drugs may be contraindicated in a patient with obstructive airway disease?

    a. Oseltamivir
    b. Peramivir
    c. Zanamivir
    d. Amantadine

Antifungal and Antiparasitic Agents

CASE STUDY

A.G. is a 29-year-old woman who returned from a military deployment in the Middle East 2 months ago. She was admitted to a military rehabilitation hospital 4 days ago for an amputee rehabilitation program. She sustained a transtibial amputation of the left lower extremity 1 week ago, secondary to a traumatic injury that occurred during a military operation. Prior to injury, A.G. was functionally independent and an avid basketball player. At admission, A.G. was noted to have several crusted raised lesions that were up to 1 inch in diameter on her face, neck, and left forearm. She reported that the lesions were much larger and painful several weeks ago. An infectious disease physician sampled skin scrapings of the lesion and diagnosed the condition as cutaneous leishmaniasis. A.G. was started on a 20-day intravenous course of sodium stibogluconate, which she receives once per day, immediately prior to afternoon physical therapy sessions. A.G. is very motivated to return to her prior level of function and has been participating in physical therapy twice per day since admission.

During the first week, she met each therapy goal regarding residual limb edema control, stretching, strengthening, and pregait activities. She was making remarkable gains in therapy until 5 days after initiation of IV sodium stibogluconate when her energy level began declining, and she was unable to complete an hour of physical therapy. Today, while exercising in the parallel bars, she had to sit down twice secondary to dizziness. A.G. complains of severe hip and knee pain, as well as gluteal, quadriceps, and back muscle soreness. Although A.G.'s symptoms may be the result of her vigorous participation in rehabilitation, the physical therapist noted that some symptoms might be adverse effects of the new drug therapy. The therapist encouraged A.G. that these symptoms were likely to dissipate once the full course of drug therapy had been completed. A.G. stated that the drug treatment "has been far worse than these little sores." She states her intention to tell the doctor that she is no longer going to take the prescribed medication, so that she can "get on with rehab."

REHABILITATION FOCUS

In the most general scientific sense, "parasites" include all of the known infectious agents such as viruses, bacteria, fungi, protozoa, and helminths (worms) that live in or on host tissue, generally at the expense of the host. Certain species of parasites cause human infections. Some infections, especially fungal, are common in both industrialized and underdeveloped nations and cause varying degrees of illness and debility. Diseases caused by protozoan and helminthic parasites are among the leading causes of disease and death in tropical and subtropical regions. Many of these infections are intensified by inadequate water sanitation and hygiene, and their management is hampered by difficulty in controlling the vector (eg, mosquito, in the case of malaria). This chapter describes the most commonly used drugs to treat fungal, protozoan, and helminthic infections.

ANTIFUNGAL AGENTS

Most human fungal infections—called mycoses—are minor or superficial. However, the incidence and severity of mycoses have increased dramatically over the last few decades. This shift largely reflects the increasing number of immunocompromised individuals (secondary to HIV, cytotoxic cancer chemotherapy, or use of immunosuppressive drugs in solid organ or bone marrow transplant recipients). The widespread use of broad-spectrum antimicrobials in critically ill patients eliminates competitive nonpathogenic bacteria, increasing the risk of invasive fungal infections in this population as well.

Fungal infections are difficult to treat for several reasons. First, selective toxicity against fungal cells (and not the human host's cells) is more difficult to achieve than for bacteria. Second, many antifungal agents suffer from problems with solubility, stability, and absorption. Third, fungi readily develop resistance, especially when single drugs are used as monotherapy.

For years, the mainstay of pharmacotherapy against *systemic* fungal infections was amphotericin B. Though effective in many serious fungal infections, amphotericin B is very toxic. Two safer antifungal drug classes have been increasingly used. The azole agents are available in both oral and parenteral formulations whereas the echinocandins are available only in parenteral formulations. Unfortunately, owing to widespread use, azole-resistant and echinocandin-resistant organisms are becoming more widespread. As a result, combination

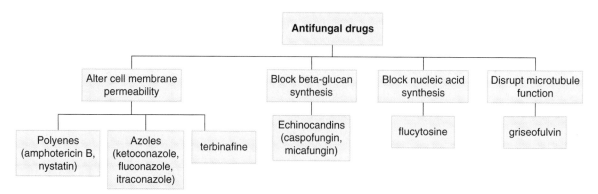

FIGURE 29-1 **Classification of antifungal drugs based on mechanism of action.** The polyenes, azoles, echinocandins, and terbinafine disrupt the fungal cell membrane, whereas flucytosine and griseofulvin interfere with fungal intracellular function. For drug classes, prototype drugs are shown in parentheses.

antifungal therapy and new formulations of old agents are being used.

Figure 29-1 classifies antifungal drugs on the basis of their target site of action. The major classes of antifungal agents—**polyenes**, **azoles**, **terbinafine**, and **echinocandins**—kill fungi by disrupting the synthesis or function of fungal cellular membranes. The antifungal activity of the less important agents, **flucytosine** and **griseofulvin**, is due to interference with intracellular functions. Clinically, antifungal drugs fall into several categories: (1) systemic drugs for systemic infections, (2) systemic drugs for mucocutaneous infections, and (3) topical drugs for mucocutaneous infections.

Systemic Drugs for Systemic Fungal Infections

The systemic drugs (oral or parenteral) available for treating systemic mycoses include amphotericin B, flucytosine, the azoles, and the echinocandins.

Amphotericin B

Amphotericin B is still one of the most important drugs for the treatment of nearly all life-threatening systemic mycoses. Amphotericin B is a polyene (containing many double bonds) agent that is available in oral, topical, and parenteral forms. Oral amphotericin B is only effective against fungi within the lumen of the gastrointestinal (GI) tract and cannot be used for treatment of systemic mycoses because it is poorly absorbed from the GI tract. Amphotericin B is generally administered intravenously as a nonlipid colloidal suspension, as a lipid complex, or in a liposomal formulation. Development of the latter form has reduced its nephrotoxicity by decreasing nonspecific binding to human cell membranes, permitting the use of larger doses. Amphotericin B is widely distributed to all tissues except the central nervous system (CNS). Therefore, treatment of certain types of fungal meningitis may necessitate intrathecal administration. Amphotericin B is primarily eliminated by

hepatic metabolism. Hepatic impairment, renal impairment, and dialysis have little effect on drug concentrations.

Amphotericin B kills fungi by binding to ergosterol. Ergosterol is a major sterol in fungal cell membranes, whereas the primary sterol found in bacteria and human cells is cholesterol. Drug binding forms pores in fungal cell membranes, causing leakage of cellular contents and fungal cell death (Figure 29-2). Some binding to human membrane sterols occurs, probably accounting for amphotericin B's serious toxicity.

Although newer and less toxic agents have replaced its use for most conditions, amphotericin B is a potent fungicidal with the widest antifungal spectrum of any agent. Thus, amphotericin B is often considered the drug (or co-drug) of choice for treating almost all life-threatening systemic infections caused by *Aspergillus, Blastomyces, Candida albicans, Cryptococcus, Histoplasma,* and *Mucor.* Amphotericin B is often used as the initial induction agent to quickly decrease fungal burden, and is then replaced by an azole agent (discussed below) for chronic treatment or relapse prevention. Amphotericin B is typically administered by slow intravenous (IV) infusion continued to a defined total dose rather than a defined time span. Doses vary depending on the particular infection, but it is not uncommon for patients to receive daily IV treatment for 6-12 weeks. Amphotericin B can also be directly injected into a joint to treat fungal arthritis or irrigated into the urinary bladder to treat candiduria. These routes have been shown to produce no serious systemic toxicity.

Toxic effects of amphotericin B are divided into two categories: immediate reactions related to drug infusion and reactions that occur more slowly. During infusion of the drug, extremely common adverse effects include fever, chills, vomiting, muscle spasms, headache, and hypotension. Slowing the infusion rate or decreasing the daily dose may reduce these effects. In addition, premedication with antipyretics, antiemetics, antihistamines, meperidine (an opioid analgesic), or glucocorticoids may be provided to partially overcome infusion-related effects.

Fungal cell

Fungal cell membrane and cell wall

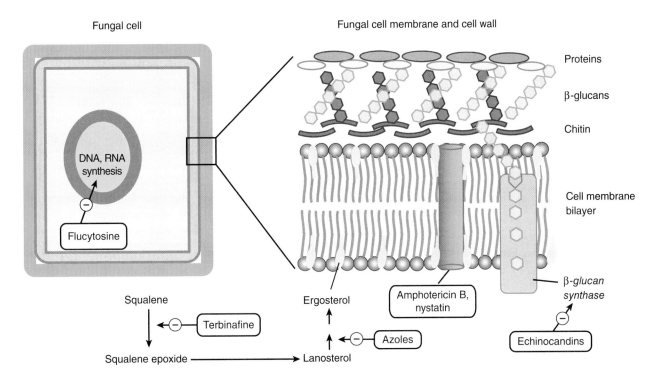

FIGURE 29-2 **Targets of antifungal drugs.** Except for flucytosine (and possibly griseofulvin, not shown), antifungal agents target the fungal cell membrane or cell wall.

The most significant toxicity associated with amphotericin B is renal damage. Nearly all patients experience some renal impairment, with reversible and irreversible components. The irreversible form of nephrotoxicity usually results from prolonged administration. Strategies to decrease nephrotoxicity include concomitant saline infusion, dose reduction (made possible by adding another antifungal agent), and the use of liposomal formulations of amphotericin B that may bind to human cell membranes less readily. Anemia may also occur due to decreased renal production of erythropoietin. Intrathecal administration may cause seizures and neurologic damage.

Flucytosine

Flucytosine (5-fluorocytosine, 5-FC) is related to the anticancer drug fluorouracil. Unlike amphotericin B, the drug is effective orally and is distributed to most body tissues, including the CNS. To avoid toxic accumulation, serum concentrations are monitored regularly and dose reductions are made for individuals with renal impairment.

Flucytosine is preferentially taken up by fungal cells, where the drug is enzymatically converted to a compound that inhibits deoxyribonucleic acid (DNA) and ribonucleic acid (RNA) synthesis, thus preventing the formation of fungal proteins (Figure 29-2). Human cells are unable to convert flucytosine to its active metabolites, which results in the drug's selective toxicity.

The antifungal spectrum of flucytosine is fairly narrow; it is active against yeasts such as *Cryptococcus neoformans*, some *Candida* species, and the molds that cause chromoblastomycosis (a chronic, localized skin and subcutaneous tissue infection that follows traumatic implantation of one of several different fungal species). When used as a single-drug therapy, resistance to flucytosine emerges rapidly. To provide optimal fungicidal effects and reduce resistance, flucytosine is given in combination with amphotericin B or fluconazole. These drug combinations may be used to treat susceptible candidal septicemia, cryptococcal meningitis (one of the most common opportunistic CNS infections in acquired immune deficiency syndrome [AIDS] patients), and chromoblastomycosis.

The most common adverse drug reactions (ADRs) result from the metabolism of flucytosine to the anticancer drug fluorouracil. Anemia, leukopenia, and thrombocytopenia result from the reversible impairment of bone marrow function. Less commonly, flucytosine causes liver dysfunction. Plasma drug concentration and renal function are monitored during drug therapy to avoid toxic accumulation.

Azoles

The azoles include eight antifungal agents named for the five-membered carbon-nitrogen ring in their structure. Six azole drugs are used for systemic fungal infections: **ketoconazole**, **fluconazole**, **itraconazole**, **posaconazole**, **voriconazole**, and **isavuconazole**. Fluconazole, posaconazole, voriconazole, and isavuconazole are more reliably absorbed than the other azoles after oral administration. The azoles are distributed to most body tissues, but drug levels achieved in the CNS are very low (with the exception of fluconazole and possibly posacon- azole). The liver metabolizes all the systemic azoles, except flu- conazole, which is eliminated by the kidneys.

The azoles disrupt membrane function of fungal cells by interfering with the synthesis of ergosterol (Figure 29-2), a process that involves fungal cytochrome P450 (CYP) enzymes similar to human CYP isoforms. Resistance to azoles has become more widespread owing to increased use of this class of drugs for long-term prophylaxis of systemic mycoses in immunocompromised and neutropenic patients.

As a group, the azoles have a broad spectrum of action, including many species of *Candida*, *Cryptococcus neoformans*, the endemic mycoses (blastomycosis, coccidioidomycosis, histo- plasmosis), and the dermatophytes. The azoles are relatively non- toxic. The most common ADRs include minor GI disturbances and rash. Varying degrees of hepatotoxicity may occur, especially in patients with impaired liver function. All azoles inhibit human hepatic CYPs to *some* extent because of their similarity to the target fungal enzymes. Thus, patients taking azoles (especially ketoconazole) in combination with other drugs may have higher plasma concentrations of drugs that are primarily metabolized by the CYP system. In addition, inhibition of human CYP (espe- cially by ketoconazole) interferes with synthesis of adrenal and other steroids, which may lead to gynecomastia, menstrual irreg- ularities, or infertility. Because ketoconazole causes more adverse effects than the other azoles, systemic ketoconazole is rarely used.

Fluconazole has the highest therapeutic index of all the azoles. This azole has high oral bioavailability, relatively good GI tolerance, and the least effect on hepatic enzymes. Flucon- azole is the drug of choice for initial treatment and secondary prophylaxis for cryptococcal meningitis, and is also used as an adjunctive drug in treating active infection due to *Cryptococ- cus neoformans*. Fluconazole is the most common drug used to treat mucocutaneous candidiasis and a single oral dose usually eradicates vaginal candidiasis. For treating candidemia, fluco- nazole is as effective as amphotericin B.

Itraconazole is effective against many systemic fungal infec- tions caused by *Blastomyces* and *Sporothrix* and for chromoblas- tomycosis. Itraconazole can be used as the primary or alternative drug for treating infections caused by *Coccidioides*, *Cryptococ- cus,* and *Histoplasma*. Itraconazole is also used extensively in the treatment of dermatophytoses and onychomycosis.

Posaconazole is a broad-spectrum azole with activity against most species of *Aspergillus* and *Candida*. This azole is recommended for prophylaxis of fungal infections during can- cer chemotherapy and as treatment in invasive aspergillosis, when preferred therapies have failed. Posaconazole and isavu- conazole are the only azoles with activity against the fungi that cause mucormycosis, aggressive and invasive infections caused by specific types of molds that can affect many organ systems.

Voriconazole is well absorbed orally and has an even wider spectrum of antifungal activity than itraconazole. Due to its greater efficacy and less toxicity, voriconazole has replaced amphotericin B as the treatment of choice for invasive aspergil- losis and some environmental molds. Voriconazole is an alterna- tive drug for treating candidemia and candidal esophagitis and

stomatitis in individuals with AIDS. In addition to the ADRs common to the azoles, voriconazole has been reported to cause transient visual disturbances in more than 30% of patients.

Echinocandins

Echinocandins represent the newest class of antifungal agents. Currently, three echinocandins are available: **caspofungin**, **micafungin**, and **anidulafungin**. These drugs are only admin- istered intravenously, distribute widely to tissues, and are mostly eliminated by hepatic metabolism. Doses are decreased in patients with severe hepatic impairment. Caspofungin does not distribute well to the cerebrospinal fluid (CSF). However, despite low CSF concentrations, positive results have been reported with caspofungin in the treatment of cerebral aspergillosis.

The echinocandins inhibit an enzyme present in fungal, but not mammalian cells. The result is impaired synthesis of β(1-3) glucan, an essential component of fungal cell walls. The echinocandins are used for treating candidemia and other forms of *Candida* infections (esophageal candidiasis, perito- nitis, and intra-abdominal abscess). This class of antifungal agents may be used as therapy in life-threatening fungal infec- tions (eg, invasive aspergillosis) with strains that are no longer susceptible to conventional antifungals such as amphotericin B and the azoles. However, clinically relevant resistance to the echinocandins is emerging. The echinocandins have excellent tolerability and safety, with infrequent reports of minor GI adverse effects and flushing.

Systemic Drugs for Mucocutaneous Fungal Infections

Superficial fungal infections include those affecting the mucous membranes (especially the oropharynx and vagina) and those affecting the skin, hair, and nails (called dermatophytoses). Typically, these superficial infections have little likelihood for systemic proliferation. Infection severity ranges from rela- tively minor cosmetic inconveniences such as onychomycosis (chronic fungal infection that commonly affects toenails more than fingernails) to oral thrush, a painful candidal infection that is often the first manifestation of local or systemic immu- nosuppression. Although these mucocutaneous infections are superficial, topical application alone is often ineffective because of insufficient penetration into the affected tissues. This is especially true with onychomycosis because topical antifungal agents are unlikely to penetrate through all nail layers to suc- cessfully eradicate the fungus. Only a few antifungal drugs have been considered safe enough to be taken orally for treat- ing superficial fungal infections: griseofulvin, terbinafine, and a select number of azole agents.

Griseofulvin

Griseofulvin's only indication is for the treatment of derma- tophytoses. Oral absorption is variable, but can be optimized when consumed with a high-fat meal. Griseofulvin interferes with microtubule formation in dermatophytes. The drug binds to keratin precursor cells. As older (infected) skin cells are gradually exfoliated, they are replaced with noninfected cells. Griseofulvin remains bound to new keratin, protecting the skin from new infection. To allow for replacement of infected keratin by newly resistant keratin, griseofulvin must be administered for long periods of time: 2-6 weeks for skin and hair infections and for at least 6 months for toenail infections. However, the use of griseofulvin is plagued by high relapse rates, especially for onychomycosis. The most common ADRs include skin rashes and urticaria (hives). Other toxic effects include GI irritation, mental confusion, headache, and photosensitivity. Terbinafine and some azoles have largely replaced griseofulvin in the treatment of dermatophytoses.

Terbinafine

Terbinafine inhibits a fungal enzyme and results in accumulation of a substance toxic to the fungus. Terbinafine offers a shorter treatment regimen, higher cure rate, lower relapse rate, and fewer adverse effects than griseofulvin. Terbinafine is available in oral and topical formulations. Daily oral treatment for 12 weeks may result in a clinical cure rate as high as 90% for onychomycosis. ADRs include GI upset, headache, rash, and taste disturbances as well as rare, though serious, hepatotoxicity. Consequently, liver enzyme levels are obtained before oral terbinafine is initiated.

Azoles

Itraconazole can be used orally for treating dermatophytoses. For onychomycosis, intermittent dosing with itraconazole (usually 1 week of dosing followed by 3 weeks without drug) is as effective as continuous dosing because the drug persists in the nails for months. Intermittent oral dosing lowers the incidence of ADRs and the financial cost of the medication. Oral fluconazole has also been used in the treatment of onychomycosis (though the drug is not labeled by the Food and Drug Administration for this indication).

Topical Drugs for Mucocutaneous Fungal Infections

A number of dermatologic fungal infections such as ringworm, jock itch, and athlete's foot as well as some localized (oral, vaginal) candidal infections may be successfully treated with antifungal agents applied topically to the affected area. Topical agents can be divided into three major categories: polyenes, azoles, and allylamines.

Nystatin is a polyene agent with a similar mechanism of action to amphotericin B (Figure 29-2). Because its toxicity precludes systemic use, nystatin is only used topically. Nystatin is not significantly absorbed from skin or mucous membranes. Nystatin (as powder, cream, ointment, or vaginal tablet) is commonly used to treat localized candidal infections in the oropharynx, in the vagina, and in areas where opposing skin surfaces may rub together, such as around the perineum or under the breasts. Localized infections can be cured rapidly, often within

24-72 hours after treatment initiation. Topical forms of amphotericin B are also used for oral or cutaneous candidiasis and topical drops are used to treat mycotic corneal ulcers.

The most common topical azole agents are **clotrimazole** and **miconazole**. Both are available as prescription and over the counter (OTC) in formulations including creams, powders, sprays, or vaginal suppositories. Clotrimazole and miconazole creams are used for the effective treatment of *tinea pedis* (athlete's foot), *tinea cruris* (jock itch), and *tinea corporis* (ringworm). Vaginal clotrimazole suppositories are used to treat vaginal yeast infections. Oral clotrimazole lozenges (called troches) are used to treat oral candidiasis infections that frequently occur in immunocompromised individuals. Systemic absorption is minimal and adverse effects are rare.

Topical allylamine creams—terbinafine and **naftifine**—are effective in the treatment of dermatologic fungal infections such as *tinea cruris* and *tinea corporis*. In the United States, these agents are prescription drugs. Table 29-1 summarizes the indications and toxicities of important antifungal agents.

ANTIPARASITIC AGENTS

A large number of protozoa and helminths (worms) are capable of infecting humans. Drugs designed to kill these parasites must take into account their complex life cycles and the differences between their metabolic pathways and those of the human host. Thus, drugs acting against protozoa are usually inactive against helminths and vice versa. Because protozoa and helminths are eukaryotes, they are metabolically more similar to humans than to bacteria. Therefore, most antibacterial drugs are ineffective against eukaryotic parasites. Key exceptions include the antibiotics metronidazole and doxycycline, which have antiprotozoal activity.

Rational approaches to antiparasitic chemotherapy use the principle of selective toxicity, which exploits the biochemical and physiologic differences between parasite and human host cells. Many antiparasitic drugs act on targets (usually enzymes) that are either unique to the parasite, or that possess sufficient differences between host and parasite to allow safe drug activity. Despite differences between host and parasite, many of the more effective antiparasitic drugs have significant toxicity and their use must balance benefit against risk.

Climatic changes and international travel have facilitated the spread of many parasitic diseases, while starvation and poor sanitation that accompany poverty and war have promoted the reemergence of others. Drug resistance has also dramatically influenced the ability to treat and control many parasitic diseases. A notable theme in treating parasitic infections is combination drug therapy, which helps decrease drug resistance and improves therapeutic efficacy.

Antiprotozoal Drugs

Protozoa are unicellular eukaryotic organisms. The parasitic protozoa that cause disease in humans either require the invasion of a suitable host to complete all or part of their life cycle, or they present as free-living protozoa that may become pathogenic in immunocompromised individuals. Figure 29-3 includes the drugs used to treat conditions malaria, amebiasis, toxoplasmosis, pnemocystosis, trypanosomiasis, and leishmaniasis.

Drugs for Malaria

In terms of annual mortality, malaria remains the most important tropical parasitic disease. In 2017, the World Health Organization (WHO) estimated approximately 219 million cases of malaria with 435,000 deaths due to the infection. Over 90% of the global malaria burden occurs in Africa, with the majority of deaths occurring in children under the age of 5 years in the sub-Saharan region of the continent. Although four *Plasmodium* species infect humans (*P falciparum, P malariae, P ovale, P vivax*), *P falciparum* is responsible for the largest burden of serious life-threatening complications and death. In 2017, over 99% of the estimated malaria cases in Africa were due to *P falciparum*, whereas *P vivax* is the predominant parasite in the Americas.

Transmission most commonly occurs when an infected mosquito injects the infectious form of the parasite, the *sporozoite*, into the individual's blood. Sporozoites circulate to the liver and infect liver cells. Here, they reproduce to form *merozoites*, which eventually leave the liver, reenter the bloodstream, and invade red blood cells (RBCs). The parasites mature within RBCs, are released, and continue infecting

TABLE 29-1 Some important antifungal drugs.

Class	Drug	Indications	Adverse Reactions
Allylamines (topical)	Terbinafine, naftifine,	*Tinea cruris, tinea corporis*	
Allylamines (oral)	Terbinafine	Onychomycosis	Rash, gastrointestinal irritation, headache, taste disturbances, rare cases of hepatic failure
Azoles (parenteral)	Fluconazole	Cryptococcal meningitis (treatment and prophylaxis) Mucocutaneous candidiasis Vaginal candidiasis	Gastrointestinal disturbances, rash, varying degree of hepatotoxicity, drug interactions, visual disturbances (voriconazole)
	Itraconazole	*Blastomyces* and *Sporothrix* infections Chromoblastomycosis Dermatophytoses, especially onychomycosis	
	Voriconazole	Invasive aspergillosis Candidemia	
	Posaconazole	Prophylaxis of fungal infections during cancer chemotherapy Invasive aspergillosis Mucormycosis	
Azoles (topical)	Clotrimazole, miconazole, ketoconazole	*Tinea pedis, tinea cruris, tinea corporis* Vaginal and oral candidal infections	Local erythema, burning/stinging, pruritus
Echinocandins	Caspofungin, micafungin, anidulafungin	*Candida* infections Infections resistant to amphotericin B and azoles	Minor gastrointestinal disturbances, flushing
Polyenes (primarily parenteral)	Amphotericin B	Almost all life-threatening systemic fungal functions	1. Infusion-related: fever, chills, muscle spasms, hypotension 2. Slower: renal damage
Polyenes (topical)	Nystatin	Localized candidal infections in oropharynx, vagina, and areas where opposing skin rub together	Local irritation
Flucytosine		*Cryptococcus neoformans* and some *Candida* species	Bone marrow impairment (anemia, leukopenia, thrombocytopenia)
Griseofulvin		Dermatophytoses	Skin rash, hives, gastrointestinal irritation

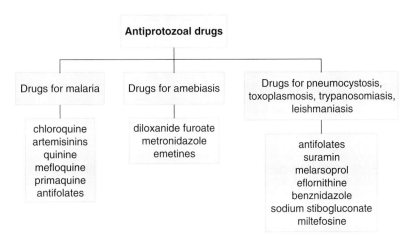

FIGURE 29-3 **Antiprotozoal drugs are used to combat malaria, amebiasis, pneumocystosis, toxoplasmosis, trypanosomiasis, and leishmaniasis.**

more RBCs. At this stage of infection, clinical disease is manifested by recurrent flu-like attacks, fever, severe anemia, and, in some cases, cerebral malaria, and death.

In both *P falciparum* and *P malariae* infections, only one cycle of liver cell invasion and multiplication occurs. Liver infection ceases spontaneously in less than 4 weeks. In this case, drugs that eliminate parasites within RBCs (blood schizonticides) can cure most of these infections if the parasite is not drug resistant. On the other hand, *P ovale* and *P vivax* can remain dormant in the liver for months or years. Subsequent malaria relapses can occur after completion of successful pharmacotherapy directed against the erythrocytic parasites. To cure these infections, drugs that eliminate liver parasites (tissue schizonticides) must be used in conjunction with blood schizonticides that eliminate erythrocytic parasites. No single available antimalarial agent can reliably bring about a "radical cure," which is the elimination of *both* hepatic and erythrocytic stages.

Table 29-2 lists the major drugs used in malarial prophylaxis and treatment. For many agents, antimalarial activity is due to either intracellular accumulation of a compound toxic to the parasite (eg, **chloroquine**), interference with parasitic DNA replication (eg, **quinine**), inhibition of critical enzymes involved in folic acid synthesis (eg, **pyrimethamine**, **proguanil**, **sulfadoxine**), inhibition of mitochondrial electron transport (eg, **atovaquone**), or production of free radicals (eg, **artemisinins**). For other drugs, the antimalarial mechanism of action is not clear (eg, **mefloquine**, **primaquine**, **halofantrine**, and **doxycycline**). Since parasites are increasingly resistant to multiple drugs, no chemoprophylactic regimen is fully protective, and treatment for malaria depends on knowledge of changing resistance patterns.

The first line of defense against malaria is limiting contact with mosquitoes by using mosquito repellent, keeping arms and legs covered, staying indoors during mosquitoes' peak feeding hours (dusk and throughout the night), and sleeping under mosquito netting. Physical therapists involved in the Peace Corps, Health Volunteers Overseas, or other international organizations are likely to practice in malaria endemic areas. Prior to leaving home, individuals should consult the Centers for Disease Control and Prevention (CDC) for current recommendations regarding specific antimalarial chemoprophylaxis, resistance patterns, and treatment, if malaria is contracted. While there are few available drugs capable of preventing erythrocytic infection, all effective chemoprophylactic antimalarials kill the erythrocytic parasites before they can reproduce and increase sufficiently in number to cause clinical disease.

Chloroquine

Chloroquine, long considered the drug of choice for prophylaxis and treatment of malaria, is no longer considered the first-line antimalarial agent in many countries owing to worldwide prevalence of chloroquine-resistant parasites. In regions where *P falciparum* is not resistant, chloroquine is used for chemoprophylaxis and treatment of acute attacks of falciparum and nonfalciparum malaria. Chloroquine is only a blood schizonticide. The drug is generally well tolerated, even with prolonged use. The most common ADRs are GI upset, skin rash or itching, and headaches. Consumption of calcium- and magnesium-containing antacids should be avoided because they significantly decrease oral chloroquine absorption. Dosing after meals may reduce some adverse effects. Long-term administration of high doses of chloroquine for rheumatologic diseases (see Chapter 34) may cause severe skin lesions, peripheral neuropathies, myocardial depression, retinal damage, auditory impairment, and toxic psychosis. Rarely, chloroquine can produce severe hemolysis in individuals with glucose-6-phosphate dehydrogenase (G6PD) deficiency.

Artemisinins

The most important newer antimalarial compounds are derivatives of artemisinin (an extract of the Chinese herbal remedy quinghaosu). **Artesunate**, **artemether**, and **dihydroartemisinin**

TABLE 29-2 Drugs used in malaria.

Drug	Use for Treatment	Use for Prophylaxis	Use for Eradication of Liver Stages
Chloroquine	Yes for *P vivax* and *P ovale* malaria, except in regions where *P falciparum* is resistant	Yes, except in regions where *P falciparum* is resistant	No
Artemisinins (artesunate, artemether, dihydroartemisinin)	Yes, for all chloroquine-resistant malaria[a]	No	No
Mefloquine	Yes, in areas with chloroquine-resistant *P falciparum* Not for severe or complicated malaria	Yes, in areas with chloroquine-resistant *P falciparum*	No
Quinine	Yes, oral for uncomplicated falciparum malaria[b]; intravenous for severe falciparum malaria	No	No
Primaquine	No	Yes, in areas of *P vivax* or *P ovale*	Yes[c]
Antifolates (pyrimethamine, proguanil, sulfadoxine)	No	Not usually advised as single agents	No
Atovaquone-proguanil (Malarone)	Yes, for uncomplicated *P falciparum* malaria	Yes, especially in areas with chloroquine-resistant *P falciparum*	No

[a]Artemisinins are usually given in combination with other antimalarial drugs.
[b]In most cases, quinine is used in combination with doxycycline, clindamycin, or an antifolate drug.
[c]Primaquine is used in conjunction with a blood schizonticide.

are blood schizonticides that have rapid antimalarial activity and are the only drugs reliably effective against quinine-resistant strains. Because of their short half-lives, the artemisinins are generally used with another antimalarial agent and are not useful in chemoprophylaxis. Artemisinin-based combination therapy is now the standard of care for treatment of uncomplicated falciparum malaria in nearly all endemic areas. The artemisinins are generally well tolerated, with common ADRs of nausea, vomiting, diarrhea, and dizziness, though these may also reflect the signs and symptoms of the underlying malaria. Treatment of uncomplicated falciparum malaria with artemisinins during pregnancy appears safe and is recommended by the WHO.

Quinine

Quinine is the original antimalarial drug that is derived from the bark of the native South American cinchona tree. The main use of quinine (and **quinidine**, its dextrorotatory stereoisomer) is in treating severe chloroquine-resistant falciparum malaria. Quinine acts rapidly against all four species of human malaria parasites in erythrocytes, but has no activity against liver stage parasites. Quinine is often used in combination with a second drug (doxycycline or **clindamycin**) to limit toxicity by shortening its duration of use (generally to 3 days). Because of its toxicity and the potential increase in parasitic resistance, quinine is generally not used in chemoprophylaxis. Therapeutic doses of quinine commonly cause cinchonism. Milder symptoms such as GI distress, headache, vertigo, blurred vision, and tinnitus do not warrant discontinuation of the drug. Higher doses of quinine result in cardiac conduction disturbances. In some individuals with hypersensitivity, severe

blood disorders can occur. Therapy is discontinued in hypersensitive patients and those with severe cinchonism.

Mefloquine

Mefloquine is a first-line chemoprophylactic drug (taken weekly) for use in most malaria-endemic regions, except those with no chloroquine resistance (where chloroquine is preferred). Mefloquine is the only chemoprophylactic other than chloroquine approved for pregnant women and children weighing less than 5 kg. Resistance is uncommon, except in parts of Southeast Asia that have high rates of multidrug resistance. For treatment of uncomplicated falciparum malaria, mefloquine is often combined with artesunate. Mefloquine causes headache and dizziness. Severe neuropsychiatric disturbances such as depression, confusion, acute psychosis, or seizures have also been reported with mefloquine.

Primaquine

Primaquine is the drug of choice to eradicate dormant liver stage parasites of *P vivax* and *P ovale* and should be used in conjunction with an antimalarial effective against parasites within RBCs (typically chloroquine). Primaquine is also an alternative chemoprophylactic regimen. The drug is generally well tolerated, but sometimes causes nausea, headache, and epigastric pain. Because primaquine can produce severe hemolysis in patients with G6PD deficiency, persons for whom this agent is being considered must be evaluated for G6PD enzyme levels and the drug should not be used in those who are G6PD deficient or pregnant females.

Antifolates

Pyrimethamine, **proguanil**, and **sulfadoxine** inhibit critical enzymes involved in folate metabolism that the malarial parasites rely on for their growth. For prevention of malaria, single antifolate agents are no longer recommended because of toxicity and frequent resistance. Instead, combination regimens (eg, **trimethoprim-sulfamethoxazole**, **sulfadoxine-pyrimethamine**) are advised. Antifolates are not recommended as therapy for malaria, though they may be used in combination with artemisinin regimens as a less preferred treatment for falciparum malaria. Toxic effects of the antifolates include GI distress, rashes, hemolysis, and kidney damage.

Other Antimalarial Drugs

Although no antibiotics are effective enough to be used as single agents in the treatment of malaria, several antibiotics are somewhat active blood schizonticides. Doxycycline or clindamycin are often used in combination with either quinine or artesunate. Doxycycline has also become a standard prophylactic drug in areas of Southeast Asia with high rates of resistance to other antimalarials, including mefloquine.

Amodiaquine is a chloroquine-like compound. Used in combination with artesunate (as a single tablet), this regimen is first-line therapy for treatment of falciparum malaria in many parts of Africa. Although long-term chemoprevention is not recommended due to toxicity, short-term seasonal prophylaxis with amodiaquine plus sulfadioxine-pyrimethamine is recommended in some parts of Africa.

Atovaquone/proguanil (Malarone) is approved for both prevention and treatment of falciparum malaria. For chemoprophylaxis, this single tablet can be taken for shorter periods before and after the period at risk for malaria transmission than either mefloquine or doxycycline. The disadvantage is that Malarone is more expensive.

Halofantrine, typically only available in malaria-endemic countries, is rapidly effective for treatment of falciparum malaria, but its use is limited by cardiac toxicity. **Lumefantrine** is a related drug with minimal cardiotoxicity that is well tolerated. Lumefantrine is used in fixed combination with artemether as first-line therapy for uncomplicated falciparum malaria in many countries. To treat falciparum and vivax malaria, **pyronaridine** is used in fixed combination with artesunate.

Drugs for Amebiasis

Amebiasis is infection with *Entamoeba histolytica*. Although amebiasis occurs worldwide, it is most prevalent in tropical and subtropical areas, especially in crowded and unsanitary living conditions. This parasitic amoeba lives and reproduces on the mucosal surface of the large intestine. Encysted forms periodically pass out in the feces, and can survive in the external environment and act as infective forms. Infection with *E histolytica* occurs as a result of inadequate sanitation, or when food or drink is contaminated by infected food handlers. Ingested cysts adhere to intestinal epithelial cells and invade the mucosal lining. *E histolytica* can cause asymptomatic intestinal infection, mild to moderate colitis, mild diarrhea, severe intestinal infection (amebic dysentery), liver abscess, and other extraintestinal infections.

Table 29-3 includes the drugs used to treat protozoal infections, including the varying forms of amebiasis. The tissue amebicides (**chloroquine**, **emetines**, **metronidazole**, **tinidazole**) are effective against the organisms in the bowel wall and

TABLE 29-3 Drugs used in the treatment of protozoal infections other than malaria.

Drugs of Choice	Primary Indications
Benznidazole or nifurtimox	Chagas disease (infection caused by *Trypanosoma cruzi*)
Diloxanide furoate	Asymptomatic intestinal amebiasis
Eflornithine	Advanced West African trypanosomiasis (infection caused by *Trypanosoma brucei gambiense*)
Melarsoprol	Advanced East African trypanosomiasis (infection caused by *Trypanosoma rhodesiense*)
Metronidazole or tinidazole plus diloxanide or iodoquinol	Mild to severe intestinal amebiasis
Pentamidine	Early stage of West African trypanosomiasis Alternative for *Pneumocystis jiroveci* pneumonia
Pyrimethamine plus sulfadiazine (or clindamycin)	Toxoplasmosis
Sodium stibogluconate or meglumine antimoniate	Leishmaniasis (cutaneous and visceral forms)
Suramin	Acute hemolymphatic stage of East African trypanosomiasis
Trimethoprim-sulfamethoxazole (TMP-SMZ)	*Pneumocystis jiroveci* pneumonia

the liver, whereas the luminal amebicides (**diloxanide furoate**, **iodoquinol**, **paromomycin**) are only effective against the organisms *within* the lumen of the bowel.

In endemic areas, asymptomatic carriers are typically *not* treated. However, in nonendemic areas, asymptomatic carriers are treated with a luminal amebicide. For asymptomatic disease (carriers with no symptoms in nonendemic areas), diloxanide furoate is the first choice single agent, though iodoquinol or paromomycin may also be used. These luminal amebicides eradicate the parasite in 80-90% of carriers. Diloxanide furoate can also be combined with other agents to treat mild intestinal disease.

For mild to severe intestinal infection, liver abscess, and other extraintestinal amebic disease, metronidazole or tinidazole is generally used in conjunction with a luminal amebicide. Efficacy after a single 10-day course of metronidazole is roughly 90%. Adverse effects of metronidazole include GI irritation, headache, and, less frequently, leukopenia, dizziness, and ataxia (Chapter 30 for further discussion of metronidazole). Tinidazole appears to have similar effectiveness and a better adverse effect profile. For rare cases in which metronidazole treatment has failed, chloroquine may be added to a second metronidazole treatment regimen. In hospitalized patients when metronidazole is ineffective or cannot be used, emetine and dehydroemetine may be used as backup drugs for treatment of severe intestinal or hepatic amebiasis. However, the emetines may cause severe toxicity including GI distress, muscle weakness, and cardiovascular dysfunction.

Drugs for Pneumocystosis

Pneumocystis jiroveci (formerly called *P carinii*) is the cause of human pneumocystosis. Although now recognized as a fungus, *P jiroveci* is responsive to antiprotozoal drugs, not to antifungal drugs. The fungus is commonly found in humans, but causes symptomatic disease only in immune-deficient individuals. Thus, there is a high incidence of *P jiroveci* pneumonia in patients receiving immunosuppressive therapy and in individuals with AIDS.

Trimethoprim plus sulfamethoxazole (**TMP-SMZ**) is the first-line therapy for *P jiroveci* pneumonia and as chemoprophylaxis in immunocompromised individuals. Chemoprophylactic dosing is generally much better tolerated than high-dose treatment for active infection. Significant toxicity occurs in up to 50% of individuals with AIDS. Important toxicities include GI distress, rash, fever, neutropenia, and thrombocytopenia. Adverse effects may be severe enough to warrant discontinuance of TMP-SMZ. Because of the high prevalence of serious adverse effects, several drugs have been used as alternative agents against *P jiroveci* infection. Notably, none is as effective as TMP-SMZ.

Pentamidine is a well-established alternative drug for *P jiroveci* infection and prophylaxis, though the drug has lower efficacy and higher toxicity than TMP-SMZ. For prophylaxis, pentamidine is administered as an inhaled aerosol. For treatment of active *P jiroveci* infection, pentamidine must be administered parenterally. Serious ADRs result from parenteral administration, including respiratory stimulation followed by respiratory depression, severe hypotension, hypoglycemia, anemia, neutropenia, hepatitis, and pancreatitis.

For mild to moderate pneumocystosis, the combination of clindamycin and primaquine is an alternative regimen offering improved tolerance compared with high-dose TMP-SMZ or pentamidine. However, the efficacy of this drug combination against severe pneumocystis pneumonia is not well studied. **Atovaquone** is an oral drug (initially developed as an antimalarial) that has also been approved for treating mild to moderate *P jiroveci* pneumonia. Although less effective than TMP-SMZ or pentamidine, this drug is better tolerated. Adverse effects include fever, rash, cough, nausea, vomiting, diarrhea, and abnormal liver function tests.

Drugs for Toxoplasmosis

Toxoplasmosis is infection with *Toxoplasma gondii*. Infection occurs by ingesting oocysts released in the feces of infected cats (the primary hosts) or by eating raw meat containing tissue cysts. Infection with this protozoan is widespread, but is not serious unless it is acquired (or reactivated) in immunosuppressed individuals or acquired during pregnancy, when the organism invades all fetal tissues, especially the CNS. Damage to the eye is the most common consequence, although the brain may also be affected.

The antifolate agents pyrimethamine with **sulfadiazine** (or with clindamycin in patients allergic to sulfonamides) are used for treatment of both congenital toxoplasmosis and acute infection in immunocompromised individuals. In AIDS-related *Toxoplasma* encephalitis, high-dose treatment must be given for many weeks and is associated with gastric irritation, neurologic symptoms (headaches, insomnia, tremors, seizures) and serious blood abnormalities. In small numbers of immunocompromised individuals with toxoplasmosis that are unresponsive to other agents, atovaquone has also been effective. **Spiramycin** is an antibiotic that is used to treat toxoplasmosis acquired during pregnancy. Treatment lowers the risk of development of congenital toxoplasmosis.

Drugs for Trypanosomiasis

The protozoan genus *Trypanosoma* contains three species that cause human disease. Infections with *T gambiense* and *T rhodesiense* cause African trypanosomiasis (African sleeping sickness), and *T cruzi* infection causes American trypanosomiasis (Chagas disease). Trypanosomiasis is transmitted by the bite of infected insect vectors. For African trypanosomiasis, the vector is the tsetse fly. For American trypanosomiasis, the vector is the reduviid bug. Currently available drugs for all forms of trypanosomiasis (Table 29-3) are seriously deficient in efficacy, safety, or both. Availability of these drugs is also a concern because they are mainly supplied by donation or nonprofit production by pharmaceutical companies.

After a bite by an infected tsetse fly, widespread lymph node enlargement occurs and the organism establishes in the blood and rapidly multiplies. **Suramin** is the first-line therapy for the acute hemolymphatic stage of East African trypanosomiasis (*T brucei rhodesiense* infection) and can also be used for chemoprophylaxis. Because suramin does not enter the CNS, it is not effective against advanced disease when the CNS becomes involved. Intravenous suramin commonly causes early adverse effects including nausea, vomiting, and fatigue as well as later reactions such as rash, neurologic and renal complications. Although pentamidine is used as an alternative to suramin for the early hemolymphatic stage of East African trypanosomiasis, pentamidine is the drug of choice to treat the early stage of West African sleeping sickness (infection caused by *T brucei gambiense*). Like suramin, pentamidine has also been used for chemoprophylaxis and should not be used to treat late trypanosomiasis with CNS involvement. Adverse effects (described above for its use in pneumocystosis) are noted in half of patients receiving therapeutic doses.

Once African trypanosomiasis has infected the CNS, drugs that cross the blood-brain barrier must be administered. Even though **melarsoprol** is extremely toxic (it is an arsenic derivative), it is still considered the drug of choice for advanced East African trypanosomiasis and second-line therapy for West African trypanosomiasis because of the consequences of advanced disease and the lack of alternative treatments. Immediate toxicity includes fever, vomiting, abdominal pain, and arthralgias. Melarsoprol may also cause a reactive encephalopathy that can be fatal. To avoid the toxicity of melarsoprol as well as increasing treatment failures that may be due to drug resistance, **eflornithine** was introduced. Eflornithine is now the drug of choice for treating advanced West African trypanosomiasis, but it is not effective for East African disease due to drug resistance. Eflornithine is available orally and intravenously, and is effective against some forms of African trypanosomiasis. For simpler and shorter treatments, eflornithine is sometimes used in combination with nifurtimox (see below). Although toxicity is markedly less than that from melarsoprol, generally reversible significant toxicities include diarrhea, vomiting, anemia, thrombocytopenia, leukopenia, and seizures.

Infection with the parasite *T cruzi* causes Chagas disease. In Latin American countries, Chagas disease is one of the main causes of death due to heart failure. *T cruzi* primarily invades cardiac muscle cells and macrophages. Initial infection usually results in a transient febrile illness. After invasion of host cells, the disease pursues a very slow course. The two major symptoms of Chagas disease—myocarditis and intestinal tract dilation—can take *years* to develop. Two orally administered drugs are available to treat Chagas disease: **nifurtimox** and **benznidazole**. Both drugs are commonly used to treat the acute infection, but benznidazole probably has better efficacy and safety. These drugs can eliminate parasites and prevent progression when used to treat acute infection, but they are often unsuccessful at complete eradication of the protozoan, thus allowing progression to the cardiac and GI syndromes. Toxicities of both drugs, including GI irritation and severe CNS effects, are a major

drawback in their use, frequently forcing discontinuation of the therapy before completion of a standard course.

Drugs for Leishmaniasis

Leishmania parasites (>20 species) are transmitted by the bite of infected sandflies (about 30 species). Infection results in cutaneous (skin), mucocutaneous (skin, nose, mouth), or visceral (liver and spleen) leishmaniasis. Millions of people are infected with leishmaniasis, with the cutaneous and mucocutaneous forms being much more prevalent than the life-threatening visceral disease. The cutaneous disease is particularly prevalent in Afghanistan, Algeria, Brazil, Columbia, Iraq, Iran, Pakistan, Peru, Saudi Arabia, and Syria. More than 90% of the world's cases of visceral leishmaniasis are in India, Bangladesh, Nepal, Sudan, and Brazil. The disease is often known by many local names (eg, Oriental sore, espundia, Baghdad boil, Delhi sore, and kala-azar). Those at increased risk of leishmaniasis (particularly cutaneous leishmaniasis) include Peace Corps volunteers, people who do research outdoors at night, and soldiers. The cutaneous and mucocutaneous leishmania infections range from localized self-healing ulcers to disseminated lesions that give rise to chronic disfiguring conditions. Lesions may eventually heal with significant scarring, but will leave the individual relatively immune to reinfection. In contrast, visceral infection develops slowly and is characterized by hepatomegaly and splenomegaly. Left untreated, visceral leishmaniasis almost always results in death.

Sodium stibogluconate and **meglumine antimoniate** are first-line agents for treatment of cutaneous and visceral leishmaniasis (except in parts of India, where the efficacy of these drugs has diminished greatly). These drugs must be administered parenterally (intravenous or intramuscular), and intramuscular injections can be very painful. Cure rates for the cutaneous and mucocutaneous forms are generally good with several weeks of therapy. However, treatment for the visceral disease is ineffective at times and has shown increasing resistance in some endemic areas (notably in India). Although few adverse effects occur initially, the toxicity of sodium stibogluconate increases over the course of therapy. The most commonly encountered adverse effects include GI symptoms, fever, headache, myalgias, arthralgias, and rash. Electrocardiographic changes (QT prolongation) may occur, but these effects are generally reversible.

Miltefosine, originally developed as an antineoplastic drug, is the first effective oral drug used in the treatment of cutaneous and visceral leishmaniasis. Miltefosine is used for the treatment of visceral leishmaniasis in India and some other countries, where it may become the treatment of choice. The drug may also have a role in treating cutaneous leishmaniasis. Advantages of miltefosine include less toxicity compared to other drugs, oral administration, and less drug resistance. Nausea and vomiting are common and short-lived ADRs. Because the drug has demonstrated teratogenicity, miltefosine should not be given to pregnant women.

Alternative drugs for visceral leishmaniasis include pentamidine, amphotericin B, and paromomycin. Paromyomycin is much less expensive than amphotericin or miltefosine. For cutaneous lesions, fluconazole or metronidazole may be used. For mucocutaneous leishmaniasis, amphotericin B has been used in some areas.

Antihelminthic Drugs

Helminths are parasitic worms. Three main groups parasitize human organs, most often the GI tract: roundworms (nematodes), flukes (trematodes), and tapeworms (cestodes). Roundworms have long cylindrical bodies and generally lack specialized attachment structures. Flukes and tapeworms are relatively flat, with specialized structures to secure attachment to the host's intestine or blood vessels. Direct transmission may occur by swallowing infective stages (eggs or larvae in water, food, or an intermediate host) or by larvae actively penetrating the skin. Indirect transmission may occur by injection from infected insect vectors. Infections are often asymptomatic. However, because worms are large and migrate throughout the body, they can directly damage almost any host tissue. Subsequently, the host's immune system can cause further damage. Figure 29-4 outlines the drugs used in helminthic infections

Drugs That Act Against Nematodes (Roundworms)

It is estimated that more than 1 billion people worldwide are infected by intestinal nematodes, with much higher prevalence in moist subtropical and tropical climates. Medically important intestinal nematodes responsive to antihelminthic drugs include *Enterobius vermicularis* (pinworm), *Trichuris trichiura* (whipworm), *Ascaris lumbricoides* (roundworm), *Ancylostoma* and *Necator* species (hookworms), and *Strongyloides stercoralis* (threadworm). Pinworms are the most common intestinal nematode in developed countries and are also the least pathogenic. Eggs that are laid on the perianal skin

cause itching, and transmission generally occurs from contaminated fingers. Hookworm infections are now rare in the United States, but threadworm infections have been identified in rural Appalachia. Though not as common as intestinal nematodes, tissue nematodes still infect over a half billion people worldwide.

In the developing world, therapy goals typically include elimination of *most* parasites, alleviating disease symptoms, and decreasing infection transmission. In endemic areas, complete elimination of parasites can be challenging with certain helminthic infections because of limited efficacy of the drugs and frequent reinfection after treatment.

Albendazole is an oral drug with a wide antihelminthic spectrum. It is the drug of choice for roundworm (ascariasis), hookworm, pinworm, and whipworm infections. It is an alternative drug for threadworm infections and filariasis (endemic in some tropical areas and responsible for elephantiasis when the lymphatics are infected). Therapy usually achieves good cure rates and dramatic decreases in egg counts in those not cured. Albendazole is also effective in treating hydatid disease (potentially fatal infection with tapeworm eggs that causes cysts to form in vital organs). Dosing depends on the parasitic infection being treated. During short courses of therapy, albendazole has relatively few adverse effects.

Mebendazole is another primary drug for ascariasis, pinworm, and whipworm infections, with cure rates of 90-100%. The drug has a low incidence of adverse effects, primarily limited to GI irritation. Its use is contraindicated in pregnancy, as it may be embryotoxic.

Diethylcarbamazine is the drug of choice for filarial infections caused by *Wucheria bancrofti*, *Brugia malayi*, *Brugia timori*, and *Loa loa*. The drug immobilizes early stages of these worms, displacing them from tissues, and making them more susceptible to host immune system destruction. Adverse reactions to proteins released from dying parasites include fever, rash, ocular damage, joint and muscle pain, and inflammation of lymphatic vessels.

Ivermectin is the drug of choice for onchocerciasis (river blindness), a chronic disease endemic in West and sub-Saharan Africa, as well Saudi Arabia and Yemen. Chronic infection often results in serious ophthalmologic complications, including blindness. Ivermectin immobilizes sensitive parasites by inhibiting their neurotransmitter function. The drug does not cross the blood-brain barrier, and does not interfere with human neurotransmission. Ivermectin is generally given as a single-dose oral therapy. Ivermectin is also an alternative drug for many other helminthic infections. Adverse effects include fever, headache, dizziness, rash, pruritus, tachycardia, hypotension, and pain in joints, muscles, and lymph glands. These reactions are often of short duration and manageable with antihistamines and nonsteroidal anti-inflammatory drugs (NSAIDs). Ivermectin should not be used in pregnancy.

By inducing depolarization-induced paralysis, **pyrantel pamoate** effectively kills adult and immature nematodes in the colon, but the drug has no activity against migratory stages in the tissues or against the eggs. Pyrantel pamoate is the drug

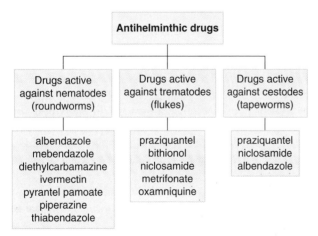

FIGURE 29-4 Antihelminthic drugs are divided into three groups on the basis of the type of worm primarily affected: nematodes, trematodes, and cestodes.

of choice against hookworm and roundworm, but is not effective against flukes or tapeworms. Adverse effects are minor, including GI distress and headache.

Piperazine and **thiabendazole** are alternative drugs for helminthic infections. Piperazine is an alternative treatment for ascariasis, with cure rates over 90% when taken over 2 days. The drug should not be given to pregnant women, those with history of epilepsy or chronic neurologic disease, or those with renal or hepatic impairment. Thiabendazole is an alternative treatment for strongyloidiasis (threadworm) and trichinosis (adult worms). Other drugs such as ivermectin are preferred because thiabendazole is much more toxic, frequently causing anorexia, nausea, and vomiting. Abdominal pain, diarrhea, headache, and neuropsychiatric symptoms may also occur. Irreversible liver failure and fatal Stevens-Johnson syndrome have been reported with use of thiabendazole.

Drugs That Act Against Trematodes (Flukes)

The medically important trematodes include several parasites that have an enormous impact on human populations, such as *Clonorchis sinensis* (human liver fluke, endemic in Southeast Asia), *Schistosoma* species (blood flukes, estimated to affect >200 million persons worldwide), and *Paragonimus westermani* (lung fluke, endemic in Asia and India).

With few exceptions, **praziquantel** is used to treat most fluke infections as well as many tapeworm infections. Praziquantel kills susceptible immature and adult worms by increasing cell membrane permeability, resulting in paralysis of their musculature, and eventual phagocytosis by human immune cells. Praziquantel is the safest and most effective drug for treating schistosomiasis (all species) and most other trematode and cestode infections. Effectiveness of praziquantel for chemoprophylaxis has not been established. Praziquantel is safe and well tolerated in children. Recent data suggest that the drug can also be given safely during pregnancy. Mild and transient ADRs that may occur within hours of oral administration include headache, dizziness, and drowsiness. Days later, individuals may experience fever, pruritus, and rashes, which may be due to the effects of proteins released from dying worms rather than directly due to praziquantel toxicity. Adverse effects are dose-dependent and generally do not require treatment, but may be more frequent or serious in patients with heavy worm burdens. In some cases, glucocorticoids may be used to limit inflammation from the acute immune response and dying worms, though this dramatically reduces praziquantel's bioavailability. Because praziquantel induces dizziness and drowsiness, patients should be warned regarding activities requiring particular physical coordination or alertness.

Alternative agents for treating fluke infections include **bithionol**, **niclosamide**, **metrifonate**, and **oxamniquine**. Choice of agent is determined by susceptiblility of the particular helminth, availability, and safety profile. Metrifonate is a safe, low-cost alternative for treating *S haematobium* infections. This drug is safe for children and has effectively been used as a chemoprophylatic in mass treatment programs in endemic areas in parts of Africa. Metrifonate and oxamniquine are contraindicated in pregnancy, whereas the safety of bithionol and niclosamide has not been established in pregnancy or in young children. The adverse effect profiles of these antihelminthics are similar, with generally minor and transient GI distress and skin rashes. Like praziquantel, bithionol, metrifonate, and oxamniquine cause dizziness.

Drugs That Act Against Cestodes (Tapeworms)

Tapeworm eggs are passed from the feces into the soil from a primary host (humans in most cestode infestations) and ingested by and hatched in an intermediate host (eg, cow, pig) in which they enter tissue and form cysts filled with eggs. Primary hosts then ingest cysts in the tissue of the intermediate host. When swallowed, the cysts pass through the stomach, attach to the lining of the small intestine, and develop into adult tapeworms over about two months. In some cestodes (*Echinococcus* and *Spirometra* species), humans are the intermediate hosts and larvae live within tissues and migrate through different organ systems. The four medically important cestodes are *Taenia saginata* (beef tapeworm), *T solium* (pork tapeworm, which can cause larval forms in the brain and eyes), *Diphyllobothrium latum* (fish tapeworm), and *Echinococcus granulosus* (dog tapeworm, which can cause cysts in the liver, lungs, and brain). The primary drugs for treatment of cestode infections are praziquantel (see above) and niclosamide. A single dose of praziquantel results in an almost 100% cure rate for most tapeworms, and niclosamide is an alternative drug for treating infections caused by beef, pork, and fish tapeworms. Niclosamide is not effective in cysticercosis, a condition in which *T solium* larval cysts infect the brain, muscle, or other tissues. Albendazole or praziquantel is used to treat cysticercosis, which is a major cause of adult onset seizures in many low-income countries. For disease caused by *E granulosus*, albendazole is used. Toxic effects of niclosamide are mild (GI distress, headache, rash, and fever), but safety has not been established in pregnancy or for very young children.

REHABILITATION RELEVANCE

This chapter includes an extremely broad spectrum of antiparasitic agents—from antifungal drugs to antimalarial and antihelminthic drugs. Most physical therapists will treat patients taking antifungal agents, whether this is the athlete using a topical antifungal ointment for athlete's foot or the person with AIDS receiving an intravenous agent to treat a systemic fungal infection. Physical therapists practicing in developed countries are less likely to come into contact with infections such as malaria and leishmaniasis that are endemic in tropical regions throughout the world. However, therapists working in these regions or in facilities with returning military personnel or recent immigrants will often encounter individuals infected with parasites. In malarial endemic regions, many people will be receiving chemoprophylaxis or treatment for active malaria while participating in rehabilitation programs. An understanding of the medications' adverse effects allows the therapist to optimize the delivery (eg, intensity and timing) of therapy sessions. In some cases, individuals suffering from advanced stages of these diseases are not appropriate rehabilitation candidates until the parasitic infection has been brought under control. In all cases, the physical therapist serves as a valuable member of the healthcare team to help provide education regarding limiting the spread of parasitic infections. Summarized below are the major classes of medications with adverse effects that may limit therapy, require additional monitoring, or entail postponement of therapy sessions.

Systemic Antifungal Drugs

- Amphotericin B almost always produces **infusion-related adverse effects** including fever, chills, vomiting, muscle spasms, headache, and significant hypotension. While slowing the infusion rate, decreasing the daily dose, and premedication with agents to partially overcome infusion-related effects may be helpful, patients' participation in rehabilitation will be limited. If a patient is receiving intravenous amphotericin B, rehabilitation services should be scheduled away from this time.
- Amphotericin B and flucytosine may cause **anemia**, and flucytosine may also cause **thrombocytopenia**. Anemia and thrombocytopenia may result in decreased capacity to exercise and to control bleeding after injury, respectively. If decreased exercise tolerance or excessive bruising is noted, alert the referring healthcare provider.
- All azole agents inhibit hepatic drug-metabolizing enzymes (cytochrome P450s) to some extent, resulting in a **potential increase or prolongation of effects of other medications**. If a patient taking an azole agent demonstrates new signs or symptoms or if a patient is considering (or currently) taking an OTC drug or herbal supplement, contact the referring healthcare provider for concerns regarding drug interactions.
- Voriconazole may cause **transient visual disturbances** that interfere with patients' functional performance in rehabilitation. Visual disturbances should be reported to the referring healthcare provider.
- The echinocandins, griseofulvin, and terbinafine produce **GI upset** and **skin reactions** such as flushing (echinocandins), photosensitivity (griseofulvin), and rash (griseofulvin,

terbinafine). If signs and symptoms are troublesome for the patient, encourage consultation with the prescribing provider.

Antimalarial Drugs

- At therapeutic doses, most antimalarial agents produce **skin rashes**, varying degrees of **GI distress**, and **headaches**. The artemisinins, quinine, and mefloquine can cause **dizziness**. For quinine, vertigo, blurred vision, and tinnitus can also occur. For mefloquine, depression, **confusion**, **acute psychosis**, or **seizures** have been reported. While these manifestations may not warrant discontinuation of drug therapy, physical therapy may not be appropriate.

Other Antiprotozoal Drugs

- Several drugs used to treat parasitic infections other than malaria may cause **varying degrees of CNS abnormalities** ranging from headaches and tremors to seizures and encephalopathies. Drugs associated with more significant CNS adverse reactions include sulfadiazine, melarsoprol, eflornithine, nifurtimox, and benznidazole. If new or increasing CNS signs and symptoms are observed, notification of the referring healthcare provider is necessary, and physical therapy may need to be postponed.
- Blood abnormalities such as **anemia**, **leukopenia**, and **thrombocytopenia** may occur with metronidazole, trimethoprim plus sulfamethoxazole (TMP-SMZ), pentamidine, eflornithine, and sulfadiazine. Therapists should assess the patient's lab values, especially the *trends*, prior to each rehabilitation session. Below critical thresholds, interventions must be appropriately decreased in intensity or therapy sessions postponed.

Antihelminthic Drugs

- These drugs tend to cause **dizziness**, **tachycardia**, **hypotension**, and **joint and muscle pain** over the course of the therapy. Since drug therapy duration is typically short (usually over one to a few days) and ADRs are reversible, rehabilitation can generally be postponed until adverse effects cease or improve.

CASE CONCLUSION

The physical therapist notified the physician of A.G.'s symptoms, as well as their limiting impact on rehabilitation goals. Over half of patients receiving IV sodium stibogluconate experience fatigue, arthralgias, and myalgias. While symptoms necessitate interruption of drug treatment in only a small percentage of cases, these adverse effects are generally *reversible*. First, the patient should be educated about the cost-benefit ratio of continuing drug therapy. Untreated cutaneous leishmaniasis lesions can leave large, unsightly scars. In some cases, localized

skin infections can spread to the mouth or nose (mucosal leishmaniasis) and cause potentially disfiguring scars. Second, attempts should be made to schedule therapy sessions as far apart from IV drug sessions as possible to determine whether timing of drug therapy attenuates symptoms during therapy sessions. Finally, the therapist can encourage and reassure the patient that the drug therapy is limited to a maximum of 20 days, and that the distressing symptoms will likely not persist or interfere with her long-term rehabilitation goals.

CHAPTER 29 QUESTIONS

1. Which of the following drugs is *not* indicated for systemic administration to treat a superficial fungal infection?

   a. Amphotericin B
   b. Terbinafine
   c. Griseofulvin
   d. Itraconazole

2. Which of the following azoles is only used topically to treat dermatophytoses?

   a. Itraconazole
   b. Ketoconazole
   c. Posaconazole
   d. Clotrimazole

3. Which of the following drugs has the broadest spectrum of antifungal activity?

   a. Flucytosine
   b. Amphotericin B
   c. Caspofungin
   d. Micafungin

4. Which of the following antimalarial drugs can be used to eradicate the liver stages of the plasmodium parasite?

   a. Chloroquine
   b. Artesunate
   c. Mefloquine
   d. Primaquine

5. Which of the following antimalarial drugs is *not* used for chemoprophylaxis against malaria?

   a. Chloroquine
   b. Mefloquine
   c. Quinine
   d. Malarone

6. Which of the following drugs would *not* be used in the treatment of amebic infection involving the bowel wall or liver?

   a. Diloxanide furoate
   b. Metronidazole
   c. Tinidazole
   d. Emetine

7. Which of the following oral drugs is used in the treatment of Chagas disease?

   a. Suramin
   b. Melarsoprol
   c. Eflornithine
   d. Benznidazole

8. Which of the following drugs is considered first-line treatment for cutaneous and visceral leishmaniasis?

   a. Eflornithine
   b. Melarsoprol
   c. Sodium stibogluconate
   d. Amphotericin B

9. Which of the following is a primary drug for tapeworm?

   a. Melarsoprol
   b. Niclosamide
   c. Diethylcarbamazine
   d. Ivermectin

10. Which of the following drugs would be the most likely to be given as therapy to a young child with a fluke infection?

   a. Praziquantel
   b. Bithionol
   c. Niclosamide
   d. Terbinafine

Miscellaneous Antimicrobial Agents: Disinfectants, Antiseptics, Sterilants, and Preservatives

CASE STUDY

E.L. is a 68-year-old woman admitted to the hospital from a skilled nursing facility with an exacerbation of chronic bronchitis. Within a few days, E.L. began having multiple bouts of diarrhea daily. Infection with *Clostridium difficile* was suspected and the patient was placed in Contact Plus Precautions isolation. Stool sample testing confirmed *C difficile* infection and the patient was immediately started on fidaxomicin. Today, the physical therapist was treating another patient on the same floor as E.L. When the therapist could not

locate a front-wheeled walker on the floor, he asked the physical therapy aide to find one. The aide recalled that E.L. had a walker in her room and decided to *borrow* this walker so that the therapist could use it for his other patient. When the aide entered the patient's room helpfully presenting the borrowed walker, the therapist requested that the aide immediately return the walker to E.L.'s room without allowing it to touch any surfaces along the way and to wash her hands with soap and water afterward.

REHABILITATION FOCUS

This chapter is divided into two distinct sections. The first includes miscellaneous antimicrobials not discussed in Chapter 27, including those specific for treating lower urinary tract infections. The second section discusses antiseptics, disinfectants, sterilants, and preservatives. Figure 30-1 outlines the categories and specific agents included in this chapter.

Like all healthcare workers, physical therapists follow standard precautions with all patients regardless of their infection status. These practices include hand hygiene before and after contact with each patient and hand drying with clean one-use towels (if washing with soap and water) and wearing appropriate personal protective equipment (PPE) when treating patients with whom there is potential to contact blood, mucous membranes, or other body fluids. If a specific diagnosis of a transmissible infection has been made, therapists follow facility guidelines regarding additional precautions that need to be taken based on how the infection is transmitted.

In outpatient and inpatient practice settings, physical therapists use therapy-related equipment (eg, gait belts, crutches, manual therapy tools) to treat *multiple* patients. Thus, it is of utmost importance to ensure that this equipment does not become an infection reservoir or transport vehicle. Therapists must know how to appropriately disinfect

treatment tables and multiple-patient use equipment to avoid the potential transfer of pathogens from one patient to another.

Disinfection procedures are chosen based upon the frequency of encountering specific pathogens. In hospital and other inpatient settings, infection control departments typically dictate the disinfectants and procedures to be used. In outpatient clinics, physical therapists are responsible for choosing suitable products that maximize infection control, while minimizing toxicity to the user and equipment. Some considerations in choosing an appropriate antiseptic or disinfectant (or when working in an environment where these agents are used) include:

- What are the active ingredients in the antiseptic or disinfectant?
- Against which microorganisms is the agent effective?
- Is the agent safe for daily use on the skin?
- Will the agent damage surfaces that it disinfects?
- When using the agent, should PPE be worn and what type?
- What conditions must be met for the agent to be the most effective antimicrobial?
- Is the agent safe to mix with another agent to maximize antimicrobial effectiveness?
- What is the cost of the product?

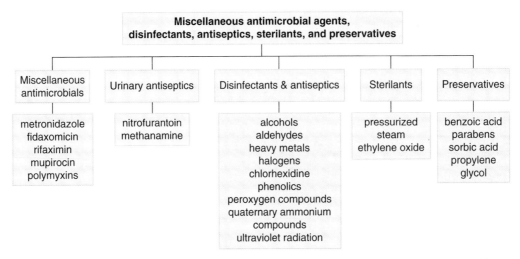

FIGURE 30-1 Agents are divided into miscellaneous antimicrobials, those specific for urinary infections, disinfectants and antiseptics, sterilants, and preservatives. Example drugs or agents are listed under each major category.

Choosing the most appropriate agent for a given application requires knowledge of the advantages and disadvantages of each antiseptic or disinfectant. Inappropriate choice, concentration, or application of agent may result in unsuccessful antimicrobial efficacy, compromised safety, or both.

MISCELLANEOUS ANTIMICROBIAL AGENTS

Metronidazole

Metronidazole is a nitroimidazole drug used primarily to treat infections caused by anaerobic bacteria and protozoa. These organisms readily take up the drug, which disrupts their DNA and inhibits nucleic acid synthesis.

When administered orally or intravenously, metronidazole penetrates readily into almost all tissues, including the cerebrospinal fluid, achieving levels similar to plasma. When administered topically, metronidazole has minimal systemic absorption.

Metronidazole is used in the treatment of anaerobic or mixed intra-abdominal infections, vaginitis, brain abscess, and anaerobic infections such as might be present in empyema, lung abscess, bone and joint infections, and diabetic foot ulcers. Metronidazole is also used to treat infections caused by *Clostridium difficile*, a gram-positive bacillus that can precipitate pseudomembranous colitis, which is clinically manifested as severe diarrhea (*C difficile*–associated diarrhea). *C difficile* is an increasingly common healthcare-associated infection that is more common in older adults, especially those who take antibiotics and are hospitalized.

Metronidazole has many other uses. As an oral tablet or topical vaginal gel, it effectively treats bacterial vaginosis. As part of a multidrug regimen, metronidazole is commonly used in the eradication of *Helicobacter pylori* in peptic ulcer disease (Chapter 36). As an antiprotozoal drug, metronidazole

is the drug of choice for treating giardiasis (one cause of traveler's diarrhea) and the common sexually transmitted disease trichomoniasis. Metronidazole is also used as a topical antibiotic for rosacea, a chronic dermatologic condition.

Adverse effects include nausea, gastrointestinal discomfort, diarrhea, headache, dizziness, dry mouth, dark coloration of urine, and altered taste sensation (especially imparting a sharp metallic taste). Because metronidazole has a disulfiram-like effect, concurrent alcohol consumption can cause stomach pain, nausea, vomiting, headache, and facial flushing. Individuals should be instructed to avoid alcohol (including alcohol-containing cough syrups) while taking metronidazole and for at least 3 days after discontinuing treatment.

Fidaxomicin

Fidaxomicin is a narrow-spectrum antibiotic that inhibits bacterial RNA synthesis. The drug is effective against gram-positive aerobic and anaerobic bacteria, but has no activity against gram-negative bacteria. When administered orally, systemic absorption is negligible, but fecal concentration is high. Fidaxomicin has been approved by the Food and Drug Administration (FDA) to treat *C difficile* in adults. For this infection, fidaxomicin is as effective as vancomycin (which also has negligible oral absorption) and may be associated with lower rates of relapsing disease.

Rifaximin

Rifaximin is a derivative of rifampin, one of the drugs used in the treatment of tuberculosis. Rifaximin inhibits protein synthesis in both gram-positive and gram-negative aerobic and anaerobic bacteria. Similar to fidaxomicin, there is minimal systemic absorption with oral administration, but fecal concentrations are high. Rifaximin is FDA-approved for the treatment of *E coli*–induced travelers' diarrhea, hepatic encephalopathy, and irritable bowel syndrome with diarrhea. Clinical effectiveness in hepatic encephalopathy is thought to be due to a reduction in ammonia production by eliminating ammonia-producing colonic bacteria.

Mupirocin

Mupirocin is an antibiotic originally isolated from the gram-negative bacterium *Pseudomonas fluorescens*. By binding to bacterial isoleucyl transfer-RNA synthetase, mupirocin prevents isoleucine incorporation into bacterial proteins, thus inhibiting bacterial protein synthesis.

Mupirocin is a topical antibiotic indicated for treatment of minor skin infections such as secondarily infected traumatic lesions and impetigo caused by gram-positive bacteria (eg, *Staphylococcus aureus*, β-hemolytic streptococci, and *Streptococcus pyogenes*). With direct application of mupirocin to the skin or mucous membranes, high local concentrations are achieved. Use of an occlusive dressing following application increases penetration 5- to 10-fold, but the absorbed amount has been estimated to be less than 0.24% of the applied amount. Systemic absorption through intact skin is minimal; however, any mupirocin reaching the systemic circulation is rapidly metabolized to an inactive metabolite that is eliminated by renal excretion. Most drug elimination is via desquamation of skin cells rather than metabolism.

Nasal carriage of *S aureus* (both methicillin-susceptible and methicillin-resistant strains) is a well-defined risk factor for subsequent nosocomial infection in hospitalized patients. Thus, intranasal application of mupirocin has been used for temporary elimination of *S aureus* in patients and healthcare workers. Patients most likely to benefit are those undergoing orthopedic or cardiothoracic procedures. Prolonged and widespread mupirocin use is associated with the development of mupirocin resistance, though most staphylococcal isolates are still susceptible. Judicious use of topical mupirocin, including limiting treatment to carriers and considering other treatment regimens, should be emphasized.

Adverse effects include local erythema, rash, stinging, and itching. In addition, prolonged usage may result in overgrowth of nonsusceptible organisms, including fungi.

Polymyxins

The polymyxins (**polymyxin B** and **polymyxin E**) are a group of cationic detergent antibiotics that kill gram-negative bacteria by disrupting their cell membranes. Owing to significant toxicity associated with systemic administration, the polymyxins have primarily been used topically and for irrigation of wounds and the urinary bladder. Ointments or drops containing polymyxin B in combination with neomycin and hydrocortisone are often used for eye or ear infections. Over-the-counter topical formulations including polymyxin B with neomycin and/or bacitracin are commonly used for infected superficial skin lesions. If systemic absorption occurs, serious adverse effects include neurotoxicity (dizziness, ataxia, paresthesias) and nephrotoxicity (acute renal tubular necrosis). Due to the emergence of several antibiotic-resistant bacterial strains (eg, *Pseudomonas aeruginosa*), there is renewed interest in parenterally administered polymyxins as salvage therapy for severe infections.

URINARY ANTISEPTICS

The urinary tract is one of most common sites of bacterial infection, especially among women. The urinary tract antiseptics include **nitrofurantoin** and two **methenamine** salts. Though administered orally, these drugs are eliminated so rapidly that they lack systemic antibacterial effects. The drugs are useful for treatment of acute lower urinary tract infections (UTIs) as well as prevention of recurrent UTIs because they are excreted into the urine in high enough concentrations to inhibit urinary pathogens. Urine pH is monitored before starting and throughout therapy because the agents' effectiveness is increased at low pH (< 5.5), and low pH is an independent inhibitor of bacterial growth in urine. Thus, these drugs are often administered with urine-acidifying agents such as ascorbic acid (4-12 g/day). Nitrofurantoin and methenamine are bactericidal for many gram-positive and gram-negative bacteria, although they have no activity against urea-splitting gram-negative bacteria (*Proteus* or *Pseudomonas* species), because these organisms increase urinary pH and thereby decrease the drugs' effectiveness. Both nitrofurantoin and methenamine have the advantage that resistance rarely or slowly develops in susceptible bacterial populations.

Nitrofurantoin

When used to treat uncomplicated acute UTI, the normal adult daily dose of nitrofurantoin is 100 mg taken four times daily, though a long-acting formulation can be taken twice daily. For prevention of chronic UTIs, a single 100-mg daily dose may be taken. To improve drug absorption and decrease adverse gastrointestinal effects (eg, vomiting, nausea, and anorexia), nitrofurantoin should be taken with food. Patients should also be informed that nitrofurantoin colors the urine dark yellowish orange or brown, which is a normal and harmless side effect.

Nitrofurantoin may cause hemolytic anemia in individuals with glucose-6-phosphate dehydrogenase (G6PD) deficiencies, the most common human enzymopathy that it is found in roughly 10% of African Americans and 60% of Kurdish Jews. Nitrofurantoin is contraindicated in women in the last month of pregnancy (38-42 weeks gestation), in nursing mothers, and in neonates less than 1 month of age because the drug may cause hemolytic anemia in neonates with immature enzyme systems within the red blood cells.

Peripheral neuropathies have been reported, and may be more likely in patients with renal impairment, diabetes mellitus, and vitamin B deficiency. Pulmonary toxicities may occur, especially with prolonged use or in those with renal impairment. In renal failure, nitrofurantoin is contraindicated because high blood levels may cause toxicity. Skin rashes and photosensitivity are common adverse effects. Finally, in people with diabetes mellitus, nitrofurantoin may cause inaccurate results with some urine glucose tests.

Methenamine

Methenamine mandelate and **methenamine hippurate** are methenamine salts. When combined with urine acidification (pH < 5.5), methenamine forms ammonia and formaldehyde. Both methenamine salts are commonly used for the prevention, but not the treatment of UTIs. The methenamines should not be taken concurrently with sulfonamide antibacterial agents because insoluble precipitates may form and increase the likelihood of crystalluria.

DISINFECTANTS AND ANTISEPTICS

Although the terms are often used interchangeably, disinfectants and antiseptics have specific definitions (Table 30-1). *Disinfectants* are chemical agents or physical procedures that inhibit or kill various microorganisms on nonliving objects in the environment. They should *not* be used on living tissue. *Antiseptics* inhibit microorganism growth and reproduction on inanimate objects, but they are also safe enough to be used on skin and mucous membranes. However, antiseptics are often avoided in cleansing wounds because they interfere with wound healing. Notably, disinfectants and antiseptics do not have selective toxicity; each agent displays a different microbicidal profile that must be considered for appropriate and effective use (Table 30-2). *Sterilization* refers to the use of physical or chemical means to destroy *all* microbial life, including highly resistant bacterial endospores.

Disinfection prevents infection by killing, removing, or diluting pathogens, thereby reducing the number of potentially infective organisms. Disinfection can be accomplished by the use of chemical agents or physical means such as ionizing radiation or dry or moist heat.

The *ideal* disinfectant would be able to kill all pathogenic microorganisms without harming healthy human tissue. Since the ideal disinfectant does not exist, a combination of agents is often used (eg, addition of a disinfectant to a detergent), and the choice of which to use depends on the particular situation.

Washing, which dilutes and partially removes potentially infectious organisms, and the use of barriers (eg, gloves, condom, respirator), which prevents pathogens from gaining entry into the host, are foremost in infection prevention and control. Hand hygiene—effective hand cleaning in the healthcare setting—is the single most important way to prevent transmission of pathogens from person to person or from regions of higher microbial load (eg, mouth, nose, gut) to potential sites of infection. Hand washing with soap and water mechanically removes and dilutes most infectious agents by trapping microorganisms and dirt in micelles and flushing them down the sink. When hands are not visibly dirty, using alcohol-based sanitizer is the preferred method because it requires less time, is more accessible than sinks, and reduces bacterial load while producing less skin irritation and dryness than soap and water. An important exception to this preferred method is when personnel are providing care for a patient infected with *Clostridium difficile*, a bacterium that produces spores that are not killed by alcohol-based sanitizers. Handwashing with soap and water is required for decontamination after caring for a patient with an infection caused by *C difficile*. For preoperative cleansing of the surgeon's hands and the patient's surgical incision site, skin antiseptics are added to detergents. For regular hand washing (ie, outside the healthcare setting), it may be preferable to create conditions that are inhospitable to bacterial reproduction rather than to kill bacteria with disinfectants or antiseptics. Because of the ability of bacteria to rapidly reproduce, it is possible that survival of bacteria following an antiseptic challenge may result in increased propagation of strains of antiseptic-resistant bacteria. For this reason and for other health safety concerns, the trend of adding antibacterial agents to regular hand soap, many household products, and impregnated cloths and fabrics has been questioned.

The choice of antiseptic, disinfectant, or sterilant (or combination) depends on several factors including, but not limited to, risk of infection associated with the use of each

TABLE 30-1 Commonly used terms related to chemical and physical killing of microorganisms.

Antisepsis	Application of an agent to living tissue for the purpose of preventing infection
Decontamination	Destruction or marked reduction in number or activity of microorganisms
Disinfection	Chemical or physical treatment that destroys most vegetative microbes and viruses, but not spores, in or on inanimate surfaces
Sanitization	Reduction of microbial load on an inanimate surface to a level considered acceptable for public health purposes
Sterilization	Process intended to kill or remove all types of microorganisms, including spores, and usually including viruses, with an acceptable low probability of survival
Pasteurization	Process that kills nonsporulating microorganisms by hot water or steam at 65-100°C

TABLE 30-2 Activities of disinfectants.

	Bacteria				Viruses			Others		
	Gram-Positive	Gram-Negative	Acid-Fast	Spores	Lipophilic	Hydrophilic	Fungi	Amebic Cysts	Prions
Alcohols (isopropanol, ethanol)	HS	HS	S	R	S	V	—	—	R
Aldehydes (glutaraldehyde, formaldehyde)	HS	HS	MS	S (slow)	S	MS	S	—	R
Chlorhexidine gluconate	HS	MS	R	R	V	R	—	—	R
Sodium hypochlorite, chlorine dioxide	HS	HS	MS	S (pH 7.6)	S	S (at high conc)	MS	S	MS (at high conc)
Hexachlorophene	S (slow)	R	R	R	R	R	R	R	R
Povidone, iodine	HS	HS	S	S (at high conc)	S	R	S	S	R
Phenols, quaternary ammonium compounds	HS	HS	MS	R	S	R	S	—	R

HS, highly susceptible; MS, moderately susceptible; R, resistant; S, susceptible; V, variable; —, no data.

agent, intrinsic resistance of the microorganisms, number of microorganisms present (microbial load), mixed populations of organisms, amount of organic material present (eg, blood, feces, tissue), stability and concentration of the agent, time and temperature of exposure, pH, and hydration and binding of the agent to surfaces.

As noted, disinfectants, antiseptics, and sterilants do not have selective toxicity. Each agent has more or less marked cytotoxic properties. All users of these agents must consider the short-term and long-term toxicities of each agent both in the body and in the environment. In the United States, the Environmental Protection Agency (EPA) regulates disinfectants and sterilants and the Food and Drug Administration (FDA) regulates antiseptics. Major classes of antiseptics, disinfectants, and sterilants are described in the text below.

Alcohols

The most frequently used alcohols for treatment table disinfection and skin antisepsis are **ethanol** and **isopropyl alcohol (isopropanol)**. Alcohols rapidly kill vegetative bacteria, *Mycobacterium tuberculosis,* many fungi, and lipophilic viruses such as HIV and hepatitis B and C viruses. Alcohol's biocidal effects are likely due to its ability to dehydrate cells, disrupt membranes, and coagulate proteins. For surface and skin disinfection and antisepsis, alcohol concentration of 60-90% (by volume in water) with exposure for several minutes (to allow complete evaporation) is optimal. Alcohols are not considered sterilants because they do not inactivate spores, penetrate protein-containing organic material, or inactivate hydrophilic viruses (eg, poliovirus). In addition, rapid evaporation prevents alcohols from having a lasting residual action. Alcohols are

useful in situations in which access to running water and soap is limited (eg, home care setting). To limit their skin-drying effect, emollients are often added to alcohol-based hand rubs. Because of their flammability, alcohols should be used and stored in cool and well-ventilated areas. Their complete evaporation must be allowed before use of any flame, cautery, or lasers.

Aldehydes

Formaldehyde and **glutaraldehyde** (sometimes called cold sterilants) are used for high-level disinfection or sterilization of medical instruments with plastic and rubber that cannot tolerate the high temperatures required for steam sterilization (autoclaving). Aldehydes inactivate a broad spectrum of microorganisms and viruses by cross-linking proteins and nucleic acids. Aldehyde disinfection or sterilization may fail if dilutions are below effective concentrations, if organic material is present, or if the liquid formulation is unable to penetrate into crevices in medical instruments. For this last reason, circulating baths can be used to increase penetration of aldehyde solutions, which also has the advantage of decreasing exposure of the operator to irritating fumes.

Formaldehyde is available as a 40% weight/volume solution in water (100% **formalin**). An 8% formaldehyde solution exhibits a broad spectrum of activity against bacteria, bacterial toxins, spores, viruses, and fungi. Destruction of spores may take up to 18 hours, but the speed of action may be increased by solution in 70% alcohol instead of water. Alcohol probably strips protective lipids, allowing formaldehyde better access to the pathogen. Formalin is used for high-level disinfection of hemodialyzers, preparation of vaccines, and embalming of tissues.

Glutaraldehyde is commonly used in 2% weight per volume solutions. To be activated, glutaraldehyde must be alkalinized to reach a pH 7.4-8.5. Specific applications for its use include disinfecting respiratory therapy equipment, physical therapy whirlpool tubs, and dialysis treatment equipment. While glutaraldehyde has greater sporicidal activity than formaldehyde, it may not be as effective at killing *M tuberculosis*. Once activated by alkali, glutaraldehyde begins to polymerize and lose its disinfectant activity. Its activated shelf life is about 2 weeks. Test strips are available to measure activity.

Formaldehyde and glutaraldehyde are highly irritating to the skin, eye, and respiratory tract even at low levels for short periods. Formaldehyde gas has a distinctive, pungent, and irritating odor that is detectable even at extremely low concentrations (<1 ppm). The Occupational Safety and Health Administration (OSHA) has declared formaldehyde a potential carcinogen and established an exposure standard that limits the 8-hour time-weighted exposure of employees to 0.75 ppm as the permissible exposure limit (PEL). Odor may not be an adequate indicator of the presence of formaldehyde and may not provide a reliable warning of hazardous concentrations. Because it is slightly heavier than air, formaldehyde vapors can result in asphyxiation in poorly ventilated, enclosed, or low-lying areas. Glutaraldehyde solutions are pale yellow liquids with a rotten-apple odor. Although OSHA does not currently have a required PEL for glutaraldehyde, the National Institute for Occupational Safety and Health (NIOSH) has established a recommended exposure limit of 0.2 ppm. There are several ways to minimize or limit occupational exposure to the aldehydes, including ensuring the agents are used in fume hoods with exhaust ventilation, using only enough to perform the required disinfecting procedure, avoiding skin contact by use of PPE such as gloves, goggles, face shields, and respirators. Gloves should be made of nitrile or butyl rubber because latex gloves do not provide adequate protection.

Heavy Metals (Mercury and Silver)

The metal salts of mercury and silver are now rarely used as disinfectants, though they still have a limited number of applications. Mercury is an environmental hazard, and many bacterial strains have developed resistance to mercurials. **Thimerosal** is a mercury-based preservative (0.001%-0.004%) used in immune sera, antitoxins, and certain vaccines. Hypersensitivity to thimerosal is common. Although a causative link between vaccines and autism was proposed by fraudulent research and has never been established, thimerosal was removed from childhood vaccines in the United States in 2001. Influenza vaccines are available in thimerosal-containing and thimerosal-free versions.

Inorganic silver salts are strongly bactericidal. Bacterial (and probably fungal) silver sensitivity relates to silver's ability to irreversibly denature key enzyme systems. **Silver nitrate** was most commonly used to prevent neonatal gonococcal ophthalmitis, but antibiotic ointments have largely replaced this use. In wound care, physical therapists may use silver nitrate sticks not as a bactericidal, but rather to chemically remove excess granulation tissue in chronic wounds. **Silver sulfadiazine** (1%) topical cream is widely used to suppress bacterial colonization in burn wounds. Over the past 15 years, silver has been incorporated as an antibacterial into a number of wound dressings. The popularity of topical silver agents and silver-impregnated dressings remains sustained despite heterogenous results regarding their effectiveness in the management of infected chronic wounds.

Halogens (Iodine, Iodophors, Chlorine)

Iodine-based antiseptics have a wide spectrum of antimicrobial and antiviral activity. Thus far, microorganisms appear unable to develop resistance. **Iodine** in a 1:20,000 solution is bactericidal within 1 minute and sporicidal within 15 minutes. **Tincture of iodine**, which is iodine in an alcohol solution, was frequently used as a preoperative antiseptic for intact skin. However, its use has decreased because of serious hypersensitivity reactions and its propensity to stain clothing and dressings.

Iodophors are mixtures of iodine with solubilizing agents such as surfactants or povidone. Povidone itself has no germicidal action; it controls the release of the inorganic iodine. Iodophors retain the activity of free iodine, but are more gentle to the skin, less likely to provoke hypersensitivity reactions, and less likely to stain fabric than tincture of iodine. **Povidone-iodine (polyvinylpyrolidone [PVP])** is the most common iodophor and marketed as Betadine. To be active, iodophors require drying time on the skin. However, unlike chlorhexidine (discussed below), they do not have persistent activity on the skin. Clinicians should be aware that povidone-iodine solutions can become contaminated with aerobic gram-negative bacteria (eg, *Pseudomonas*).

Chlorine is a fairly universal and inexpensive disinfectant. It is typically found as a 5.25% **sodium hypochlorite** solution in the form of household bleach. The Centers for Disease Control and Prevention (CDC) recommends a 1:10 dilution of 5.25% household bleach (5000 ppm of available chlorine) for disinfection of blood spills. At this concentration, most pathogens including HIV, hepatitis B and C viruses, fungi, antibiotic-resistant strains of staphylococci, enterococci and bacterial spores are killed or inactivated. The exception is that a concentration range of 1000-10,000 ppm is required to kill mycobacteria. Dilutions of sodium hypochlorite in water (pH 7.5-8.0) will retain antimicrobial activity for months if kept in tightly closed opaque containers. However, frequent opening and closing markedly reduces its efficacy.

Chlorine is inactivated by blood, serum, feces, and protein-containing materials. Thus, organic material must be removed from surfaces *prior* to disinfection with sodium hypochlorite. After cleaning, a 1:10 solution is effective simply by being wiped on and left to dry. Sodium hypochlorite solutions are known to be corrosive to some plastics and metals such as aluminum, silver, and stainless steel. Thus, there is potential for corrosive damage to multipatient use equipment such as treatment tables and walkers with repetitive use of bleach solutions (or wipes).

Extreme caution must be taken not to combine sodium hypochlorite with either ammonia (which can be found in many household glass cleaners and in urine) or with any acid because irritating chlorine gas evolves. If sodium hypochlorite solution contacts a product containing formaldehyde, a carcinogenic compound results. The best practice is not to add *anything* to sodium hypochlorite except water. Sodium hypochlorite solutions are caustic to the skin and eyes, so users should wear rubber gloves and—if ventilation is not ideal—goggles.

Chlorhexidine

Chlorhexidine is an antiseptic whose bacteriostatic and bactericidal properties arise from its ability to disrupt bacterial membranes. It is more effective against gram-positive cocci (eg, *Staphylococcus*) and mycobacteria and less effective against gram-positive and gram-negative rods. It also has moderate activity against fungi and viruses. Chlorhexidine inhibits spore germination (unlike alcohol-based antiseptics), and is effective in the presence of blood and organic materials (unlike sodium hypochlorite). Chlorhexidine binds strongly to the skin and mucosa. This significant residual activity inhibits the proliferation or survival of microorganisms after application. However, since some agents in neutral soaps and moisturizers may neutralize its action, these should not be used after hand washing with chlorhexidine immediately prior to patient care.

Chlorhexidine may be used as a preoperative skin preparation (Hibiclens: 4% chlorhexidine gluconate). Chlorhexidine gluconate in combination with 70% alcohol is often preferred over povidone-iodine for skin antisepsis in many surgical and percutaneous procedures for several reasons. Chlorhexidine has a rapid action after application, retains its activity with exposure to body fluids, has persistent activity on the skin, and has very low skin-sensitizing capacity. Chlorhexidine is not safe for use during middle ear or neurosurgery and eye contact should be avoided because it can cause corneal damage.

Phenolics

Phenol was the first disinfectant to be used in clinical medical practice. Although effective, it is highly corrosive, toxic upon absorption, and carcinogenic. Many less toxic derivatives of phenol have been developed, but these are only used as disinfectants for hard surface decontamination in hospitals (eg, floors, counters, beds). Phenolics are bactericidal (including mycobacteria), fungicidal, and capable of inactivating many viruses such as HIV and herpes simplex types 1 and 2. Phenolics do not destroy spores. **Hexachlorophene** was once widely used in surgical scrub routines and was an ingredient in deodorant soaps. It is no longer available in the United States because of neurotoxicity.

Peroxygen Compounds

When used at appropriate concentrations, the peroxygen compounds **hydrogen peroxide** and **peracetic acid** are useful disinfectants and sterilants. Their advantages include effectiveness against a wide variety of organisms (bacteria, yeast, fungi, viruses, and spores) and the fact that their decomposition products (oxygen and water) are nontoxic. The primary disadvantage is a rather short-lived antimicrobial effect.

Hydrogen peroxide's killing ability is due to the hydroxyl radical, which is one of the strongest oxidants known. It is an effective disinfectant when used for inanimate objects with low water content. Anaerobes are most sensitive because they do not produce catalase, which breaks down peroxide. Household hydrogen peroxide is typically in a diluted form (3-10%) whereas industrial hydrogen peroxide is in more concentrated solutions (30% or greater). To be an effective sporicidal, concentrations of 10-25% are required. Hydrogen peroxide is not stable; it must be protected from light and kept in a cool place because light and heat exposure cause degradation.

Hydrogen peroxide is used as a mouthwash, for cleaning wounds, and for disinfecting soft contact lenses. As a mouthwash, dilute hydrogen peroxide may help control plaque, although it has not been proven to be effective in critically ill patients. When applied to a wound, hydrogen peroxide combines with catalase produced in tissues, decomposing into oxygen and water and producing effervescence. It was rationalized that this process helped loosen necrotic or inorganic material that might inhibit wound healing. However, hydrogen peroxide is no longer recommended for wound care because it damages healthy cells (keratinocytes and fibroblasts), which may delay healing.

Peracetic acid is a mixture of hydrogen peroxide and acetic acid in a watery solution. Since it is explosive in pure form, it is used in dilute solution and transported in vented containers to prevent increased pressure as oxygen is released. As with hydrogen peroxide, the hydroxyl radical released from peracetic acid is the lethal species. Peracetic acid is a stronger bactericidal and sporicidal agent than hydrogen peroxide. At room temperature, peracetic acid (250-500 ppm) is effective against most bacteria when applied to contaminated surfaces for 5 minutes. Destruction of spores is increased with both a rise in temperature and an increase in concentration (500-300,000 ppm). Effectiveness is slightly decreased by the presence of organic matter, but can be maintained by an increase in concentration. Peracetic acid may be formulated as a liquid spray or mop-on solution. Automatic sterilization systems using low concentrations of peracetic acid (0.1-0.5%) have been designed to sterilize medical and dental instruments and hemodialyzers. Peracetic acid is also extensively used by food processing and beverage industries to control microbial contamination of food contact surfaces. Peracetic acid offers the advantage that it breaks down into harmless byproducts of water, oxygen, and acetic acid.

Quaternary Ammonium Compounds

Quaternary ammonium compounds ("quats") are cationic surface-active detergents widely used in hospitals for disinfection of noncritical hard surfaces such as bench tops and floors (similar to uses of the phenolics). **Benzalkonium chloride** and **cetylpyridinium chloride** are most likely to be encountered by healthcare workers in central supply, housekeeping, and patient and surgical services areas.

Quaternary ammonium compounds are mostly bacteriostatic, sporistatic, and fungistatic, although they are microbicidal against certain pathogens at higher concentrations. They are ineffective against mycobacteria and spores. Presence of organic material, soaps, many nonionic detergents, and sometimes the cotton fibers in mops and cloths used to apply them can inactivate the disinfectant by removing the quaternary ammonium compound from solution. Low toxicity has led to their use in food production facilities. However, several infection outbreaks resulting from contamination of stock solutions with gram-negative bacteria (eg, *Pseudomonas*) led the CDC to recommend that benzalkonium chloride not be used as an antiseptic.

Ultraviolet Radiation

Short-wavelength ultraviolet light (UVC) can be used to disinfect surfaces, water, and air. Some healthcare facilities have added UVC delivery systems to the disinfection procedures of patient care areas. The effectiveness of germicidal UVC depends on intensity and wavelength of the UV radiation and duration of exposure. Decontamination for most bacteria takes less than 25 minutes, whereas decontamination for *C difficile* takes less than 1 hour. Automated systems claim 99.9% efficacy in eradication of pathogens.

STERILANTS

When it is essential that all microbial life—including highly resistant bacterial endospores—is destroyed, sterilization is required. Sterilization can be performed by physical or chemical means. The classic method of sterilization for biohazardous material has been **autoclaving**—the use of pressurized steam at a temperature of 120°C for a minimum of 30 minutes. Autoclaving medical and surgical instruments can only be done when materials do not contain plastic or rubber. When autoclaving is not possible, gas sterilization may be performed. **Ethylene oxide** gas (diluted with either carbon dioxide or a fluorocarbon to decrease its extreme flammability) is a highly effective sterilant and kills spores rapidly. However, ethylene oxide is mutagenic and carcinogenic, with a permissible exposure level of 1 ppm as a time-weighted measure. Alternative sterilants (some discussed above) are increasingly being employed, such as vapor phase hydrogen peroxide, peracetic acid, ozone, gas plasma, chlorine dioxide, formaldehyde, and propylene oxide.

PRESERVATIVES

Preservatives are required to prevent microbial growth and contamination in many pharmaceutical, cosmetic, and therapy-related products in multiple-use containers such as ultrasound gel or friction massage cream. The ideal preservative must be sufficiently soluble and stable, effective against a broad spectrum of microorganisms, and nonirritating to skin.

Commonly used preservatives include **benzoic acid** and salts, **parabens**, **sorbic acid** and salts, **propylene glycol**, phenolic compounds, quaternary ammonium salts, alcohols, and mercurials such as thimerosal. To inhibit *S aureus* and *Escherichia coli*, the concentration of propylene glycol must exceed 10%. At this concentration, propylene glycol is a skin sensitizer (ie, a chemical that causes a large proportion of exposed individuals to develop an allergic reaction after repeated exposure). Although rare, cases of contact dermatitis from preservatives in ultrasonic gels have been reported. Therapists should be aware of the type and concentration of preservatives in any product prior to patient application, inquire about known sensitivities, and have alternative products or strategies available.

REHABILITATION RELEVANCE

Physical therapists may under-appreciate the importance of their active participation in infection control. In hospitals and skilled nursing facilities, physical therapists often move among floors, treating patients with various infections and variable degrees of immunosuppression. Therapy equipment such as walkers, crutches, and gait belts are frequently moved around the hospital. Without knowledge and execution of appropriate disinfection procedures, this equipment can serve as the perfect transportation vehicle for pathogens. In situations in which patients have been identified as having a readily transmissible pathogen, therapists must follow appropriate isolation precautions. Ideally, the therapy equipment should be dedicated to that particular patient for the entire length of stay. If equipment *must* be used with other patients, facility infection control policies should be consulted to determine what type of disinfectant and procedure must be used to eradicate the particular pathogen. If appropriate disinfection cannot take place inside the patient's room, infection control specialists at the facility should be consulted regarding the safest way to transport equipment to the location where it can be cleaned to decrease the potential of pathogen transmission en route. In outpatient physical therapy clinics, individual treatment tables and mats can be protected with clean single-use sheets. Between patients, these surfaces should be wiped down with a broad-spectrum spray disinfectant (eg, Matt-Kleen, Whizzer) active against many fungi, viruses, and strains of *Streptococcus* and *Staphylococcus*.

Of course, inhibiting or destroying pathogens on the skin and on therapy equipment must also be performed while providing adequate protection for the patient and the healthcare professional. Patients and therapists should be asked about potential sensitivities to agents used to disinfect patient-interface surfaces and therapists must recognize signs and symptoms of allergy or sensitivities to agents.

Some of the antimicrobial drugs described in the first section of the chapter have potential adverse effects that may negatively impact a patient's rehabilitation progress. In addition, each of the disinfectants and antiseptics discussed in the latter section of the chapter can cause potentially toxic reactions or sensitivities that may affect the patient and the physical therapist using or coming into contact with them.

- **Dizziness** is a common adverse effect of metronidazole, which may limit patients' ability to change positions abruptly and participate in aerobic exercise.
- **Peripheral neuropathies** may occur with nitrofurantoin. Peripheral neuropathies may be purely sensory or mixed sensorimotor, manifested by numbness, tingling, or pinprick sensation (paresthesias) in fingers and toes.
- Especially when used frequently, **alcohols and chlorhexidine can produce excessive drying of the skin** that can lead to skin irritation or breakdown. For therapists who consistently use alcohol-based hand antiseptics, choose products with added emollients rather than separate hand creams to ameliorate the skin-drying effect. Be aware that hand creams can become reservoirs for pathogens.
- **Flammability of alcohol-based** hand antiseptics limits their use to cool, well-ventilated areas free of sparks or flames, which may prevent their use during certain home-based rehabilitation treatments. Ensure that the agent has completely evaporated before the use of any equipment that could potentially create a spark.
- **Quaternary ammonium compounds and chlorhexidine** are **rendered ineffective in the presence of soaps and many nonionic detergents**. Avoid hand moisturizers after washing hands with chlorhexidine because some agents in moisturizers may neutralize its action.

- Inquire about **allergies or sensitivities to silver** prior to the use of silver-impregnated wound care products or silver sulfadiazine cream. Recognize and report any adverse reaction and ensure that the patient's medical record reflects the silver allergy or sensitivity since many wound care and medical products contain silver.
- **Iodine and iodophors** may cause serious **hypersensitivity reactions**.
- **Sodium hypochlorite (bleach)** is **inactivated by organic material**. To disinfect a surface effectively, body fluids must be removed first, creating twice the work for the healthcare professional responsible for cleaning and disinfecting biologic spills. In the presence of organic material, chlorhexidine is still an effective disinfectant. If sporicidal effects are required, an additional disinfectant must be chosen since chlorhexidine is only sporistatic.
- Before choosing bleach as a disinfectant, determine whether the chemical used to initially clean the area is safe to use since **bleach reacts with other chemicals and urine to create toxic gases**.
- Alcohol-based disinfectants are reasonably inexpensive and safe and can be used if the **corrosive effects of bleach** are to be avoided. These agents may be used to disinfect treatment tables and rehabilitation equipment between every patient. However, alcohols do not inactivate spores; if the presence of spores is suspected (ie, patient with diagnosed *C difficile*), sodium hypochlorite-based disinfection is necessary.
- **Hydrogen peroxide damages healthy keratinocytes and fibroblasts**. Iodine, iodophors, and hydrogen peroxide should not be used to disinfect or debride wounds.
- **Some preservatives** contained in products used in the rehabilitation setting (eg, ultrasound gel, friction massage cream) have the potential to **cause allergic skin reactions such as contact dermatitis**. Know the ingredients in products applied to patients' skin and inquire whether patients have known sensitivities or allergies to specific preservatives, be able to recognize skin reactions, and discontinue use immediately.

CASE CONCLUSION

It has been shown that patients receiving rehabilitation services in a hospital setting have a 2.6-fold higher chance of developing *C difficile*–associated diarrhea (CDAD), a potentially fatal infection, compared to patients not receiving such services. However, appropriate infection control measures can decrease the incidence of CDAD by 50%. The therapist's instructions to the aide to return the borrowed walker without touching any surfaces and to wash her hands with soap and water are in line with strategies designed to decrease the nosocomial transmission of *C difficile*. Preventing the spread of *C difficile* spores among patients in institutional settings requires isolation of the

C difficile–infected patient, use of barrier precautions, appropriate hand hygiene, and use of appropriate sporicidal agents on environmental surfaces. Physical therapists can reduce the incidence of CDAD associated with rehabilitation by handwashing with soap and water since alcohol-based hand cleaners are ineffective against *C difficile* spores. Therapy-related equipment that has come in contact with *C difficile*–infected patients should be dedicated to that patient for the duration of the hospital stay. If the equipment is not discharged with that patient, it should be disinfected with bleach or bleach wipes with high levels of chlorine, which effectively inactivate *C difficile* spores.

CHAPTER 30 QUESTIONS

1. Which of the following agents is effective in the treatment of acute lower urinary tract infections?

    a. Mupirocin
    b. Nitrofurantoin
    c. Isopropyl alcohol
    d. Metronidazole

2. Which of the following conditions is *not* an indication for treatment with metronidazole?

    a. Rosacea
    b. Anaerobic bacterial joint infection
    c. Infection caused by *Clostridium difficile*
    d. Viral upper respiratory tract infection

3. Which of the following disinfectants is effective against pathogens, including bacterial spores?

    a. Isopropyl alcohol
    b. Silver sulfadiazine
    c. Sodium hypochlorite
    d. Phenolics

4. Which of the following is *not* a reason that chlorhexidine is often preferred over povidone-iodine for surgical skin antisepsis?

    a. Chlorhexidine acts rapidly after application.
    b. Chlorhexidine retains its activity with exposure to body fluids.
    c. Chlorhexidine lacks persistent activity on the skin.
    d. Chlorhexidine has low skin-sensitizing capacity.

5. Which of the following methods or disinfectants cannot effectively eradicate bacterial spores?

    a. Pressurized steam
    b. Peracetic acid
    c. Hexachlorophene
    d. Ethylene oxide gas

6. Which of the following agents is most likely to be used as a preservative in a product such as ultrasound gel?

    a. Parabens
    b. Formaldehyde
    c. Sodium hypochlorite
    d. Hydrogen peroxide

7. Gram-negative bacteria have been shown to contaminate containers containing which of the following?

    a. Formalin
    b. Povidone-iodine
    c. Sodium hypochlorite
    d. Isopropyl alcohol

8. The user should wear a respirator when applying which of the following agents?

    a. Isopropyl alcohol
    b. Hydrogen peroxide
    c. Glutaraldehyde
    d. Silver sulfadiazine

9. Which of the following methods is recommended to disinfect equipment that has been used by a patient with a *C difficile* infection?

    a. Wipe down the surfaces with 3% hydrogen peroxide.
    b. Wipe down the surfaces with 1:10 dilution of 5.25% sodium hypochlorite.
    c. Wipe down the surfaces with a mixture of sodium hypochlorite and formaldehyde.
    d. Throw away all equipment that this individual has touched.

10. Which federal agency in the United States regulates disinfectants and sterilants?

    a. Environmental Protection Agency (EPA)
    b. Food and Drug Administration (FDA)
    c. Department of Health and Human Services (HHS)
    d. Department of Commerce

Cancer Chemotherapy

P.Y. is a 42-year-old man diagnosed with chronic myelogenous leukemia (CML) in the chronic phase. He has been taking the tyrosine kinase inhibitor imatinib daily for the past 3 months. At a scheduled evaluation with his oncologist, it was discovered that the leukemia was not responding well. As a first option, the oncologist decided to increase the imatinib dose. Within a couple weeks, P.Y. began experiencing significant muscle pain and difficulty breathing. On a Friday night, his breathing became so labored and difficult that P.Y.

went to the emergency department. He was admitted to the hospital for evaluation of these new symptoms. As part of the admission, a physical therapy consult was automatically ordered. On Saturday, the physical therapist reviewed the patient's electronic medical record and discussed the case with the on-call oncology fellow before seeing the patient. After discussion with the physician, they decided that the physical therapy evaluation should be deferred for a few days.

REHABILITATION FOCUS

Cancer is among the leading causes of death worldwide and the second most common cause of death in the United States, resulting in over half a million fatalities annually. The most common cancers are breast, lung, prostate, colorectal, melanoma, bladder, non-Hodgkin lymphoma, kidney, endometrium, leukemia, pancreas, thyroid, and liver. Although the rate of smoking—a major cause of several cancers—has declined in the United States, two other important risk factors are increasing. The American population is aging and cancer rates rise with age. Another risk factor for cancer is obesity. Rates continue to rise, with the most recent estimate of over 39% of American adults being classified as obese.

Since the early 1990s, the *overall* cancer death rate has declined 26% in the United States. This trend highlights both the progress that has been made in treating cancer and that the number of cancer survivors has increased. Physical therapists are likely to be treating individuals receiving cancer therapies in inpatient settings, but are even more likely to be treating cancer survivors in outpatient settings. Individuals may seek physical therapy specifically for the adverse effects of cancer treatments, such as lymphedema secondary to removal of affected lymph nodes. More commonly, patients are seeking physical therapy for another condition that may be impacted by the long-term consequences of chemotherapy. For example, a patient that had been successfully treated for testicular cancer may suffer from breathing difficulties related to the lung toxicity that is associated with bleomycin. The patient that is in remission of chronic myelogenous leukemia (CML) may

suffer from significant peripheral neuropathy secondary to the specific chemotherapeutic regimen. Physical therapists must recognize that the delayed toxicities of many chemotherapeutic agents are typically irreversible. Thus, an aerobic exercise program must be adapted and combined with energy conservation principles for the person who has bleomycin-induced lung damage. Likewise, balance training and fall risk reduction strategies for the person with peripheral neuropathy may need to emphasize enhancing the visual and vestibular systems.

The primary goals of this chapter are to provide physical therapists with a broad understanding of the different chemotherapy modalities, basic mechanisms by which anticancer drugs have their effects, underlying reasons for combination chemotherapy regimens, and general adverse reactions of chemotherapeutic agents. This chapter does *not* discuss the use of specific cytotoxic and biologic agents for each cancer for two reasons. First, the precise biochemical mechanisms of action are beyond the typical therapists' knowledge base and practice expectation. Second, cancer chemotherapy is a highly active field, with implementation of new combination protocols and sometimes the development of new agents. Physical therapists should understand the *principle* of why combination chemotherapy is the treatment standard for many cancers, but not the *choice* of particular agents.

BACKGROUND

Cancer is a disease characterized by a shift in the control mechanisms that govern cell proliferation and differentiation. Cells that have undergone neoplastic transformation often express normal *fetal* cell surface antigens or display other signs of apparent immaturity. Cancer cells may also exhibit qualitative or quantitative chromosomal abnormalities, including translocations and amplified gene sequences. Cancer cells proliferate excessively and form local tumors that can compress or invade adjacent normal structures. Within local tumors, there is a small subpopulation of cells that can be described as tumor stem cells. These cells retain the ability to undergo repeated cycles of proliferation and can migrate to distant sites in the body to colonize various organs in the process called metastasis. Tumor stem cells can express clonogenic (colony-forming) capabilities. Chromosomal abnormalities in tumor stem cells reflect their genetic instability, which leads to progressive selection of subclones that can survive more readily in the host's multicellular environment. Abnormalities in various metabolic pathways and cellular components (eg, expression of cell-surface drug transporters) accompany neoplastic progression. The invasive and metastatic processes, as well as metabolic abnormalities resulting from the cancer, cause illness and eventual death unless the neoplasm can be eradicated with treatment.

CAUSES OF CANCER

The incidence, geographic distribution, and behavior of specific types of cancer are related to multiple factors, including sex, age, race, genetic make-up, and exposure to environmental carcinogens. Of these, environmental exposure is likely the most important and also the only *modifiable* risk factor. Ionizing radiation is a major risk factor for cancers including acute leukemias, thyroid cancer, and skin cancer. Chemical carcinogens, particularly those in tobacco smoke, as well as azo dyes, aflatoxins (produced by certain fungi found on agricultural crops), asbestos, and benzene have been clearly implicated in a wide variety of cancers. Potential environmental carcinogens can be identified in the laboratory by microbial mutagenesis and animal testing.

Certain viruses have been implicated in the etiology of several cancers. For example, human papillomavirus (HPV) is associated with cervical, anal, and penile cancers as well as oropharyngeal head and neck cancer; hepatitis B virus (HBV) and hepatitis C virus (HCV) are associated with liver cancer; and, Epstein-Barr virus (EBV) is associated with nasopharyngeal cancer, Burkitt lymphoma, and Hodgkin lymphoma. The expression of virus-induced neoplasia depends on host and environmental factors that modulate the transformation process. Certain cellular genes, known as oncogenes, are homologous to the transforming genes of retroviruses and induce neoplastic transformation. Oncogenes code for specific growth factors and their corresponding receptors. Oncogenes may be amplified (increased number of gene copies) or modified (mutated). The result of either of these processes can be constitutive *overexpression* of these genes in cancerous cells.

Another class of genes, called tumor suppressor genes, plays an important role in *suppressing* neoplastic transformation. If a tumor suppressor gene is mutated, deleted, or damaged, neoplastic change is likely to occur. The best-established tumor suppressor gene is the *p53* gene. In its normal form, *p53* plays a key role in inhibiting malignant transformation. Mutations of *p53* are evident in up to 50% of solid tumors including liver, breast, colon, lung, cervix, bladder, prostate, and skin. Such mutations may be inherited, occur spontaneously, or may be acquired through exposure to exogenous carcinogens.

CANCER THERAPEUTIC MODALITIES

Currently, about one-third of cancer patients are cured with *local* modalities (surgery or radiation therapy), which are quite effective when the tumor has not metastasized by the time of treatment. In the remaining cases, early micrometastasis is a characteristic feature of the tumor and a *systemic* approach such as chemotherapy is required (often in conjunction with surgery or radiation) for effective cancer management. At present, about 50% of individuals with cancer can be cured. However, chemotherapy *alone* cures less than in 10% of all cancer patients when the tumor is diagnosed at an advanced stage.

There are three main approaches to the use of chemotherapy: primary, neoadjuvant, and adjuvant. *Primary* chemotherapy refers to the administration of chemotherapy as the main treatment in patients who present with advanced cancer for which there is no alternative treatment. In most cases, the goals are to relieve tumor-related symptoms, improve quality of life, and prolong time to tumor progression in patients that present with metastatic disease. Primary cancer chemotherapy can be curative in only a small subset of these individuals. In adults, these curable cancers include Hodgkin and non-Hodgkin lymphoma, acute myelogenous leukemia, and choriocarcinoma. In children, curable cancers include acute lymphoblastic leukemia, Burkitt lymphoma, and Wilms tumor. *Neoadjuvant* chemotherapy is the use of chemotherapy in patients who present with localized cancer for which surgery and/or radiation are less than completely effective. For some cancers (eg, anal, nonsmall cell lung cancer [NSCLC]), the optimal benefit is when chemotherapy is administered with radiation therapy either concurrently or sequentially. The goal of this neoadjuvant approach is to reduce the size of the primary tumor so that surgical resection is easier and more effective, or to spare more of the surrounding tissue (eg, breast). Last, adjuvant chemotherapy represents one of the most important roles for cancer chemotherapy. *Adjuvant* chemotherapy refers to the use of chemotherapy *after* local methods of treatment such as surgery. The goal of the chemotherapy is to reduce the incidence of local and systemic recurrence and improve patient survival. Adjuvant chemotherapy has improved overall survival rates in patients with many different types of cancer including breast, colon, and gastric cancers, as well as NSCLC and Wilms tumor. The antihormonal agent tamoxifen (Chapter 22) is an example of adjuvant therapy that is effective in the treatment of postmenopausal women with early-stage breast cancer whose tumors express the estrogen receptor.

ROLE OF CANCER CELL CYCLE AND POPULATION KINETICS

Two important determinants of the actions of anticancer drugs are the cancer cell cycle and cancer cell population kinetics. Figure 31-1 is a schematic summary of the cell cycle phases that all cells—normal and neoplastic—go through before and during cell division. This basic cellular biology is relevant because some anticancer drugs are most effective when cells are in a particular phase of the cell cycle (cell cycle-specific [CCS] drugs). Other cell cycle-nonspecific (CCNS) anticancer drugs kill tumor cells in *both* cycling and resting phases of the cell cycle (although cycling cells are more sensitive). It is common to follow treatment with a CCNS drug with a CCS drug, so that cancer cells are recruited into the cell cycle, where CCS drugs can be more effective. Examples of drugs falling into these two major classes are summarized in Table 31-1.

In general, CCS drugs are most effective in hematologic malignancies and in solid tumors in which a relatively large proportion of the cells are proliferating or are in the growth fraction. The growth fraction represents the number of cells within the malignant tumor that are at some stage of division (ie, other than G_0) compared to the total number of malignant cells (ie, those in division plus those in G_0; Figure 31-1). The CCNS drugs (many of which bind to and damage cellular DNA) are useful for treating solid tumors with both low and high growth fractions. In all instances, effective agents inactivate tumor stem cells, which are often only a small fraction of the cells within a tumor. Nonstem cells (ie, those that have

TABLE 31-1 Cell cycle effects of major classes of anticancer drugs.

Cell Cycle-Specific (CCS) Agents	Cell Cycle-Nonspecific (CCNS) Agents
Antimetabolites (S phase)	**Alkylating agents**
Capecitabine	Altretamine
Cladribine	Bendamustine
Clofarabine	Busulfan
Cytarabine	Carmustine
Fludarabine	Chlorambucil
Fluorouracil	Cyclophosphamide
Gemcitabine	Dacarbazine
Mercaptopurine	Lomustine
Methotrexate	Mechlorethamine
Nelarabine	Melphalan
Pralatrexate	Temozolomide
Thioguanine	Thiotepa
Antitumor antibiotic	**Anthracyclines**
Bleomycin (G_2-M phase)	Daunorubicin
Podophyllotoxins	Doxorubicin
Etoposide (G_1-S phase)	Epirubicin
Teniposide (G_2-S phase)	Idarubicin
Taxanes (M phase)	Mitoxantrone
Cabazitaxel	**Antitumor antibiotics**
Docetaxel	Mitomycin
Paclitaxel	**Platinum analogs**
Vinca alkaloids (M phase)	Carboplatin
Vinblastine	Cisplatin
Vincristine	Oxaliplatin
Vinorelbine	
Camptothecins (G_2-M phase)	
Irinotecan	
Topotecan	

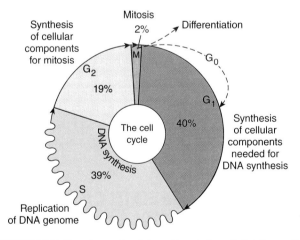

FIGURE 31-1 Schematic of the cell cycle for all dividing cells. The percentages given represent the approximate percentage of time spent in each phase by a typical malignant cell. However, the duration of G_1 can vary dramatically. Drugs that exert their actions on cells traversing the cell cycle are called cell cycle-specific (CCS) drugs (Table 31-1). Cell cycle-nonspecific (CCNS) drugs act on tumor cells while they are actively cycling and while they are in the resting phase (G_0). G_1, gap or growth; G_2, gap 2; M, mitosis; S, synthesis.

irreversibly differentiated) are not a significant component of the cancer problem.

The second important determinant of the use and actions of anticancer drugs is the *growth rate* of cancer cells. The key principle for understanding cancer cell growth was originally outlined in an experimental mouse model of leukemia. In this model system, in which all the cells are actively progressing through the cell cycle, a cytotoxic drug acts with *first-order kinetics*. That is, a given dose kills a constant *proportion* of a

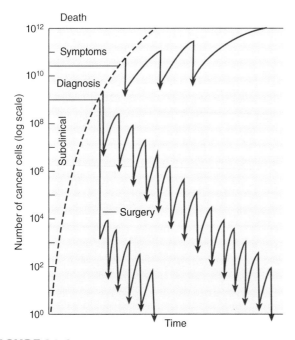

FIGURE 31-2 **The log-kill hypothesis.** Relationship of tumor cell number to time of diagnosis, symptoms, treatment, and death. Three approaches to drug treatment (*indicated by three red lines with arrows*) are shown in comparison with the course of tumor growth when no treatment is given (*dashed line*). In the protocol diagrammed at the top, treatment is given infrequently (3 times) and the result is increased survival, but with recurrence of symptoms between courses of treatment, and eventual death of the patient. In the middle protocol, the cancer is diagnosed earlier. Treatment begins earlier and is given more frequently. Tumor cell kill exceeds regrowth, drug resistance does not develop, and "cure" results. Treatment is continued long after clinical evidence of cancer has disappeared (1-3 years). This approach has been established as effective in the treatment of childhood acute leukemia, testicular cancer, and Hodgkin lymphoma. In the bottom protocol, early surgery removes the primary tumor, and intensive adjuvant chemotherapy has been administered long enough (up to 1 year) to eradicate remaining tumor cells that comprise the occult micrometastases.

cell population rather than a constant number of cells. The log-kill hypothesis proposes that the magnitude of tumor cells killed by anticancer drugs is a logarithmic function. To illustrate what this means, consider that patients with widespread cancer may have up to 10^{12} tumor cells throughout the body at the time of diagnosis (Figure 31-2). If an effective anticancer drug kills 10^3-fold (99.9%) of these tumor cells, treatment would induce a clinical remission associated with major symptomatic improvement and the number of tumor cells would be reduced 1000-fold from 10^{12} to 10^9 (ie, a 3-log-kill dose), resulting from a total kill of 999×10^9 cells. The same dose would reduce a starting population of 10^6 cells to 10^3 cells. This would represent a kill of 999×10^3 cells. In both cases, the dose reduces the numbers of cells by three orders of magnitude, or "3 logs." The remaining cells might be inherently resistant to the drug, may reside in a pharmacologic sanctuary such as the central nervous system (CNS), or may have been in an insensitive stage of the cell cycle.

Figure 31-2 shows the relationship between the number of tumor cells and the time of diagnosis, symptoms, treatment, and death. This schematic highlights the value of repeated courses of anticancer treatment at intervals shorter than the time for tumor regrowth (comparison of middle treatment regimen to upper treatment regimen). The middle treatment regimen also illustrates the value of earlier diagnosis, when there are fewer cancer cells. Finally, the lower treatment regimen illustrates the value of combining various therapeutic modalities such as surgery and anticancer drug regimens to decrease the number of neoplastic cells.

The log-kill hypothesis based on the mouse leukemia model that displays exponential cell kinetics has been applicable to chemotherapy for hematologic cancers such as acute leukemias and lymphomas. However, mathematical modeling data have suggested that most human *solid* tumors do not grow in an exponential manner. Rather, the growth fraction of the tumor decreases over time because of limited blood supply and other factors. In drug-sensitive solid tumors, response to chemotherapy depends on where the tumor is in its growth curve.

ROLE OF COMBINATION DRUG THERAPY

With very few exceptions, single cytotoxic drugs cannot cure cancers that are in advanced stages. Effective combination regimens typically include a number of active drugs from different classes. Combination chemotherapy has three main advantages. First, it usually increases log-kill markedly, and in some cases synergistic effects are achieved. Second, drug combinations are often cytotoxic to a heterogeneous population of cancer cells, and may prevent development of resistant clones. Third, combination chemotherapy may prevent or slow the development of cellular drug resistance (see below). Four principles are important for selecting appropriate drugs to use in combination chemotherapy. First, each drug should be active when used alone against the particular cancer. Second, the drugs should have different mechanisms of action. Third, cross-resistance between drugs should be minimal. Finally, the drugs should have different toxic effects. Although such selection leads to a wider range of adverse effects, it minimizes damage to the same organ system by different drugs to allow dose intensity to be maximized.

STRATEGIES USED IN CANCER CHEMOTHERAPY

Anticancer drugs are administered in prescribed doses and times. The scheduling of chemotherapy is specific to the type of cancer, the drugs used, and the individual. Intervals of drug infusions and in-between periods are called *cycles*. The time between drug infusions (1 day up to several weeks) allows individuals to recover from drug-induced toxicities. A *course* of chemotherapy is often comprised of several cycles.

Pulse therapy involves intermittent treatment with high doses of an anticancer drug—doses that are too toxic to be used continuously. Intensive pulse therapy every 3-4 weeks allows for maximum effects on neoplastic cells, with hematologic and immunologic recovery between courses. Although this strategy is still used, it is employed less often as studies have shown that pulse therapy does not result in clinically significant results compared with continuous chemotherapy delivery.

The strategy of *recruitment therapy* involves the initial use of a CCNS drug to achieve a significant log-kill, which results in recruitment into cell division of cells previously resting in the G_0 phase of the cell cycle. Subsequent administration of a CCS drug that is active against dividing cells may then achieve maximal cell kill. *Synchrony therapy* is a similar approach that uses a combination regimen to pull malignant cells into the same part of the cell cycle. One example is the use of vinca alkaloids to hold cancer cells in the M phase. Subsequent treatment with another CCS drug, such as the S phase-specific agent cytarabine, may result in a greater killing effect on the neoplastic cell population.

Toxic effects of anticancer drugs can sometimes be alleviated by a *rescue strategy*. This involves the administration of essential metabolites to counteract the effects of anticancer drugs on normal (nonneoplastic) cells. For example, high doses of methotrexate may be given for 36-48 hours and terminated before severe toxicity occurs in cells of the gastrointestinal tract and bone marrow. **Leucovorin**, which is accumulated more readily by normal than by neoplastic cells, is then administered. This results in rescue ("*leucovorin rescue*") of the normal cells because leucovorin bypasses the dihydrofolate reductase step in the folic acid cycle. **Mercaptoethanesulfonate** (mesna) "traps" acrolein released from cyclophosphamide and thus reduces the incidence of hemorrhagic cystitis. **Dexrazoxane** inhibits free radical formation and affords protection against the cardiac toxicity of the anthracyclines.

RESISTANCE TO ANTICANCER DRUGS

Drug resistance is a major problem in cancer chemotherapy. Primary resistance or inherent resistance refers to drug resistance in the *absence* of prior exposure to the drug. For example, loss of function of the *p53* tumor suppressor gene leads to resistance to a wide range of anticancer drugs (as well as radiation therapy). In contrast to primary resistance, acquired resistance develops in response to exposure to a chemotherapeutic agent. Mechanisms of acquired resistance include, but are not limited to, the following examples:

1. Cancer cells may increase their rate of DNA repair. This mechanism is particularly important in the case of resistance to alkylating agents and cisplatin.
2. Tumor cells may increase their production of thiol-trapping agents (eg, glutathione), which inactivate certain anticancer drugs. This mechanism of resistance is seen with several of the alkylating agents, cisplatin, and the anthracyclines.

3. Cancer cells may alter target enzymes. For example, changes in dihydrofolate reductase and increased synthesis of this enzyme are mechanisms of resistance of tumor cells to methotrexate.
4. Cancer cells may decrease conversion of a prodrug into the active form of the drug. Resistance to the purine antimetabolites (mercaptopurine, thioguanine) and the pyrimidine antimetabolites (cytarabine, fluorouracil) can result from decreased activity of tumor cell enzymes required to convert these prodrugs to their cytotoxic metabolites.
5. Cancer cells may increase the inactivation of certain cancer drugs. Increased activity of enzymes that inactivate anticancer drugs is a mechanism of tumor cell resistance to most of the purine and pyrimidine antimetabolites.
6. Cancer cells may decrease intracellular drug concentration by accelerating the efflux of anticancer drugs. This form of multidrug resistance (MDR) involves increased expression of a normal gene (*MDR1*) that codes for a cell surface glycoprotein. This transport protein is normally present in various cells throughout the body. In intestinal cells, the transporter is involved in moving the drugs back into the lumen. In some multidrug-resistant malignancies, the activity of this transporter is increased, and the accelerated efflux of many anticancer drugs provides resistance for these cells.

ANTICANCER DRUGS

Figure 31-3 outlines the major classes of anticancer drugs divided on the basis of their mechanism of action, chemical structure, or source. As a group, anticancer drugs are more toxic than any other drugs, so their benefits must be carefully weighed against their risks. The majority of currently available chemotherapeutic drugs act on all dividing cells—regardless of whether they are malignant or normal.

Alkylating Agents

The alkylating agents are CCNS drugs that are classified into several different groups based on their chemical structure. They include nitrogen mustards (**cyclophosphamide**, **chlorambucil**, **mechlorethamine**, **melphalan**), nitrosoureas (**carmustine**, **lomustine**), ethylamine and methylamine derivatives (**altretamine**, **thiotepa**), and alkyl sulfonates (**busulfan**). Other drugs that act in part as alkylating agents include the platinum analogs (**cisplatin**, **carboplatin**, **oxaliplatin**), **dacarbazine**, and **procarbazine**. By definition, an alkylating agent is one that replaces a hydrogen atom with an alkyl group (a chain with only carbon and hydrogen atoms). When alkylating drugs substitute alkyl groups for the hydrogen atoms normally linking DNA strands in the double helix, the two DNA strands become cross-linked. The resulting cross-linked DNA cannot be separated and replicated in mitosis, thus halting cell division. Alkylation of DNA also results in abnormal base pairing and DNA strand breakage. Alkylating agents may also exert cytotoxic effects by forming covalent bonds

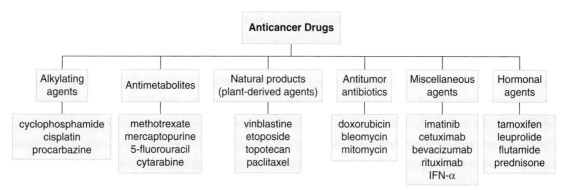

FIGURE 31-3 **Classification of anticancer drugs based on mechanism of action or chemical structure.** Only select example agents are listed below the major classes.

with other cellular constituents such as proteins. While these actions occur in *all* cells, alkylating drugs have their primary effect on rapidly dividing cells that do not have time for DNA repair. Since cancer cells are among the most rapidly dividing cells, they are among the most affected. Predictably, the common adverse drug reactions (ADRs) are the result of the drugs' effects on other rapidly dividing cells such as hematopoietic, reproductive, and endothelial cells (Table 31-2). Last, the alkylating drugs are themselves carcinogenic; their use is associated with an increased risk of secondary malignancies, especially acute myelogenous leukemia.

Cyclophosphamide is one of the most widely used alkylating agents. One of its significant advantages is high oral bioavailability. Cyclophosphamide is a prodrug that is converted to one or more highly reactive metabolites by hepatic cytochrome P450 (CYP) enzymes. Clinical uses include non-Hodgkin lymphoma, breast and ovarian cancers, soft tissue sarcoma, and neuroblastoma. In addition to the toxicities listed in Table 31-2, cyclophosphamide may cause cardiac dysfunction, pulmonary toxicity, and a syndrome of inappropriate antidiuretic hormone (ADH) release.

The two nitrosourea drugs carmustine and lomustine are highly lipid-soluble drugs that readily cross the blood-brain barrier. As such, they are common adjuncts in the management of malignant brain tumors. These drugs appear to be non-cross-resistant with other alkylating agents.

TABLE 31-2 Alkylating agents and toxicities.

Alkylating Agent	Acute Toxicity	Delayed Toxicity
Mechlorethamine Chlorambucil Cyclophosphamide Melphalan Thiotepa	Nausea and vomiting, myelosuppression[a]	Moderate depression of peripheral blood count; excessive doses produce severe myelosuppression with leukopenia, thrombocytopenia, and bleeding; alopecia and hemorrhagic cystitis occasionally occur with cyclophosphamide; cystitis can be prevented with adequate hydration plus mesna[b]
Busulfan	Nausea and vomiting, myelosuppression	Busulfan is associated with skin pigmentation, pulmonary fibrosis, and adrenal insufficiency
Carmustine[c] Lomustine[c]	Nausea and vomiting	Myelosuppression; rarely: interstitial lung disease and interstitial nephritis
Altretamine		Myelosuppression, peripheral neuropathy
Procarbazine	CNS depression	Myelosuppression, hypersensitivity reactions
Dacarbazine	Nausea and vomiting	Myelosuppression, CNS toxicity with neuropathy, ataxia, lethargy, confusion
Cisplatin	Nausea and vomiting, myelosuppression	Nephrotoxicity, peripheral sensory neuropathy, ototoxicity, nerve dysfunction
Carboplatin	Nausea and vomiting	Myelosuppression; rarely: peripheral neuropathy, renal toxicity, hepatic dysfunction
		Drug-induced renal damage may be reduced by use of mannitol (osmotic diuretic) and forced hydration
Oxaliplatin	Nausea and vomiting, laryngopharyngeal dysesthesias	Peripheral sensory neuropathy, diarrhea, myelosuppression

[a]Myelosuppression is the depression of bone marrow activity, with reduction of mature blood cells such as erythrocytes, leukocytes, and platelets in the circulating blood.
[b]Mesna prevents urotoxic effects of cyclophosphamide.
[c]If a tumor is resistant to one alkylating agent, it will usually be relatively resistant to other agents of this class except for nitrosoureas such as those presented.

The platinum analogs cisplatin, carboplatin, and oxaliplatin are rarely used alone, but rather as part of a combination chemotherapy regimen for a broad range of solid tumors. Their mechanism of action is not completely understood, but they are thought to act like alkylating agents. These drugs are used intravenously, distribute to most tissues, and are cleared in unchanged form by the kidney. Cisplatin is commonly used as a component of regimens for cancers of the testicle, bladder, lung, and ovary. Carboplatin has similar uses. Since carboplatin causes significantly less renal and gastrointestinal toxicity than cisplatin, this drug has replaced cisplatin in various combination chemotherapy regimens. Carboplatin's dose-limiting toxicity is myelosuppression. Oxaliplatin has activity against colorectal cancer that is resistant to the other platinum analogs, making it the first-line treatment of advanced colorectal cancer. Oxaliplatin's dose-limiting toxicity is neurotoxicity that presents as peripheral sensory neuropathy.

Procarbazine is often used as a component of chemotherapy regimens for Hodgkin and non-Hodgkin lymphomas and for some brain tumors. The drug is orally active and penetrates into most tissues, including the cerebrospinal fluid (CSF). Procarbazine has several mechanisms of action that extend beyond alkylation of DNA. Procarbazine inhibits DNA, RNA, and protein synthesis. In addition, procarbazine forms hydrogen peroxide, which generates free radicals that cause DNA strand breaks. Procarbazine has multiple toxicities (Table 31-2) including myelosuppression, peripheral neuropathy, and skin reactions. Its carcinogenic potential is likely higher than that of other alkylating agents, especially with respect to increased risk of acute leukemia. Procarbazine also inhibits many enzymes, including monoamine oxidase and those involved in hepatic drug metabolism. Alcohol should be avoided when taking procarbazine as disulfiram-like reactions have occurred.

Antimetabolites

Antimetabolites used in cancer are structurally similar to endogenous compounds that are important in rapidly dividing cells. Drugs within this class have been designed to interrupt specific critical cellular processes that are required for DNA synthesis. The antimetabolites include antagonists of folic acid (**methotrexate**), purines (**mercaptopurine**, **thioguanine**), or pyrimidines (**fluorouracil**, **cytarabine**, **gemcitabine**). Antimetabolites are CCS drugs that act primarily in the S phase of the cell cycle (Figure 31-1). In addition to cytotoxic effects on neoplastic cells, the antimetabolites also have immunosuppressant effects (Chapter 32). Clinical applications and toxicities of these drugs are presented in Table 31-3. Select commonly used antimetabolites are discussed in more detail below.

Methotrexate (MTX) inhibits dihydrofolate reductase, an enzyme that is essential for cell proliferation and growth. Inhibition of this enzyme decreases synthesis of thymidylate, purine nucleotides, and several amino acids. Inhibition of these processes interferes with the formation of DNA, RNA, and cellular proteins. The formation and accumulation of polyglutamate derivatives of MTX inside cancer cells appears to be important for its slight preference to kill cancer cells instead of normal cells. Oral and intravenous administration of MTX affords good tissue distribution except to the CNS. For MTX to penetrate into the CNS, intrathecal or very high intravenous doses must be given. Methotrexate is not metabolized. The main route of elimination is renal excretion via glomerular filtration and secretion. Adequate hydration is needed to prevent crystallization in renal tubules. In individuals with renal impairment, doses must be reduced. Tumor cells have developed several resistance mechanisms to MTX, including decreased drug accumulation, changes in the activity of dihydrofolate reductase or its drug sensitivity, and decreased formation of polyglutamates. Clinically, MTX is effective in

TABLE 31-3 Antimetabolites and toxicities.

Antimetabolite Agent	Toxicity
Capecitabine	Diarrhea, hand-foot syndrome,[a] myelosuppression, nausea and vomiting
Cladribine	Myelosuppression, nausea, vomiting, immunosuppression
Cytarabine	Nausea and vomiting, bone marrow depression, cerebellar ataxia
Fludarabine	Myelosuppression, immunosuppression, nausea and vomiting, fever, myalgias, arthralgias
Fluorouracil (5-FU)	Nausea, mucositis, diarrhea, myelosuppression, neurotoxicity
Gemcitabine	Nausea and vomiting, diarrhea, myelosuppression
Mercaptopurine (6-MP)	Myelosuppression, immunosuppression, hepatotoxicity
Methotrexate (MTX)	Mucositis, diarrhea, myelosuppression with leukopenia and thrombocytopenia
Pemetrexed	Myelosuppression, skin rash, mucositis, diarrhea, fatigue, hand-foot syndrome
Thioguanine (6-TG)	Myelosuppression, immunosuppression, hepatotoxicity

[a]Hand-foot syndrome is a form of erythromelalgia manifested as tingling, numbness, pain, swelling, and redness of the palms of the hands and/or soles of the feet.

choriocarcinoma, acute leukemias, non-Hodgkin and primary CNS lymphomas, and several solid malignant tumors, including those of the breast, head and neck, and bladder. Methotrexate is also used as an immune suppressant in rheumatoid arthritis, psoriasis, and transplant rejection (Chapters 32, 34, and 36). Typically given as a single intramuscular or intravenous injection, MTX is an effective early abortifacient used for ectopic pregnancy. In addition to the most common toxicities (Table 31-3), long-term use of MTX has caused hepatotoxicity and pulmonary infiltrates and fibrosis. Salicylates, nonsteroidal anti-inflammatory drugs, sulfonamides, and sulfonylureas enhance the toxicity of MTX. To limit the toxicity of MTX on normal cells, leucovorin (folinic acid) can be given. This "leucovorin rescue" strategy is used in conjunction with high-dose MTX to rescue normal cells from excessive damage.

Mercaptopurine and thioguanine act as purine antimetabolites. Both are prodrugs that are activated by hypoxanthine-guanine phosphoribosyltransferases (HGPRTases) to toxic nucleotides that inhibit several enzymes involved in de novo purine synthesis. Although both drugs are given orally, they have low oral bioavailability because of first-pass metabolism. Resistant tumor cells may have decreased HGPRTase activity (causing less production of the toxic nucleotides) or increased production of alkaline phosphatases that inactivate the toxic nucleotides. Clinical uses of purine antimetabolites are mainly in the acute leukemias and chronic myelocytic leukemia. Bone marrow suppression is the dose-limiting toxicity. Hepatic dysfunction includes cholestasis, jaundice, and necrosis. The metabolism of mercaptopurine by xanthine oxidase is inhibited by allopurinol, a drug frequently given to patients with acute leukemia to prevent development of hyperuricemia that often occurs with tumor cell lysis. This is clinically relevant because doses of mercaptopurine must be significantly reduced (by 50-75%) to prevent excess toxicity. This interaction does not occur with thioguanine.

Each of the pyrimidine antagonists acts in slightly different ways, but ultimately these drugs inhibit DNA synthesis and function. In tumor cells, resistance mechanisms to the pyrimidine antagonists include decreased drug uptake, decreased conversion to the toxic metabolite, and decreased target enzyme sensitivity to the drug. 5-Fluorouracil (5-FU) is a prodrug that requires activation via several enzymatic reactions. When given intravenously, 5-FU is widely distributed, including into the CSF. Because of its very short half-life (10-15 minutes), the drug is typically given via infusion versus bolus administration. Elimination is mainly by metabolism. 5-FU is the most widely used chemotherapy agent for colorectal cancer, and also has activity against many solid tumors, including cancers of the anus, breast, head and neck, liver, stomach and esophagus. In addition to the toxicities listed in Table 31-3, alopecia may occur. Topically, 5-FU is used to treat keratoses and superficial basal cell carcinoma.

Cytarabine (cytosine arabinoside, ara-C) is only used parenterally and (with slow intravenous infusion) may reach appreciable levels in the CSF. Its half-life is also short, so administration is typically via continuous infusion over 5-7 days. Cytarabine is eliminated via hepatic metabolism. Of all the antimetabolites, cytarabine is the most specific for the S phase of the tumor cell cycle. Clinically, cytarabine is exclusively used for hematologic malignancies (cancers derived from blood cell lines) and has no activity in solid tumors. When high doses are used, neurotoxicity occurs which includes cerebellar dysfunction and peripheral neuritis. In contrast to cytarabine, gemcitabine has broad-spectrum activity against both hematologic and solid cancers. Gemcitabine is widely used to treat NSCLC, bladder cancer, soft tissue sarcoma, and non-Hodgkin lymphoma. Myelosuppression in the form of neutropenia is the dose-limiting toxicity.

Natural Products: Plant-Derived Agents

Important plant-derived chemotherapeutic drugs include the vinca alkaloids (**vinblastine**, **vincristine**, **vinorelbine**), the podophyllotoxins (**etoposide**), the camptothecins (**topotecan**, **irinotecan**), and the taxanes (**paclitaxel**, **docetaxel**). These CCS drugs act in S, G_2, and M phases of the cell cycle (Figure 31-2). Table 31-4 summarizes the acute and delayed toxicities associated with these drugs.

Vinblastine and vincristine are natural alkaloids derived from the periwinkle plant (but are available in synthesized forms), whereas vinorelbine is semisynthetic. These agents act primarily in the M phase of the cell cycle, blocking mitotic spindle formation by preventing the assembly of tubulin dimers into microtubules. Because microtubules are critical for maintenance of cell shape and intracellular protein transport, inhibition of their formation can lead to cell death. The vinca alkaloids are given parenterally and they penetrate most tissues, except for the CSF. The drugs are cleared mainly via biliary excretion, so doses must be decreased in patients with liver dysfunction. Resistance can occur from increased drug efflux from tumor cells via overexpression of membrane drug transporters. Clinically, vinblastine is used for Hodgkin and non-Hodgkin lymphomas, breast cancer, and germ cell cancer. Vincristine, which has a higher affinity for microtubules, possesses a different clinical and ADR profile than vinblastine. Vincristine is used in several acute leukemias and lymphomas, as well as several pediatric cancers including Wilms tumor, Ewing sarcoma, and neuroblastoma. Vincristine myelosuppression tends to be less than that of vinblastine. However, neurotoxicity is dose-limiting. Symptoms include peripheral sensory neuropathy, urinary retention, constipation, cranial nerve palsies, and ataxia. Vinorelbine is used mainly in lung, breast, and ovarian cancers.

Etoposide is a semisynthetic derivative of podophyllotoxin extracted from the root of the mayapple plant (*Podophyllum peltatum*). The drug is usually given parenterally, but can be given orally, although oral dosage typically must be twice that of intravenous administration. Elimination is mainly via the kidneys, so dose reductions are required in those with renal impairment. Etoposide inhibits the enzyme necessary for cutting and religating (ie, joining) double-stranded DNA, thus inhibiting DNA synthesis and function.

TABLE 31-4 Natural product anticancer drugs and toxicities.

Drug	Acute Toxicity	Delayed Toxicity
Docetaxel	Hypersensitivity, rash	Neurotoxicity, fluid retention, neutropenia
Etoposide	Nausea and vomiting, hypotension	Alopecia, myelosuppression
Irinotecan	Diarrhea, nausea, and vomiting	Diarrhea, myelosuppression, nausea and vomiting
Paclitaxel	Nausea and vomiting, hypotension, arrhythmias, hypersensitivity	Myelosuppression, peripheral sensory neuropathy
Topotecan	Nausea and vomiting	Myelosuppression
Vinblastine	Nausea and vomiting	Myelosuppression, mucositis, alopecia, SIADH, vascular events
Vincristine	None	Neurotoxicity, peripheral neuropathy, paralytic ileus, myelosuppression, alopecia, SIADH
Vinorelbine	Nausea and vomiting	Myelosuppression, constipation, SIADH

SIADH, syndrome of inappropriate secretion of antidiuretic hormone.

Clinically, etoposide is used in combination drug regimens for small cell and NSCLC, Hodgkin and non-Hodgkin lymphomas, and gastric cancer.

The camptothecins are derived from the *Camptotheca acuminata* tree native to southern China and Tibet. Although the precise enzyme that these drugs inhibit is different than that of etoposide, the result is similar in that these agents inhibit cells' ability to cut and religate single DNA strands, processes that are essential for normal DNA replication and repair. Topotecan is second-line treatment for advanced ovarian cancer after initial treatment with platinum-based chemotherapy and as second-line treatment for small cell lung cancer. The main route of elimination is renal excretion. Irinotecan is a prodrug converted by the liver into the active antimetabolite. In combination chemotherapy regimens, irinotecan is first-line therapy to treat metastatic colorectal cancer. Diarrhea associated with irinotecan therapy can be severe, leading to significant electrolyte imbalance and dehydration.

The taxanes were originally extracted from the bark of yew trees in the *Taxus* genus. Now, paclitaxel and docetaxel are produced synthetically. These drugs are mitotic spindle poisons that work in the M phase of the cell cycle to inhibit cell division by preventing microtubule disassembly into tubulin monomers. Paclitaxel and docetaxel are given intravenously.

Their clinical uses overlap and include treatment for several solid tumors, including advanced breast and ovarian cancers, head and neck cancers, and lung cancers. The toxicities of these two taxanes are not identical to each other (Table 31-4).

Antitumor Antibiotics

Screening of microbial agents led to the discovery of many growth-inhibiting agents that are useful as anticancer drugs. This category of antineoplastic drugs comprises several structurally dissimilar agents. The anthracyclines represent a group of drugs extracted from the *Streptomyces peucetius* (variant *caesius*) bacterium. These include **doxorubicin**, **daunorubicin**, **idarubicin**, **epirubicin**, and **mitoxantrone**. **Bleomycin** and **mitomycin** are antibiotics isolated from *Streptomyces*, though from different species than that of the anthracyclines. A major mechanism of action of these antibiotics is binding to DNA through intercalation between specific bases. They block synthesis of DNA and/or RNA and cause DNA strand scission, thus interfering with cell replication. Acute and delayed toxicities associated with these anticancer drugs are listed in Table 31-5.

The anthracyclines must be given intravenously. They are metabolized in the liver, and the products are excreted in the bile and urine. Although anthracyclines are usually

TABLE 31-5 Antitumor antibiotics and toxicities.

Drug	Acute Toxicity	Delayed Toxicity
Bleomycin	Allergic reactions, fever, hypotension	Skin toxicity, pulmonary fibrosis, mucositis, alopecia
Daunorubicin	Nausea and vomiting, fever, red urine (not hematuria)	Cardiotoxicity, alopecia, myelosuppression
Doxorubicin	Nausea, red urine (not hematuria)	Cardiotoxicity, alopecia, myelosuppression, stomatitis
Idarubicin	Nausea and vomiting	Myelosuppression, mucositis, cardiotoxicity
Mitomycin	Nausea and vomiting	Myelosuppression, mucositis, anorexia and fatigue, hemolytic-uremic syndrome

administered on an every-3-week schedule, low-dose weekly or continuous infusions over a few days have been shown to have equivalent efficacy with reduced toxicity. Doxorubicin is one of the most important anticancer drugs currently used. Its clinical applications include many solid cancers, soft tissue cancers, and several childhood cancers. Daunorubicin is mainly used in the treatment of acute myeloid leukemia, and idarubicin is used in combination regimens as induction therapy for acute myeloid leukemia. Epirubicin is a component of adjuvant therapy for early-stage, node-positive breast cancer, metastatic breast cancer, and gastroesophageal cancer. Mitoxantrone is used for treating advanced, hormone-insensitive prostate cancer, low-grade non-Hodgkin lymphoma, breast cancer, and acute myeloid leukemias in adults and children. The primary dose-limiting toxicity of the anthracyclines is myelosuppression; sometimes, mucositis is dose-limiting. Cardiotoxicity is the most distinctive ADR of the anthracyclines. Within the first few days, transient arrhythmias, pericarditis, and myocarditis occur, though these are usually asymptomatic. Dose-dependent chronic cardiotoxicity includes a slowly developing cardiomyopathy and heart failure. Dexrazoxane is an inhibitor of iron-mediated free radical generation that may be used in some patients to protect against anthracycline-induced cardiotoxicity.

Bleomycin is a CCS drug that generates free radicals that bind to DNA, causing strand breaks and inhibiting DNA replication in the G_2 phase of the tumor cell cycle. Bleomycin is given parenterally (intramuscular, intravenous, or subcutaneous). The drug is inactivated by tissue aminopeptidases, but renal clearance of the intact drug also occurs. Bleomycin is an important component of drug regimens for Hodgkin and non-Hodgkin lymphomas, germ cell tumors, head and neck cancer, and squamous cell cancer of the skin, cervix, and vulva. Pulmonary fibrosis develops slowly, but is the dose-limiting toxicity. The incidence of pulmonary toxicity increases with larger cumulative doses and in persons over 70 years, those with underlying pulmonary disease, and those who have received chest irradiation.

Mitomycin is a CCNS agent that is converted by liver enzymes to an alkylating agent that cross-links DNA. The drug is given intravenously and is rapidly cleared via hepatic metabolism. Mitomycin's main use is in combination anticancer regimens for treatment of squamous cell cancer of the anus. In addition, mitomycin is used as intravesicular treatment of superficial bladder cancer, a route that is not associated with systemic toxicity. Systemic mitomycin produces severe myelosuppression.

Miscellaneous Anticancer Agents

Many anticancer drugs do not fit within the traditional categories described above. Table 31-6 lists the acute and delayed toxicities of the tyrosine kinase inhibitors (**imatinib, dasatinib, nilotinib, bosutinib, ponatinib**), the epidermal growth factor receptor inhibitors (**cetuximab, panitumumab, necitumumab**), the vascular endothelial growth factor inhibitors (**bevacizumab, ziv-aflibercept, ramucirumab, sorafenib, sunitinib, pazopanib**), other important monoclonal antibodies (**rituximab, trastuzumab**), and **alfa interferon**.

TABLE 31-6 Miscellaneous anticancer drugs and toxicities.

Drug	Acute Toxicity	Delayed Toxicity
Tyrosine kinase inhibitors (TKIs)		
Imatinib		Fluid retention, diarrhea, myalgia, congestive heart failure
Dasatinib	Nausea and vomiting	Fluid retention, diarrhea, myelosuppression, myalgia, pleural effusion
Bosutinib		Diarrhea, fluid retention, skin rash, myelosuppression, hepatotoxicity
Epidermal growth factor receptor (EGFR) inhibitors		
Cetuximab	Infusion reaction	Skin rash, hypomagnesemia, fatigue, interstitial lung disease
Panitumumab	Infusion reaction (rare)	
Vascular endothelial growth factor (VEGF) inhibitors		
Bevacizumab	Hypertension, infusion reaction	Arterial thromboembolic events, gastrointestinal perforations, wound healing and bleeding complications, proteinuria
Ziv-aflibercept	Hypertension	Arterial thromboembolic events, gastrointestinal perforations, wound healing and bleeding complications, proteinuria, diarrhea, mucositis
Sorafenib	Hypertension, nausea	Skin rash, fatigue, weakness, bleeding complications, hypophosphatemia
Sunitinib or pazopanib	Hypertension	Skin rash, fatigue, weakness, bleeding complications, cardiac toxicity (rarely, congestive heart failure)
Additional monoclonal antibodies		
Rituximab	Headache, nausea, fever, infusion reaction	Anemia, neutropenia
Trastuzumab	Infusion reaction, pain, weakness	Cardiomyopathy
Interferons		
Alfa interferon	Flu-like symptoms	Myelosuppression, neurologic dysfunction

Imatinib is a classic example of an anticancer drug whose development was guided by knowledge of a specific oncogene. Imatinib inhibits the tyrosine kinase activity of the protein product of the *bcr-abl* oncogene that is commonly expressed in chronic myelogenous leukemia (CML). Durable remissions and apparent cures have occurred in patients treated with this drug. Imatinib is also effective for treatment of gastrointestinal stromal tumors that express the *c-kit* tyrosine kinase. The other four tyrosine kinase inhibitors (TKIs) are used to treat different phases of CML or individuals with CML that are intolerant or resistant to imatinib or specific other inhibitors. Resistance may occur due to mutation of the *bcr-abl* gene. The TKIs are administered orally (and thus can be taken at home) and metabolized primarily by the CYP3A4 family of liver enzymes. Since many other drugs are metabolized by the CYP3A4 system, patients must be counseled and monitored for drug-drug interactions. In particular, consumption of grapefruit products should be avoided, as this can lead to increased drug toxicities.

The epidermal growth factor receptor (EGFR) regulates signaling pathways involved in cell proliferation, invasion and metastasis, and angiogenesis. Activation of EGFR is also implicated in inhibiting the cytotoxic effects of some anticancer drugs and radiation therapy. EGFR is overexpressed in many solid tumors. Thus, drugs have been developed to inhibit activation of the EGFR. Cetuximab, panitumumab, and necitumumab are monoclonal antibodies directed against specific domains of the EGFR. Cetuximab and panitumumab are used in combination chemotherapy regimens to treat metastatic colon cancer, whereas necitumumab is used in combination with other drugs to treat squamous NSCLC.

Vascular endothelial growth factor (VEGF) is one of the most important angiogenic growth factors. Both primary and metastatic tumors require vasculature. Inhibition of VEGF results in decreased tumor growth and cancer progression by starving tumors of blood supply. Currently, many drugs (six listed above) are available that either inhibit the ability of VEGF to bind to its receptor or prevent its downstream signaling. VEGF inhibitors are used to treat several solid tumors, including metastatic colorectal cancer, NSCLC, and advanced renal and liver cancers.

Many monoclonal antibodies have been developed that bind to specific proteins that are often overexpressed in particular cancer cells. Only a couple examples will be covered here. **Rituximab** is a monoclonal antibody with high affinity for a surface protein (CD20) in non-Hodgkin lymphoma cells. The drug is currently used with conventional anticancer drugs (eg, cyclophosphamide plus vincristine plus prednisone) in CD20-positive lymphomas. Rituximab is also used as an immunosuppressant in the treatment of severe rheumatoid arthritis (Chapter 32). Use of rituximab is associated with hypersensitivity reactions and myelosuppression. **Trastuzumab** is a monoclonal antibody directed against the human epidermal growth factor receptor-2 (HER2). Binding of trastuzumab to the HER2 receptor causes receptor uptake into the tumor cells, thereby preventing receptors from being activated by the circulating ligand. Addition of trastuzumab to adjuvant combination chemotherapy benefits women with HER2 overexpressing breast cancer with respect to disease free and overall survival. Acute toxicity includes nausea and vomiting, chills, fevers, and headache.

The interferons are endogenous glycoproteins with antineoplastic, immunosuppressive, and antiviral actions. The use of alpha-interferons (IFN-α; Chapter 32), often in combination chemotherapy regimens, is effective against a number of neoplasms, including hairy cell leukemia, Kaposi sarcoma, melanoma, and non-Hodgkin lymphoma. Toxic effects of interferons include myelosuppression and neurologic dysfunction.

Hormonal Agents

Many hormonal agents that are used in cancer chemotherapy have been discussed in other chapters. In this chapter, the use of gonadal hormone antagonists and aromatase synthesis inhibitors (Chapter 22) and glucocorticoids (Chapter 23) is discussed only in relation to their clinical application in cancer chemotherapy.

Two of the most common cancers—breast cancer and prostate cancer—are often present in a hormone dependent form. Agents that inhibit estrogen or progesterone synthesis or the receptors for these ligands are extremely useful in many women with breast cancer. Similarly, antiandrogenic drugs are useful in men with advanced prostate cancer.

Tamoxifen, a selective estrogen receptor modulator (Chapter 22), acts as an estrogen antagonist in estrogen-sensitive breast cancer cells. For *postmenopausal* women with estrogen receptor-positive breast cancer, tamoxifen is beneficial when used alone or in combination with cytotoxic chemotherapy. Typically, women are advised to take daily oral tamoxifen for 5 years after surgical resection of the tumor. After tamoxifen therapy is completed, treatment with a drug that inhibits aromatase, the enzyme that converts precursor steroids into estrogens is recommended. Treatment with **anastrozole**, a common aromatase inhibitor, is recommended for years, though the ideal duration is unknown. For stage I (node-negative) breast cancer (ie, localized cancer that has not invaded the lymph nodes), adjuvant chemotherapy for premenopausal women and adjuvant tamoxifen for postmenopausal women after surgery further decreases the risk of recurrence.

Prostate cancer was the second cancer (after breast cancer) shown to be responsive to hormonal manipulation. In this case, the goal is to eliminate testosterone, the androgenic steroid hormone that stimulates growth of prostate cells. For men with metastatic prostate cancer, the treatment of choice is to eliminate testosterone production by either surgical castration (removal of the testes) or chemical castration. A preferred approach is the use of a gonadotropin-releasing hormone (GnRH) agonist (eg, **leuprolide**, **goserelin**) alone or in combination with an androgen receptor antagonist (eg, **flutamide**, **bicalutamide**, **nilutamide**). When GnRH agonists are administered in constant doses, they inhibit pituitary release of luteinizing hormone (LH) and follicle-stimulating hormone (FSH). As a result, androgen production drops to castration levels and tumor growth may be slowed. The advantages of hormonal treatment are reduction of symptoms (especially bone pain) and a reduction in the level of prostate-specific antigen (PSA), which is a surrogate marker for response to treatment in prostate cancer. Second-line hormonal therapies include **aminoglutethimide** plus **hydrocortisone** (see below), the antifungal agent **ketoconazole** plus hydrocortisone, or hydrocortisone alone. Aminoglutethimide is a nonselective inhibitor of *all* steroidal hormones; as such, the drug's effects have sometimes been described as that of a chemical adrenalectomy. Unfortunately, hormonal therapy typically only controls symptoms for up to 2 years and nearly all those with advanced prostate cancer eventually become refractory to hormone therapy. For men with hormone-refractory prostate cancer, docetaxel (a taxane CCS agent discussed above) plus **prednisone** is one of the regimens of choice.

Glucocorticoids such as hydrocortisone and prednisone have been useful in the treatment of several hematologic malignancies as well as in advanced breast and prostate cancer. Anticancer actions probably involve multiple mechanisms. In addition, glucocorticoids are effective as supportive therapy in the management of cancer-related hypercalcemia.

REHABILITATION RELEVANCE

Integration of physical therapy and conditioning programs into overall cancer treatment regimens has increased over the past decade. Research has documented that exercise programs benefit all participants, regardless of the type of cancer, sex, or age of the patients. Rehabilitation programs help maintain cardiovascular and pulmonary function, improve quality of life, and also improve cancer-related fatigue, a common side effect of cancer or cancer treatment.

Cancer-related fatigue may fluctuate in intensity and duration, but is characterized as an extreme tiredness that does not abate with rest. There are likely multiple causes of cancer-related fatigue, including endogenous cytokines released from malignant cells and immune cells, anemia, radiation treatment, chemotherapy, and deconditioning. If a particular cause can be identified (eg, anemia), then it is usually treated (eg, by a blood transfusion or drugs to increase red blood cell formation). However, in most cases, cancer-related fatigue is not easily treatable.

Many recent studies have supported the effectiveness of incorporating a formal aerobic exercise program during the inpatient treatment of individuals with cancer. Compared to those who received usual cancer care, adults receiving chemotherapy and/or radiation that participated in a walking program (total of 3 to ≥ 24 hours) demonstrated clinical improvements in quality of life and cancer-related fatigue, and statistically improved their aerobic functional capacity. Most studies have used walking interventions performed at moderate intensity (50-70% of age-predicted heart rate maximum,

or at an RPE of 12-13). Walking should be encouraged daily with a goal of at least 60 minutes of walking per week *during* cancer treatment.

Physical therapists in outpatient settings should ask patients whether they are currently receiving anticancer treatments or if they are cancer survivors. Most outpatient orthopedic therapists perform a medical screening to assess the potential for metastatic bone lesions masquerading as straightforward musculoskeletal impairments. Therapists must also ask cancer survivors about previous anticancer treatments, with particular focus on agents or interventions (eg, radiation) that have the potential to induce long-term complications. The ultimate goal of cancer chemotherapy is to be able to selectively target and destroy specific cancer cells. While a few such agents are in clinical use, most anticancer drugs have broad cytotoxic effects. Common adverse effects are discussed below.

- **Nausea** and **vomiting**, **fatigue**, and **myelosuppression** are almost universal adverse effects of anticancer drugs. If these manifestations are profound (especially nausea and vomiting), physical therapy interventions may have to be deferred. For fatigue, physical therapists should educate individuals that participation in an aerobic exercise program even *during* chemotherapy has many documented physical and psychological benefits. To prescribe safe and appropriate exercise intensity, the therapist must determine whether the patient's hematological values (eg, hemoglobin, platelet count) are above critical cut-off levels. Due to patients' immunosuppression, vigilance in standard precautions cannot be overemphasized. If sick, the therapist should not work with immunocompromised patients.

- **Pulmonary fibrosis** (or, interstitial lung disease) is a recognized delayed toxicity associated with several chemotherapy drugs, especially cyclophosphamide, methotrexate, busulfan, carmustine, bleomycin, and cetuximab. Lung damage is irreversible, though in some cases may be *slowed* with medications. Patients may experience dyspnea at rest or with exertion. Physical therapists should closely monitor respiratory rate, pulse oximetry, and ratings of perceived exertion during activity. Exercise intensity must be adjusted appropriately to prevent oxygen desaturation. In cases where patients desaturate at rest or with exercise, this information must be relayed to the referring provider to determine whether and when oxygen supplementation is indicated.

- Several plant-derived chemotherapeutic drugs induce **sensory peripheral neuropathy** that can present as pain, paresthesias, or reduced sensation in the hands and feet. Symptoms range in severity and duration. Sometimes, the symptoms cease within months after chemotherapy cessation. In other cases, the symptoms may last for years or indefinitely.

- **Cardiotoxicity** ranging from arrhythmias to cardiomyopathy has been associated with the anthracyclines, paclitaxel, tyrosine kinase inhibitors, and VEGF inhibitors. Close monitoring of hemodynamics during activity is especially warranted. For individuals taking tyrosine kinase inhibitors, **fluid retention** can occur. If new or exacerbated dyspnea is noted, this information should be relayed to the referring provider. In some cases, the dyspnea may be due to pleural or pericardial effusion.

CASE CONCLUSION

Due to its efficacy and mild toxicity, imatinib has been the standard therapy for CML. However, some patients do not respond completely to the drug. In such cases, several options are available including increasing the imatinib dose or switching to another tyrosine kinase inhibitor. In this case, P.Y.'s oncologist chose to increase the imatinib dose. Common adverse effects of imatinib include muscle pain and fluid retention. Sometimes, the fluid retention can result in pleural effusion or pulmonary edema, causing difficulty breathing. The oncology fellow suspected that P.Y.'s current symptoms may have been the result of the increasing dosage of imatinib over the past couple weeks. The oncology team decided to discontinue the imatinib, determine the etiology of the patient's dyspnea, and investigate other CML treatment options for P.Y. After relaying these suspicions to the physical therapist, the pair decided to hold the physical therapy evaluation until Tuesday. By this time, much of the imatinib would have been eliminated (half-life of imatinib's active metabolite is 40 hours), with the potential that at least some of P.Y.'s symptomology may be improved.

CHAPTER 31 QUESTIONS

1. Which of the following statements regarding the log-kill hypothesis is true?

   a. A 2-log-kill dose represents a decrease in tumor cells from 1000 cells to 10 cells.
   b. A 2-log-kill dose represents a decrease in tumor cells from 1000 to 500 cells.
   c. A 2-log-kill dose represents a decrease in tumor cells from 10^{12} to 10^8.
   d. The log-kill hypothesis is most applicable to the treatment of human solid tumors.

2. Which of the following refers to adjuvant chemotherapy?

   a. The use of chemotherapy as the main cancer treatment
   b. The use of chemotherapy after local methods of cancer treatment
   c. The use of chemotherapy in people who present with cancer for which local cancer treatment has not been completely effective
   d. The use of only one cytotoxic drug

3. Which of the following anticancer drugs does *not* have its effect by alkylation?

   a. Bleomycin
   b. Cyclophosphamide
   c. Carboplatin
   d. Procarbazine

4. Which of the following statements is true regarding antimetabolite chemotherapy agents?

   a. Antimetabolites are CCNS agents.
   b. Methotrexate is a classic antimetabolite that acts by inhibiting an enzyme required for cell proliferation and growth.
   c. Antimetabolites are CCS drugs that act primarily in the M phase of the cell cycle.
   d. The toxicities associated with antimetabolites can be avoided with adequate hydration.

5. Which of the following drugs would *not* be considered a plant-derived anticancer agent?

   a. Topotecan
   b. Vinblastine
   c. Vincristine
   d. 5-fluorouracil

6. Which of the following statements is true regarding the anthracyclines?

   a. Gastrointestinal distress is the primary dose-limiting toxicity of the anthracyclines.
   b. The only cardiac toxicity associated with the anthracyclines is transient arrhythmias.
   c. Anthracyclines are a class of antibiotics that must be given intravenously.
   d. The anthracyclines are antibiotics derived from bacteria within the *Staphylococcus* genus.

7. Which of the following is true regarding the epidermal growth factor receptor (EGRF)?

   a. Epidermal growth factor receptors are often overexpressed in many solid tumors.
   b. Drugs that stimulate epidermal growth factor receptors represent an important class of anticancer agents.
   c. Antibodies that stimulate epidermal growth factor receptors are used to treat many cancers.
   d. Drugs that inhibit signaling pathways associated with epidermal growth factor receptors are important in the treatment of acute leukemias.

8. Which of the following is an anticipated delayed toxicity of bleomycin?

   a. Nausea
   b. Tachycardia
   c. Pulmonary fibrosis
   d. Valvular stenosis

9. Which of the following is an anticipated delayed toxicity of the vinca alkaloids?

   a. Diarrhea
   b. Arrhythmias
   c. Gynecomastia
   d. Peripheral neuropathy

10. All of the following agents have been used in drug regimens for the treatment of breast cancer, except for:

   a. Prednisone
   b. Flutamide
   c. Tamoxifen
   d. Anastrozole

Immunopharmacology

J.M. is 66-year-old man with a history of three myocardial infarctions within the last decade. Over that time, his ejection fraction fell to less than 40% and he demonstrated symptom-limited exercise tests with a decline in sustainable workload of less than 5 metabolic equivalents (METs). J.M. qualified for a heart transplant and was enrolled in an outpatient precardiac transplant rehabilitation program to help prevent further functional decline. Two months ago, J.M. received a heart transplant. His post-transplant immunosuppressant maintenance medication includes oral cyclosporine, mycophenolate mofetil, and prednisone. In addition, J.M. is taking other drugs to maintain cardiovascular hemodynamics and improve his plasma lipid profile. After surgery, J.M. spent 14 days in the hospital: 4 days in the cardiac intensive care unit and 10 days on the cardiac telemetry floor. On post-transplant day 18, a cardiologist performed a symptom-limited stress test to determine J.M.'s readiness for a 12-week Phase II outpatient cardiac rehabilitation program. On day 21, J.M. began a physical therapist-supervised and monitored aerobic training by walking on the treadmill. Five minutes of low intensity warm-up were followed by 20 minutes at a sustained Borg rating of perceived exertion (RPE) of 11, and then 5 minutes of cool-down exercise. By day 28, J.M. had progressed to sustained aerobic exercise for 35 minutes at an RPE of 13. At 42 days post-transplant, resistance training was incorporated into the program with alternating upper and lower body exercises and 2 minutes of walking between exercises to prevent hypotension. One week ago (post-transplant day 48) at his regularly scheduled cardiac rehabilitation session, J.M. complained of chest pain and fatigue. The physical therapist noted that J.M.'s blood pressure was low and also observed that the patient's feet were swollen. The therapist called the referring cardiologist's office to report J.M.'s symptoms and vital signs. Shortly after, a medical diagnosis of rejection-induced coronary artery vasculitis was made. Cyclosporine and mycophenolate mofetil were continued and prednisone was discontinued. J.M. was placed on antithymocyte globulin and bolus intravenous methylprednisolone.

REHABILITATION FOCUS

Drugs that modulate the immune system can be broadly divided into two major classifications: immunosuppressants and immune enhancers (Figure 32-1). Drugs that *suppress* the immune system play an important role in preventing tissue or organ transplant rejection and in treating certain diseases that arise from dysregulation of the immune response. Drugs that *augment* the immune response or selectively alter the balance of various components of the immune system are also important in the management of certain diseases such as cancer and autoimmune or inflammatory diseases.

While immunosuppressant therapy has significantly reduced the morbidity and mortality associated with organ transplantation, the adverse effects associated with these drug classes may limit the rate of rehabilitation or the quality of life after transplantation. In addition to causing organ dysfunction, these drugs have significant detrimental effects on musculoskeletal function. Glucocorticoids such as prednisolone cause both muscle atrophy and osteoporosis. Calcineurin antagonists such as cyclosporine decrease the concentration of oxidative enzymes in skeletal muscle, and thus aerobic capacity.

Prior to transplantation, instituting a rehabilitation program can slow the decrement in pulmonary, cardiovascular, and skeletal muscle function. *After* transplantation, participation in rehabilitation programs has been shown to reduce morbidity and mortality. In heart transplant recipients that began rehabilitation programs with both aerobic and resistance components immediately post-transplant, long-term outcomes approach 95% of the functional parameters for age-matched norms. Even at 5 years post-transplant, a 1-year rehabilitation program begun immediately after transplant improves cardiovascular and skeletal muscle function. Challenges specific to post-transplant rehabilitation are related to surgical procedure, previous deconditioned state of the individual, pharmacologic regimen, and specific organ transplanted. For example, heart transplant recipients have limited chronotropic and inotropic responses to exercise. This is due in part to organ denervation, but also to immunosuppressants

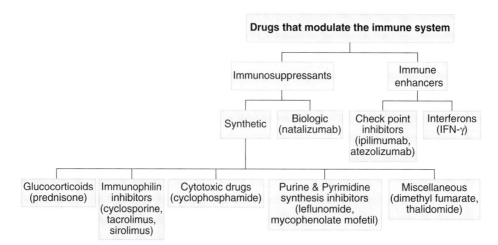

FIGURE 32-1 **Initial classification of immune system modulators is based on whether drugs suppress or enhance immune function.** Classification of immunosuppressants is based on mechanism of action with five classes of small molecular weight synthetic drugs and larger molecular weight biologic agents. Immune enhancers presented in this chapter include large molecular weight biologic agents divided into check point inhibitors and interferons. Select example drugs are shown in parentheses.

and the use of other drugs to control cardiovascular dynamics. These individuals require an extended warm-up phase, several minutes between resistance exercise sets, and longer cool-down periods to prevent hypotension.

Although much research regarding rehabilitation prior to and following transplantation has focused on heart transplantation, rehabilitation programs for people receiving other solid organ transplants and autologous stem cell transplants may also reduce morbidity and mortality. This beneficial effect is not limited to the adult population, because children who receive transplants also appear to benefit.

NORMAL IMMUNE RESPONSES

The immune system evolved to protect the host from invading pathogens. When functioning optimally, the immune system is exquisitely responsive to invading pathogens while retaining the capacity to recognize and tolerate (ie, not attack) the host's own tissues. Protection from infection and disease are provided by the collaborative efforts of the innate and adaptive immune systems. Recognition of normal cells from transformed cells, such as cancer cells, is an additional important role for the immune system.

Innate Immune System

The innate immune system is the first line of defense against invading bacteria, viruses, fungi, or parasites. The system consists of mechanical, biochemical, and cellular components. Mechanical components include physical barriers such as the skin and mucus. The biochemical components include antimicrobial peptides and proteins, the complement system, lytic enzymes, interferons, acidic pH, and free radicals. Key cells of the innate immune system include neutrophils, monocytes, macrophages, natural killer (NK) cells and natural killer T (NKT) cells. Table 32-1 lists common acronyms used in

immunology. In contrast to adaptive immune responses, the innate immune response exists and acts prior to infection, is *not* enhanced by repeated infection, and is generally *not* antigen specific. Intact skin or mucosa is the first barrier to pathogenic

TABLE 32-1 **Common acronyms used in immunology.**

APC	Antigen-presenting cell
CD	Cluster of differentiation
CTLA-4	T-lymphocyte-associated antigen 4
DTH	Delayed-type hypersensitivity
FKBP	FK-binding protein
GVH	Graft-versus-host
HVG	Host-versus-graft
IFN	Interferon
ICAM	Intercellular adhesion molecule-1
IVIG	Intravenous immune globulin therapy
IL	Interleukin
MAB	Monoclonal antibody
MHC	Major histocompatibility complex
NK cell	Natural killer cell
NKT cell	Natural killer T cell
PD	Programmed cell death protein
PD-L1	Programmed cell death protein-ligand 1
TCR	T-cell receptor
TGF-β	Transforming growth factor-β
TH1, TH2	T helper cell types 1 and 2
TNF	Tumor necrosis factor

entry into the host. When this barrier is breached, an immediate innate immune response, referred to as "inflammation," is provoked and ultimately leads to destruction of the pathogen. The pathogen can be destroyed by lysosomal components that break down bacterial peptidoglycan cell walls and by activation of complement. The complement system (Figure 32-2) enhances macrophage and neutrophil phagocytosis by acting as opsonins and chemoattractants, which recruit immune cells from the bloodstream to the site of infection. The activation of complement eventually leads to pathogen lysis via the generation of a membrane attack complex that creates holes in the pathogen membrane, killing it.

When infection triggers the inflammatory response, neutrophils and monocytes from the peripheral circulation must find their way to the infected tissue. The chemicals that attract these phagocytes to the precise location are chemoattractant cytokines (chemokines) such as interleukin(IL)-8 that are released from activated endothelial cells and tissue macrophages at the inflammatory site. Movement of the immune cells from blood vessels into the inflammatory site is mediated by adhesive interactions between cell surface

receptors—integrins on the immune cells and intercellular adhesion molecule-1 (ICAM-1) on the activated endothelial cells. Tissue macrophages and other antigen-presenting cells (APCs) such as dendritic cells express pattern recognition receptors (eg, Toll-like receptors) that recognize key evolutionarily conserved pathogen components. Recognition of these various pathogen components stimulates the release of proinflammatory cytokines, chemokines, and interferons. If the innate immune response is successfully executed, the invading pathogen is ingested, degraded, and eliminated, and disease is either prevented or is of short duration.

Various immune cell types recruited to the inflammatory site contribute to the innate response by secreting interferon-gamma (IFN-γ) and interleukin-17 (IL-17). These chemical mediators activate resident tissue macrophages and dendritic cells and recruit neutrophils to successfully destroy the pathogens. NK cells are called "natural" because they are able to recognize and destroy virus-infected normal cells as well as tumor cells *without* prior stimulation. This activity is regulated by "killer cell immunoglobulin-like receptors" on the surface of NK cells that are specific for major histocompatibility complex

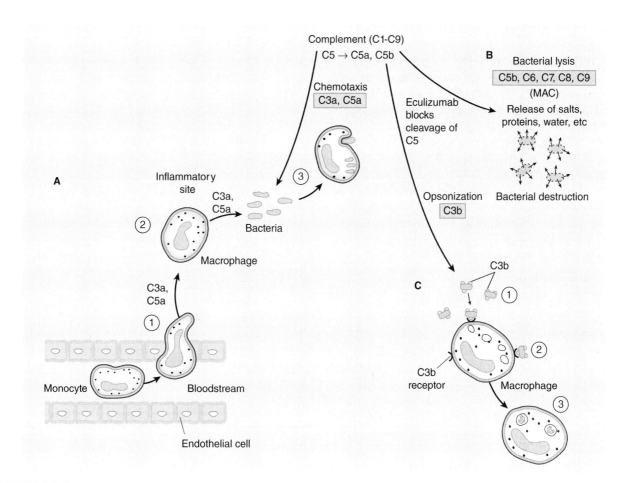

FIGURE 32-2 Role of complement in innate immunity. Complement is comprised of nine proteins (C1-C9) that are split into fragments during activation. (**A**) Via chemotaxis, complement components C3a and C5a attract phagocytes (1) to inflammatory sites (2), where they ingest and degrade pathogens (3). (**B**) Complement components C5b, C6, C7, C8, and C9 associate to form a membrane attack complex (MAC) that lyses bacteria, causing their destruction. (**C**) Complement component C3b is an opsonin that coats bacteria (1) and facilitates their ingestion (2) and digestion (3) by phagocytes.

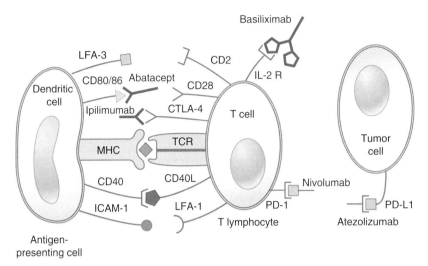

FIGURE 32-3 **T-cell activation by an antigen-presenting cell (APC) requires engagement of the T-cell receptor (TCR) by the MHC-peptide complex (signal 1) and binding of the costimulatory molecules (CD80/86) on the dendritic cell to CD28 on the T cell (signal 2).** The activation signals are strengthened by CD40/CD40L and ICAM-1/LFA-1 interactions. In a normal immune response, T-cell activation is regulated by T-cell–derived CTLA-4 and PD-1. CTLA-4 binds to CD80 or CD86 with higher affinity than CD28 and sends inhibitory signals to the nucleus of the T cell. Ligation of PD-1 to PD-L1 or -L2 also inhibits T cell proliferation. Abatacept prevents T-cell CD28 from binding APC CD80/86. Basiliximab inhibits the IL-2 receptor on the T cell. Ipilimumab helps maintain T-cell activation by inhibiting CTLA-4 interaction with CD80/86. Atezolizumab and nivolumab maintain T-cell activation by binding to the PD-L1 receptor and PD-1 receptor, respectively.

(MHC) class I molecules (present on all nucleated cells). When NK cells bind to self MHC class I proteins, these receptors on the NK cells deliver inhibitory signals, preventing them from killing normal host cells. Tumor cells or virus-infected cells that have down-regulated MHC class I expression do not engage the surface receptors on the NK cells. This failure results in activation of the NK cells, and subsequent destruction of the virally infected or tumor cell. NK cells kill target cells by releasing cytotoxic granules that induce programmed cell death. Natural killer T (NKT) cells share properties of both NK cells and T cells. The NKT cells recognize microbial lipid antigens presented by a unique class of MHC-like molecules known as CD1 and have been implicated in host defense against microbial agents, autoimmune diseases, and tumors.

Adaptive Immune System

When the innate immune processes are incapable of coping with an infection, the adaptive immune system is mobilized by signals from the innate response. The adaptive immune system has a number of characteristics that contribute to its success in eliminating pathogens. These include the ability to: (1) respond to a variety of antigens, each in a specific manner; (2) discriminate between foreign antigens (ie, pathogens) and host self-antigens; and (3) respond to a previously encountered antigen in a learned way by initiating a vigorous memory response. This adaptive response culminates in the production of antibodies (the effectors of humoral immunity) and the activation of T lymphocytes (the effectors of cell-mediated immunity).

The induction of specific adaptive immunity requires the participation of APCs, which includes dendritic cells,

macrophages, and B lymphocytes. The APCs play critical roles in the adaptive immune response because of their capacity to phagocytize particulate antigens or endocytose protein antigens and enzymatically digest them to generate peptides. The peptides are then loaded onto class I or class II MHC proteins and *presented* to the cell surface T-cell receptor (TCR) (Figure 32-3). CD8 T cells (cytotoxic or killer T cells) recognize class I–MHC peptide complexes, while CD4 T cells (helper T cells) recognize class II–MHC peptide complexes. At least two signals are necessary for the activation of T cells. The first signal is the engagement of the TCR with peptide-bound MHC molecules. In the absence of a second signal, the T cells become unresponsive or undergo apoptosis. The second signal involves binding of costimulatory molecules on the APC (either CD40, CD80, or CD86) to their respective ligands on the T-cell surface (CD40L for CD40, CD28 for CD80/CD86).

Activation of T cells is also regulated via a negative feedback loop involving another molecule known as T-lymphocyte–associated antigen 4 (CTLA-4). After CD28 binds with CD80 or CD86, CTLA-4 in the cytoplasm moves to the T-cell surface where, because of its higher affinity of binding to CD80 and CD86, it outcompetes or displaces CD28, resulting in suppression of T-cell activation and proliferation. Another negative regulator of T cells is programmed cell death protein-1 (PD-1). Binding of PD-1 with its ligands (PD-L1 or PD-L2) suppresses T-cell activity. Both CTLA-4 and PD-1 are considered immune checkpoints. Blockade of these ligands results in sustained T-cell activation. This has been exploited as a strategy for *sustaining* a desirable immune response such as that directed against cancer.

T lymphocytes develop and learn to recognize self from non-self antigens. In animal studies, T-cell clones have

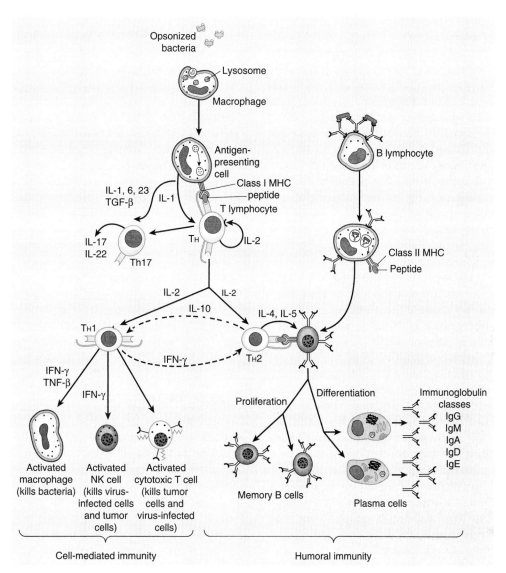

FIGURE 32-4 **Scheme of cellular interactions during the generation of cell-mediated and humoral immune responses.** The cell-mediated arm of the immune response involves the ingestion and digestion of antigen by antigen-presenting cells. The processed peptides are bound to MHC surface proteins that are recognized by the TCR on T helper cells, resulting in T-cell activation. Activated T_H cells secrete IL-2, which causes proliferation and activation of cytotoxic T cells as well as T_H1 and T_H2 cell subsets. T_H1 cells produce IFN-γ and TNF-β, which can directly activate macrophages and NK cells. T_H17 cells may be induced by IL-1, -6, -23, or TGF-β secretion by antigen-presenting cells. The T_H17 cells secrete the proinflammatory cytokines IL-17 and -22. The humoral response is triggered when B lymphocytes bind antigen via their surface immunoglobulin. They are then induced by T_H2-derived IL-4 and IL-5 to proliferate and differentiate into memory cells and antibody-secreting plasma cells. Regulatory cytokines such as IFN-γ and IL-10 (dashed arrows) downregulate T_H2 and T_H1 responses, respectively.

demonstrated the presence of two subsets of T helper lympho-cytes (T_H1 and T_H2) based on the cytokines they secrete after activation (Figure 32-4). The T_H1 subset characteristically produces IFN-γ, IL-2, and IL-12 and induces cell-mediated immunity by activating macrophages, cytotoxic T cells, and NK cells. The T_H2 subset produces IL-4, IL-5, IL-6, and IL-10, and sometimes IL-13, which induce B-cell proliferation and differentiation into antibody-secreting plasma cells. IFN-γ produced by T_H1 cells inhibits the proliferation of T_H2 cells. Conversely, IL-10 produced by T_H2 cells inhibits cytokine pro-duction by T_H1 cells via the downregulation of MHC expres-sion by APCs. *Extracellular* bacteria typically cause the T_H2

cells to release their cytokines, ultimately resulting in the production of neutralizing or opsonic antibodies. In contrast, *intracellular* organisms such as mycobacteria or viruses elicit the production of T_H1 cytokines, which lead to the activation of effector cells such as macrophages.

Another subset of CD4 T cells that secrete IL-17 (T_H17) is important in leukocyte recruitment to sites of bacterial and fungal pathogens. T_H17 cells also contribute to the pathogen-esis of autoimmune diseases such as psoriasis, inflammatory bowel disease, rheumatoid arthritis (RA), and multiple sclero-sis (MS). To treat some of these diseases, the Food and Drug Administration (FDA) has approved monoclonal antibodies

(MABs) that neutralize IL-17 by binding to the cytokine itself or to its receptor (Chapter 34).

There are additional important T-cell populations for which there are currently no targeted drugs. These cells include regulatory T cells that constitute a population of CD4 T cells essential for preventing autoimmunity and allergy as well as homeostasis and tolerance to self-antigens. CD8 T cells recognize endogenously processed peptides presented by virus-infected cells or tumor cells. These peptides are derived from virus or protein tumor antigens in the cytoplasm and are loaded onto MHC class I molecules. Upon activation, CD8 T cells induce target cell death via lytic granule enzymes, perforins, or apoptosis pathways.

B lymphocytes undergo selection in the bone marrow, during which self-reactive B lymphocytes are clonally deleted, while B-cell clones specific for foreign antigens are retained and expanded. The repertoire of antigen specificities by T cells is genetically determined and arises from *T-cell receptor* gene rearrangement, while the specificities of B cells arise from *immunoglobulin* gene rearrangement; for both T cells and B cells, these determinations occur *prior* to encounters with antigen. Upon an encounter with antigen, a mature B cell binds the antigen, internalizes and processes it, and presents its peptide—bound to class II MHC—to CD4 helper cells, which in turn secrete IL-4 and IL-5 (Figure 32-4). These interleukins stimulate B-cell proliferation and differentiation into memory B cells and antibody-secreting plasma cells. The antibodies also undergo affinity maturation, which allows them to bind more efficiently to the antigen. With the passage of time, this results in accelerated elimination of microorganisms in subsequent infections. Antibodies mediate their functions by acting as opsonins to enhance phagocytosis and cellular cytotoxicity and by activating complement to elicit an inflammatory response and induce bacterial lysis.

ABNORMAL IMMUNE RESPONSES

The normally functioning immune response successfully neutralizes toxins, inactivates viruses, destroys transformed cells, and eliminates pathogens. Inappropriate immune responses can lead to extensive tissue damage (hypersensitivity) or reactivity against self-antigens (autoimmunity). In contrast, states of immunodeficiency result in impaired reactivity to appropriate targets, which disrupts essential defense mechanisms.

Hypersensitivity

Hypersensitivity can be classified as antibody-mediated or cell-mediated. Three types of hypersensitivity are antibody-mediated (types I-III), while the fourth is cell-mediated (type IV). Hypersensitivity occurs in two phases: the sensitization phase and the effector phase. Sensitization occurs upon initial encounter with an antigen, whereas the effector phase involves immunologic memory and results in tissue pathology upon a subsequent encounter with that antigen. Type I, or immediate hypersensitivity, is mediated by IgE and may include both

atopic (eg, asthma; Chapter 35) and systemic (anaphylaxis) reactions. Anaphylaxis is the most severe type I hypersensitivity and requires immediate medical intervention. Both type II and III hypersensitivity disorders are mediated by IgG or IgM. In type II hypersensitivity, antigen-antibody complexes initiate the pathophysiologic events. Examples of type II hypersensitivities include red blood cell ABO mismatching in which antibodies bind to the red blood cell surface and mediate cell destruction, and Graves' disease in which antibodies bind and activate thyroid stimulating hormone receptors resulting in hyperthyroidism. In type III hypersensitivity disorders, antigen-antibody complexes precipitate out of the circulation and into the tissues, resulting in subsequent complement activation and inflammation. This hypersensitivity mechanism accounts in part for glomerulonephritis in systemic lupus erythematosus (SLE). Last, type IV, or delayed hypersensitivity disorders are mediated by antigen-specific T cells. Unlike the other hypersensitivity disorders, responses occur 2-3 days after exposure to the sensitizing antigen. Widely recognized examples include contact hypersensitivity associated with poison ivy and latex. Hypersensitivity disorders are discussed in relation to drug allergies later in the chapter.

Autoimmunity

Autoimmune disease arises when the body mounts an immune response against its *own* tissues. This phenomenon derives from the activation of self-reactive T and B lymphocytes that generate cell-mediated or humoral immune responses directed against self-antigens. The consequences of this reactivity include several types of autoimmune diseases, including RA, psoriasis, and SLE (Chapter 34), type 1 diabetes mellitus (Chapter 24) and multiple sclerosis.

Immunodeficiency Diseases

Immunodeficiency diseases result from inadequate function in the immune system that can be due to congenital causes or arise from extrinsic factors such as bacterial or viral infections or drug treatment. The consequences of immunodeficiency include increased susceptibility to infections and prolonged duration and severity of disease. Affected individuals frequently succumb to infections caused by opportunistic organisms of low pathogenicity for the immunocompetent host.

IMMUNOMODULATORY THERAPIES

Modulation of the immune system—either by suppressing or enhancing its responsivity—can be done with small molecular weight synthetic chemicals and larger molecular weight biologic agents such as MABs and fusion proteins (Figure 32-1). Both immunosuppressants and immune enhancers are also discussed in other chapters within this textbook (Chapters 28, 31, 34, 35, 36). The drugs discussed in this chapter represent

TABLE 32-2 Small molecular weight drugs used as immunosuppressive agents.

Drug	Characteristics and Clinical Uses
Azathioprine	Prodrug of the anticancer drug mercaptopurine, which interferes with purine nucleic acid metabolism. Used to prevent transplantation rejection[a] and for treating rheumatic diseases (Chapter 34).
Cyclophosphamide	Anticancer alkylating agent used in cancer chemotherapy and to prevent transplant rejection (Chapter 31).
Dimethyl fumarate	Appears to activate the nuclear factor (erythroid-derived)-like-2 (NFR-2) transcriptional pathway. Reduces oxidative stress, demyelination, and nerve cell inflammation. Used in multiple sclerosis (MS).
Fingolimod hydrochloride	Prodrug metabolized to fingolimod phosphate, which binds the sphingosine 1-phosphate S1P receptor and decreases the number of circulating lymphocytes in the periphery and central nervous system. Used in MS.
Glatiramer acetate	Mixture of synthetic polypeptides and four amino acids (L-glutamic acid, L-alanine, L-lysine, and L-tyrosine) in a fixed ratio. Used in MS, but mechanism of immunomodulation is unknown.
Hydroxychloroquine	Antimalarial drug with immunosuppressive activity used to prevent transplant rejection and to treat rheumatoid arthritis and SLE (Chapter 34).
Leflunomide	Inhibitor of dihydroorotate dehydrogenase, enzyme involved in de novo pyrimidine synthesis. Used in relapsing MS and rheumatoid arthritis (Chapter 34).
Methotrexate	Anticancer drug with multiple mechanisms of action. Used for hematopoietic stem cell transplantation and in rheumatoid arthritis. (Chapters 31 and 34).
Thalidomide	Originally used as sedative and antiemetic, but withdrawn from the marketplace due to teratogenicity. Multiple immunosuppressive mechanisms may be useful in transplant rejection[a].

[a]Transplantation rejection includes solid organ allograft and autologous stem cells. Types of rejection include graft-versus-host and host-versus-graft.

those used in transplantation and in the treatment of MS that are not discussed elsewhere.

Immunosuppressive drugs are used to lower the risk of transplant rejection. Transplanted tissue includes organs from donor(s) (allograft) or autologous tissue in the form of skin or stem cell transplants. Rejection may be divided into two broad categories. Host-versus-graft (HVG) disease occurs when the immune system of the host attacks the transplanted tissue. Graft-versus-host (GVH) disease occurs when the host is immune-suppressed and the transplanted tissue is immunocompetent and mounts an attack against the host's tissues. Although immunosuppressive agents have proven very useful in minimizing the occurrence and impact of exaggerated or inappropriate immune responses, these agents also have the potential to cause disease and increase risk of infection and malignancies.

Enhancing the immune system has benefit in clinical situations such as cancer and potentially other immunosuppressed states. At present, biologics such as MABs, fusion proteins, or interferons and CAR T-cell are clinically used. MABs are used to prevent the downregulation of the immune system mediated by certain cancers. This pharmaceutical prevention allows antitumor T cells to mediate cytotoxic destruction of the neoplastic cells. Interferons find clinical application in some immunodeficiency states and as adjuvants to some therapies for viral liver infections (Chapter 28). CAR T-cell therapy involves harvesting a patient's T cells, changing them in vitro to attack tumor cells, and then reinfusing them back into the patient.

Table 32-2 summarizes the mechanisms of action and clinical uses for several small molecular weight drugs used as immunosuppressive agents. Table 32-3 lists the mechanisms of action and clinical uses of select immunoglobulin-based agents; both immunosuppressants and immune-enhancing agents are presented.

TABLE 32-3 Characteristics of select biologic immunoglobulin-based agents used as immunosuppressants and immune enhancers.

Drug	Characteristics and Clinical Uses
Alemtuzumab	Binds to CD52 receptor on multiple different immune cells, resulting in cell lysis. Used in treatment of relapsing remitting multiple sclerosis (MS).
Atezolizumab	Binds to PD-L1 on tumor cells, preventing suppression signal to antitumor T cells. Used in treatment of multiple cancers.
Basiliximab	Binds to α chain on IL-2 receptor on lymphocytes, inhibiting immune response. Used to prevent transplant rejection.
Ipilimumab	Binds to CTLA-4 receptor on T cells, preventing suppressive signal. Used in treatment of multiple cancers.
Natalizumab	Binds to integrin receptors on leukocytes, preventing emigration of cells from vasculature. Used in treatment of relapsing remitting MS.
Nivolumab	Binds to PD-1 receptor on antitumor T cells, allowing cells to remain active. Used in treatment of multiple cancers.

SYNTHETIC IMMUNOSUPPRESSANTS

Glucocorticoids

Glucocorticoids are a subclass of corticosteroid hormones released from the adrenal gland. Glucocorticoids have significant anti-inflammatory and immunosuppressive effects that account for their beneficial effects in diseases like asthma, inflammatory bowel disease, and autoimmune diseases such as RA. Glucocorticoids are also first-line immunosuppressive therapy for both solid organ and hematopoietic stem cell transplant recipients, with variable results. The mechanisms of action of glucocorticoids are described in Chapter 23, and discussion of their use in a wide variety of clinical applications is presented in multiple chapters (Chapters 23, 34, 35, 36). Glucocorticoids are recognized as having lympholytic properties, reducing the size and lymphoid content of the lymph nodes and spleen. Glucocorticoids are quite toxic to certain subsets of T cells, but their immunologic effects are probably due to their ability to modify cellular functions. Although cellular immunity is more affected than humoral immunity, the primary antibody response can be diminished. However, these drugs have no toxic effect on proliferating myeloid or erythroid stem cells in the bone marrow. The toxicities of long-term systemic glucocorticoid therapy can be severe (Chapter 23).

Immunophilin Inhibitors

Cyclosporine and **tacrolimus** represent a group of immunophilin inhibitors that inhibit the activation of T cells. Cyclosporine is a peptide antibiotic that appears to act at an early stage in the antigen receptor-induced differentiation of T cells. Cyclosporine binds to cyclophilin, a member of a class of intracellular proteins called immunophilins. Cyclosporine and cyclophilin form a complex that inhibits calcineurin, the cytoplasmic phosphatase that is necessary for activation of a transcription factor specific to T cells (NF-AT). NF-AT is involved in the synthesis of IL-2 (and possibly IL-3 and IFN-γ) by activated T cells. Cyclosporine does not block the effect of such chemokines on primed T cells, nor does it block interaction with antigen. Tacrolimus (FK 506) is not chemically related to cyclosporine, but their mechanisms of action are similar. While cyclosporine binds to cyclophilin, tacrolimus binds to another immunophilin called FK-binding protein (FKBP). The tacrolimus-FKBP complex also inhibits calcineurin, and thus prevents activation of NF-AT. On a weight basis, tacrolimus is 10-100 times more potent than cyclosporine in inhibiting immune responses.

Cyclosporine may be given orally, though it is slowly and incompletely absorbed (20-50%), or intravenously. The absorbed drug is primarily metabolized in the liver, with resultant multiple drug interactions which results in the propensity for significant interpatient variability in bioavailability. Cyclosporine half-life varies (8-19 hours) based on formulation. Tacrolimus may be administered orally or intravenously. The

half-life of the intravenous form is approximately 9-12 hours. Like cyclosporine, tacrolimus is metabolized in the liver, and there is potential for drug interactions. The dosage is determined by trough blood level at steady state. Newer formulations of cyclosporine are improving patient compliance (smaller, better-tasting tablets) and increasing bioavailability.

Cyclosporine has therapeutic value in human organ transplantation, in the treatment of GVH disease after hematopoietic stem cell transplantation, and in the treatment of certain autoimmune diseases. Cyclosporine may be used alone or in combination with other immunosuppressants, particularly glucocorticoids. Tacrolimus is utilized for the same indications as cyclosporine, particularly in organ and stem cell transplantation. The drug has proven to be effective therapy for preventing rejection in solid organ transplant recipients even after failure of standard rejection therapy. Tacrolimus is now considered part of a standard prophylactic therapy for GVH disease. Tacrolimus ointment is also currently used in the therapy of atopic dermatitis and psoriasis. Cyclosporine toxicities are numerous and include nephrotoxicity, hypertension, hyperglycemia, liver dysfunction, hyperkalemia, altered mental status, seizures, and hirsutism. Cyclosporine causes very little bone marrow toxicity. An increased incidence of lymphoma and other cancers, such as Kaposi sarcoma, have been observed in transplant recipients receiving cyclosporine. Other immunosuppressive agents may also predispose recipients to cancer. The toxic effects of tacrolimus are similar to those of cyclosporine and include nephrotoxicity, neurotoxicity, hyperglycemia, hypertension, hyperkalemia, and gastrointestinal complaints.

A newer class of immunosuppressive agents called proliferation signal inhibitors (PSI) includes **sirolimus** (rapamycin) and its derivative **everolimus**. PSIs inhibit the activation of T cells and B cells by binding to circulating immunophilin FK506-binding protein 12 (FKBP12) to form an active sirolimus-FKBP12 complex. This complex binds to and inhibits a kinase called mTOR (molecular target of rapamycin). mTOR is a key component of a complex intracellular signaling pathway involved in cell growth, proliferation, angiogenesis, and metabolism. Thus, PSI-induced blockade of mTOR ultimately can lead to inhibition of interleukin-driven T-cell proliferation. Everolimus and sirolimus may also inhibit B-cell proliferation and immunoglobulin production. Sirolimus is available only as an oral drug. Its half-life is about 60 hours, while that of everolimus is about 43 hours. Both drugs are rapidly absorbed. Elimination and drug interactions are similar to that of the calcineurin inhibitors.

Sirolimus has been used effectively alone and in combination with other immunosuppressants to prevent rejection of solid organ allografts. The drug may be used as prophylaxis or as therapy for acute and chronic GVH disease in hematopoietic stem cell transplant recipients. Topical sirolimus is used in some dermatologic disorders. Recently, sirolimus-eluting coronary stents have been shown to reduce restenosis, due to the drug's antiproliferative effects. Everolimus is a newer drug that has shown clinical efficacy similar to sirolimus in solid organ transplant recipients, and possibly to prevent restenosis in coronary stents. Toxicities of the PSIs can include profound myelosuppression (especially thrombocytopenia), hepatotoxicity, diarrhea, hypertriglyceridemia, pneumonitis, headache, and delayed wound healing. Increased use of PSIs to prevent GVH disease in stem cell transplantation regimens has revealed an increased incidence of hemolytic-uremic syndrome, particularly when combined with tacrolimus.

Cytotoxic Drugs

The alkylating agent **cyclophosphamide** is one of the most efficacious immunosuppressive drugs available. Cyclophosphamide destroys proliferating lymphoid cells but also appears to alkylate some resting cells. Very large doses (eg, >120 mg/kg intravenously over several days) may induce an apparent specific tolerance to a new antigen if the drug is administered simultaneously with, or shortly after, the antigen. In smaller doses, the drug has been effective in treating some autoimmune disorders, individuals with acquired factor XIII antibodies and bleeding syndromes, autoimmune hemolytic anemia, and antibody-induced pure red cell aplasia. Treatment with large doses of cyclophosphamide carries considerable risk of pancytopenia and therefore is generally combined with stem cell rescue (transplant) procedures. Although cyclophosphamide appears to induce tolerance for marrow or immune cell grafting, its use does not prevent the subsequent GVH disease, which may be serious or lethal if the donor is a poor histocompatibility match (despite the severe immunosuppression induced by high doses of cyclophosphamide). The drug may also cause hemorrhagic cystitis, which can be prevented or treated with **mesna**. Other adverse drug reactions (ADRs) of cyclophosphamide include nausea, vomiting, cardiac toxicity, and electrolyte disturbances.

Other cytotoxic drugs include **pentostatin** and **azathioprine**. Pentostatin is an adenosine deaminase inhibitor, which results in increased extracellular adenosine levels that inhibits immune responsiveness. Pentostatin produces a profound lymphocytopenia. The main use of the drug is as an antineoplastic agent for lymphoid malignancies. It is also frequently used for steroid-resistant GVH disease after allogeneic stem cell transplantation, as well as in preparative regimens prior to those transplants to provide severe immunosuppression to prevent allograft rejection. Azathioprine is a prodrug of mercaptopurine and functions as an antimetabolite. Although its action is presumably mediated by conversion to mercaptopurine and further metabolites, it has been more widely used than mercaptopurine for immunosuppression in humans. Azathioprine and mercaptopurine appear to be of definite benefit in maintaining renal allografts and may be of value in transplantation of other tissues. The drugs have been of occasional use in prednisone-resistant antibody-mediated idiopathic thrombocytopenic purpura and autoimmune hemolytic anemias. Azathioprine is also used in the treatment of rheumatic diseases (Chapter 34). Other cancer chemotherapeutic agents (Chapter 31) such as vincristine, cytarabine, and vinblastine,

can be used for immunosuppression. However, their use has not been as widespread and their indications for immunosuppression are less certain.

Purine and Pyrimidine Inhibitors

Leflunomide is a prodrug that inhibits pyrimidine synthesis. **Teriflunomide** is the principal active metabolite of leflunomide. Teriflunomide is FDA-approved for the treatment of relapsing-remitting MS, though its exact mechanism of action is unclear. Teriflunomide is hypothesized to decrease the number of activated lymphocytes in the central nervous system (CNS). The drug is a once-daily oral drug that, unlike leflunomide, does not require a loading dose. The adverse effect profile for teriflunomide is similar to that of leflunomide. Both drugs are contraindicated in pregnancy and severe liver disease. The incidence of neutropenia in patients taking teriflunomide is 15% and 10% of patients have a decrease in platelet counts. Leflunomide is also clinically effective in the treatment of rheumatic diseases (Chapter 34).

Mycophenolate mofetil (MMF) is a semisynthetic derivative of mycophenolic acid. Mycophenolic acid is the active immunosuppressive moiety. MMF is used in solid organ transplant recipients for refractory rejection and, in combination with prednisone, as an alternative to cyclosporine or tacrolimus in patients who do not tolerate those drugs. The antiproliferative properties make MMF the first-line drug for preventing or reducing chronic allograft vasculopathy in cardiac transplant recipients. MMF is used to prevent and treat both acute and chronic GVH disease in hematopoietic stem cell transplant recipients. Newer immunosuppressant applications for MMF include lupus nephritis and RA (Chapter 34). The drug's mechanism of action and ADRs are discussed in chapter 34.

Methotrexate has been used in the treatment of GVH disease. Methotrexate is used in the treatment of cancer (Chapter 31) and rheumatic diseases (Chapter 34). The mechanisms of action and ADRs are extensively discussed in these chapters.

Miscellaneous Drugs

Several synthetic immunosuppressants do not fall into the previously discussed categories. Three are FDA-approved immunomodulators (**dimethyl fumarate**, **glatiramer acetate**, **fingolimod hydrochloride**) used exclusively in the treatment of relapsing-remitting MS. These drugs have different mechanisms of action, but all share one uncommon adverse effect—increased risk of progressive multifocal leukoencephalopathy (PML)—which results in damage to the white matter in the brain. It has been proposed that PML is caused by the common JC virus, but PML only occurs in immunosuppressed individuals.

Dimethyl fumarate (DMF) is the methyl ester of fumaric acid. The drug appears to activate the nuclear factor (erythroid-derived 2)-like 2 (NRF-2) transcriptional pathway. Activation of the NRF-2 pathway reduces the oxidative stress that contributes to demyelination and also appears to help protect the nerve cells from inflammation. DMF is given orally. Lymphocytopenia may be significant, so blood counts must be monitored regularly and the drug may be withheld if active infection is present. Flushing is common with treatment initiation and usually improves with time. Other less common ADRs include nausea, diarrhea, abdominal pain, increased hepatic enzymes, and eosinophilia.

Glatiramer acetate (GA) is a mixture of synthetic polypeptides and four amino acids (L-glutamic acid, L-alanine, L-lysine, and L-tyrosine) in a fixed molar ratio. The mechanism of immunomodulation in MS may be via downregulation of the immune response to myelin antigens. Induction and activation of suppressor T cells that migrate to the CNS appear to play a key role. GA is given as a subcutaneous injection in variable dosages and schedules. Toxicities include skin hypersensitivity, and rarely lipoatrophy and skin necrosis at the injection site. Other ADRs include flushing, chest pain, dyspnea, throat constriction, and palpitations, all of which are usually mild and self-limited.

Fingolimod hydrochloride (FH) is an orally active sphingosine 1-phosphate (S1P) receptor modulator. The S1P receptor (subtype 1) controls the release of lymphocytes from lymph nodes and the thymus. FH is metabolized to fingolimod phosphate, which subsequently binds the S1P receptor and ultimately decreases circulating lymphocyte numbers in the periphery and CNS. S1P receptors are also expressed on neurons. Thus, FH may modify disease activity in MS by affecting neurodegeneration, gliosis, and endogenous repair mechanisms in addition to causing lymphocytopenia. The drug is metabolized primarily by the cytochrome P450 (CYP) system; thus, caution is needed when FH is used in combination with other drugs metabolized by the same CYP family. FH can cause serious cardiac toxicity including bradycardia, prolongation of the QT interval, and other arrhythmias. Because of these potential complications, the drug requires cardiac monitoring for 6 hours after the first dose is given. FH is contraindicated in patients with preexisting conditions such as second- or third-degree atrioventricular block, prolonged QTc, recent myocardial infarction, or heart failure. Less common ADRs include macular edema, elevated hepatic enzymes, headache, diarrhea, and cough.

Thalidomide was originally developed as an oral sedative/hypnotic, and subsequently prescribed for morning sickness in pregnancy. The drug was withdrawn from the market in the 1960s due to high rates of phocomelia, a birth defect resulting from retardation of limb bud growth in utero. Use of thalidomide has resurged because of its significant immunomodulatory actions. The drug is currently in active use and in clinical trials for more than 40 different illnesses. Thalidomide inhibits angiogenesis and has multiple anti-inflammatory and immunomodulatory effects. These effects include inhibiting tumor necrosis factor-alpha (TNF-α), reducing phagocytosis by neutrophils, increasing production of IL-10, altering adhesion molecule expression, and enhancing cell-mediated immunity via interactions with T cells. As its clinical uses evolve, the complex actions of thalidomide continue to be studied. Thalidomide is undergoing clinical investigation for GVH disease and as a chemotherapeutic agent in multiple different cancers. The drug is also being used to treat some of the clinical manifestations of both leprosy and skin manifestations of SLE. The adverse effect profile of thalidomide is extensive. In addition to phocomelia, other ADRs include peripheral neuropathy, constipation, rash, fatigue, hypothyroidism, and increased risk of deep vein thrombosis. Thrombosis is sufficiently frequent that many patients are placed on some type of anticoagulant when thalidomide treatment is initiated. Owing to thalidomide's serious toxicity profile, considerable effort has been expended in the development of safer analogs. Immunomodulatory derivatives of thalidomide (IMiDs) are much more potent than thalidomide in regulating cytokines and affecting T-cell proliferation. **Lenalidomide** and **pomalidomide** are newer oral IMiDs. Both drugs have clinical applications as anticancer chemotherapeutics, but not as immunosuppressants in transplantation or rheumatic diseases. Both lenalidomide and pomalidomide have ADR profiles similar to that of thalidomide.

Hydroxychloroquine is an antimalarial drug that has clinical efficacy in prevention of organ transplant rejection and in the treatment of rheumatic diseases (Chapter 34). The drug is concentrated in lysosomes and increases the pH of lysosomal and endosomal compartments within APCs. This action results in decreased intracellular antigen processing and loading of peptides onto MHC class II molecules, which leads to decreased antigen presentation to T cells and decreased T-cell activation. Because of these immunosuppressant activities, hydroxychloroquine is used to prevent and treat GVH disease after allogeneic stem cell transplantation.

BIOLOGIC IMMUNOSUPPRESSANTS

Many immunosuppressive biologic agents find clinical application in both transplantation and treatment in various rheumatic diseases (Chapter 34). Other biologics are finding clinical application in the immunosuppressive treatment of asthma (Chapter 35) and autoimmune inflammatory bowel diseases (Chapter 36).

One of the earliest major advances in immunopharmacology was the development of a technique for preventing Rh hemolytic disease of the newborn. Sensitization of Rh-negative mothers to the D antigen occurs usually at the time of birth of an $Rh_o(D)$-positive or D^u-positive infant. During birth (or sometimes with a miscarriage or ectopic pregnancy), fetal red cells leak into the mother's bloodstream, which presents the opportunity for the mother to make antibodies against the D antigen. In subsequent pregnancies, maternal antibodies against Rh-positive cells are transferred to the fetus during the third trimester, leading to the development of erythroblastosis fetalis (hemolytic disease of the newborn). If an injection of $Rh_o(D)$ **antibody** is administered to the Rh-negative mother within 24-72 hours after the birth of an Rh-positive infant, the mother's own antibody response to the foreign $Rh_o(D)$-positive cells is suppressed because the infant's red cells are cleared from circulation before the mother can generate a B-cell response against $Rh_o(D)$. The technique is based on the observation that a *primary* antibody response to a foreign antigen can be blocked if specific antibody to that antigen is administered passively at the time of exposure to antigen. $Rh_o(D)$ immune globulin is a concentrated (15%) solution of human IgG containing high-titer antibodies against the $Rh_o(D)$ antigen of the red cell. When the mother has been treated in this fashion, Rh hemolytic disease of the newborn has not been observed in subsequent pregnancies.

Alemtuzumab is a humanized IgG that binds to CD52 found on normal and malignant B and T cells, NK cells, monocytes, macrophages, and a small population of granulocytes (neutrophils, eosinophils, basophils). Alemtuzumab appears to deplete leukemic (and normal) cells by direct antibody-dependent lysis. Alemtuzumab was previously approved for the treatment of B-cell chronic lymphocytic leukemia. In 2014, the FDA approved alemtuzumab for the treatment of individuals diagnosed with relapsing remitting MS. In MS, alemtuzumab depletes autoimmune inflammatory T and B cells when the drug is in the circulation. Repopulating lymphocytes appear to temporarily rebalance the immune system. Patients receiving this antibody become lymphopenic and may also become neutropenic, anemic, and thrombocytopenic. As a result, patients should be closely monitored for opportunistic infections and hematologic toxicity.

Basiliximab is an immunosuppressive antibody because it functions as an IL-2 antagonist. Basiliximab is a chimeric mouse-human IgG. Basiliximab binds to the α subunit of the IL-2 receptor on activated T cells, preventing the binding of IL-2. The drug is indicated for prophylaxis of acute organ rejection in renal transplant recipients. The drug may be used as part of an immunosuppressive regimen that also includes glucocorticoids and cyclosporine.

Natalizumab is a humanized IgG monoclonal antibody that binds to the α4-subunit of α4β1 and α4β7 integrins expressed on the surfaces of all leukocytes except neutrophils. Integrin molecules are critical in allowing the movement of immune cells out of the vascular compartment and into the tissues. Natalizumab inhibits the α4-mediated adhesion of leukocytes to their cognate receptor on endothelial cells. Natalizumab is indicated for individuals with MS who have not tolerated or have had inadequate responses to conventional treatments. As with many other immunosuppressive biologics, risk of infection is always a potential adverse effect. Due to inhibited immune cell immigration into the CNS, natalizumab increases the risk of PML caused by the JC virus. Natalizumab is also approved for the treatment of inflammatory bowel disease, but has been replaced by **vedolizumab** (Chapter 36) for this clinical application due to the above stated risk.

Prior to the development of MABs presented above, pools of antibodies directed to related, but different antigens (ie, polyclonal antibodies), were clinically used for immunosuppression. To obtain these antibodies, horses, pigs, or rabbits were immunized with human lymphoid cells. The resulting antisera are directed against lymphocytes in the form of heterologous **antilymphocyte globulin** (ALG) or T lymphocytes as **antithymocyte globulin** (ATG). With repeated administration, ALG results in destruction or inactivation of T cells, and impairment of delayed hypersensitivity and cellular immunity. Humoral antibody formation remains relatively intact. Only ATG is in clinical use in many medical centers, especially in transplantation programs for the management of solid organ and bone marrow transplantation. The adverse effects are mostly those associated with injection of a foreign protein. Local pain and erythema often occur at the injection site (type III hypersensitivity). Anaphylactic and serum sickness reactions have been observed, and usually require cessation of therapy. Complexes of host antibodies with horse ALG may precipitate and localize in the glomeruli of the kidneys causing kidney damage.

A different approach to immunomodulation is the intravenous use of polyclonal *human* immunoglobulin. This immunoglobulin preparation (usually IgG) is prepared from pools of thousands of healthy donors, and no single, specific antigen is the target of the "therapeutic antibody." Rather, one expects that the pool of different antibodies will have a normalizing effect upon the patient's immune networks. These polyclonal antibodies are given intravenously—and aptly named **intravenous immune globulin (IVIG) therapy**. Possible mechanisms of action of IVIG include a reduction of T helper cells, an increase in regulatory T cells, decreased spontaneous immunoglobulin production, Fc receptor blockade, or increased antibody catabolism. IVIG clinical applications include immunoglobulin deficiencies, transplantation, and some autoimmune diseases.

IMMUNE ENHANCERS

The development and use of drugs that can *selectively* enhance or modulate the immune system has added a vital tool to the treatment of cancer and chronic infectious diseases. Many biologic agents used in cancer chemotherapy are discussed in Chapter 31. Therefore, only the checkpoint inhibitors are discussed here. Checkpoint inhibitors are a class of drugs that enhance the immune system's ability to attack cancer cells. As previously discussed, both CTLA-4/(CD80/86) and PD-1/PD-L1 are considered immune checkpoints (Figure 32-3). That is, these proteins suppress the ability of T cells to kill cancer cells. When these proteins or ligands are blocked, this essentially releases the natural "brake" on the immune system, resulting in sustained T-cell activation that can allow them to destroy tumor cells more effectively. Clinical use of MABs blocking immune checkpoints has changed cancer chemotherapy. **Ipilimumab** binds to CTLA-4 on T cells, preventing CD80/86 from delivering a suppressive signal to T cells. Ipilimumab is approved for the treatment of unresectable or metastatic melanoma and treatment of cutaneous melanoma with regional nodes in the adjuvant surgical setting. **Nivolumab** is an antibody directed against the PD-1 receptor on *T cells,* whereas **atezolizumab** binds to PD-L1 on *tumor cells.* Both serve as immune checkpoint inhibitors by blocking the PD-1 pathway-mediated antitumor immune response inhibition. Nivolumab is approved for Hodgkin lymphoma, renal cell carcinoma, non-small cell lung cancer, and melanoma. Atezolizumab is approved for bladder cancer and is in late-stage clinical trials for several other cancer types.

Interferons are proteins grouped into three families: **IFN-α**, **IFN-β**, and **IFN-γ**. IFN-α and IFN-β constitute type I IFNs. IFN-γ is called a type II IFN because it binds to a separate receptor on target cells than that of the type I IFNs. Leukocytes produce IFN-α and fibroblasts and epithelial cells produce IFN-β. IFN-γ is usually the product of activated T cells. For the most part, IFNs act through activation of cell surface receptors to produce a wide variety of effects that depend on the cell and IFN type. IFNs, particularly IFN-γ, display immune-enhancing properties, which include increased antigen presentation, enhancement of macrophage action, and activation of NK cells and cytotoxic T cells. Another striking IFN action is increased expression of MHC molecules on cell surfaces. While all three types of IFN induce MHC class I molecules, only IFN-γ induces class II expression. IFN-α is approved for treating several neoplasms including chronic myelogenous leukemia, malignant melanoma, Kaposi sarcoma and hepatitis B and C infections. IFN-β is approved for use in relapsing-type MS. IFN-γ is approved for the treatment of chronic granulomatous disease. The ADRs of IFNs can severely restrict their clinical use. The toxicities include fever, chills, malaise, myalgia, myelosuppression, headache, and depression.

IMMUNOLOGIC MECHANISMS OF DRUG ALLERGY

Adverse drug reactions have multiple mechanisms. Some adverse reactions to drugs may be mistakenly classified as allergic reactions when they are actually due to genetic deficiency states or are idiosyncratic and not mediated by immune mechanisms. When drugs activate the immune system in an undesired way, these reactions are often classified as "drug allergy." Drug reactions mediated by immune responses can have several different mechanisms. In some immune drug reactions, several hypersensitivity responses may occur simultaneously. Thus, any of the four major types of hypersensitivity discussed earlier in this chapter can be associated with allergic drug reactions.

Type I (Immediate) Drug Allergy

Type I (immediate) allergy occurs when the drug—not capable of inducing an immune response by itself—covalently links to a host carrier protein. When this happens, the immune system detects the drug-protein complex as "modified self." Tн2 cells produce interleukins and B cells respond by generating polyclonal IgE antibodies specific for the drug-protein complex. Why some individuals mount an IgE response to a drug while others mount IgG responses is currently unknown.

Following initial sensitization, when the offending drug is *reintroduced* into the body, it binds and cross-links basophil and mast cell-surface IgE to signal release of mediators such as histamine or leukotrienes from their granules. Other vasoactive substances such as kinins may also be generated during histamine release. Manifestations of type I hypersensitivity include urticaria, bronchoconstriction, edema, and vascular hypotension, depending in part upon whether the response is atopic or anaphylactic. Both **penicillin** and sulfonamide antimicrobial drugs have been documented to initiate type I hypersensitivity reactions, though the incidence is less than 5% for either drug. These drugs are associated with a higher incidence of the other hypersensitivity disorders.

Type II (Cytotoxic) Drug Allergy

Drugs often modify host proteins, thereby eliciting antibody responses to the modified protein. These responses involve IgG or IgM antibodies that bind to drug-modified tissue and are destroyed by the complement system or by phagocytic cells with Fc receptors. Examples of these drug-induced autoimmune states include systemic lupus erythematosus following hydralazine or procainamide therapy, autoimmune hemolytic anemia resulting from methyldopa administration, thrombocytopenic purpura due to quinidine, and agranulocytosis due to a variety of drugs. Fortunately, autoimmune reactions to drugs usually subside within several months after the offending drug is withdrawn. Immunosuppressive therapy is warranted only when the autoimmune response is unusually severe.

Type III (Immune Complex) Drug Allergy

Drugs may cause serum sickness, which is a multisystem complement-dependent vasculitis initiated by immune complexes containing IgG or IgM complexed with a foreign antigen. The immune complexes deposit on basement membranes in tissues such as the lung or kidney. This is followed by complement activation and infiltration of leukocytes, causing tissue destruction. Immunologic reactions to drugs resulting in serum sickness are more common than type I immediate anaphylactic responses, but type II and type III hypersensitivities often overlap. Drugs or drug classes that have been associated with this type of reaction include the sulfonamides, penicillin, and anticonvulsants. Clinical manifestations of serum sickness include urticarial and erythematous skin eruptions, arthralgia or arthritis, lymphadenopathy, glomerulonephritis, peripheral edema, and fever. The reactions generally last 6-12 days and usually subside once the offending drug is eliminated. More severe reactions include hypersensitivity angiitis. Erythema multiforme is a relatively mild vasculitic skin disorder that may be secondary to drug hypersensitivity. Stevens-Johnson syndrome is probably a more severe form of this hypersensitivity reaction and consists of erythema multiforme, arthritis, nephritis, CNS abnormalities, and myocarditis. This pathophysiologic disorder has frequently been associated with sulfonamide therapy.

Type IV (Delayed) Drug Allergy

Type IV hypersensitivity occurs 24-48 hours after exposure to the allergen and therefore is called delayed type hypersensitivity (DTH). Like other drug hypersensitivities, the drug may chemically react with host tissue to create a new antigen. Upon first exposure to the allergen (ie, the drug), APCs stimulate a T-cell response specific for that allergen (Figure 32-4). This takes 1-2 weeks. Following sensitization, and during all subsequent exposures, tissue-derived APCs that come in contact with the new allergen-modified host protein secrete chemokines and cytokines that attract memory T cells to the site of allergen reexposure. This process takes only 24-48 hours. Lymphocytes and APCs such as macrophages accumulate at the site, cause induration, erythema, and swelling. Contact hypersensitivity is a form of DTH and occurs when an allergen elicits DTH on the skin, resulting in spongiosis such as when an ointment containing an allergen is applied to skin.

REHABILITATION RELEVANCE

Transplantation procedures and the associated pharmacotherapy will continue to have an expanding influence on rehabilitation and physical therapy practice. This relationship is multifaceted. First, the number of solid organ and stem cell transplantations is increasing. As such, practicing therapists will interact with these patients more often in rehabilitation in every practice setting. Therapists may be seeing transplantation recipients for dysfunction not directly related to transplantation. However, this medical history will have a significant influence on patient assessment and therapy outcomes. Second, the inclusion of conditioning programs both pre- and post-transplantation has resulted in more professional opportunities to specifically work with this population. Thus, physical therapists need to recognize not only the benefits of their interventions, but also some limitations of transplant recipients and the effect of their drug regimens. Highlighted below are ADRs that have a significant effect on physical therapy outcomes and are common to more than one drug, or represent significant ADRs for a single drug. For the ADRs associated with glucocorticoids, see Chapter 23.

- To some extent, all of these drugs **increase infection risk**. Infections may be local (eg, respiratory or skin), but there is also a potential for severe life-threatening systemic bacterial, viral, or fungal opportunistic infections. Thoughtful considerations regarding patient scheduling include avoidance of crowded waiting rooms and rescheduling when either the patient or therapist is ill. Extra attention should be paid to standard precautions and infection control procedures.

- Many of these drugs are bone marrow depressants that decrease hematopoiesis, resulting in an **increased risk of leukopenia, anemia, and thrombocytopenia**. Therapists should review hematologic values prior to therapy sessions (or ask patients of recent known values, if lab values are not available in the patient's medical record). Leukopenia may be the underlying mechanism for increased infection risk discussed above. Anemia may result in a clinically relevant decrease in oxygen-carrying capacity of the blood. Aerobic interventions and goals should be reduced and hemoglobin and hematocrit levels closely monitored. Thrombocytopenia may increase the risk of bleeding. Patients should be monitored for excessive bleeding that can manifest in many ways, including, but not limited to severe bruising, prolonged nosebleeds, bleeding gums, coughing up blood, passing blood in urine or stool, or hemarthrosis.

- Because many of these drugs decrease immune surveillance, there is an increased **cancer risk**. Various forms of cancer may include Kaposi sarcoma, lymphomas, and others. As some of these cancers have cutaneous manifestations, the therapist should be particularly observant for abnormal skin lesions and recommend the patient contact the referring healthcare professional for medical follow-up, if new skin growths are noted.

- Cardiovascular ADRs (**arrhythmias**, **deep vein thrombosis, pulmonary embolism**) are significant risks associated with several drugs. Fingolimod hydrochloride increases arrhythmia risk to the extent that monitoring is required following drug initiation. Increased monitoring of vital signs and assessment of signs and symptoms of exercise intolerance is indicated. Thalidomide increases the risk of deep vein thrombosis and pulmonary embolism. Therapists should be vigilant at recognizing early manifestations of these conditions. When detected in a nonemergency situation, the referring healthcare professional should be contacted.

- **Peripheral sensory and motor neuropathy** is an ADR associated with thalidomide. Therapists should incorporate regular sensory and motor screening to detect peripheral neuropathy. If observed, the referring healthcare professional should be contacted immediately since early recognition may help prevent further motor or sensory damage by discontinuing the medication. If benefits of the medication outweigh the risk, or if the patient already presents with neuropathy, fall risk reduction strategies should be incorporated into the treatment plan.

- Proliferation signal inhibitors such as sirolimus and everolimus **delay wound healing**. As anticipated, integumentary wounds will heal slower. In addition, muscle strains and ligament sprains will also heal slower. This latter effect should be considered when working with patients on aerobic or resistance training programs.

If J.M. is medically cleared to return to Phase II cardiac rehabilitation during the period of rejection-induced coronary artery vasculitis, aerobic activities should be significantly reduced based on the patient's exercise tolerance. However, all resistance training should be eliminated for two reasons. First, there is an increased risk of a coronary event during bolus administration of glucocorticoids (methylprednisolone in this case). Second, the potential benefits of resistance training are overwhelmed by the catabolic influence of immunosuppressive steroids on muscle and bone. When the acute rejection phase passes, J.M. may return toward achieving target aerobic goals and restart resistance activities.

CHAPTER 32 QUESTIONS

1. Which of the following drugs binds to FK506-binding protein and inhibits the molecular target of rapamycin?

   a. Sirolimus
   b. Tacrolimus
   c. Cyclosporine
   d. Azathioprine

2. Which of the following drug's immunosuppressant action results from increasing extracellular adenosine levels?

   a. Everolimus
   b. Pentostatin
   c. Teriflunomide
   d. Thalidomide

3. Which of the following monoclonal antibodies is an immune enhancer that binds to CTLA-4 receptor on T cells?

   a. Atezolizumab
   b. Nivolumab
   c. Ipilimumab
   d. Antithymocyte globulin

4. Which of the following drugs is a monoclonal antibody that may cause progressive multifocal leukoencephalopathy?

   a. Glatiramer acetate
   b. Basiliximab
   c. Alemtuzumab
   d. Natalizumab

5. Which of the following hypersensitivity responses is mediated by IgE?

   a. Type 1 hypersensitivity
   b. Type 3 hypersensitivity
   c. Type 4 hypersensitivity
   d. Type 2 hypersensitivity

6. Which of the following hypersensitivity responses is mediated by T cells?

   a. Type I hypersensitivity
   b. Type IV hypersensitivity
   c. Type III hypersensitivity
   d. Type II hypersensitivity

7. Which of the following drugs has been associated with the adverse effect of inhibition of limb bud development in utero?

   a. Mycophenolate mofetil
   b. Dimethyl fumarate
   c. Thalidomide
   d. Hydroxychloroquine

8. Which of the following cell types is responsible for antibody production in the immune response?

   a. T cells
   b. NK cells
   c. Macrophages
   d. B cells

9. Which of the following monoclonal antibodies acts as a checkpoint inhibitor by binding to the PD-1 receptor on T cells?

   a. Nivolumab
   b. Ipilimumab
   c. Atezolizumab
   d. Vedolizumab

10. Which of the following drug's immunosuppressant actions is mediated in part by cross-linking (alkylating) DNA strands?

    a. Azathioprine
    b. Cyclophosphamide
    c. Cyclosporine
    d. Pentostatin

Skeletal Muscle Relaxants

CASE STUDY

S.E. is a 54-year-old man with relapsing remitting multiple sclerosis (RR-MS) diagnosed 12 years ago. He lives in a single-level home with his wife and two teenage children. S.E. is able to perform stand-pivot transfers independently and can sometimes ambulate limited household distances with a four-wheeled walker. His major mode of mobility is an electric wheelchair; however, he states that he would like to stand and walk more if possible. He is self-employed as an architect and works approximately 30 hours per week. S.E. is slightly overweight (BMI 25 kg/m^2) but has no other comorbidities. He is currently taking oral baclofen and tizanidine for bilateral lower extremity spasticity. S.E. was referred to physical therapy for evaluation of his ambulatory skills and assessment of

assistive devices. Upon initial evaluation, the patient had limited movement and volitional activity of his lower extremities, but upper extremity strength was normal. He has significant functional strength, as he is able to lift himself into and out of his vehicle daily. The physical therapist initially fitted S.E. with custom molded ankle-foot orthoses and began a neuromuscular re-education program to improve his ambulatory skills. S.E. had significant spasticity in his lower extremities, which was exacerbated with transfers and lower extremity weight-bearing activity. Because spasticity was limiting his ability to make functional improvements, S.E.'s baclofen was increased to a maximum tolerated oral dose along with a slight increase in his oral dose of tizanidine.

REHABILITATION FOCUS

Drugs that affect skeletal muscles fall into two major therapeutic groups: neuromuscular blockers and skeletal muscle relaxants, or spasmolytics. Neuromuscular blockers are used primarily as adjuncts to general anesthesia to produce the muscle paralysis necessary for surgery, tracheal intubation, and control of ventilation. These compounds are nicotinic antagonists at the neuromuscular junction and lack central nervous system (CNS) activity. Neuromuscular blockers were discussed in Chapter 5.

Figure 33-1 broadly categorizes the diverse class of skeletal muscle relaxants into two groups: agents more commonly used to reduce spasticity in a variety of neurologic conditions and those agents used to reduce muscle spasm following

muscle injury or inflammation. Spasmolytic drugs have traditionally been called *centrally acting* skeletal muscle relaxants because almost all act at multiple sites in the CNS rather than at the neuromuscular end plate—a fact that has significant clinical ramifications. Only two spasmolytic drugs—**dantrolene** and **botulinum toxin**—act in or near skeletal muscle with no significant central effects.

PATHOPHYSIOLOGY OF SPASTICITY AND MUSCLE SPASM

Spasticity is characterized by an increase in tonic stretch reflexes and flexor muscle spasms (ie, increased basal muscle tone), together with muscle weakness and a reduction in

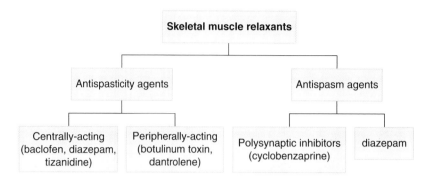

FIGURE 33-1 **Skeletal muscle relaxants may be divided into antispastic agents that are used chronically to treat central nervous system (CNS) associated spasticity and agents used acutely to reduce muscle spasms following muscle injury or inflammation.** Prototype drugs are in parentheses.

viscoelastic muscle properties. Spasticity is frequently associated with cerebral palsy, multiple sclerosis, spinal cord injury, and stroke. These conditions often involve abnormal function of the bowel and bladder as well as skeletal muscle. The mechanisms underlying spasticity in these types of neurologic injury involve the stretch reflex arc itself (Figure 33-2) and higher centers in the CNS.

After an upper motor neuron (UMN) lesion, damage to descending pathways in the spinal cord results in loss of supraspinal inhibition to alpha and gamma motor neurons in the anterior horn of the spinal cord. When UMNs from the cerebral cortex and brainstem nuclei are no longer able to modulate spinal reflexes or activate spinal cord inhibitory interneuron pools, decreased activity of inhibitory interneurons results in increased excitability of alpha motor neurons in the spinal cord. Figure 33-3 illustrates descending polysynaptic input onto alpha motor neurons from many CNS centers, drawing attention to the normal considerable *inhibitory* input.

Some of the signs and symptoms of neurologic injury spasticity may be improved by pharmacologically modifying the stretch reflex or by interfering directly with skeletal muscle (ie, excitation-contraction coupling). Drugs that modify the reflex arc may modulate excitatory or inhibitory synapses (Chapter 12). To reduce the hyperactive stretch reflex, it is desirable to reduce the activity of Ia sensory afferent fibers providing information from the muscle spindle, enhance the activity of the inhibitory interneurons, and/or directly decrease the activity of alpha motor neurons. Figure 33-4 illustrates select sites of action for various skeletal muscle relaxants.

Muscle spasms are distinct from spasticity in that these localized tonic contractions result from a *peripheral* injury rather than an UMN injury. Muscle spasms are sustained contractions of specific muscles that often occur after

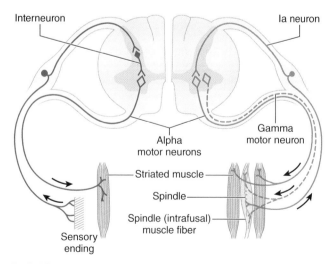

FIGURE 33-2 **Schematic of structures involved in the stretch reflex arc.** The right half of the diagram illustrates innervation of extrafusal skeletal muscle fibers by an alpha motor neuron (solid line) and innervation of an intrafusal muscle fiber (within the muscle spindle) by a gamma motor neuron (dashed line). The left half of the diagram shows an inhibitory reflex arc that includes an inhibitory interneuron.

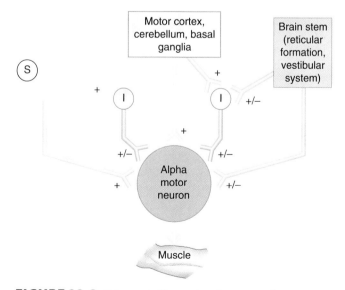

FIGURE 33-3 **Schematic illustrating the converging polysynaptic input that determines whether an individual alpha motor neuron will fire an action potential.** I, brain stem interneuron; S, sensory primary afferent; "+," excitatory synapse; "−," inhibitory synapse.

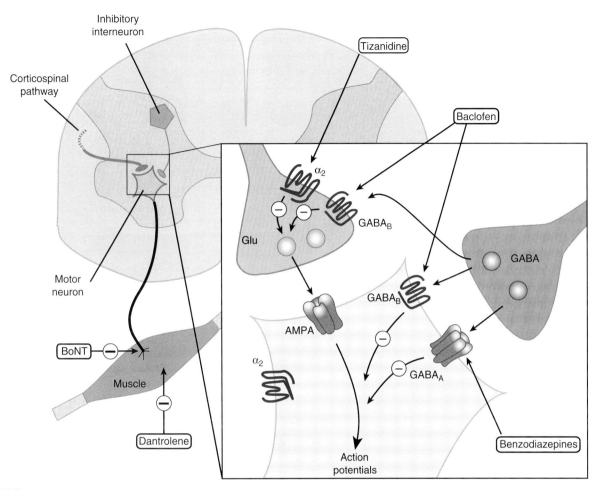

FIGURE 33-4 Postulated sites of spasmolytic drug action in the spinal cord and muscle. Inset shows: axon terminal of a glutamatergic (Glu) neuron in green; axon terminal of a GABAergic neuron in mustard yellow; and, cell body of an alpha motor neuron in peach. Tizanidine activates presynaptic α_2 receptors to decrease glutamate release onto the alpha motor neuron. Baclofen is an agonist at GABA$_B$ receptors. Presynaptic activation of GABA$_B$ receptors decreases glutamate release onto the alpha motor neuron, while postsynaptic activation of GABA$_B$ receptors hyperpolarizes the alpha motor neuron. Benzodiazepines (eg, diazepam) are agonists at GABA$_A$ receptors. Dantrolene acts within the sarcoplasmic reticulum to decrease calcium release in skeletal muscle cells. Botulinum toxin (BoNT) inhibits acetylcholine release from the presynaptic nerve terminal at the neuromuscular junction.

musculoskeletal injuries and inflammation secondary to nerve impingement, muscle strains, or muscle overuse. They may also result from chemical or mechanical stimuli in the peripheral nervous system. Noxious nociceptive stimuli set in motion a pain-spasm-pain cycle that can be interrupted by enhancing the activity of inhibitory interneurons to promote muscle relaxation.

Regardless of whether the origin of hyperexcitable skeletal muscle is neurologic spasticity or muscle spasm, skeletal muscle relaxants have the overall effect of decreasing the activity of skeletal muscle. Some skeletal muscle relaxants such as baclofen or tizanidine are used more frequently to decrease spasticity or spasm associated with *chronic* conditions. Other agents such as cyclobenzaprine are typically used to relieve the *acute* muscle spasm associated with musculoskeletal injury. However, these "rules" are not set in stone. For example, **diazepam** and botulinum toxin may be used to treat either spasticity or localized muscle spasms.

For both spasticity and muscle spasms, the pharmacotherapeutic goal is to *normalize* muscle excitability. However, skeletal muscle relaxants produce a nonspecific depression of all synapses involved in the stretch reflex—reducing not only the undesirable excitatory transmission, but also the desired inhibitory input transmission (Figure 33-3). In addition, excessive depression of synapses at the level of the spinal cord segments can result in a loss of voluntary muscle activity. Thus, selective *enhancement* of inhibitory or selective *depression* of excitatory transmission is needed. Unfortunately, selective agents have yet to come to fruition.

Currently available drugs can provide significant relief from spasticity (antispasticity drugs) as well as painful muscle injury spasms (antispasm drugs). In spite of this, the ultimate goal of normalizing muscle excitability *without* a significant decrease in voluntary muscle activity and patient function is largely unfulfilled. This challenge can be partially met by effective communication between the healthcare providers

TABLE 33-1   **Characteristics of several skeletal muscle relaxants.**

Generic Name	Elimination Half-Life (h)	Spasticity	Muscle Spasm	Other Uses
		Common Indications		
Baclofen	4.9 ± 1.9	Yes	No	Intractable hiccups, intractable low back pain, trigeminal neuralgia, cluster headache, drug and alcohol dependence
Botulinum toxin	—[a]	Yes	Yes	Migraine headache, torticollis, overactive bladder, axillary hyperhidrosis, cosmetic appearance
Cyclobenzaprine	18 ± 9.1	No	Yes	Fibromyalgia
Dantrolene	8.7	Yes	No	Malignant hyperthermia
Diazepam	43 ± 13	Yes	Yes	Anxiety, preoperative or procedural sedation, alcohol withdrawal, seizures
Gabapentin	6 ± 1	Yes	No	Partial seizures, postherpetic neuralgia, neuropathic pain, fibromyalgia
Tizanidine	~2	Yes	No	Cluster headache

[a]Botulinum toxin's physiologic effect, lasting 1-3 months, is not related to pharmacokinetic half-life.

(often physical and occupational therapists) observing effects on patients' function and the prescribers that can make appropriate adjustments in medications, dosages, and/or methods of administration. Table 33-1 lists characteristics of several skeletal muscle relaxants.

ANTISPASTICITY DRUGS

Diazepam

As described in Chapter 13, benzodiazepines facilitate the action of γ-aminobutyric acid (GABA), the primary inhibitory neurotransmitter in the CNS. Diazepam (Valium) is the benzodiazepine most commonly used as a spasmolytic agent. Diazepam acts at all $GABA_A$ synapses, but its action in reducing spasticity is at least partly mediated in the spinal cord (Figure 33-4). It is somewhat effective in treating spasticity resulting from cord transection and spasticity due to cerebral palsy. Diazepam is also used to treat muscle injury spasm of almost any origin, including local muscle trauma. However, diazepam produces sedation in most patients at the dose required to significantly reduce muscle tone. Other benzodiazepines have been used as spasmolytics, but experience with them is much more limited.

Baclofen

Baclofen (p-chlorophenyl-GABA) is an orally active GABA-mimetic agent and exerts its spasmolytic activity at $GABA_B$ receptors. Activation of central $GABA_B$ receptors by baclofen results in hyperpolarization by increasing K^+ conductance in postsynaptic neurons. Hyperpolarization of presynaptic terminals reduces calcium influx, which decreases release of excitatory transmitters in the brain and spinal cord (Figure 33-4). Baclofen inhibits activity of Ia sensory afferents

in muscle spindles, spinal interneurons, and motor neurons. Baclofen may also reduce pain in individuals with spasticity, perhaps by inhibiting the release of substance P in the spinal cord.

Baclofen is at least as effective as diazepam and tizanidine (discussed below) in reducing spasticity due to neurologic injury and it produces much less sedation and weakness than diazepam. Baclofen is rapidly and completely absorbed after oral administration. Adverse effects include drowsiness (to which patients may become tolerant with chronic administration) and generalized muscle weakness at higher doses. Increased seizure activity has been reported in epileptic patients, especially upon withdrawal of the drug. Therefore, withdrawal of baclofen must be done very slowly.

Chronic infusion of baclofen via an implantable intrathecal pump can control severe spasticity for individuals unresponsive to oral baclofen or those who experience intolerable adverse effects at effective spasmolytic doses. Intrathecal administration is becoming more widely used for two main reasons. First, baclofen does not readily leave the spinal canal, so the frequency of systemic adverse effects is lower. However, cases of excessive somnolence, respiratory depression, and even coma have been reported with high doses. Second, the intrathecal catheter can be placed to more selectively target baclofen delivery to appropriate spinal cord segments. Partial tolerance to the antispastic effect of the drug may occur after several months of therapy but can be overcome by upward dosage adjustments. A major disadvantage of this therapeutic approach is the difficulty of maintaining the drug-delivery catheter in the subarachnoid space. Recently, it has been noted that the observed partial tolerance to baclofen may be due to unrecognized catheter malfunction. To address this concern, instructions provided to patients include the avoidance of sudden, excessive, or repeated movements such as bending, twisting, bouncing, or stretching. These movements may interrupt or stop drug delivery by damaging the pump (located subcutaneously in the anterior abdominal wall) or dislodging, kinking or blocking the intrathecal catheter. Long-term intrathecal baclofen therapy can improve the quality of life for patients with severe spasticity associated with multiple sclerosis, stroke, and cerebral palsy.

Oral baclofen has been studied in several other medical conditions. Off-label uses (uses outside of what is approved by the Food and Drug Administration [FDA]) include intractable hiccups, intractable low back pain, trigeminal neuralgia, cluster headache, and the management of drug and alcohol dependence.

Tizanidine

As noted in Chapter 6, α-adrenoceptor$_2$ agonists (eg, clonidine) have a variety of CNS effects that are not fully understood. Among these effects is the ability to reduce muscle spasm. Tizanidine (Zanaflex) has significant α$_2$-adrenoceptor agonist effects, but lacks the antihypertensive efficacy of clonidine. Studies in animals and humans suggest that tizanidine reinforces both presynaptic and postsynaptic inhibition in the spinal cord (Figure 33-4). Tizanidine also inhibits nociceptive transmission in the spinal dorsal horn.

Oral tizanidine is just as effective in relieving spasticity as diazepam, baclofen, and dantrolene, but produces significantly less muscle weakness. For this reason, tizanidine may be a better choice for reducing spasticity while maintaining adequate muscle strength for transfers, ambulation, and general activity. In addition, tizanidine is relatively short acting, so individuals may reserve dosing for activities of daily living and times when relief of spasticity is most important. However, since tizanidine induces drowsiness that may impair function, some individuals take the drug at night. Dry mouth and asthenia are also common. Hypotension is a less frequent adverse reaction.

Other Centrally Acting Spasmolytic Drugs

Gabapentin (Neurontin) and its newer analog **pregabalin** (Lyrica) have no activity at GABA$_A$ or GABA$_B$ receptors. These drugs bind to a subunit of voltage-gated calcium channels, though their exact mechanism of action is unknown. Gabapentin has traditionally been used as an antiepileptic drug (Chapter 14), but both gabapentin and pregabalin have shown considerable promise as antispasticity agents in individuals with multiple sclerosis. Both drugs are also recommended as first-line therapy in the pharmacological management of neuropathic pain. Though not a federally scheduled drug, gabapentin has been added to the list of Schedule V controlled substances by several states due to its potential abuse by individuals misusing opioids.

Preliminary studies have shown that **progabide** and **glycine** reduce spasticity. Progabide is a GABA$_A$ and GABA$_B$ agonist and has active metabolites, including GABA itself.

Glycine, the principal inhibitory neurotransmitter in the spinal cord (Chapter 12), appears to possess pharmacologic activity when given orally and readily passes the blood-brain barrier. **Idrocilamide** and **riluzole** are newer drugs for the treatment of amyotrophic lateral sclerosis that appear to have spasm-reducing effects, possibly through inhibition of glutamatergic transmission in the CNS.

Peripherally Acting Spasmolytic Drugs

Botulinum Toxin

When *Clostridium botulinum* bacteria are exposed to anaerobic conditions that allow the spores to germinate, botulinum toxin (BoNT) is produced as an exotoxin. There are seven immunologically distinct toxins, though only two strains—BoNT-A and BoNT-B—are used therapeutically. After injection into a muscle, BoNT blocks acetylcholine release at the neuromuscular junction (Figure 33-4), causing paralysis of muscles within the diffusion distance of the injected toxin (~ 1 inch). The localized paralysis is dose dependent and transient, with recovery occurring within 1-3 months. Because muscle function returns in approximately 3 months, BoNT injections into affected muscles needs to be ongoing.

BoNT has been FDA-approved for at least nine indications, including blepharospasm, strabismus, cervical dystonia, migraine prophylaxis, overactive bladder, upper limb spasticity, and improvement in the appearance of wrinkles around the eyes and forehead. There has also been tremendous expansion of BoNT's off-label uses. These include many conditions frequently treated by physical therapists such as focal dystonias, spastic conditions, and disorders of localized muscle spasms. Several studies have evaluated the efficacy of combining physical and occupational therapy with BoNT injection of carefully selected muscles to manage spasticity. Although these studies have shown benefit of regaining function and independence and reduced risk of long-term complications like contractures, study heterogeneity limits the ability to demonstrate the overall impact of adjunctive rehabilitative therapy to BoNT injections. Future investigations are needed to determine the best parameters for combined treatment.

Dantrolene

Dantrolene is a drug related to phenytoin, an antiseizure medication. In contrast to the centrally active muscle relaxants, dantrolene acts directly at the level of skeletal muscle cells. By binding to a specific calcium channel in the sarcoplasmic reticulum, dantrolene decreases the release of calcium necessary for excitation-contraction coupling. Cardiac and smooth muscle fibers are minimally affected because calcium release from their sarcoplasmic reticulum involves a different calcium channel.

Because there are more effective skeletal muscle relaxants with better safety profiles, dantrolene is neither advocated for use in treating muscle injury spasms nor is it a first-line agent for treating spasticity. For example, tizanidine, baclofen, and gabapentin are first-line options for pharmacologically managing spasticity due to multiple sclerosis. Dantrolene is usually reserved to treat severe spasticity when no clinical improvement has been observed with other agents.

Dantrolene's most common adverse effects are drowsiness and generalized muscle weakness. Rarely, dantrolene may cause hepatotoxicity; dantrolene is recognized as a well-established cause of clinically apparent liver injury.

A special application of dantrolene is in the treatment of malignant hyperthermia (Chapters 5 and 15), a rare heritable disorder characterized by often-fatal hyperthermia due to a sudden and prolonged release of calcium, with massive muscle contraction, lactic acid production, and increased body temperature. Dantrolene inhibits skeletal muscle contraction throughout the body, thus reducing excessive body temperature generated by massive, repetitive muscle contractions.

ANTISPASM DRUGS

Polysynaptic Inhibitors

A large number of drugs (eg, **carisoprodol**, **chlorzoxazone**, **cyclobenzaprine**, **metaxalone**, **methocarbamol**, and **orphenadrine**) are promoted for the relief of acute muscle spasm caused by local tissue trauma or muscle strains. All of these agents are centrally acting skeletal muscle relaxants that are thought to act primarily at the levels of the brainstem and spinal cord. Although their mechanisms of action are not well understood, animal research suggests that some of these drugs interfere with the polysynaptic transmission of neuronal impulses within the spinal cord, thus reducing alpha motor neuron excitability and activity (Figure 33-3). Table 33-2 describes the onset and duration of action of the polysynaptic inhibitors.

Polysynaptic inhibitors are often used as adjuncts to rest and physical therapy for relief of painful muscle spasm associated with musculoskeletal injuries. They are often prescribed in combination with nonsteroidal anti-inflammatory agents or analgesics. These agents are ineffective in treating spasticity caused by cerebral palsy, multiple sclerosis, or spinal cord injury. Major adverse effects of these drugs are generalized sedation, confusion, headache, and nausea and vomiting. This drug class is also associated with abuse potential. Cyclobenzaprine, the prototype agent in this class, also has strong antimuscarinic actions, with manifestations of sedation that potentially increase fall risk.

REHABILITATION RELEVANCE

Skeletal muscle relaxants are prescribed for many patients involved in rehabilitation programs. These drugs are used for both neurologic injury spasticity and for muscle injury spasms; concurrent physical and occupational therapy are important adjuncts to improve function. For example, the implementation of therapeutic interventions may facilitate more normal physiologic motor control and functioning to replace previously used spastic tone. Localized injections of BoNT in spastic muscles may be combined with stretching of these muscles and strengthening of antagonist muscle groups, which may improve self-care or nursing care and spastic contractures. Similarly, skeletal muscle relaxants are frequently used in conjunction with nonpharmacologic interventions (eg, modalities, manual therapy) to acutely reduce muscle spasm following strains or nerve root impingement. While these medications are helpful to acutely interrupt the pain-spasm-pain cycle, they do not remove the inciting *cause* of the muscle spasm. Therapeutic programs to improve strength, flexibility, posture, relaxation, and body mechanics are often essential to healing. One of the clinical challenges is encouraging patients to appreciate that such active therapy interventions may be necessary to make lasting changes and ultimately decrease the need for skeletal muscle relaxants.

- All but two skeletal muscle relaxants (dantrolene and BoNT) act centrally to decrease the activity of alpha motor neurons. Thus, almost all drugs in this class have fairly predictable CNS effects such as **sedation**, **dizziness**, and **ataxia**. If these adverse effects affect functional outcomes, potential solutions include coordinating physical therapy sessions at a time of day when sedative effects are less marked and alerting the prescribing practitioner to initiate discussion of other therapeutic options.
- Many centrally acting skeletal muscle relaxants are associated with **tolerance** and **risk of physical dependence**, **abuse**, and **misuse**. In addition, these agents should not be combined with other CNS depressants (eg, alcohol, barbiturates, opioids), which can lead to profound sedation, respiration depression, and death.
- **Weakness** is an inherent complication of all skeletal muscle relaxants. If muscle weakness prevents attainment of therapeutic goals, therapists must assess patient performance with functional or quality-of-life outcome measures and communicate these results to other team providers and prescribers.

TABLE 33-2 Polysynaptic inhibitors used as antispasm agents.

Generic Drug (Brand Name)	Onset of Action (min)	Duration of Action (hr)
Carisoprodol (Soma)	30	4-6
Chlorzoxazone (Lorzone)	< 60	3-4
Cyclobenzaprine (Flexeril, Amrix)	< 60	12-24
Metaxalone (Skelaxin)	< 60	4-6
Methocarbamol (Robaxin)	< 30	24
Orphenadrine (Norflex)	< 60	12

CASE CONCLUSION

Soon after the increased dosage in oral medications, S.E. noted significant upper extremity weakness. He was experiencing difficulty transferring into and out of his vehicle and ambulating within his home. Although his spasticity was now well controlled, it left him with limited functional ability. The patient, physician, and physical therapist decided that an intrathecal baclofen pump (with catheter placement near the lumbar spinal cord segments) might make it possible to control his lower extremity spasticity without drastically reducing his upper extremity strength. After recovery from the surgery and titration of the intrathecal baclofen dose, S.E. returned to physical therapy. The patient was well maintained with this drug-delivery system and was able to improve his ambulatory ability within several weeks.

CHAPTER 33 QUESTIONS

1. Which of the following skeletal muscle relaxants does *not* act in the central nervous system?

   a. Diazepam
   b. Cyclobenzaprine
   c. Botulinum toxin
   d. Baclofen

2. Which of the following skeletal muscle relaxants is *not* indicated for relief of acute muscle spasm?

   a. Dantrolene
   b. Cyclobenzaprine
   c. Diazepam
   d. Carisoprodol

3. Which of the following drugs is injected directly into the hyperexcitable muscle to have its therapeutic effect?

   a. Botulinum toxin
   b. Glycine
   c. Dantrolene
   d. Baclofen

4. Which of the following skeletal muscle relaxants is commonly used to treat *both* spasticity and acute muscle spasm?

   a. Dantrolene
   b. Baclofen
   c. Diazepam
   d. Cyclobenzaprine

5. Which of the following drugs is given intrathecally for optimal therapeutic effect?

   a. Dantrolene
   b. Baclofen
   c. Tizanidine
   d. Diazepam

6. Which of the following drugs is used to treat spasticity, but produces the *least* muscle weakness?

   a. Gabapentin
   b. Diazepam
   c. Oral baclofen
   d. Tizanidine

7. Which of the following skeletal muscle relaxants can also be used to treat malignant hyperthermia?

   a. Diazepam
   b. Dantrolene
   c. Baclofen
   d. Tizanidine

8. Which of the following drugs is *not* considered a first-line option for treating spasticity associated with multiple sclerosis?

   a. Baclofen
   b. Gabapentin
   c. Tizanidine
   d. Dantrolene

9. Which of the following drugs does *not* have sedation as an adverse effect?

   a. Baclofen
   b. Botulinum toxin
   c. Diazepam
   d. Cyclobenzaprine

10. Which of the following drugs is an agonist at $GABA_B$ receptors?

   a. Tizanidine
   b. Diazepam
   c. Baclofen
   d. Glycine

Drugs Affecting Eicosanoid Metabolism, Disease-Modifying Antirheumatic Drugs, and Drugs Used in Gout

CASE STUDY

T.C. is a 54-year-old postal worker with a long history of bilateral knee pain who self-referred to outpatient physical therapy. The patient's current medication includes daily ezetimibe (for hyperlipidemia) and over-the-counter acetaminophen and ibuprofen. During the initial patient interview, T.C. tells the therapist that his knee pain has been increasing over the past several months to the extent that he is concerned he will not be able to make it to his goal retirement age of 65 years. As T.C. is talking, the therapist observes bilateral ulnar deviation of T.C.'s metacarpophalangeal joints and Swan-neck deformities of the first two fingers. When the therapist notes her observation, T.C. adds that his hands are also stiff and painful, especially for long periods in the morning, and that he has had progressive difficulty quickly moving envelopes and packages in and out of his carrier bag. Upon closer examination of T.C.'s wrists, the therapist observes radial deviation with swelling that feels "boggy" on palpation. Examination of T.C.'s lower extremities reveals mild valgus deformities, no edema, and no loss of motion around the knee. The only positive findings are decreased strength in bilateral hamstrings, quadriceps, and hip abductors. The physical therapist provides T.C. with a lower extremity strengthening home exercise program. She asks T.C. to follow up with his primary care physician or a rheumatologist for further evaluation. T.C. says that he does not want to take time off to see more healthcare providers and does not see why this is necessary. T.C. feels that these new leg exercises will help him get stronger, and that he may just try to "power through" the pain with his current medication regimen.

REHABILITATION FOCUS

Inflammation is a complex response to cell injury that occurs in vascularized tissues. The chemical and cellular mediators of inflammation attempt to eliminate the cause of cell injury and clear away debris in preparation for tissue healing (regeneration and/or repair). Several inflammatory mediators also cause pain. In autoimmune rheumatic diseases such as rheumatoid arthritis or metabolic arthropathies, the cause of cell injury cannot be eliminated and the result is a chronic condition of pain and tissue damage. Several classes of anti-inflammatory drugs decrease *both* inflammation and pain. Other drugs such as glucocorticoids and disease-modifying antirheumatic drugs are more directly targeted at reducing inflammation via modifying immune processes. In contrast, analgesic drugs only decrease pain, without affecting the inflammatory process. In gout, a metabolic disease associated with precipitation of uric acid crystals in the joints, drug treatment of acute episodes targets the inflammation, whereas treatment of chronic gout targets both inflammatory processes and the production and elimination of uric acid.

Drug classes discussed in this chapter relieve pain and decrease inflammation, which are almost universal conditions shared by patients seen by physical therapists, regardless of their diagnosis. Some drugs or drug classes are more generally aimed at inhibiting inflammation, while others are targeted against specific inflammatory mediators that are elevated in patients with autoimmune or metabolic conditions.

INFLAMMATION AND PAIN

Inflammation is a common nonspecific manifestation of injury, infection, and many diseases. Inflammation occurs in acute or chronic forms that are usually characterized by typical timeframes, but they are distinguished by the presence and activity of particular cell types and mediators. Acute and chronic inflammation may occur independently or overlap. The primary initial characteristics of acute inflammation are vasodilation and extravasation of white blood cells to the injured or infected area with the hallmark clinical manifestations of redness, heat, swelling, pain, and loss of function.

Inflammation also involves the activation and proliferation of the immune system. Immune responses are regulated in part by cytokines (Chapter 32), and in part by eicosanoids, a group of endogenous 20-carbon (eicosa = 20) compounds that are synthesized from arachidonic acid, a fatty acid lipid liberated from cell membranes. Inflammation and the immune response often benefit the host because invading organisms are phagocytosed or neutralized and cellular debris is removed, thus setting the stage for healing. However, these processes may be deleterious if they lead to *chronic* inflammation without resolution of the underlying injurious agent or agents.

The pain associated with inflammation is also mediated in part by eicosanoids both in peripheral tissues at the inflammatory sites and within the central nervous system (CNS). In the peripheral tissues, two key prostaglandins (a subgroup of eicosanoids)—prostaglandin E_2 (PGE_2) and prostaglandin I_2 (PGI_2)—*sensitize* nociceptive nerve endings. In the CNS, PGE_2 and leukotriene B_4 (LTB_4) (another arachidonic acid metabolite) may modulate pain perception.

EICOSANOIDS

Synthesis and Classification

The eicosanoids are endogenous chemical compounds that are synthesized in response to a variety of stimuli (eg, physical injury, immune reactions). These stimuli activate phospholipases in the cell membrane or cytoplasm to release arachidonic acid from the cell membrane. Figure 34-1 outlines the enzymatic cascade that starts with liberation of arachidonic acid from the membrane and leads to production of each primary eicosanoid subgroups: leukotrienes, prostaglandins, prostacyclin, and thromboxane. Arachidonic acid is metabolized by one of several mechanisms. Metabolism to straight-chain products is performed by lipoxygenase (LOX), ultimately

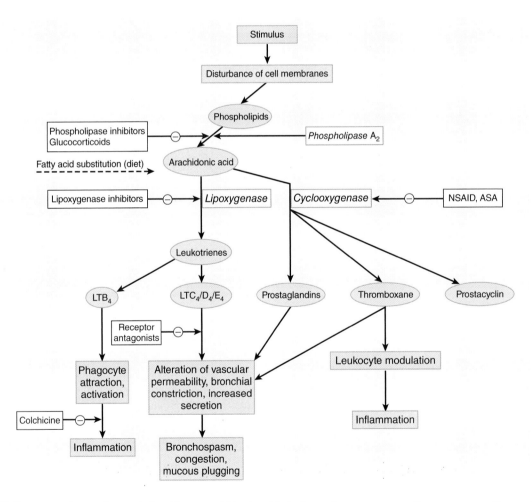

FIGURE 34-1 Scheme for mediators derived from arachidonic acid via the cyclooxygenase- or lipoxygenase pathways. Inhibitory sites of action are presented with solid arrow and circle enclosing a "minus" sign. Aspirin and the nonselective NSAIDs inhibit, to varying degrees, all COX isozymes. The COX-2 selective inhibitors preferentially inhibit COX-2. The lipoxygenase pathway may be inhibited at an enzymatic level or receptor level. Colchicine, which is used in the treatment of gout, prevents amplification of inflammation by inhibiting leukocyte functions. Abbreviations are within the text.

producing the leukotrienes (LT). Alternatively, cyclization by the enzyme cyclooxygenase (COX) results in the production of the other three major eicosanoid subgroups: prostacyclin (PGI_2), prostaglandins (PG), and thromboxane (TX). For most of the cyclized subgroups, there are several series of compounds based on different substituents (indicated by letters A, B, etc) and different numbers of double bonds (indicated by a subscript number) in the molecule (eg, PGE_2). *Naturally* occurring eicosanoids have very short half-lives (seconds to minutes) and are inactive when given orally. Figure 34-1 highlights the sites of action of drug classes that inhibit enzymatic production of various eicosanoids or their subgroups.

Two unique COX isoforms—COX-1 and COX-2—convert arachidonic acid into prostanoid products. There are many physiologic and pathophysiologic processes in which these enzymes function together and others in which COX-1 or COX-2 is uniquely involved. The COX-1 enzyme is sometimes referred to as a "housekeeping enzyme" because it is expressed constitutively in most cells and often generates the prostanoids for "housekeeping" functions. For example, certain prostanoids produced by COX-1 are involved in maintaining the mucosal layer in the gastric epithelium that helps protect against ulceration. In contrast, COX-2 is readily inducible by particular stimuli and is primarily expressed in activated lymphocytes, polymorphonuclear cells (neutrophils, eosinophils, basophils), and other inflammatory cells. COX-2 is an immediate early-response gene product that is markedly up-regulated by shear stress, growth factors, tumor promoters, and cytokines. More recently, it has been appreciated that activation of COX-2 also participates in beneficial tissue function and maintenance. For instance, endothelial COX-2 is the primary source of vascular prostacyclin (PGI_2) that helps maintain patency in various vascular beds. Renal COX-2-derived prostanoids are important for normal renal development and maintenance of function. However, inducible activation of COX-2 results in production of the majority of the prostanoids involved in inflammation and cancer. Genetic variations in human COX-2 have been linked with increased risk of coronary heart disease and certain cancers, and reduced pain perception.

Mechanism of Action and Physiologic Effects

Most eicosanoid effects appear to be brought about by activation of cell surface receptors that are coupled by G proteins to second messenger systems. Activation of receptors coupled by the G_s protein activates adenylate cyclase and produces the second messenger cyclic adenosine monophosphate (cAMP). Activation of receptors coupled by the G_q protein activates the phosphatidylinositol cascade and produces inositol 1,4,5-trisphosphate (IP_3) and diacylglycerol (DAG) second messengers.

Table 34-1 outlines a few physiologic effects of seven important eicosanoids in smooth muscle, platelets, the CNS, and other tissues. The three prostaglandins PGE_1, PGE_2, and PGI_2 play important roles as endogenous vasodilators. PGE_1 and its derivatives have significant protective effects on the gastric mucosa by increasing secretion of bicarbonate and mucus, decreasing acid secretion, or both. PGE_2 is one of the most widely investigated prostaglandins. PGE_2 appears to be the natural vasodilator that maintains patency of the ductus arteriosus during fetal development and also appears to be involved in the physiologic changes of the cervix at term. PGE_2 and prostaglandin $F_{2\alpha}$ ($PGF_{2\alpha}$) are released in large amounts from the endometrium during menstruation and may play a physiologic role in labor. Menstrual cramps caused by uterine contractions are induced by prostaglandins, especially $PGF_{2\alpha}$. In contrast, PGE_2 and PGE_1 relax nonvascular smooth muscle. Exogenous $PGF_{2\alpha}$ reduces intraocular pressure, but it is not known whether this is a physiologic effect of the endogenous substance. In response to shear stress on the walls of blood vessels, endothelial cells release prostacyclin (PGI_2). Prostacyclin causes vasodilation and prevents formation of the platelet plug by inhibiting platelet activation. Prostacyclin's actions serve to counteract the vasoconstriction and platelet aggregation actions of thromboxane A_2 (TXA_2). Two products of the COX cascade—$PGF_{2\alpha}$ and TXA_2—are most directly involved in pathologic processes. From the LOX cascade, LTB_4 is a chemotactic factor important in inflammation. The leukotrienes C_4 and D_4 (LTC_4 and LTD_4) are important mediators of

---

TABLE 34-1 Physiologic effects of some important eicosanoids.

Effect	PGE_2	$PGF_{2\alpha}$	PGI_2	TXA_2	LTB_4	LTC_4	LTD_4
Vascular tone	↓	↑ or ↓	↓↓	↑↑↑	?	↑ or ↓	↑ or ↓
Bronchial tone	↓↓	↑↑	↓	↑↑↑	?	↑↑↑↑	↑↑↑↑
Uterine tone	↑, ↓[a]	↑↑↑	↓	↑↑	?	?	?
Platelet aggregation	↑ or ↓		↓↓↓	↑↑↑	?	?	?
Leukocyte chemotaxis	?	?	?	?	↑↑↑↑	↑↑	↑↑

LTB_4, leukotriene B_4; LTC_4, leukotriene C_4; LTD_4, leukotriene D_4; PGE_2, prostaglandin E_2; $PGF_{2\alpha}$, prostaglandin $F_{2\alpha}$; PGI_2, prostaglandin I_2; TXA_2, thromboxane A_2; ?, unknown effect.
[a]Low concentrations cause contraction; higher concentrations cause relaxation.

bronchoconstriction and are secreted in asthma and anaphylaxis (Chapter 35).

ARTHRITIS-ASSOCIATED DISEASES

Arthritis refers to *any* type of inflammation and damage to a joint. The term is applied to more than 100 rheumatic diseases, oversimplifying the nature of the various disease processes. Rheumatic disease describes a disease process associated with joints, bones, connective tissues, muscles, bursae, and ligaments. The etiologies of arthritis and musculoskeletal disorders may be classified into three broad categories: those associated with immune complex disorders such as rheumatoid arthritis (RA), those associated with degeneration of the joints such as osteoarthritis (OA), and those associated with metabolic disorders and crystal deposition in joints.

Chronic autoimmune-mediated inflammation is the underlying mechanism of tissue damage in several diseases (eg, RA, ankylosing spondylitis, systemic lupus erythematosus). In RA, the main sites of tissue damage are the synovial joints. In ankylosing spondylitis, the attachments of tendons and ligaments at bones are the sites of chronic inflammation. In systemic lupus erythematosus (SLE), a multitude of targets (eg, skin, joints, and kidneys) are potential sites of inflammation and tissue damage. In the infectious arthropathies, inflammation is the result of the immune response when infective agents are concentrated in connective tissues. The roles of cell- and humoral-mediated immune responses in these processes are discussed in Chapter 32.

Osteoarthritis (previously known as degenerative joint disease) is the most prevalent arthritic disease. This "wear and tear" arthritis results from mechanical overloading with subsequent loss of hyaline cartilage and bony deformation of affected joints. Besides aging, other recognized causes of OA

include previous trauma or infection at the affected joint, obesity (for lower limb weightbearing joints), and genetic predisposition. Osteoarthritis is a major cause of morbidity in older adults, and increasingly for younger obese individuals.

The last broad type of arthritis is that associated with metabolic dysfunction. This type of arthritis may be typified by gout, whose arthritic component is the result of crystalline-induced synovial joint inflammation.

DRUG CLASSES USED TO TREAT RHEUMATIC DISEASES AND GOUT

Treatment of individuals with rheumatic diseases involves two primary goals. The first is pain relief, which is often the major complaint of the patient. The second goal is to slow or potentially arrest the tissue-damaging process.

Figure 34-2 outlines the drugs used in the treatment of arthritic diseases. Some of these treatment strategies involve inhibiting the formation of eicosanoid products with NSAIDs or glucocorticoids. Reduction of inflammation with NSAIDs or glucocorticoids often results in relief of pain for significant periods. Glucocorticoids represent the most powerful anti-inflammatory drugs that inhibit the formation of all eicosanoid products by several mechanisms, including inhibition of phospholipase A_2 activity. Glucocorticoids are discussed in Chapter 23; their use in treating rheumatic diseases is discussed later in this chapter. Acetaminophen may relieve pain associated with rheumatic diseases, but does *not* affect the underlying inflammatory process initiating the pain. The disease-modifying antirheumatic drugs (DMARDs) are a unique group of diverse drugs that modify the cellular and humoral immune responses in some autoimmune-mediated rheumatic diseases. These drugs slow the tissue damage associated with inflammation and are thought to affect more basic inflammatory

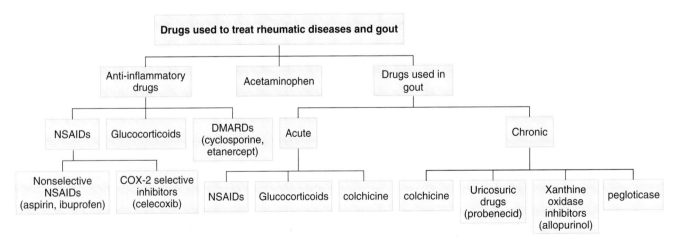

FIGURE 34-2 **Drug classes used in the treatment of rheumatic diseases and gout.** Anti-inflammatory drugs are divided into nonsteroidal anti-inflammatory drugs (NSAIDs), glucocorticoids, and disease-modifying antirheumatic drugs (DMARDs). Acetaminophen is an analgesic with no anti-inflammatory effect. The drugs used in the treatment of gout are divided based on whether the gouty inflammation is in an acute or chronic phase. In the acute phase, NSAIDs, glucocorticoids, and colchicine may be used. In the chronic phase, drugs may be classified based on whether they inhibit inflammatory cell function (colchicine), increase the excretion of uric acid (uricosurics), inhibit the formation of uric acid (xanthine oxidase inhibitors), or metabolize uric acid (pegloticase). Prototype drugs are in parentheses.

mechanisms than do the NSAIDs. Unfortunately, they are also more toxic. In gout, several anti-inflammatory classes are used to inhibit the inflammatory process. In addition, prophylaxis includes use of xanthine oxidase inhibitors to prevent formation of uric acid, or uricosuric drugs to increase uric acid excretion.

ASPIRIN AND NONSELECTIVE NONSTEROIDAL ANTI-INFLAMMATORY DRUGS (NSAIDs)

Classification and Mechanism of Action

Aspirin (acetylsalicylic acid) is the prototype of the nonselective NSAIDs. The classification of these drugs as "nonselective" refers to their relatively equivalent inhibition of *both* COX-1 and COX-2. Thus, nonselective NSAIDs decrease the production of prostaglandins, prostacyclin, and thromboxane necessary for homeostatic function (generally attributed to inhibition of COX-1) as well as those inducible prostaglandins involved in inflammation (generally attributed to inhibition of COX-2). The major distinction between the mechanism of action of aspirin and that of other NSAIDs is that aspirin *irreversibly* inhibits COX (via acetylation), whereas other NSAIDs *reversibly* inhibit COX. Salicylate is a metabolite of aspirin; in contrast to aspirin, salicylate is a reversible inhibitor of COX.

Pharmacokinetics

Aspirin and the other nonselective NSAIDs vary primarily in their potency and duration of action. Table 34-2 lists their half-lives and recommended anti-inflammatory dosages. Aspirin is readily absorbed and hydrolyzed in blood and tissues to acetate and salicylate. Elimination of salicylate follows first order kinetics at low doses, with a half-life of 3-5 hours. At high (anti-inflammatory) doses, the half-life increases to 15 hours or more and elimination follows zero order kinetics. The other NSAIDs are also well absorbed after oral administration. **Ibuprofen** has a half-life of about 2 hours, is relatively safe, and is the least expensive of the older, nonselective NSAIDs. **Indomethacin** is a potent NSAID with increased toxicity. **Oxaprozin** and **piroxicam** are noteworthy because of their longer half-lives (>50 hours), which permit once-daily dosing. All of the nonselective NSAIDs are weak organic acids except **nabumetone**, which is a ketone prodrug that is metabolized to an acidic form of the active drug. The long half-life of nabumetone also permits once-daily dosing. While renal excretion is the most important route for final elimination of all the nonselective NSAIDs, nearly all undergo varying degrees of biliary excretion and reabsorption (enterohepatic circulation). In fact, the degree of lower gastrointestinal (GI) tract irritation correlates with the amount of enterohepatic circulation.

Physiologic Effects and Clinical Uses

The name of this class of drugs—nonsteroidal anti-inflammatory drugs—encompasses only *one* of the four main effects of

TABLE 34-2 Properties of aspirin and other nonsteroidal anti-inflammatory drugs.

Drug	Half-Life (hr)	Urinary Excretion of Unchanged Drug	Recommended Anti-Inflammatory Dosage
Aspirin	0.25	< 2%	1200-1500 mg tid
Salicylate[a]	2-19	2%-30%	See footnote[b]
Celecoxib	11	27%	100-200 mg bid
Diclofenac	1.1	< 1%	50-75 mg qid
Diflunisal	13	3%-9%	500 mg bid
Etodolac	6.5	< 1%	200-300 mg qid
Fenoprofen	2.5	30%	600 mg qid
Flurbiprofen	3.8	< 1%	300 mg tid
Ibuprofen	2	< 1%	600 mg qid
Indomethacin	4-5	16%	50-70 mg tid
Ketoprofen	1.8	< 1%	70 mg tid
Meloxicam	20	< 1%	7.5-15 mg qd
Nabumetone[c]	26	1%	1000-2000 mg qd[d]
Naproxen	14	< 1%	375 mg bid
Oxaprozin	58	1%-4%	1200-1800 mg qd[d]
Piroxicam	57	4%-10%	20 mg qd[d]
Sulindac	8	7%	200 mg bid
Tolmetin	1	7%	400 mg qid

bid, twice a day; qd, once a day; qid, four times a day; tid, three times a day.
[a]Major anti-inflammatory metabolite of aspirin.
[b]Salicylate is usually given in the form of aspirin.
[c]Nabumetone is a prodrug; half-life and urinary excretion are for its active metabolite.
[d]A single daily dose is sufficient because of the long half-life.

these drugs. Aspirin and the NSAIDs possess anti-inflammatory, antithrombotic, antipyretic, and analgesic actions. Aspirin has three oral optimal therapeutic dose ranges. The low range (81-325 mg once per day) is effective in thromboembolus prevention. The intermediate range (600-650 mg/day) has antipyretic and analgesic effects. Aspirin is rarely used clinically as an anti-inflammatory drug. The other nonselective NSAIDs share similar dose-dependent actions as antithrombotic, antipyretic, analgesic, and anti-inflammatory agents. For most agents, anti-inflammatory actions require the *highest* dosages.

Aspirin and the nonselective NSAIDs have their antithrombotic effect by inhibiting platelet aggregation. These drugs inhibit COX-1 in platelets, which reduces the synthesis of TXA_2, an essential platelet aggregation component. Aspirin is the *optimal* antithrombotic drug to minimize the risk of coronary occlusion and heart attacks because of its prolonged antiplatelet action compared to the other nonselective

NSAIDs (Chapter 11). Aspirin's irreversible inhibition of COX-1 in platelets is essentially permanent because platelets lack a nucleus and thus the machinery for new COX-1 synthesis. In contrast, aspirin-mediated inhibition of COX-2 and prostacyclin synthesis in the vascular endothelium is temporary because these cells can synthesize new COX-2. However, concomitant administration of nonselective NSAIDs with aspirin may diminish the irreversible platelet inhibition induced by aspirin. This is because the nonselective NSAIDs and aspirin compete for binding to COX-1 in platelets. Binding of the nonselective NSAID to COX-1 prevents aspirin from binding and irreversibly inhibiting the enzymatic site. When plasma levels of both drugs fall, the COX-1 with a nonselective NSAID bound to it will become enzymatically active again when the nonselective NSAID dissociates. To avoid this interaction between aspirin and the other nonselective NSAIDs, dosing recommendations are to take the aspirin for its antiplatelet effect at least 1 hour prior to taking any of the nonselective NSAIDs.

Although NSAIDs reduce the manifestations of inflammation, they have no effect on underlying tissue damage or immunologic reactions. These drugs decrease the sensitivity of blood vessels to bradykinin and histamine, affect lymphokine production from T lymphocytes, and reverse the vasodilation of inflammation. Fever is caused by exogenous or endogenous substances called pyrogens that stimulate prostaglandin synthesis in the CNS (primarily PGE_2) to upregulate the set point for body temperature. Aspirin and other NSAIDs suppress central PGE_2 synthesis, thereby reducing fever.

The analgesic effect, or the ability of these drugs to relieve pain, is less well understood. Drug-mediated reduction of prostaglandin production in injured tissue may decrease activation of peripheral nociceptors. In addition, a central COX mechanism is operative which provides analgesia. NSAIDs are used to treat *mild* to *moderate* pain. Common indications include alleviating the pain associated with OA and musculoskeletal overuse injuries. Less frequently, the NSAIDs are used to decrease the pain associated with inflammatory arthropathies (RA, gout, and others). Aspirin and selected NSAIDs are also commonly used to treat non-musculoskeletal conditions such as dysmenorrhea, dental pain, and headache. Ibuprofen and **naproxen** have both moderate analgesic and anti-inflammatory efficacy. Other NSAIDs such as indomethacin may sometimes be chosen because of greater anti-inflammatory effectiveness. For severe pain, these drugs are often combined with opioid analgesics (Chapter 20). **Ketorolac** is an NSAID clinically used as a short-term analgesic (not longer than 1 week), but not as an anti-inflammatory agent. The half-life is 4-10 hours with 58% of the unchanged drug excreted in the urine. Ketorolac has been used successfully to replace morphine in some situations involving mild to moderate postsurgical pain. The drug is administered either intramuscularly or intravenously, but an oral formulation is available. When used in conjunction with an opioid, ketorolac may decrease the opioid requirement by 25-50%.

The nonselective NSAIDs have additional clinical uses. For example, indomethacin or ibuprofen can be used to accelerate closure of a patent ductus arteriosus in an otherwise normal infant. Long-term use of aspirin and several of the nonselective NSAIDs also reduces the incidence of colon cancer. Several large epidemiologic studies have shown a 50% reduction in relative risk for this neoplasm when the drugs are taken for 5 years or longer. The mechanism for this protective effect is unclear.

All these drugs interfere with the homeostatic functions that prostaglandins serve in many tissues. Most importantly, these drugs reduce prostaglandin-mediated cytoprotection in the GI tract and autoregulation of renal function, which contributes to their GI and renal toxicities, respectively. Because many of the nonselective NSAIDs are available over-the-counter (without a prescription), they are widely used and clinicians must be aware of their adverse effect profile.

Adverse Effects

Adverse drug reactions (ADRs) are usually similar for aspirin and all the nonselective NSAIDs. ADRs are listed or discussed below by organ system.

1. Central nervous system: Headaches, tinnitus, vertigo, and rarely, aseptic meningitis.
2. Cardiovascular: Fluid retention, hypertension, edema, and rarely, myocardial infarction and congestive heart failure (CHF). In 2005, the United States Food and Drug Administration (FDA) required a black box warning on labels for *prescription* nonaspirin NSAIDs concerning the increased risk of heart attack and stroke with their use. In 2015, after a comprehensive review of newer data, the FDA strengthened the existing warning that NSAIDs (with the exception of aspirin)—*including those available over-the-counter*—can cause heart attacks or strokes.
3. Gastrointestinal: Abdominal pain, dyspepsia, nausea, vomiting, and rarely, ulcers or bleeding. Chronic use can result in gastric ulceration and upper GI bleeding, though the potential is lower with the COX-2 inhibitors (see below) compared to nonselective NSAIDs.
4. Hematologic: Rare thrombocytopenia, neutropenia, or even aplastic anemia. These ADRs are more common with indomethacin.
5. Hepatic: Abnormal liver function test results and rarely, liver failure.
6. Pulmonary: When prostaglandin synthesis is inhibited by even small doses of aspirin, persons with aspirin hypersensitivity may experience asthma. Some cases of aspirin allergy result from diversion of arachidonic acid to the leukotriene pathway when the COX-catalyzed prostaglandin pathway is blocked. The resulting increase in leukotriene synthesis causes the bronchoconstriction that is typical of aspirin allergy. For unknown reasons, this form of aspirin allergy is more common in individuals with nasal polyps. This type of hypersensitivity to aspirin precludes treatment with any of the nonselective NSAIDs.
7. Skin: Rashes (all types) and pruritus.

8. Renal: Renal insufficiency, acute tubular necrosis, interstitial nephritis, renal failure, hyperkalemia, and proteinuria. Renal toxicity is more common with chronic use of ketorolac than with that of other NSAIDs. Since the kidneys eliminate these drugs, preexisting renal dysfunction results in higher, more toxic drug serum concentrations.

9. At high doses of aspirin, hyperventilation and respiratory alkalosis occur. At very high doses, aspirin causes metabolic acidosis, dehydration, hyperthermia, cardiovascular collapse, coma, and death. Aspirin should not be used to treat fever-producing illness in children younger than 19 years of age because of increased risk of Reye's syndrome, a rare but serious condition that causes liver dysfunction and encephalopathy.

COX-2-SELECTIVE INHIBITORS

COX-2 inhibitors, or "-coxibs," were developed in an attempt to more selectively inhibit prostaglandin synthesis induced by activation of the COX-2 isozyme. The goal of COX-2-selective inhibitors is to reduce inflammation *without* affecting the action of the constitutively active "housekeeping" COX-1 necessary for normal function in the GI tract, kidneys, and platelets (and thus avoid or limit some of the ADRs of nonselective NSAIDs). As previously discussed, nonselective NSAIDs inhibit both COX-1 and COX-2 equally (**diclofenac**, **flurbiprofen**, ibuprofen, indomethacin, **ketoprofen**, **meclofenamate**, piroxicam, **tenoxicam**, and **tolmetin**). In contrast, **celecoxib**'s selectivity for inhibiting COX-2 is 10-20 times that for COX-1. The inhibition of COX-1 compared to COX-2 by aspirin, nonselective NSAIDs, and COX-2 inhibitors varies with each drug. For example, **meloxicam** is considered a "preferential" COX-2 inhibitor because this nonselective NSAID has a slightly higher selectivity for COX-2 compared to COX-1 (though not as selective as celecoxib).

Theoretically, COX-2-selective inhibitors should have less effect on the prostaglandins involved in homeostatic function, particularly those in the GI tract. The evidence has shown that COX-2 inhibitors cause a lower incidence of GI effects, (including gastric ulcers and serious GI bleeding) compared to nonselective NSAIDs. COX-2 inhibitors have analgesic, antipyretic, and anti-inflammatory effects similar to those of the nonselective NSAIDs, though they are primarily used in inflammatory disorders. COX-2-selective and nonselective NSAIDs also reduce colonic polyp formation in people with primary familial adenomatous polyposis. Due to increased cardiovascular risks associated with the use of COX-2 inhibitors (see below), celecoxib is the only COX-2 inhibitor available in the United States.

Adverse Effects

The COX-2-selective inhibitors are not recommended for use in individuals with renal dysfunction since COX-2 is constitutively active in the kidney. Because celecoxib is a sulfonamide, the drug may cause a hypersensitivity reaction.

In contrast to aspirin and nonselective NSAIDs, COX-2 inhibitors at usual doses have no impact on platelet aggregation, which is mediated by TXA_2 produced by the COX-1. However, these drugs inhibit COX-2-mediated prostacyclin (PGI_2) synthesis in the vascular endothelium. Since prostacyclin is an effective vasodilator and inhibits platelet activation, drugs that inhibit its production would not offer protection in individuals at high-risk of myocardial infarction or stroke. In fact, clinical investigations have documented an *increased* risk of adverse cardiovascular events in people taking COX-2 inhibitors. This increased risk is not equivalent across the spectrum of COX-2 inhibitors, which resulted in the voluntary withdrawal of two COX-2-selective inhibitors (rofecoxib and valdecoxib) by their manufacturers from the United States market in 2004 and 2005. The FDA required celecoxib, the last available COX-2 inhibitor in the United States, to display a black box warning concerning the risk of cardiovascular thrombotic events. Following scrutiny of data from many randomized controlled trials, the FDA concluded that increased risk of cardiovascular events may be a class effect and extended this black box warning for all *nonaspirin* NSAIDs. Recommended dosages of COX-2 inhibitors also cause renal toxicities similar to those associated with aspirin and the nonselective NSAIDs.

ACETAMINOPHEN

Acetaminophen is not an NSAID. The drug is available over-the-counter and is also often found in many combination drug products such as cold remedies. **Phenacetin**, a toxic prodrug that is metabolized to acetaminophen, is still available in some countries. Acetaminophen is well absorbed orally and metabolized in the liver. Peak blood concentrations are usually reached in 30-60 minutes. The half-life is 2-3 hours in persons with normal hepatic function and is unaffected by renal disease. Acetaminophen is poorly bound to plasma proteins and is partially metabolized by hepatic microsomal enzymes to the inactive metabolites. Less than 5% is excreted unchanged.

Mechanism of Action and Clinical Uses

Acetaminophen is an analgesic and antipyretic agent lacking anti-inflammatory or antithrombotic effects. The analgesic mechanism of action is unclear. Acetaminophen is only a weak COX-1 and COX-2 inhibitor in peripheral tissues, which accounts for its lack of anti-inflammatory effect. The analgesic and antipyretic properties of the drug occur through a CNS mechanism not well defined at present.

Acetaminophen is effective for the same indications as intermediate-dose aspirin. Acute pain and fever may be effectively treated with 325-500 mg four times daily and proportionately less for children. Acetaminophen is preferred to aspirin in children with viral infections because its use is not associated with Reye's syndrome. Acetaminophen is also preferable to aspirin in people with a history of peptic ulcer, in individuals that have experienced aspirin-induced bronchospasm, and in people with hemophilia (since aspirin and the nonselective NSAIDs inhibit platelet activity and increase bleeding risk). Unlike aspirin, acetaminophen does not antagonize the effects of uricosuric agents used to treat gout.

Adverse Effects

In therapeutic dosages, acetaminophen has negligible toxicity in *most* individuals. In larger doses, a minor but highly reactive metabolite is important because it is toxic to both liver and kidney. The mechanism of toxicity requires oxidation to cytotoxic intermediates by phase I cytochrome P450 (CYP) enzymes. This occurs if substrates for phase II conjugation reactions (acetate and glucuronide) are lacking (Chapter 3). Even 4 gm of acetaminophen is associated with increased liver function test abnormalities. However, the dosage at which acetaminophen is toxic also depends upon additional factors and comorbidities. Because acetaminophen toxicity is among the most common causes of *acute* liver failure in the United States, in 2014 the FDA required manufacturers of prescription combination drug products to limit the amount of acetaminophen to no more than 325 mg in each tablet or capsule. Cases of severe injury have occurred in those who took more than the prescribed dose in a 24-hour period, took more than one acetaminophen-containing product at the same time, or drank alcohol while taking acetaminophen products.

GLUCOCORTICOIDS

The NSAIDs have assumed a major role in the long-term treatment of arthritis because many are effective in relieving inflammation and associated pain in rheumatic diseases. However, these drugs do not alter the long-term morbidity or mortality associated with these diseases. Glucocorticoids are a group of corticosteroids that play a vital role in inhibiting inflammation. The term "corticosteroids" refers to *all* steroid hormones produced by the adrenal cortex (ie, glucocorticoids and mineralocorticoids). However, when most clinicians discuss the use of therapeutic corticosteroids to treat inflammation, they are technically referring only to the glucocorticoids. Glucocorticoids (Chapter 23) inhibit the release of arachidonic acid by phospholipases in the membrane (Figure 34-1). This effect is mediated by intracellular steroid receptors that increase the expression of specific proteins capable of inhibiting phospholipase A_2. In addition, glucocorticoids inhibit the synthesis of COX-2. Thus, glucocorticoids are potent anti-inflammatory drugs because they inhibit production of *all* the arachidonic acid metabolites. Both oral administration and intra-articular injections can be used in treatment. The latter is often preferable to avoid or limit the adverse effects of systemic administration. When first introduced, glucocorticoids were considered to be the ultimate answer to the treatment of inflammatory arthritis. Unfortunately, toxicity associated with chronic systemic glucocorticoid therapy restricts their use to the control of acute severe exacerbations and long-term low-dose use in individuals with severe disease not controlled by other agents.

DISEASE-MODIFYING ANTIRHEUMATIC DRUGS (DMARDs)

This heterogeneous group of drugs is called *disease-modifying* because evidence shows that they slow or even reverse damage to cartilage and bone in autoimmune rheumatic diseases, an effect never seen with NSAIDs or glucocorticoids. DMARDs are slow-acting because it may take 2 weeks to 6 months for their benefits to become apparent. Among the major groups of anti-inflammatory agents, the NSAIDs have the quickest rate of action, glucocorticoids have an intermediate rate, and the DMARDs have the slowest rate. Table 34-3 outlines the major clinical uses and toxicities of several common DMARDs.

The DMARD therapies include conventional synthetic (cs) and biologic (b) disease-modifying antirheumatic drugs (recently designated csDMARDs and bDMARDs, respectively). The csDMARDs include small molecule drugs such as **azathioprine**, **chloroquine** and **hydroxychloroquine**, **cyclosporine**, **leflunomide**, **methotrexate**, **mycophenolate mofetil**, and **sulfasalazine**. **Tofacitinib**, though marketed as a biologic, is actually a targeted synthetic DMARD (tsDMARD). The bDMARDs are large-molecule therapeutic agents (usually proteins) that are often produced by recombinant DNA technology. There are multiple bDMARD therapies focusing on different aspects of the autoimmune disease process. These bDMARDs are further divided into biological original products and biosimilar DMARDs (boDMARDs and bsDMARDs, respectively). In the past decade, the number of csDMARDs and bDMARDs clinically used in the treatment of rheumatic diseases has increased exponentially. As such, only representatives of the various DMARDs will be presented. In the following section, the csDMARDs and tsDMARDs are discussed alphabetically and the bDMARDs are grouped by major mechanism of action.

Drug combinations are commonly used to treat moderately aggressive RA. Combinations of DMARDs can be designed rationally on the basis of complementary mechanisms of action, nonoverlapping pharmacokinetics, and nonoverlapping toxicities. While combination therapy might be anticipated to result in more toxicity, this is often not the case. Combination therapy for individuals not responding adequately to monotherapy is now the rule in the treatment of RA.

csDMARDs AND tsDMARDs

Azathioprine

Azathioprine is a csDMARD that may be given orally or parenterally. Its metabolism is bimodal in humans, with rapid metabolizers clearing the drug four times faster than slow metabolizers. Azathioprine acts through its major metabolite, 6-thioguanine, which suppresses inosinic acid synthesis, B-cell and T-cell function, immunoglobulin production, and

TABLE 34-3 Select disease-modifying antirheumatic drugs.

Drug	Other Clinical Uses	Toxicity When Used for Rheumatoid Arthritis
csDMARDs and tsDMARD		
Azathioprine	Tissue transplantation	Bone marrow suppression, GI disturbances
Cyclosporine	Tissue transplantation	Nephrotoxicity, hypertension, liver toxicity
Hydroxychloroquine, chloroquine	Antimalarial[a]	Rash, GI disturbance, myopathy, neuropathy, ocular toxicity
Leflunomide		Teratogen, hepatotoxicity, GI disturbance, skin reactions
Methotrexate	Anticancer	Nausea, mucosal ulcers, hematotoxicity, hepatotoxicity, teratogenicity
Mycophenolate mofetil	Tissue transplantation	Bone marrow suppression, GI disturbances, infection
Sulfasalazine	Inflammatory bowel disease	Rash, GI disturbance, dizziness, headache, leukopenia
Tofacitinib (Janus kinase inhibitor)		Infection, neutropenia, anemia, and increases in LDL and total cholesterol
bDMARDs		
TNF-α inhibitors (infliximab, etanercept, adalimumab, golimumab, certolizumab)	Inflammatory bowel disease, other rheumatic disorders	Infection, lymphoma, hepatotoxicity, hematologic effects, hypersensitivity reactions, cardiovascular toxicity
Abatacept (T-cell modulator)		Infection, exacerbation of COPD, hypersensitivity reactions
Anti-IL-1 drugs (anakinra, rilonacept, and canakinumab)		Injection-site reaction, infection, neutropenia
Anti-IL-6 drug (tocilizumab)		Upper respiratory tract infections, headache, hypertension, and elevated liver enzymes
Anti-IL-12 and -23 drug (ustekinumab)	Psoriatic arthritis, Crohn's disease	Respiratory infection, malignancy
Anti-IL-17A3 drug (secukinumab)	Psoriatic arthritis	Infection
Anti-CD-20 drug (rituximab)	Autoimmune vasculitis, non-Hodgkin lymphoma	Infusion reaction, rash, cardiac toxicity, infection risk
Belimumab (inhibits B-lymphocyte stimulator [BLyS])	Systemic lupus erythematosus	Nausea, diarrhea, and respiratory tract infection

COPD, chronic obstructive pulmonary disorder; GI, gastrointestinal; LDL, low density lipoprotein.
[a]See Chapter 29.

IL-2 secretion (Chapter 32). Production of 6-thioguanine is dependent on thiopurine methyltransferase (TPMT). Individuals with low or absent TPMT activity are at very high risk of myelosuppression due to excessive concentration of the parent drug, if dosage is not adjusted.

Azathioprine is approved for use in RA and for the prevention of kidney transplant rejection (in combination with other immune suppressants). Controlled trials show efficacy in RA, reactive arthritis, polymyositis, SLE, and maintenance of remission in vasculitis. Azathioprine toxicity includes bone marrow suppression, GI disturbances, and some increase in infection risk. Lymphomas may be increased with azathioprine use. Rarely, fever, rash, and hepatotoxicity signal acute allergic reactions.

Chloroquine and Hydroxychloroquine

Chloroquine and hydroxychloroquine were originally developed and primarily used for treating malaria (Chapter 29).

They are also used as csDMARDs in rheumatic diseases. Both drugs are rapidly absorbed, and 50% protein-bound in the plasma. They are very extensively tissue-bound, particularly in melanin-containing tissues such as the eyes. The drugs are deaminated in the liver and have blood elimination half-lives of up to 45 days. The following mechanisms have been proposed: suppression of T-cell responses to mitogens, inhibition of leukocyte chemotaxis, stabilization of lysosomal enzymes, processing through the Fc receptor (an antibody receptor on the surface of certain immune cells that is involved in antigen recognition; Chapter 32), inhibition of DNA and RNA synthesis, and the trapping of free radicals.

Although these antimalarials are approved for RA, they are not considered very effective as DMARDs. There is no evidence that these drugs alter bony damage in RA at their usual dosages, but dose-loading—in which an initial higher dose is given at the beginning of a treatment regimen—may increase the rate of response. Treatment usually requires 3-6 months to obtain a response. In SLE, chloroquine and hydroxychloroquine are commonly used because they decrease mortality and the skin manifestations, serositis, and joint pains characteristic of this disease. Ocular toxicity may occur at higher dosages. Even at lower dosages, ophthalmologic monitoring every 12 months is advised. Other toxicities include dyspepsia, nausea, vomiting, abdominal pain, rashes, and nightmares.

Cyclosporine

Cyclosporine is a peptide antibiotic, but is considered a csDMARD. Cyclosporine absorption is incomplete and somewhat erratic, although a microemulsion formulation improves its consistency and provides 20%-30% bioavailability. Cyclosporine is metabolized by CYP3A and consequently is subject to a large number of drug interactions. Grapefruit juice (a CYP3A inhibitor) increases cyclosporine bioavailability by as much as 62%. Through regulation of gene transcription, cyclosporine inhibits IL-1 and IL-2 production (Chapter 32). In addition, cyclosporine inhibits interactions between macrophages and T cells and T-cell responsiveness and T-cell-dependent B-cell function.

Cyclosporine is approved for use in RA and retards the appearance of new bony erosions. Anecdotal reports suggest that it may be useful in SLE, polymyositis and dermatomyositis, and juvenile chronic arthritis. Adverse effects include leukopenia, thrombocytopenia, and to a lesser extent, anemia. High doses may be cardiotoxic, nephrotoxic, and neurotoxic. Bladder cancer is very rare but must be looked for, even 5 years after cessation of use.

Leflunomide

Leflunomide is an oral csDMARD that is completely absorbed from the gut. Both in the intestine and plasma, leflunomide undergoes rapid conversion to its active metabolite, **teriflunomide**. Leflunomide's mean plasma half-life is 19 days; teriflunomide has approximately the same half-life and is subject to enterohepatic recirculation. The active metabolite inhibits dihydroorotate dehydrogenase, which decreases de novo pyrimidine synthesis, leading to a decrease in ribonucleotide synthesis and the arrest of stimulated cells in the G1 phase of cell growth. Consequently, leflunomide inhibits T-cell proliferation and reduces production of autoantibodies by B cells. Other mechanisms of action include increasing IL-10 receptor mRNA, decreasing IL-8 receptor type A mRNA, and decreasing tumor necrosis factor-alpha-dependent nuclear factor kappa B (NF-κB) activation.

Leflunomide is as effective as methotrexate in RA, including inhibition of bony damage. Teriflunomide is also FDA-approved for the treatment of relapsing-remitting multiple sclerosis (Chapter 32). Adverse effects include diarrhea in approximately 25% of patients. Elevation in liver enzymes may also occur. Decreasing the dose of leflunomide may reduce both of these effects. Other ADRs associated with leflunomide are mild alopecia, weight gain, and increased blood pressure. Leukopenia and thrombocytopenia occur rarely.

Methotrexate

Methotrexate is a csDMARD that may be administered orally or parentally via either subcutaneous or intramuscular routes. The drug is approximately 70% absorbed after oral administration. Both the parent compound and the metabolite are polyglutamated within cells where they stay for prolonged periods. Methotrexate's serum half-life is 6-9 hours. Methotrexate is excreted principally in the urine, but up to 30% may be excreted in bile. At the low doses used in the rheumatic diseases, methotrexate's mechanism of action probably relates to inhibition of amino-imidazolecarboxamide ribonucleotide (AICAR) transformylase and thymidylate synthetase. AICAR accumulates intracellularly and competitively inhibits AMP deaminase, which leads to an accumulation of AMP. The AMP is released and converted extracellularly to adenosine, which is a potent inhibitor of inflammation. As a result, the inflammatory actions of neutrophils, macrophages, dendritic cells, and lymphocytes are suppressed. Methotrexate has secondary effects on the chemotaxis of polymorphonuclear leukocytes. There is also some effect on dihydrofolate reductase, which affects lymphocyte and macrophage function. Methotrexate directly inhibits proliferation and stimulates apoptosis in immune-inflammatory cells. Last, the drug inhibits proinflammatory cytokines linked to rheumatoid synovitis.

Methotrexate is recommended to start treatment in patients with RA. The drug decreases the rate of appearance of new erosions. Evidence supports its use in juvenile chronic arthritis, psoriasis, polymyositis, dermatomyositis, SLE, and vasculitis. Increases in dosage increase toxicity risk. The most common ADRs are nausea and mucosal ulcers. Other ADRs such as leukopenia, anemia, stomatitis, GI ulcerations, and alopecia are probably due to inhibition of cellular proliferation. Progressive dose-related hepatotoxicity in the form of enzyme elevation occurs frequently, but cirrhosis is rare. A rare hypersensitivity-like lung reaction with acute shortness of breath has been documented, as have pseudo-lymphomatous reactions. Leucovorin (folinic acid) administered 24 hours after each weekly methotrexate dose reduces the incidence of GI and liver function test abnormalities. Folinic acid is metabolized to various folic acid derivatives. Alternatively, folic acid may be administered following methotrexate, although this may decrease the efficacy of the methotrexate by about 10%.

Mycophenolate Mofetil

Mycophenolate mofetil is a csDMARD, and a prodrug that is converted to its active form, mycophenolic acid. The active product inhibits inosine monophosphate dehydrogenase and decreases de novo purine biosynthesis, which leads to suppression of T- and B-lymphocyte proliferation. Downstream, mycophenolic acid interferes with leukocyte adhesion to endothelial cells through inhibition of E-selectin and P-selectin (cell adhesion molecules), and intercellular adhesion molecule.

Mycophenolic acid is effective for the treatment of renal disease due to SLE and may be useful in vasculitis. Although the drug is occasionally used to treat RA, there are no well-controlled data regarding its efficacy in this disease. The ADRs include nausea, dyspepsia, abdominal pain, leukopenia (with increased risk of infections), thrombocytopenia, and anemia. Like azathioprine, mycophenolate mofetil may cause hepatotoxicity.

Sulfasalazine

Sulfasalazine is a csDMARD whose mechanisms of action may include suppression of T-cell responses, inhibition of B-cell proliferation, and decreased release of inflammatory cytokines (IL-1, IL-6, IL-12, and tumor necrosis factor-alpha [TNF-α]) produced by monocytes or macrophages. Only 10-20% of orally administered sulfasalazine is absorbed, although a fraction undergoes enterohepatic recirculation into the bowel where it is reduced by intestinal bacteria to liberate sulfapyridine and 5-aminosalicylic acid. Sulfapyridine is well absorbed, but 5-aminosalicylic acid remains unabsorbed. Some sulfasalazine is excreted unchanged in the urine whereas sulfapyridine is excreted after hepatic acetylation and hydroxylation. Sulfasalazine's half-life is 6-17 hours.

When sulfasalazine is used to treat RA, sulfapyridine is probably the active moiety, whereas 5-aminosalicylic acid is the active component when the drug is used to treat inflammatory bowel disease (IBD, Chapter 36). Sulfasalazine itself may also have a therapeutic effect. Sulfasalazine is effective in RA and reduces radiologic disease progression. The drug is used in juvenile chronic arthritis, IBD, and ankylosing spondylitis. Common ADRs include nausea, vomiting, headache, rash, and hemolytic anemia. Neutropenia occurs in 1-5% of patients, while thrombocytopenia is very rare. Pulmonary toxicity is occasionally seen, but drug-induced lupus is rare. Reversible infertility occurs in men, but sulfasalazine does not affect fertility in women. The adverse effects of sulfasalazine cause roughly 30% of patients to discontinue its use.

Tofacitinib

Tofacitinib is a targeted synthetic small molecule (tsDMARD) that selectively inhibits all members of the Janus kinase family to varying degrees (Chapter 2). At therapeutic doses, tofacitinib exerts its effect mainly by inhibiting JAK3, and to a lesser extent JAK1, interrupting the JAK-STAT signaling pathway. This pathway plays a major role in the pathogenesis of autoimmune diseases, including RA. The JAK3/JAK1 complex is responsible for signal transduction from the common γ-chain receptor (IL-2RG) for IL-2, IL-4, IL-7, IL-9, IL-15, and IL-21, which subsequently influences transcription of several genes critical for the differentiation, proliferation, and function of T cells, B cells, and natural killer (NK) cells. In addition, JAK1 controls signal transduction from IL-6 and interferon receptors.

Tofacitinib has an absolute oral bioavailability of 74%, high-fat meals do not affect the area under the curve, and the half-life is about 3 hours. Metabolism for 70% of the drug occurs in the liver, mainly by CYP3A4 and to a lesser extent by CYP2C19. The remaining 30% is excreted unchanged by the kidneys. People with moderate hepatic or renal impairment require dose reduction. The drug should not be given to individuals with severe hepatic disease.

Tofacitinib was originally developed to prevent solid organ allograft rejection. Tofacitinib is approved in the United States for the treatment of adults with moderately to severely active RA who have failed or are intolerant to methotrexate. Tofacitinib rapidly reduces C-reactive protein in this population. The drug may be used as monotherapy or in combination with other csDMARDs, including methotrexate. The drug has also been tested for the treatment of IBD, spondyloarthritis, and psoriasis. Thus far, tofacitinib has not been used with potent immunosuppressants (eg, azathioprine, cyclosporine, or bDMARDs) due to fears of additive immunosuppression.

Adverse effects include slightly increased risk of infection, particular those of the upper respiratory tract and urinary tract. More serious infections including pneumonia, cellulitis, esophageal candidiasis, and other opportunistic infections have been reported. Before initiation of treatment with tofacitinib, all patients should be screened for latent or active tuberculosis (TB). Lymphoma and other malignancies such as lung and breast cancer have been reported in patients taking tofacitinib, although some studies discuss the potential use of JAK inhibitors to treat certain lymphomas. Plasma lipid levels should be monitored during the initial 6 weeks of treatment because patients may experience dose-dependent increases in plasma low-density lipoprotein (LDL) and total cholesterol. Other ADRs include headache, diarrhea, elevation of liver enzymes, and GI perforation. Blood clots may occur with high doses. If drug-related thrombosis or neutropenia and anemia occur, tofacitinib must be discontinued.

bDMARDs

Biologic DMARDs represent another class of medications used to treat RA and related inflammatory rheumatic diseases. The bDMARDs are based on proteins made by living cells. The bDMARDs include TNF-α inhibitors, a T-cell modulator (**abatacept**), B-cell modulators, interleukin-1 (IL-1) inhibitors, and other proinflammatory interleukin inhibitors.

To understand how these drugs are made and have their action, antibody structure must be reviewed (Figure 34-3). The classic antibody structure consists of four polypeptides—two heavy (H) chains and two light (L) chains that join to form a "Y"-shaped structure. There is a constant region (C) of the antibody that is conserved within each immunoglobulin class (ie, IgG, IgA, IgD, IgE, IgM). The constant region of the antibody contains three components of the heavy chain (C_{H1}, C_{H2}, C_{H3}) and one component of the light chain (C_L). The variable (V) region of the antibody has both heavy (V_H) and light (V_L) chain components. It is this variable region of the antibody that provides its *specificity* for binding a particular antigen. The "tips" of the "Y" contain amino acid sequences that vary dramatically among different antibodies, and allow binding to a specific antigen epitope. The base of the "Y" is called the Fc

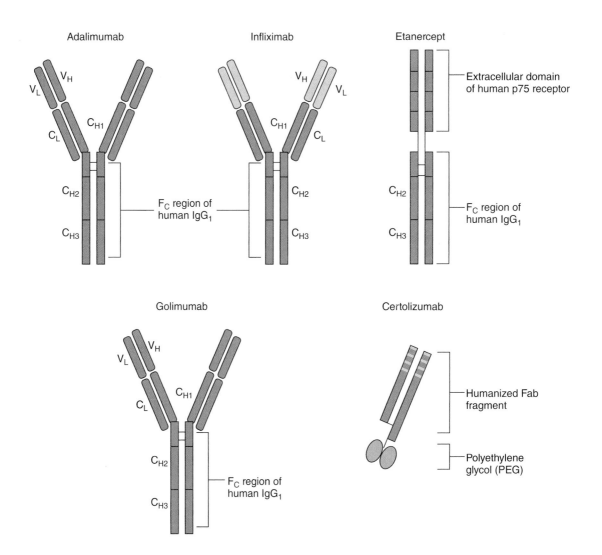

FIGURE 34-3 **Structures of TNF-α inhibitors used in rheumatoid arthritis.** CH, constant heavy chain; CL, constant light chain; Fc, complex immunoglobulin region (consisting of C_{H2} and C_{H3}); VH, variable heavy chain; VL, variable light chain. Red regions, human derived; blue regions, mouse derived; green regions, polyethylene glycol (PEG). All monoclonal antibodies end in the suffix "–mab." All fusion proteins end in the suffix "–cept."

portion, which binds to Fc receptors on the surface of target cells. Treating the antibody with a protease can cleave the variable region, producing an antigen-binding fragment (Fab). This modification allows the Fab to bind to an antigen epitope, but does not bind to the Fc cell receptor or result in activation of the immune system discussed below.

Monoclonal antibodies that bind to a unique epitope on the target ligand can be manufactured in mass. These monoclonal antibodies (MAB) are used therapeutically and can be easily identified because the generic drug names end in "-mab." After binding to the target, monoclonal antibodies can initiate destruction of the target by one of several mechanisms. For instance, after the Fab portion of the MAB binds to its target, the Fc portion subsequently binds to an Fc cell surface receptor of the same immunoglobulin class. The target ligand and bound MAB are then internalized into the cell, and the

target ligand-MAB complex degraded. Alternatively, for MAB directed against cell surface epitopes, the binding of the MAB may initiate activation of complement (with subsequent cell destruction), immune-mediated apoptosis, or other immune-mediated mechanisms of destruction. Another mechanism of action for a bDMARD is that of a "dummy receptor" for the target ligand. In this mechanism, the external portion of a cell surface receptor for the target ligand is fused to the Fc portion of an antibody, thus the term "fusion protein" (Figure 34-3, **etanercept**). The mechanisms of action of the fusion proteins etanercept and abatacept are discussed below.

Since these drugs are proteins, they typically cannot be taken orally because ingested proteins are digested by proteases in the stomach and intestine. Therefore, they are administered parenterally. Infusion reactions are a potential adverse effect for all bDMARDs. Pretreatment with acetaminophen, an antihistamine, and/or intravenous glucocorticoids 30 minutes prior to infusion decreases the incidence and severity of infusion reactions.

TUMOR NECROSIS FACTOR-ALPHA (TNF-α) INHIBITORS

Cytokines play a central role in the immune response (Chapter 32) and in RA. Although many different cytokines are expressed in the joints of individuals with RA, TNF-α appears to be particularly important in the inflammatory process. TNF-α affects cellular function via activation of specific membrane-bound TNF-1 and TNF-2 receptors. Five "legacy" bDMARDs interfering with TNF-α are approved for RA and other rheumatic diseases. Figure 34-3 outlines the structures of **adalimumab**, **certolizumab**, etanercept, **golimumab**, and **infliximab**. Each of these agents is specific for a unique epitope on the target ligand (ie, TNF-α). Though some agents can be used as monotherapy, they are often used in combination with a csDMARD—usually methotrexate. The advantages of combined therapy include increased efficacy and decreased formation of antibodies. Lower-cost biosimilar drugs (bsDMARDs) are available in some countries. To date, the efficacy, toxicity, and immunogenicity of the biosimilars are equivalent to the legacy compounds.

Adalimumab

Adalimumab is a fully human IgG anti-TNF monoclonal antibody (Figure 34-3) injected subcutaneously, with a half-life of 10-20 days. Clearance is decreased by more than 40% in the presence of methotrexate. When methotrexate is given at the same time, the formation of human anti-monoclonal antibody (which would decrease the drug's efficacy) is also decreased. Adalimumab complexes with soluble TNF-α and prevents its interaction with p55 and p75 cell surface receptors. This results in down-regulation of macrophage and T-cell function. The compound is approved for RA and other autoimmune rheumatic diseases, Crohn's disease, and ulcerative colitis. Adalimumab decreases the rate of formation of new erosions, and is effective both as monotherapy and in combination with csDMARDs.

Certolizumab

Certolizumab is a recombinant, humanized antibody Fab fragment conjugated to a polyethylene glycol (PEG) with specificity for human TNF-α (Figure 34-3). The drug is administered subcutaneously and has a half-life of 14 days. Methotrexate decreases the appearance of anti-certolizumab antibodies. Certolizumab neutralizes membrane-bound and soluble TNF-α in a dose-dependent manner. Certolizumab does not contain the Fc region found on a complete antibody and does not fix complement or cause antibody-dependent cell-mediated cytotoxicity. Certolizumab is indicated for the treatment of adults with moderately to severely active RA. The MAB may be used

as monotherapy or in combination with csDMARDs. Certolizumab is also approved in adults with Crohn's disease, active psoriatic arthritis, and active ankylosing spondylitis.

Etanercept

Etanercept is given subcutaneously once or twice weekly. The drug is slowly absorbed, with peak concentration 72 hours after drug administration, and a mean serum elimination half-life of 4.5 days. Etanercept is a recombinant fusion protein consisting of two soluble TNF p75 receptor moieties linked to the Fc portion of human IgG (Figure 34-3). This fusion protein binds to both soluble and membrane-associated TNF-α molecules, and also inhibits lymphotoxin α (TNF-β). Binding to TNF-α or TNF-β decreases the availability for these molecules in subsequent biologic responses.

Etanercept is approved for the treatment of RA, juvenile arthritis, psoriasis, psoriatic arthritis, and ankylosing spondylitis. Etanercept may be used as monotherapy, although over 70% of patients taking etanercept are also using methotrexate. Etanercept decreases the rate of formation of new erosions relative to methotrexate alone. The drug is also being used in other rheumatic syndromes such as scleroderma and giant cell arteritis.

Golimumab

Golimumab is a human IgG monoclonal antibody with a high affinity for soluble and membrane-bound TNF-α (Figure 34-3). The drug is administered subcutaneously and has a half-life of approximately 14 days. Concomitant use with methotrexate increases golimumab serum levels and decreases anti-golimumab antibodies. Golimumab effectively neutralizes the inflammatory effects produced by TNF-α seen in diseases such as RA. Golimumab with methotrexate is indicated for the treatment of moderately to severely active RA in adults. The drug is also indicated for the treatment of psoriatic arthritis, ankylosing spondylitis, and moderate to severe ulcerative colitis.

Infliximab

Infliximab (Figure 34-3) is a chimeric (25% mouse, 75% human) IgG monoclonal antibody that binds with high affinity to soluble and possibly membrane-bound TNF-α. Mechanism of action is likely the same as that of adalimumab. Infliximab is given as an intravenous infusion with "induction" at 0, 2, and 6 weeks and maintenance every 8 weeks thereafter. There is a relationship between serum concentration and effect, although individual clearances vary markedly. The terminal half-life is 9-12 days without accumulation after repeated dosing at the recommended interval of 8 weeks. The clinical recommendation is that methotrexate be used in conjunction with infliximab. However, several other csDMARDs (eg, antimalarials, azathioprine, leflunomide, cyclosporine) may also be used as background therapy with this drug. Alternatively, infliximab may be used as monotherapy. Infliximab is approved for use in

RA, ankylosing spondylitis, psoriatic arthritis, Crohn's disease, ulcerative colitis, and psoriasis. In RA, infliximab plus methotrexate decreases the rate of formation of new erosions. After intermittent therapy, infliximab elicits human anti-chimeric antibodies in up to 62% of patients. Concurrent therapy with methotrexate markedly decreases the prevalence of human anti-chimeric antibodies.

Adverse Effects of TNF-α Inhibitors

TNF-α inhibitors share multiple adverse effects. The risk of bacterial (including TB), fungal, and other opportunistic infections is increased although it remains very low. Activation of latent TB is lower with etanercept than with other TNF-α inhibitors. Nevertheless, all patients should be screened for latent or active TB before starting TNF-α inhibitors. Use of TNF-α inhibitors is also associated with increased risk of activation of latent hepatitis B virus (HBV); screening for HBV is important before starting the treatment. TNF-α inhibitors increase the risk of skin cancers such as melanoma, which necessitates periodic skin examination, especially in high-risk individuals. On the other hand, there is no clear evidence of increased risk of solid organ malignancies or lymphomas with TNF-α inhibitors, and their incidence may not be different compared with other bDMARDs or active RA itself. In people with borderline or overt heart failure, TNF-α inhibitors can exacerbate the disease process. TNF-α inhibitors may increase the risk of GI ulcers and large bowel perforation including diverticular and appendiceal perforation. Rare toxicities include nonspecific interstitial pneumonia, psoriasis, sarcoidosis-like syndrome, leukopenia, neutropenia, thrombocytopenia, pancytopenia, cutaneous pseudolymphomas (especially with infliximab). The precipitating drug should be discontinued in such cases. Cases of alopecia areata, hypertrichosis, and erosive lichen planus have also been reported. Clinical lupus is extremely rare. TNF-α inhibitors can induce the immune system to develop anti-drug antibodies in about 17% of cases. These antibodies may interfere with drug efficacy and correlate with infusion site reactions, although they rarely result in discontinuation of therapy.

T-CELL MODULATOR

Abatacept is a fusion protein that selectively inhibits the activation of T cells (see also Chapter 32, Figure 32-3). After a T cell has engaged an antigen-presenting cell (APC), a second signal is produced by CD28, one of the surface proteins expressed on the T cell that is required for T-cell activation and survival. The CD28 interacts with CD80 or CD86 proteins on the surface of the APC, leading to T-cell activation. Abatacept contains the endogenous ligand CTLA-4 that binds to CD80 and 86, thereby inhibiting the binding to CD28 and preventing the activation of T cells.

The recommended dosage of abatacept for the treatment of adults with RA is three intravenous infusion "induction" doses (day 0, week 2, and week 4), followed by monthly infusions. Abatacept is also available as a subcutaneous formulation that is given weekly. The terminal serum half-life is 13-16 days. Most patients respond to abatacept within 12-16 weeks after the treatment initiation. However, some patients can respond in as few as 2-4 weeks. Abatacept can be used as monotherapy or in combination with methotrexate or other DMARDs in individuals with moderate to severe RA. The drug has been tested in combination with methotrexate in early rapidly progressing RA. This combination was superior to methotrexate in achieving minimal disease activity as early as 2 months, significantly inhibiting radiographic progression at 1 year and improving patients' physical function and symptoms. Abatacept has been tested in other rheumatic diseases like SLE and psoriatic arthritis. The drug has also been tested in autoimmune diseases such as type 1 diabetes to determine whether it can delay or prevent progression of insulin loss.

As with other bDMARDs, there is a slightly increased risk of infection, predominantly of the upper respiratory or urinary tracts. Concurrent use with TNF-α inhibitors or other biologics is not recommended due to the increased incidence of serious infection. All patients should be screened for latent TB and viral hepatitis before starting this medication. Live vaccines should be avoided in individuals while taking abatacept and up to 3 months after discontinuation. Infusion-related reactions and hypersensitivity reactions, including anaphylaxis, have been reported, but are rare. Anti-abatacept antibody formation is infrequent (< 5%). There is a possible increase in lymphomas but not other malignancies when using abatacept.

B-CELL MODULATORS

Belimumab

Belimumab is an antibody that specifically inhibits B lymphocyte stimulator (BLyS), a soluble ligand of the TNF cytokine family that is critical for B-cell differentiation, homeostasis, and selection. High levels of BLyS contribute to autoantibody production by enhancing survival and decreasing selective apoptosis of autoantibody-producing B cells. Belimumab is administered as an intravenous infusion, at weeks 0, 2, and 4, and every 4 weeks thereafter. Belimumab has a distribution half-life of 1.75 days and a terminal half-life of 19.4 days.

Belimumab is approved only for the treatment of adults with active SLE who are receiving standard treatment. The place of this drug in the SLE armamentarium is not clear. Belimumab should not be used in individuals with active renal or neurological manifestations of SLE because there are no data for these conditions. In addition, the efficacy of belimumab has not been tested in combination with other bDMARDs. As with other bDMARDs, there is a slight increase in the risk of infection, including serious infections. The most common ADRs are nausea, diarrhea, and respiratory tract infection. Cases of depression and suicide have been reported in people taking belimumab, although these individuals may have had neurologic SLE, which confounds a causal relationship. Infusion reactions including anaphylaxis are among the other adverse effects. A very small percentage of patients develop antibodies toward belimumab, though the clinical significance of this is unclear.

Rituximab

Rituximab is a chimeric monoclonal antibody that binds to the CD20 surface marker on B cells. After binding to rituximab, B cells die by cell-mediated cytotoxicity, complement-dependent cytotoxicity, and stimulation of cell apoptosis. The ultimate result is a depletion of B cells from the circulation, which reduces inflammation by decreasing the presentation of antigens to T lymphocytes and inhibiting the secretion of proinflammatory cytokines.

Rituximab is given as intravenous infusions, separated by 2 weeks. Injections may be repeated every 6-9 months, as needed. Repeated courses remain effective. Rituximab was originally used to treat lymphomas and leukemias (Chapter 31), but its use is increasing in the treatment of certain autoimmune diseases. Rituximab is indicated for the treatment of moderately to severely active RA in combination with methotrexate in patients with an inadequate response to one or more TNF-α inhibitors.

About 30% of patients develop rash with the first treatment. This incidence decreases to about 10% with the second infusion and progressively decreases with each course of therapy thereafter. Rashes do not usually require discontinuation of therapy, although an urticarial or anaphylactoid reaction precludes further therapy. With repeated courses of therapy, immunoglobulins (in particular IgG and IgM) may decrease. However, repeated infections do not seem to be directly associated with the decreases in these immunoglobulins. Serious, and sometimes fatal, bacterial, fungal, and viral infections are reported for up to 1 year of the last dose of rituximab. Individuals with severe and active infections should not receive rituximab. Rituximab is associated with activation of latent HBV infection, which requires monitoring before and several months after initiating rituximab treatment. Rituximab has not been associated with either activation of latent TB or the occurrence of lymphomas or other tumors. Fatal mucocutaneous reactions have been reported in some individuals receiving rituximab. Different cytopenias can occur, which require complete blood cell monitoring every 2-4 months in RA patients. Other ADRs, such as cardiovascular events, are rare.

INTERLEUKIN-1 INHIBITORS

IL-1α plays a major role in the pathogenesis of several inflammatory and autoimmune diseases including RA. IL-1α, IL-1β, and IL-1 receptor antagonist (IL-1RA) are other members of the IL-1 family. All three bind to IL-1 receptors in the same manner. However, IL-1RA does not initiate the intracellular signaling pathway and thus acts as a competitive inhibitor of the proinflammatory IL-1α and IL-1β. The IL-1 inhibitors

are all administered by subcutaneous injection. They include **anakinra**, **canakinumab**, and **rilonacept**. In addition to the clinical use in rheumatic diseases, these drugs are used in the treatment of gout.

Anakinra is a recombinant protein of IL-1RA and the oldest IL-1 inhibitor. The drug reaches a maximum plasma concentration after 3-7 hours. The absolute bioavailability of anakinra is 95%, and it has a 4- to 6-hour terminal half-life. For individuals with renal insufficiency, it is recommended that the frequency of administration be decreased from daily to every other day. Anakinra is rarely used for RA, but has clinical use in other rheumatic diseases.

Canakinumab is a human IgG monoclonal antibody against IL-1β. The drug forms a complex with IL-1β, preventing its binding to IL-1 receptors. Canakinumab reaches peak serum concentrations 7 days after a single subcutaneous injection, has an absolute bioavailability of 66% and a 26-day mean terminal half-life. The drug is indicated for active juvenile arthritis.

Rilonacept is a fusion protein with the ligand-binding domain of the IL-1 receptor. The drug binds primarily to IL-1β, neutralizing IL-1β and preventing its attachment to IL-1 receptors. Rilonacept binds with lower affinity to IL-1α and IL-1RA. Rilonacept is administered weekly and the steady-state plasma concentration is reached after 6 weeks. Rilonacept was originally developed for RA, but was found to be of limited clinical benefit. In 2008, the drug received orphan drug approval for other rheumatic pathophysiologies. Rilonacept is also used to treat gout.

The most common ADRs associated with IL-1 inhibitors are injection site reactions (up to 40%) and upper respiratory tract infections. Serious infections rarely occur. Headache, abdominal pain, nausea, diarrhea, arthralgia, and flu-like illness all have been reported, as have hypersensitivity reactions. Patients taking IL-1 inhibitors may experience transient neutropenia, which requires regular monitoring of neutrophil counts.

OTHER PROINFLAMMATORY INTERLEUKIN INHIBITORS

Secukinumab

Secukinumab is a human IgG monoclonal antibody that selectively binds to the IL-17A cytokine, inhibiting its interaction with the IL-17A receptor. IL-17A is involved in normal inflammatory and immune responses. Elevated concentrations of IL-17A are found in psoriatic plaques and psoriatic arthritis. The initial subcutaneous loading dose of secukinumab is administered at weeks 0, 1, 2, 3, and 4, followed by monthly maintenance. The elimination half-life of the drug is 22-31 days. The drug is indicated for individuals with moderate to severe plaque psoriasis and active psoriatic arthritis and ankylosing spondylitis. Infection is a common ADR (28.7%). Nasopharyngitis occurs in about 12%. TB status should be evaluated prior to therapy. Secukinumab may exacerbate Crohn's disease.

Tocilizumab

Tocilizumab is an antibody that binds to soluble and membrane-bound IL-6 receptors, inhibiting IL-6-mediated signaling. IL-6 is a proinflammatory cytokine produced by different cell types including T cells, B cells, monocytes, fibroblasts, and synovial and endothelial cells. IL-6 is involved in a variety of physiologic processes such as T-cell activation, hepatic acute-phase protein synthesis, as well as stimulation of the inflammatory processes involved in diseases such as RA.

The half-life of tocilizumab is approximately 11-13 days. Higher doses result in longer half-lives. Dosage modifications are recommended on the basis of certain laboratory changes such as elevated liver enzymes, neutropenia, and thrombocytopenia. The IL-6 cytokine may suppress several CYP isoenzymes. Thus, inhibition of IL-6 by tocilizumab may restore CYP activity to higher levels. This may be clinically relevant for drugs that are CYP substrates and have a narrow therapeutic window, such as cyclosporine or warfarin. In these cases, dosage adjustment of these medications may be needed.

Tocilizumab may be used in combination with nonbiologic DMARDs or as monotherapy. In the United States, the drug is administered intravenously every 4 weeks. Tocilizumab is indicated for adults with moderately to severely active RA who have had an inadequate response to one or more DMARDs. The most common ADRs are upper respiratory tract infections, headache, hypertension, and elevated liver enzymes. Serious infections including TB, fungal, viral, and other opportunistic infections have occurred. Screening for TB should be done prior to beginning tocilizumab. Neutropenia and reduction in platelet counts occur occasionally, and the plasma lipid profile should be monitored. GI perforation has been reported when using tocilizumab in patients with diverticulitis and in those using glucocorticoids, although it is not clear that this adverse effect is more common than with TNF-α inhibitors. Demyelinating disorders including multiple sclerosis are rarely associated with tocilizumab use. Fewer than 1% of those taking tocilizumab develop an anaphylactic reaction. Anti-tocilizumab antibodies develop in 2% of patients, and these can be associated with hypersensitivity reactions requiring discontinuation.

Ustekinumab

Ustekinumab is an IL-12 and IL-23 antagonist. The drug is a fully human IgG monoclonal antibody to the p40 protein subunit, which is part of both IL-12 and IL-23. These two cytokines are important contributors to the chronic inflammation in psoriasis plaques and psoriatic arthritis. Ustekinumab prevents the binding of the p40 subunit of both IL-12 and IL-23 to the IL-12 receptor β1 found on the surface of CD4 T cells and NK cells. This interruption interferes with IL-12 and IL-23 signal transduction and suppresses the formation of proinflammatory T_H1 and T_H17 cells.

After subcutaneous injection, ustekinumab has a bioavailability of 57%, with a time to peak plasma concentration of 7-13.5 days and elimination half-life of 10-126 days.

Ustekinumab is indicated for treatment of adults with psoriatic arthritis. For adults with psoriatic arthritis, a loading dose at 0 and 4 weeks is followed by maintenance doses once every 12 weeks. The drug may be used as monotherapy or in combination with methotrexate. Upper respiratory tract infection is the most common adverse effect, but rare severe infection, malignancy, and reversible posterior leukoencephalopathy syndrome have been reported. Ustekinumab should be discontinued at least 15 weeks before live vaccines are administered and can be resumed at least 2 weeks after.

DIETARY MANIPULATION OF INFLAMMATION

Given growing patient interest in lifestyle interventions beyond pharmacotherapy and increased research into the influence of diet on inflammation, clinicians should be aware of the use of diets and dietary supplementation designed to suppress the activity of inflammatory mediators. Much effort to modify inflammation by altering specific nutrients in the diet has concentrated on fats—specifically, the absolute amount and/or the ratio of omega-6 polyunsaturated fatty acids (found in vegetable oils, nuts, seeds) to omega-3 polyunsaturated fatty acids such as eicosapentaenoic acid (EPA) and docosahexaenoic acid (DHA). EPA and DHA are found naturally in fish, fish oils, and krill oils and as dietary supplements. Some of these fatty acids increase inflammation, while others inhibit inflammation. In *general*, the eicosanoids derived from omega-6 fatty acids are more potent mediators of different aspects of the inflammatory response. Dietary manipulation that substitutes EPA or DHA for omega-6 fatty acids causes these alternative fatty acids to be metabolized by COX and LOX (Figure 34-1), changing the final prostaglandin and leukotriene products. The omega-3 unsaturated fatty acid metabolites are less potent than the corresponding eicosanoid products derived from arachidonic acid, sometimes by several orders of magnitude. The omega-3 products diminish the activities of the eicosanoid mediators by competing with them for shared target-cell receptors. Ultimately, higher concentrations of EPA and DHA than arachidonic acid shift the eicosanoid balance toward *less* inflammation.

The impact of dietary interventions in RA has received increased attention in recent years. Clinical studies suggest that consumption of omega-3 unsaturated fatty acids decreases both morning stiffness and the number of tender joints in individuals with RA as well as erythema associated with psoriasis. The efficacy of dietary omega-3 unsaturated fatty acids approximates that of the NSAIDs. Preliminary results and the near absence of significant adverse effects suggest that dietary alteration or supplementation may be a beneficial addition to conventional treatment of RA. This area of research is evolving rapidly. Specific recommendations for supplementation should be done in consultation with a prescribing healthcare provider because omega-3 fatty acids exert an antiplatelet effect and thus increase risk of bleeding.

DRUGS USED IN THE TREATMENT OF GOUT

Gout is a metabolic disease usually associated with elevated blood levels of monosodium urate or uric acid (ie, hyperuricemia). Uric acid is a breakdown product of purines that are naturally found in the body and also in high concentration in certain foods (eg, organ meats, alcoholic beverages, some fish). Uric acid is poorly soluble and thus precipitates out of solution in the form of crystals. Humans (unlike most mammals) lack uricase, the enzyme that converts uric acid to the more soluble allantoin. Gout is characterized by recurrent episodes of acute arthritis due to urate crystals in joints and cartilage. Individuals with gout may also experience uric acid kidney stones, tophi (deposits in skin and soft tissue), and interstitial nephritis. The disease may also be associated with adverse cardiovascular outcomes. While gouty "flare-ups" are associated with hyperuricemia, most individuals with hyperuricemia never develop a clinical event associated with urate crystal deposition.

Gout treatment aims to relieve acute gouty attacks and prevent recurrent gouty episodes and urate crystal formation. Therapies for acute gout are based on our current understanding of the pathophysiologic events that occur in this disease (Figure 34-4).

Urate crystals activate NLRP3 (a macromolecular complex of proteins) in specialized cells inside the synovium called synoviocytes. Activation of NLRP3 causes the synoviocytes to release prostaglandins and lysosomal enzymes. Attracted by these mediators, polymorphonuclear leukocytes migrate into the joint space and amplify the ongoing inflammatory process.

In the later phases of the attack, increased numbers of mononuclear phagocytes (macrophages) appear, ingest the urate crystals, and release more inflammatory mediators.

Asymptomatic hyperuricemia is common and should not ordinarily be treated because the efficacy of long-term drug treatment in asymptomatic hyperuricemic individuals has not been proven. In people that are asymptomatic, efforts should be made to lower urate levels with lifestyle interventions. Several different agents have been used to treat acute and chronic gout. However, nonadherence to these drugs is exceedingly common. Healthcare providers should be aware that medication adherence has been documented to be 18-26% in younger individuals. Treatment strategies for gout are twofold. The first is to reduce inflammation during acute attacks. NSAIDs like indomethacin, **colchicine**, or glucocorticoids may be used to decrease inflammation during the acute episode (Figure 34-2). Second, after the acute gouty flare-up is controlled, three types of drugs may be used to reduce the likelihood of recurrent episodes. Uricosuric drugs accelerate renal excretion of uric acid. Xanthine oxidase inhibitors reduce the conversion of purines to uric acid. Last, pegloticase is the newest urate-lowering therapy that works by converting insoluble uric acid to soluble allantoin.

DRUGS USED IN ACUTE GOUT

NSAIDs

NSAIDs are the preferred therapy for treatment of gout in individuals without complications. In addition to inhibiting prostaglandin synthase, NSAIDs inhibit urate crystal phagocytosis. All NSAIDs except aspirin, salicylates, and tolmetin have been successfully used to treat acute gouty episodes. Aspirin is not used because it causes renal retention of uric acid at low doses (≤ 2.6 gm/day) and is only uricosuric at doses greater than 3.6 gm/day. Indomethacin is commonly used in the initial treatment of gout. Oxaprozin is theoretically a good choice because it lowers serum uric acid. These agents appear to be as effective and safe as the older drugs. The ADRs of NSAIDs were discussed previously in this chapter.

Colchicine

Colchicine is an antimitotic drug that is the oldest treatment for gout. Colchicine may be used for treating acute gout, during the intercritical period between acute attacks, and for prolonged prophylaxis (at low doses). Colchicine is absorbed readily after oral administration, reaches peak plasma levels within 2 hours, and is eliminated with a serum half-life of 9 hours. Metabolites are excreted in the intestinal tract and urine. Colchicine relieves the pain and inflammation of acute gouty arthritis in 12-24 hours without altering the metabolism or excretion of urates and without other analgesic effects. Colchicine produces its anti-inflammatory effects by binding to intracellular tubulin. This action prevents the polymerization of tubulin into

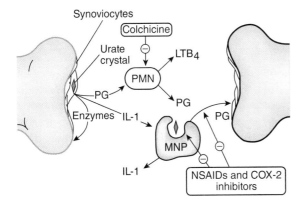

FIGURE 34-4 Sites of action of some anti-inflammatory drugs in a gouty joint. Synoviocytes damaged by urate crystals release prostaglandins (PG), interleukins (eg, IL-1), and other mediators of inflammation. Polymorphonuclear leukocytes (PMN), macrophages, and other inflammatory cells enter the joint and also release inflammatory substances, including leukotrienes (eg, LTB₄), which attract additional inflammatory cells. Colchicine acts on microtubules in the inflammatory cells. Nonselective NSAIDs and COX-2 inhibitors act on cyclooxygenase-2 (COX-2) to inhibit PG formation in all of the cells of the joint. MNP, mononuclear phagocytes.

microtubules and leads to the inhibition of leukocyte migration and phagocytosis. Colchicine also inhibits formation of the inflammatory mediators LTB_4 (Figure 34-4) and IL-1β.

Several of colchicine's ADRs are the direct result of its inhibition of tubulin polymerization and cell mitosis. Colchicine frequently causes GI disturbances such as diarrhea, nausea, vomiting, and abdominal pain. Hepatic necrosis, acute renal failure, disseminated intravascular coagulation, and seizures have also been observed. Rarely, colchicine may cause hair loss, bone marrow depression, peripheral neuropathy, myopathy, and death in some cases. The more severe ADRs have been associated with intravenous administration of higher doses of colchicine, which resulted in intravenous formulations being discontinued in the United States.

Glucocorticoids

The physiologic effects, clinical uses, and ADRs of glucocorticoids are discussed in Chapter 23. For monoarticular gouty attacks, an intra-articular injection of a glucocorticoid may be used because it is as effective and less toxic than systemic administration. If high doses of NSAIDs fail to provide analgesia and minimize inflammation, systemic high-dose glucocorticoids may be used.

DRUGS USED IN CHRONIC GOUT

Uricosuric Drugs

Lesinurad, **probenecid**, and **sulfinpyrazone** are uricosuric drugs used to decrease the body pool of urate in individuals with increasingly frequent gouty attacks or those with tophaceous gout. Tophaceous gout is a form of chronic gout associated with nodular masses of urate crystals called tophi that are deposited in soft tissues. Uricosuric therapy should be initiated in gouty patients with *underexcretion* of uric acid, when **allopurinol** or **febuxostat** is contraindicated, or when tophi are present. The uricosuric agents should not be used in patients who excrete large amounts of uric acid.

All uricosuric drugs inhibit active transport sites for reabsorption and secretion of uric acid in the proximal renal tubules so that net reabsorption of uric acid is decreased. Uricosuric agents may also reduce the secretion of other weak acids like penicillin. As urinary excretion of uric acid increases, the total amount of uric acid in the body decreases, although the plasma concentration may not be greatly reduced. In people who respond favorably, tophaceous deposits of urate are *reabsorbed*, with relief of arthritis and remineralization of bone. However, the resulting increase in uric acid excretion predisposes individuals to forming uric acid kidney stones. Therefore, urine volume should be maintained at a high level. At least early in treatment with uricosuric drugs, urine acidification should also be minimized.

Uricosuric drugs are organic acids and, as such, act at the anion transport sites of the renal tubule. Probenecid is completely reabsorbed by the renal tubules and is metabolized slowly with a terminal serum half-life of 5-8 hours.

Sulfinpyrazone (or its active hydroxylated metabolite) is excreted by the kidneys. Even so, the duration of its effect after oral administration is almost as long as that of probenecid, which is given once or twice daily. Lesinurad has a terminal serum half-life of approximately 5 hours, and is metabolized by the liver.

All these drugs, but especially sulfinpyrazone, cause some degree of GI irritation. A rash may appear after the use of either probenecid or sulfinpyrazone. Nephrotic syndrome has occurred after the use of probenecid. Rarely, sulfinpyrazone and probenecid may cause aplastic anemia.

Xanthine Oxidase Inhibitors

Figure 34-5 illustrates the biochemical synthesis of uric acid and steps at which the two drugs allopurinol and febuxostat inhibit its formation. Allopurinol is an isomer of hypoxanthine that is metabolized by xanthine oxidase. The resulting metabolite, alloxanthine, inhibits xanthine oxidase. Febuxostat is a nonpurine that inhibits xanthine oxidase.

Dietary purines are not the most important source of uric acid. Quantitatively, important amounts of purine are formed from metabolism of endogenous amino acids, formate, and carbon dioxide. The purine ribonucleotides that are not incorporated into nucleic acids and those derived from nucleic acid degradation are converted to hypoxanthine or xanthine and oxidized to uric acid. Allopurinol inhibits this last step, resulting in lowered plasma urate level and decreased total body urate. Allopurinol (or, more specifically, its metabolite alloxanthine) increases plasma levels of the more soluble hypoxanthine or xanthine that are excreted in the urine. Similarly, febuxostat is a potent and selective inhibitor of xanthine oxidase, thereby reducing the formation of xanthine and uric acid without affecting other enzymes in the purine or pyrimidine metabolic pathway. The efficacy of febuxostat's ability to lower uric acid is comparable regardless of whether hyperuricemia is due to overproduction or underexcretion of uric acid.

Allopurinol is often the first-line agent for the treatment of chronic gout in the period between attacks and it tends to prolong the intercritical period. As with uricosuric agents, allopurinol is initiated with the expectation that the drug will be continued for years, if not for life. When initiating allopurinol, colchicine or an NSAID should be used until steady-state serum uric acid is normalized or decreased to less than 6 mg/dL and the drug combination should be continued for 6 months or longer to avoid acute gout flares. Thereafter, colchicine or the NSAID can be cautiously stopped while continuing allopurinol therapy. Allopurinol is approximately 80% absorbed after oral administration and has a terminal serum half-life of 1-2 hours. Because allopurinol is an irreversible inhibitor of xanthine oxidase with a long enough duration of action, the drug is given only once a day. Common ADRs of allopurinol include GI intolerance (nausea, vomiting, and diarrhea). Rarely, peripheral neuropathy, necrotizing vasculitis, bone marrow suppression, and aplastic anemia occur.

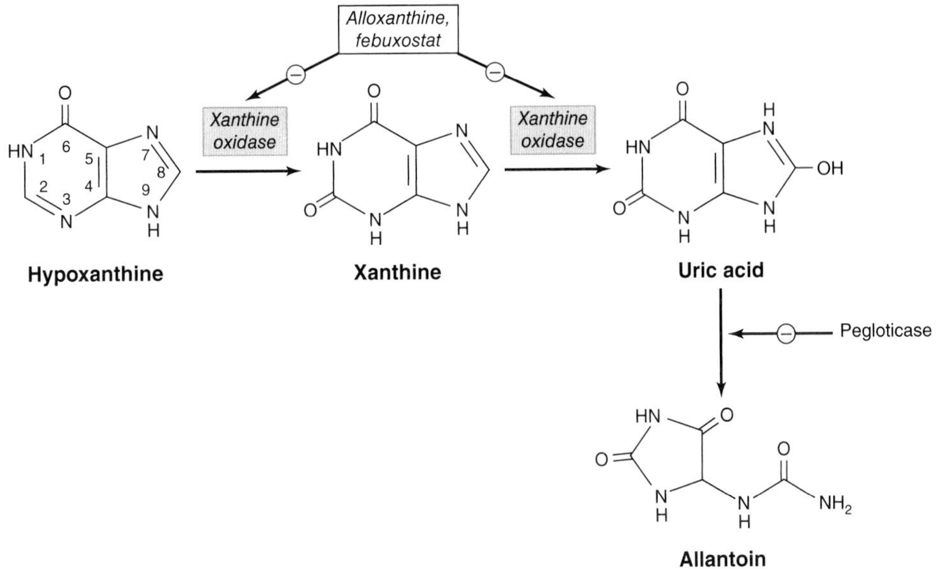

FIGURE 34-5 **The action of xanthine oxidase in uric acid synthesis.** Pharmacologic inhibition of the process occurs by either alloxanthine or febuxostat. Allopurinol is converted to alloxanthine by xanthine oxidase. Pegloticase converts the less soluble uric acid into allantoin, which is a more soluble product that can be excreted in the urine.

Hepatic toxicity and interstitial nephritis have been reported. Isolated cases of exfoliative dermatitis have also been reported. In very rare cases, allopurinol has become bound to the lens, resulting in cataracts. Drug interactions are varied and depend upon the mechanisms. When chemotherapeutic purines (eg, azathioprine) are given concurrently with allopurinol, dosage reductions must be made because their metabolism may be reduced, increasing active drug levels and risk of toxicity. Allopurinol inhibits the metabolism of probenecid and oral anticoagulants and may increase hepatic iron concentration. Safety in children and during pregnancy has not been established.

Febuxostat is approved for the treatment of chronic hyperuricemia in individuals with gout. Febuxostat is more than 80% absorbed after oral administration. With maximum concentration achieved in roughly 1 hour and a half-life of 4-18 hours, once-daily dosing is effective. Febuxostat is extensively metabolized in the liver. The parent drug and its inactive metabolites appear in the urine, although less than 5% appears as unchanged drug. As with allopurinol, prophylactic treatment with colchicine or NSAIDs should be started at the beginning of febuxostat therapy. The dose equivalence of allopurinol and febuxostat is unknown. The most frequent ADRs of febuxostat are liver function abnormalities, diarrhea, headache, and nausea. Febuxostat is well tolerated in patients with a history of allopurinol intolerance. There does not appear to be an increased risk of cardiovascular events.

Pegloticase

Pegloticase is the newest urate-lowering therapy approved for the treatment of refractory chronic gout. The drug is a recombinant mammalian uricase that is covalently attached to methoxy polyethylene glycol (mPEG) to prolong the circulating half-life and diminish immunogenic response. Uricase converts uric acid to the soluble product allantoin (Figure 34-5). The recommended dosing interval for pegloticase is every 2 weeks administered as an intravenous infusion. The drug acts rapidly, achieving a peak decline in uric acid level within 24-72 hours. Pegloticase has been shown to maintain low urate levels for up to 21 days after a single dose. The drug is highly soluble and can be easily eliminated by the kidney. The serum half-life ranges from 6 to 14 days. As with the xanthine oxidase inhibitors, gout flare can occur, especially during the first 3-6 months of pegloticase treatment, requiring prophylaxis with NSAIDs or colchicine. Large numbers of patients show immune responses to pegloticase. The presence of anti-pegloticase antibodies is associated with shortened circulating half-life, loss of response (leading to a rise in plasma urate), and a higher rate of infusion reactions and anaphylaxis. Nephrolithiasis, arthralgia, muscle spasm, headache, anemia, and nausea may occur. Other less frequent ADRs include upper respiratory and urinary tract infections, peripheral edema, and diarrhea. There is some concern for hemolytic anemia in patients with glucose-6-phosphate dehydrogenase deficiency because of the formation of hydrogen peroxide by uricase; therefore, pegloticase should be avoided in these individuals.

Interleukin-1 Inhibitors

Drugs targeting the IL-1 pathway (anakinra, canakinumab, rilonacept) that were previously discussed for their use in inflammatory rheumatic diseases may also be used in the treatment of gout. Although data are limited, these agents may provide a promising treatment option for acute gout in individuals who are refractory to traditional therapies like NSAIDs or colchicine or in those for whom these agents are contraindicated. IL-1 inhibitors may provide rapid and sustained pain relief during acute gouty flares and their use is being evaluated for prevention of gout flares while initiating urate-lowering therapy.

REHABILITATION RELEVANCE

The drug classes discussed in this chapter have a high impact and strong association with physical therapy practice. Many patients receiving physical therapy are taking these drugs. Several of these drug classes increase function by minimizing musculoskeletal pain. Some drug classes retard the rate of functional loss by inhibiting the pathophysiologic processes of immune-mediated rheumatic diseases. An important point for the therapist to remember is that the analgesic and/or anti-inflammatory effects of many of these drugs are maximized at peak plasma levels. Thus, if the clinician is familiar with the pharmacokinetic profiles of these drugs, therapy appointment times scheduled around the expected peak plasma levels may decrease pain, improve function, and increase participation during therapy. Clinical studies have demonstrated that combining drug therapy with rehabilitation optimizes functional improvements and decreases pain. These functional improvements may decrease length of hospital stay, shorten the time to return to work, or delay or decrease disability in people with chronic rheumatic autoimmune-mediated diseases. These drugs are among those with the highest potential for improving rehabilitation outcomes. No other drug classes are likely to have such a significant influence on musculoskeletal function. The ADRs and risks highlighted below are those that have both a significant effect on physical therapy outcomes and are common to more than one drug. (For the common ADRs associated with glucocorticoids, see Chapter 23.)

- Many of the DMARDs **increase infection risk**, especially in the respiratory and urinary tracts. There is also a potential for severe life-threatening systemic bacterial, viral, or fungal opportunistic infections. Clinicians should consider this potential when scheduling these patients for physical therapy sessions and reschedule when either the patient or the therapist is ill.
- Multiple classes of DMARDs increase the risk of **leukopenia**, **anemia**, and **thrombocytopenia**. Therapists should review hematologic values prior to therapy sessions (or ask patients of known values, if not available in the patient's

medical record). Leukopenia may be the underlying mechanism for increased infection risk discussed above. Anemia may result in a clinically relevant decrease in oxygen-carrying capacity of the blood. Aerobic interventions and goals should be reduced and hemoglobin and hematocrit levels closely monitored. Thrombocytopenia may increase the risk of bleeding, which will be exacerbated with concurrent administration of aspirin or the nonselective NSAIDs. Patients should be monitored for excessive bleeding that can manifest in many ways, including, but not limited to severe bruising, prolonged nosebleeds, bleeding gums, coughing up blood, passing blood in urine or stool, or hemarthrosis.

- **Gastrointestinal distress** and **ulceration** are increased with aspirin and the nonselective NSAIDs.
- **Bleeding** as a result of GI ulcerations or within the vasculature is also increased with the nonselective NSAIDs, although aspirin carries the highest risk due to the irreversible inhibition of platelet COX-1. Bleeding risk is increased when patients take multiple agents or with anticoagulants (eg, warfarin). This risk is especially relevant since aspirin and many of the nonselective NSAIDs are available over-the-counter. Therapists should review the accuracy of patients' medication lists to determine potential risk and consult the patient's primary care provider in the context of relevant presenting signs and symptoms.
- There is an **increased risk of heart attack**, **stroke**, and **peripheral thrombosis** in individuals taking COX-2 selective inhibitors, though this risk is also present for the nonselective NSAIDs. Careful monitoring for clinical manifestations of these events is prudent. In addition, therapists should continue to promote and use nonpharmacologic interventions to decrease pain and inflammation, which increases the potential to lower the total pharmacological armamentarium.
- Common drugs for gout—colchicine and allopurinol—may cause **peripheral neuropathy**. Because patients may be taking these drugs for extended periods of time, examination for peripheral sensory or motor deficits should be assessed more frequently. If deficits are suspected to be drug-associated, the referring or prescribing healthcare provider should be informed.

CASE CONCLUSION

The physical therapist recognized several classic rheumatoid arthritic deformities in T.C.'s wrists and hands. T.C.'s complaint of prolonged morning joint stiffness, the "bogginess" at his wrist joints suggestive of synovitis, and symmetrical joint involvement are also characteristic of RA. While RA affecting the knees is slightly less common, and T.C.'s knee symptoms may be osteoarthritic in nature, the therapist appreciated the need for T.C. to get a medical diagnosis. The physical therapist carefully explained to T.C. that his knee symptoms might be related to

his wrist and hand symptoms and deformities. She expressed her concerns that self-medication may be alleviating some of his pain and inflammation, but that an accurate diagnosis might allow more appropriate and potentially more effective pharmacologic intervention. If testing confirmed a diagnosis of rheumatoid arthritis, T.C. could start taking DMARDs to treat the autoimmune disease and potentially slow or halt the progression of his joint deformities.

CHAPTER 34 QUESTIONS

1. Which of the following drugs is an irreversible inhibitor of cyclooxygenase?

    a. Aspirin
    b. Ibuprofen
    c. Acetaminophen
    d. Allopurinol

2. Which of the following drugs is a nonsteroidal anti-inflammatory drug that is clinically used as an analgesic?

    a. Aspirin
    b. Ketorolac
    c. Celecoxib
    d. Acetaminophen

3. Which of the following drugs is a selective type 2 cyclo-oxygenase inhibitor?

    a. Cyclosporine
    b. Ketorolac
    c. Celecoxib
    d. Probenecid

4. Which of the following drugs is a fusion protein that binds to tumor necrosis factor-alpha?

    a. Adalimumab
    b. Rituximab
    c. Certolizumab
    d. Etanercept

5. Which of the following is a Fab fragment of a monoclonal antibody that binds to TNF-α?

    a. Certolizumab
    b. Cyclosporine
    c. Adalimumab
    d. Etanercept

6. Which of the following drugs suppresses inflammation by increasing adenosine levels?

    a. Leflunomide
    b. Methotrexate
    c. Celecoxib
    d. Cyclosporine

7. Which of the following drugs inhibits uric acid reabsorption from the proximal renal tubule?

    a. Allopurinol
    b. Colchicine
    c. Probenecid
    d. Pegloticase

8. Which of the following nonsteroidal anti-inflammatory drugs has a half-life that would allow for once-a-day dosing?

    a. Indomethacin
    b. Ibuprofen
    c. Diclofenac
    d. Piroxicam

9. Which of the following drugs does *not* have anti-inflammatory effects?

    a. Acetaminophen
    b. Aspirin
    c. Celecoxib
    d. Naproxen

10. Which of the following drugs is a monoclonal antibody that binds to the cluster of differentiation (CD) on B lymphocytes and results in apoptosis of these cells?

    a. Adalimumab
    b. Rituximab
    c. Etanercept
    d. Infliximab

Drugs Affecting the Respiratory System

CASE STUDY

L.B. is a 54-year-old man who works in the shipping and receiving department at a state university. His job entails transporting mail and equipment to and from various locations around the campus. Two days ago, he strained his back while moving several boxes. Because the pain has prevented him from doing his job, L.B. was referred to the university-associated rehabilitation clinic. His medical chart states that he had asthma in childhood, and that he is a current smoker with a 30-pack-year history of smoking. His medication includes nadolol combined with bendroflumethiazide (Corzide) for essential hypertension and ipratropium combined with albuterol (Combivent) as needed for dyspnea. At the initial physical therapy evaluation, L.B.'s blood pressure and heart rate were 138/82 mm Hg and 79 bpm, respectively. The therapist chose to use the university pool, kept at 34°C, to initiate functional pain-reduced movement. A small pool to the side of the main pool has a shallow end with a depth of 2-4 ft and a deeper end at 6-10 ft. On his way from the rehabilitation clinic to the pool, the therapist observed L.B. smoking a cigarette. The

therapist wanted to start the treatment session with spinal traction, using the buoyancy of the water with strategic placement of weights. In the shallow end of the pool, the therapist attached a float to the L.B.'s upper chest under his axillae to keep his head out of the water. Next, the therapist attached a 4-kg weight to each ankle and gently guided the patient toward the deeper end of the pool until his feet did not touch the bottom. The therapist asked L.B. to relax, allowing the weight on the ankles to provide gentle spinal traction. After 10 minutes, the patient stated that the pain decreased and the therapist instructed him to begin slowly walking in place. Approximately 4 minutes into this part of the therapy, L.B. complains of shortness of breath. He becomes pale and frantically attempts to reach the shallow end of the pool. The therapist quickly assists L.B. to the side of the pool and a therapist's aide helps get him out of the water. Once safely at the edge of the pool, the therapist takes his vital signs; blood pressure and heart rate are 153/90 mm Hg and 89 bpm, respectively.

REHABILITATION FOCUS

Patients may be taking over-the-counter (OTC) drugs for respiratory disorders without consulting healthcare professionals, and some of these drugs can have significant interactions with rehabilitation therapy. For example, decongestants such as oxymetazoline, a common nasal spray, can increase blood pressure and cardiac workload. Clinically, these effects may manifest as exertional angina during aerobic activities or painful procedures. In addition, decongestants may cause

orthostatic hypotension, though this adverse effect is more common with opioid antitussives and antihistamines. Opioid antitussives may also depress respiratory drive, resulting in hypercapnia during aerobic activity. Last, antihistamines and opioid antitussives also cause sedation, which may impair psychomotor skills and increase risk of falls.

Individuals with obstructive airway disorders are often in rehabilitation. Some may be in rehabilitation for nonpulmonary therapy, but their pulmonary disorders and the drugs used to treat them can have significant effects on rehabilitation outcomes.

Other patients will be in pulmonary rehabilitation programs for obstructive airway disorders. Exercise therapy has proven beneficial in patients with chronic obstructive pulmonary disease (COPD). There is less clear evidence for the benefits of exercise therapy in individuals with asthma. Some asthmatics experience exercise-induced bronchospasm for which medication prior to aerobic activity may be beneficial. These patients may also benefit from resistance exercises to improve aerobic conditioning.

Drugs used to treat COPD reduce the effort of respiration and improve aerobic capacity during treatment sessions. When developing aerobic programs, physical therapists should understand the pharmacokinetics of inhaled short-acting bronchodilators, specifically the time to peak bronchodilation in order to optimize patient performance. Patients should also be educated regarding the benefits of maintaining their respiratory prescription regimen for rehabilitation activities.

Optimal pulmonary rehabilitation programs include exercise therapy, patient education, and psychosocial/behavioral training. These programs use a combination of classes provided in group settings as well as individualized exercise training. The same drugs that benefit the person with COPD may also precipitate adverse drug reactions (ADRs) during the rehabilitation process. Bronchodilators such as β_2 agonists and methylxanthines can cause cardiac disturbances, which are exacerbated during aerobic activities in rehabilitation. When administered systemically, airway anti-inflammatory glucocorticoids may result in insulin resistance. Administration for prolonged periods may result in osteoporosis.

BACKGROUND

The respiratory tract may be divided into upper and lower portions. The upper portion consists of the nose, sinuses, oropharynx, and larynx. The lower portion comprises the trachea and lungs. Disorders and drug therapy of the upper respiratory system differ from those of the lower respiratory tract.

Most disorders of the upper respiratory tract are infections (eg, uncomplicated viral rhinosinusitis and pharyngitis) and seasonal allergies (eg, allergic rhinoconjunctivitis). Chapter 27 discusses treatment of infections in all parts of the respiratory tract. For the most part, these dysfunctions are self-limiting and drug classes used to treat them may be obtained without a prescription (ie, OTC). Disorders of the lower respiratory tract may be broadly classified as parenchymal infections (eg, pneumonia) and obstructive airway (bronchial) conditions. In general, the latter disorders limit expiratory airflow.

Obstructive airway conditions are divided into bronchial asthma, which is characterized by acute episodes, and chronic obstructive airway disorders—COPD. Classic terminology has subdivided COPD into chronic bronchitis, emphysema, bronchiectasis, and cystic fibrosis. The Global Initiative for Chronic Obstructive Lung Disease (GOLD) broadly defines COPD as a common preventable and treatable disease characterized by airflow limitation that is usually progressive and associated with enhanced chronic inflammation in the airways and lungs in response to noxious particles and gases. Emphysema is described as chronic airflow limitation due to small airway disease and parenchymal destruction. Chronic bronchitis is manifested by cough and sputum production for at least 3 months in each of 2 consecutive years that may precede or follow the development of airflow limitation.

DISORDERS OF THE UPPER RESPIRATORY TRACT

Common manifestations of upper respiratory tract dysfunctions include vasodilation and mucus and watery discharge from the nose. These effects are mediated in part through histamine and other substances released from mast cells. Mast cells are important "gate-keeper" cells concentrated in the skin and other tissues near external body surfaces. Histamine is produced from the amino acid histidine and is stored in vesicles within mast cells. Four histamine receptor subtypes are designated H_1-H_4. The H_1 receptors mediate mucus discharge and vasodilation; H_2 receptors are important in gastric acid secretion (Chapter 36); H_3 receptors are found in the central nervous system (CNS); H_4 receptors likely modulate inflammatory reactions by chemotactic effects on eosinophils and mast cells. Secretion of histamine and other mast cell mediators causes vasodilation and increased permeability of the nasal vasculature, leading to the nasal congestion and "runny nose" commonly associated with seasonal allergies and viral infections. Drugs used to treat these manifestations include H_1 antihistamines, which decrease mucus production, vasodilation, and permeability and nasal decongestants, which decrease vasodilation.

Bronchial congestion and excessive mucus production are additional manifestations frequently associated with viral infections. Antitussives may suppress coughing, while expectorants may assist in clearance of mucus from larger airways. Figure 35-1 outlines major drug classes used in the treatment of upper respiratory tract disorders. Many of the OTC drugs for these conditions are presented in Table 35-1.

DRUGS USED IN UPPER RESPIRATORY TRACT DISORDERS

Antihistamines

Two major subgroups or "generations" of H_1 blockers have been developed (Table 35-1). Older members of the first-generation agents, typified by **diphenhydramine**, are highly sedating agents with significant muscarinic receptor-blocking effects. **Chlorpheniramine**, the prototype of a newer subgroup of first-generation agents, is less sedating and has fewer autonomic effects. The second-generation H_1 blockers, typified by **fexofenadine**, **loratadine**, and **cetirizine**, are far less lipid soluble than first-generation agents, and are largely free of sedative and autonomic effects. Because they have been developed for use in chronic conditions, all H_1 blockers are active by the oral route. Most are metabolized extensively in the liver. Half-lives of the

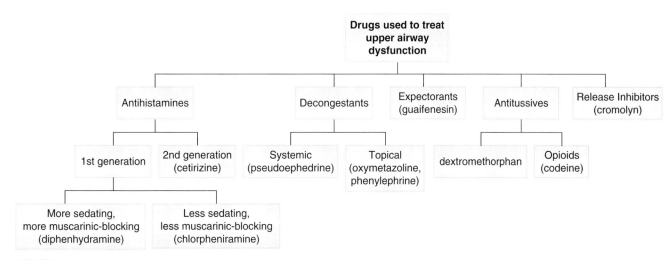

FIGURE 35-1 Broad classification of drugs used to treat upper airway dysfunction includes antihistamines (histamine type 1 receptor antagonists; H$_1$ blockers), decongestants, expectorants, antitussives, and release inhibitors. Antihistamines are divided into first and second generations. Decongestants include those taken systemically and those applied topically to the nasal mucosa. Antitussives include dextromethorphan and opioid analgesics with addictive properties. Prototype drugs are in parentheses.

TABLE 35-1 Ingredients of known efficacy for select over-the-counter (OTC) drug classes.

OTC Category	Generic Drug (Brand Name Example)	Comments
Allergy and "cold" preparations	cetirizine (Zyrtec) chlorpheniramine (Chlor-Trimeton) clemastine (Tavist Allergy, Dayhist Allergy 12-h relief) diphenhydramine (Benadryl Allergy) fexofenadine (Allegra) loratadine (Alavert, Claritin)	Antihistamines alone relieve most symptoms associated with allergic rhinitis or hay fever. Chlorpheniramine and clemastine cause less drowsiness than diphenhydramine. Occasionally, symptoms unrelieved by antihistamines respond to the addition of a sympathomimetic. Avoid use in children under 2 yr of age. Avoid combination with other sedatives or alcohol because sedative effects may be potentiated. Use caution when driving or operating machinery.
Decongestants, topical (intranasal)	oxymetazoline (Afrin) phenylephrine (Neo-Synephrine)	Topical sympathomimetics are effective for acute, temporary management of rhinorrhea associated with common colds and allergies. Oxymetazoline is long-acting, though phenylephrine is equally effective. Topical decongestants should not be used for longer than 3 days to prevent rebound nasal congestion.
Decongestants, systemic	phenylephrine (Sudafed PE) pseudoephedrine (Sudafed)[1]	Orally administered decongestants are often combined with other drugs in OTC cold and seasonal allergy formulations. Systemic administration often results in longer duration of action, but also increases the incidence of adverse effects.
Antitussives	codeine dextromethorphan (Robitussin 12-h cough) hydrocodone	Codeine and hydrocodone have been rescheduled to Schedule II and are not available OTC. Dextromethorphan is a nonanalgesic nonaddicting congener of levorphanol. Dextromethorphan is often used with antihistamines, decongestants, and expectorants in combination products.
Expectorants	guaifenesin (Mucinex)	The only OTC expectorant recognized as safe and effective by the FDA. Often used with antihistamines, decongestants, and antitussives in combination products.
Release Inhibitors	cromolyn (NasalCrom) nedocromil (Alocril)	Stabilizes mast cells and prevents degranulation.

FDA, Food and Drug Administration.

[1]Pseudoephedrine no longer available OTC; available "behind the counter" or with prescription.

older H_1 blockers vary from 4 to 12 hours, whereas those of most second-generation agents are 12-24 hours.

H_1 blockers are competitive antagonists or inverse agonists at the H_1 receptor. Therefore, these drugs have no effect on histamine release from storage sites and are more effective if given *before* histamine release occurs. Because their chemical structure closely resembles that of muscarinic antagonists and alpha (α) adrenoceptor antagonists, many first-generation agents are potent pharmacologic inhibitors at these autonomic receptors. A few agents also block serotonin receptors. Most of the older first-generation agents are sedating, and some have anti-motion sickness effects. Several first-generation H_1 blockers are potent local anesthetics. Cetirizine and several other second-generation H_1 blockers inhibit mast cell release of histamine and several other mediators of inflammation by a mechanism not fully understood, but do not involve blockade of H_1 receptors. H_1-blocking drugs have negligible antagonistic effects at H_2 receptors (Chapter 36).

H_1 blockers have major applications in treating type 1 hypersensitivity responses such as hay fever and urticaria. These immediate allergic responses are caused by antigens acting on IgE antibody-sensitized mast cells. H_1 blockers are often formulated into OTC combination preparations, and are listed in Table 35-1 under "allergy and cold preparations." **Scopolamine**, **meclizine**, **promethazine** and several other drugs in this class are used in the treatment of motion sickness. Diphenhydramine is also used for management of chemotherapy-induced vomiting.

Sedation and antimuscarinic effects such as dry mouth and blurred vision occur with some first-generation drugs, especially diphenhydramine, doxylamine, and promethazine. Because of their highly anticholinergic effects, it has been recommended that older adults avoid use of the first-generation antihistamines. For the second-generation agents, sedation is much less common partly due to less complete distribution into the CNS. Drugs with α adrenoceptor-blocking actions may cause orthostatic hypotension.

When older antihistamines are taken with drugs that cause sedation (eg, benzodiazepines and alcohol), the sedative effects are additive. If drugs that inhibit hepatic metabolism are taken concurrently, dangerously high levels of certain antihistamines may result. The sedative effect of older antihistamines has also been exploited therapeutically (eg, often used as hypnotics in institutions and in OTC sleep aids).

Decongestants

Nasal decongestants are used to ease the discomfort of hay fever and, to a lesser extent, the common cold. These drugs are agonists at α adrenoceptors. Blood vessels of the nasal mucosa express a high density of $α_1$ receptors. Receptor stimulation causes vasoconstriction with resultant decreased volume of inflamed nasal mucosa. (Chapters 4 and 6 discuss α adrenoceptors and physiologic effects of their stimulation).

Nasal decongestants may be classified by whether they are delivered systemically or topically (Figure 35-1). Several OTC formulations are available (Table 35-1). **Ephedrine** was the first orally active sympathomimetic drug. Despite its long history of use for conditions such as asthma, obesity, and nasal congestion, ephedrine has not been extensively studied in humans. Use of the drug is associated with significant cardiac and nervous system adverse effects. **Pseudoephedrine**, one of four ephedrine enantiomers, is used in orally administered nasal decongestants. Although oral versus topical administration is convenient and associated with a longer duration of action, this route provides lower local drug concentration in the nasal mucosa with greater potential for cardiac and CNS adverse effects. Restrictions on the sale of pseudoephedrine-containing products have been implemented because pseudoephedrine is a precursor in the illicit manufacture of methamphetamine. **Oxymetazoline**, an $α_1$ and $α_{2A}$ agonist, is classified as a long-acting topical decongestant. **Phenylephrine**, an $α_1$ agonist, can be taken orally or topically applied as a nasal spray.

Ephedrine, pseudoephedrine, and phenylephrine have many sympathomimetic effects. Pseudoephedrine also activates β receptors, which probably accounts for its earlier use in asthma. Because pseudoephedrine gains access to the CNS, it is a mild stimulant. The duration of action of these drugs is dependent on the individual compound and the route of administration.

The adverse effects of adrenoceptor agonists are primarily extensions of their pharmacologic effects in the cardiovascular system and CNS (Chapter 6). Ephedrine is one of the active components of "ma-huang," a popular herbal supplement taken for appetite suppression and weight reduction. Ingestion of ephedrine contained in ma-huang has been associated with hypertension, arrhythmias, myocardial infarction, and stroke. Repeated topical use of nasal decongestants causes rebound hyperemia—an *increase* in blood flow (and symptomatic congestion) to the nasal mucous membranes. High local drug concentrations may result in ischemic changes in nasal membranes, probably due to vasoconstriction of nutrient arteries. Cardiovascular effects include elevated blood pressure and resulting increased cardiac workload. The latter may result in manifestations of cardiac ischemia such as angina pectoris. Stimulatory CNS effects may present as insomnia, nervousness, tremor, and anxiety. When taken in large doses, oxymetazoline may cause hypotension through activation of $α_{2A}$ receptors.

Antitussives and Expectorants

Natural opioids and their derivatives suppress the cough center in the medulla oblongata. Drug suppression increases the stimulatory threshold required to initiate the coughing reflex. **Codeine** and **hydrocodone** are opioids that may be included in antitussive formulations. Because these drugs are listed in Schedule II by the Drug Enforcement Agency, they require a prescription by a provider with a DEA license. (Detailed discussion of opiates is in Chapter 20.) **Dextromethorphan**, an opioid derivative, lacks direct analgesic and addictive properties. However, this derivative increases the analgesic properties of morphine. **Guaifenesin** is the most common expectorant formulated in both OTC and prescription medications.

Guaifenesin assists expectoration of respiratory mucus by stimulating respiratory tract secretion, resulting in increased airway fluid volume and decreased mucus viscosity. Antitussives and expectorants may be formulated alone, with each other, or in combinations with decongestants or antihistamines (Table 35-1). Except for the opioids, many are available OTC.

Adverse effects of opioids include decreased respiratory drive due to inhibition of brainstem respiratory mechanisms. This may result in hypercapnia, which may not be tolerated in patients with obstructive airway disorders. Dextromethorphan can also cause gastrointestinal (GI) distress. Dextromethorphan has recently received attention as a drug of abuse among adolescents due to its hallucinogenic effects at dosages significantly exceeding that of the recommended antitussive dose. Hallucinogenic effects may result from noncompetitive inhibition of central N-methyl-D-aspartate receptors (which are also antagonized by phencyclidine or "PCP"; Chapter 21). Additional toxic manifestations of dextromethorphan include tachycardia, hypertension, lethargy, psychomotor delay, and seizures. Dextromethorphan inhibits biotransformation of some monoamine oxidase inhibitors, increasing the potential of ADRs with concurrent administration of these drugs (Chapter 19). Guaifenesin may cause GI distress, dizziness, and drowsiness.

Release Inhibitors

Cromolyn (disodium cromoglycate) and **nedocromil** are unusual chemicals. When insufflated topically into the nasal passages or swallowed, these drugs have minimal systemic absorption because they are extremely insoluble. Because they are not absorbed from the site of administration, cromolyn and nedocromil have only local effects. Although originally developed and used for asthma management, the primary current indications are allergic rhinoconjunctivitis.

Their precise mechanism of action is poorly understood, but these agents are thought to act by inhibiting mast cell degranulation and subsequent inflammation. As such, these drugs are effective for *prophylaxis* of inflammation. When administered orally, cromolyn has some efficacy in preventing food allergy. Oral administration is also used in the treatment of systemic mastocytosis, where these drugs help control abdominal cramping and diarrhea due to an overabundance of mast cells in the GI mucosa.

Except for rare instances of drug allergy, these drugs demonstrate minimal ADRs when nasally insufflated or swallowed.

PATHOPHYSIOLOGY OF OBSTRUCTIVE AIRWAY DISORDERS

Obstructive airway disorders include those traditionally considered under the umbrella term of COPD (chronic bronchitis, emphysema, and bronchiectasis) as well as asthma. The term asthma has been applied to a variety of disorders that share clinical features, but have distinct pathophysiologic mechanisms. The classic asthma model is a chronic episodic bronchospastic disorder characterized by an early-phase response and a late-phase response. The early phase begins 15-45 minutes following the binding of an allergen to IgE bound to mast cells in the airway mucosa (Figure 35-2). Subsequent release of eicosanoids and other inflammatory mediators results in the initial *reversible* bronchospasm, vasodilation, and increased vascular permeability. Bronchospasm decreases the airway diameter and limits expiratory airflow. Mediators released during the early phase also result in a later influx of additional inflammatory cells.

The late-phase response begins 4-8 hours after allergen exposure. The hallmark of this phase is airway inflammation with interstitial airway edema, invasion of inflammatory cells, epithelial injury with decreased mucociliary function, and *sustained* bronchoconstriction. This late phase response is partly due to cytokines produced by T_H2 cells that are derived from CD4$^+$ T cells (Figure 35-3). These T cells are thought to play an essential role in the increased expression of IgE and interleukins (eg, IL5 and IL13), increased mucus production, and influx of inflammatory cells such as eosinophils. The combination of these processes that occurs during the late-phase response further decreases airway diameter and limits expiratory airflow. Both the early and late phases are associated with increased airway responsiveness to subsequent allergen challenges. Examples of allergen triggers that initiate the complex immunologic response include house dust mites, cockroach detritus, animal dander, pollens, and molds.

There are major limitations to the classic asthma model previously described. Foremost, the pathogenesis includes many pathways and mechanisms *other than* production of IgE and activation of mast cell degranulation. There are also many well-recognized *nonallergen* triggers that provoke asthmatic responses, including viral respiratory tract infections, inhaled irritants (eg, smoke), strong emotions, exercise, and cold air. Last, the bronchoconstriction characteristic of an asthmatic attack also results from the direct effect of mediators on cholinergic neural pathways (Figure 35-4).

For COPD, common characteristics include chronic and repeated airway obstruction and inflammation. The main risk factor for COPD is tobacco smoking, but other environmental exposures may contribute. Emphysema is characterized by a loss of lung elasticity and parenchymal (alveoli and alveolar walls) destruction. The former inhibits expiratory airflow and the latter results in a loss of surface area available for gas exchange. In contrast, chronic bronchitis is caused by inflammation that results in submucosal hyperplasia and edema, along with excessive mucus secretion. Airway narrowing and mucus plugs inhibit expiratory airflow. Bronchiectasis is a chronic condition resulting from repeated cycles of bacterial infection and subsequent inflammation. This process destroys the elastic support of the airways, anatomically distorting medium-sized bronchi and bronchioles. Secretions that

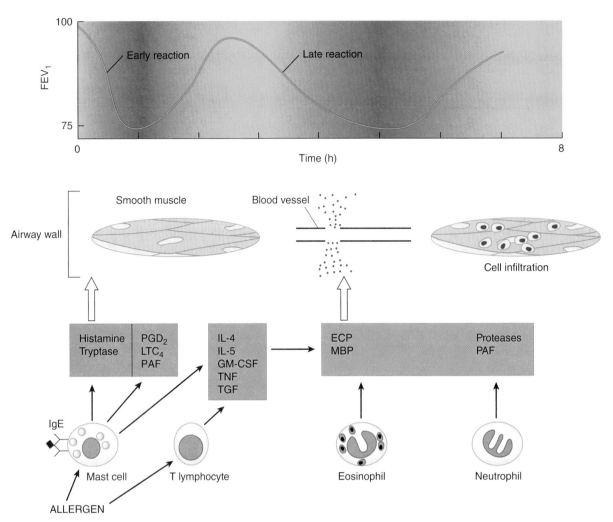

FIGURE 35-2 **Conceptual model for the immunopathogenesis of asthma.** Exposure to allergen causes synthesis of IgE, which binds to mast cells in the airway mucosa. On re-exposure to allergen, antigen-antibody interaction on the surfaces of mast cells triggers release of mediators of anaphylaxis: histamine, tryptase, prostaglandin D2 (PGD_2), leukotriene (LT) C_4, and platelet-activating factor (PAF). These agents provoke airway smooth muscle contraction, causing the immediate fall in forced expiratory volume in 1 second (FEV_1). Re-exposure to allergen causes synthesis and release of a variety of cytokines: interleukins (IL) 4 and 5, granulocyte-macrophage colony-stimulating factor (GM-CSF), tumor necrosis factor (TNF), and tissue growth factor (TGF) from T cells and mast cells. These cytokines in turn attract and activate eosinophils and neutrophils, whose products include eosinophil cationic protein (ECP), major basic protein (MBP), proteases, and platelet-activating factor. These mediators cause the smooth muscle contraction, mucus hypersecretion, and edema (ie, spasm, secretions, and swelling) as well as the increased bronchial reactivity associated with the late asthmatic response, indicated by a second fall in FEV_1 3-6 hours after the exposure.

collect in the dilated and distorted airways become chronically infected. Mucus plugs form that decrease expiratory airflow.

DRUGS USED IN OBSTRUCTIVE LUNG DISEASES

The drug classes used in the treatment of asthma and other obstructive airway disorders are presented in Figure 35-5. Therapeutic interventions may be divided into two categories: "short-term relievers" and "long-term controllers." The former drugs *relieve* acute bronchospasm associated with obstructive airway diseases, and the latter drugs minimize—or,

control—the associated inflammation to decrease the frequency of subsequent acute bronchospastic attacks.

Acute bronchospasm can usually be treated promptly and effectively with bronchodilators. Short-acting beta$_2$ (β_2)-selective agonists and muscarinic antagonists are available for this indication. Late response inflammation and bronchial hyper-reactivity can be treated with inhaled glucocorticoids, theophylline and its derivatives, roflumilast, and leukotriene antagonists. These drugs either inhibit release of mediators from mast cells and other inflammatory cells or block their effects. The leukotriene antagonists may have inhibitory effects on both bronchoconstriction and inflammation, but are prescribed only for prophylaxis due to the oral route of administration and

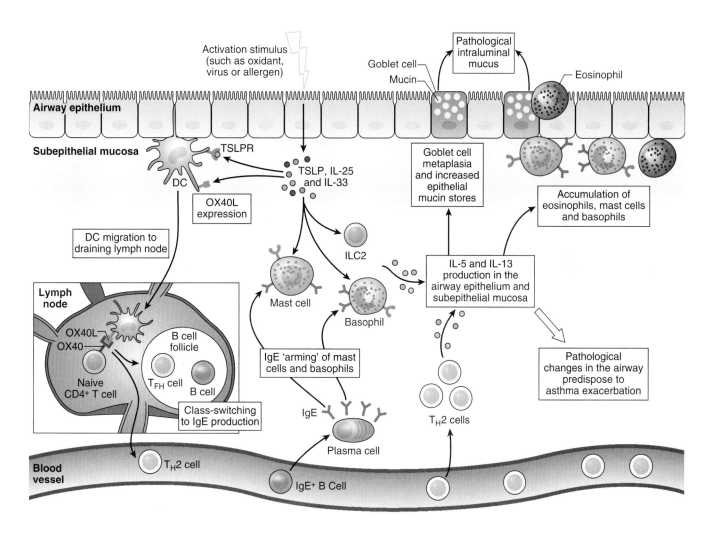

FIGURE 35-3 **Inflammatory mechanism of asthma.** Airway epithelial cells exposed to activation stimuli (allergens, viruses, and irritants) release cytokines that promote dendritic cell (DC) mobilization to draining lymph nodes, where they present antigens and thereby activate naive CD4 T cells. These T cells then induce B-cell class switching and maturation into plasma cells, which produce IgE. T$_H$2 cells also migrate into the airway subepithelial mucosa, where they release inflammatory cytokines such as IL-5 and IL-13, which induce goblet cell metaplasia and mucus production, and act as a chemokine for eosinophils, mast cells, and basophils. Unbound IgE secreted by plasma cells binds the Fcε-R1 receptor on submucosal mast cells and basophils and, when crosslinked by an antigen, induces the release of preformed mediators such as histamine and leukotrienes, as well as the release of inflammatory cytokines.

resulting delayed onset of action. In maintenance therapy, drugs in multiple classes are used. For example, monoclonal antibodies directed against IgE and the IL-5 system have a significant role in chronic maintenance therapy.

BRONCHODILATOR DRUGS

β-Adrenoceptor Agonists

The β$_2$-selective agonists are the most important drugs used to reverse asthmatic bronchoconstriction. In the United States, **albuterol**, **terbutaline**, **metaproterenol**, and **pirbuterol** are the key short-acting β$_2$ agonists. These drugs should be used only for acute episodes of bronchospasm—*not* for prophylaxis. In contrast, long-acting and ultra-long acting β$_2$ agonists

are used for prophylaxis (not acute relief) of bronchospasm because they are effective in improving asthmatic control when taken regularly. **Salmeterol** and **formoterol** are long-acting β$_2$ agonists. **Indacaterol**, **olodaterol**, **vilanterol**, and **bambuterol** are ultra-long acting β$_2$ agonists taken once a day. Because of their potential to mask bronchial inflammation, ultra-long acting drugs are only taken by individuals with asthma if they are concurrently taking inhaled glucocorticoids. However, these agents are used as a monotherapy in COPD. Beta-2 agonists are given almost exclusively by inhalation, usually from a metered dose inhaler (MDI), but occasionally via a nebulizer that dispenses the drug in the form of a vapor. The inhalational route decreases the systemic dose (and ADRs), while delivering an effective dose locally to the airway smooth muscle.

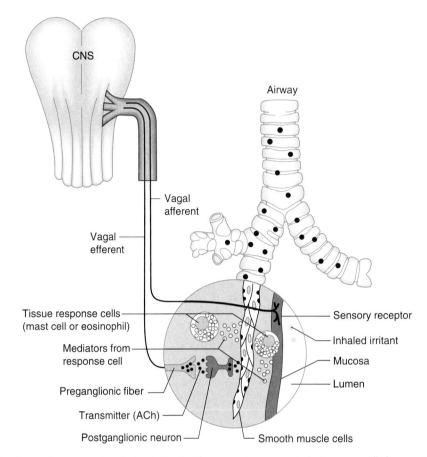

FIGURE 35-4 **Mechanisms of response to inhaled irritants.** The airway is represented microscopically by a cross section of the wall with branching vagal sensory endings lying adjacent to the lumen. Afferent pathways in the vagus nerves travel to the CNS; efferent pathways from the CNS travel to efferent ganglia. Postganglionic fibers release acetylcholine (ACh), which binds to muscarinic receptors on airway smooth muscle. Inhaled materials may provoke bronchoconstriction by several possible mechanisms. First, they may trigger release of chemical mediators from mast cells. Second, they may stimulate afferent receptors to initiate reflex bronchoconstriction or to release tachykinins (eg, substance P) that directly stimulate smooth muscle contraction. CNS, central nervous system.

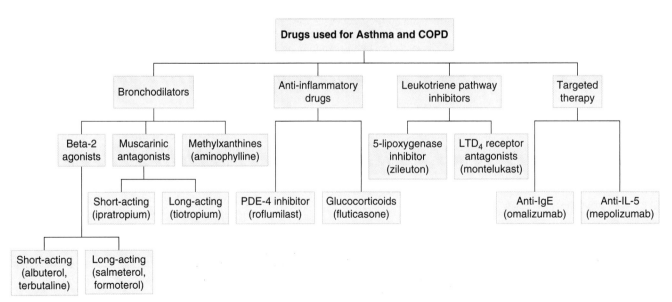

FIGURE 35-5 **Drug classes useful in obstructive airway disorders include bronchodilators (smooth muscle relaxants) and anti-inflammatory drugs.** Bronchodilators include β_2-selective agonists, muscarinic antagonists, and methylxanthines. Anti-inflammatory drugs include phosphodiesterase-4 (PDE-4) inhibitors and glucocorticoids. Leukotriene antagonists have both bronchodilator and anti-inflammatory mechanisms of action. Biologic drugs include monoclonal antibodies directed at IgE and interleukin 5 (IL-5). Prototype drugs are in parentheses.

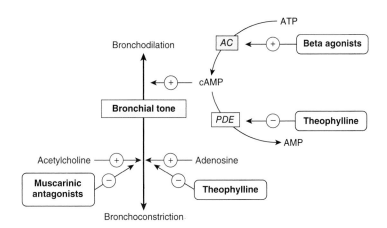

FIGURE 35-6 **Bronchodilation is promoted by cAMP.** Intracellular cAMP concentration can be increased by β-adrenoceptor agonists, which increase the rate of its synthesis by adenylate cyclase (AC), or by phosphodiesterase (PDE) inhibitors such as theophylline, which slow the rate of its degradation. Bronchoconstriction can be inhibited by muscarinic antagonists and possibly by adenosine antagonists such as theophylline.

Detailed discussion of β adrenoceptors and physiologic effects of their stimulation is in Chapters 4 and 6. Briefly, activation of β receptors stimulates adenylate cyclase activity, increasing intracellular cyclic adenosine monophosphate (cAMP) in smooth muscle cells. This causes a decrease in smooth muscle tone and a powerful bronchodilator response (Figure 35-6). Beta-2 agonist preparations are a mixture of R (levo) and S (dextro) isomers. Only the R isomer acts as an agonist on the β_2 receptor. The shorter-acting drugs are hydrophilic, cause maximal bronchodilation within 15 minutes, and have a duration of action of 3-4 hours. The longer acting drugs are more hydrophobic and dissolve in high concentrations into the smooth muscle cell membrane near the beta adrenergic receptor or "moor" next to molecules near the receptor. This allows these drugs to have durations of action of 12 hours (for long-acting agents) or up to 24 hours (for the ultra-long acting agents).

A common ADR of β-adrenergic agonists is skeletal muscle tremor. The β_2 selectivity of these drugs is relative. At high clinical dosage, these agents have significant β_1-receptor mediated cardiac effects. Even when given by inhalation, tachycardia is common. However, the concern that these agents precipitate cardiac arrhythmias appears unsubstantiated. After several days of regular use of short-acting β_2 agonists, loss of responsiveness (ie, tolerance or tachyphylaxis) can be shown. Adverse effects resulting from this tolerance has not been demonstrated in clinical trials. Individuals with COPD and concurrent cardiac disease may have limited benefit from use of these drugs.

Muscarinic Antagonists

For many years, atropine and other naturally occurring belladonna alkaloids were used in the treatment of asthma. Now, **ipratropium**, a quaternary antimuscarinic agent, has replaced these agents. Ipratropium is taken by inhalation via MDI.

Tiotropium, **aclidinium**, and **umeclidinium** are newer, longer-acting analogs also taken by inhalation using a dry powder inhaler (DPI).

Muscarinic antagonists competitively block muscarinic receptors in the airways and effectively prevent bronchoconstriction mediated by vagal discharge (Figures 35-4 and 35-6). These drugs bind to three muscarinic (M) receptor subtypes with equal affinity, but dissociate from M_2 receptors located on presynaptic nerve endings more rapidly compared to the others. This effect means that the drugs do not inhibit the M_2 receptor-mediated inhibition of acetylcholine release.

These drugs only inhibit the parasympathetic role in asthma; they have no effect on the inflammatory aspects of asthma. As such, ipratropium is only useful in one-third to two-thirds of asthmatic patients. For comparison, β_2 agonists are effective in almost all. Therefore, β_2 agonists are usually preferred for acute bronchospasm. However, in COPD, which is often associated with acute episodes of bronchospasm, antimuscarinic agents may be more effective and less toxic than β_2 agonists.

Because ipratropium is delivered directly to the airway and is poorly absorbed, there are minimal systemic effects. When given in excessive dosage, minor atropine-like toxic effects may occur (Chapter 5). In contrast to β_2 agonists, ipratropium does not cause tremors or arrhythmias.

Methylxanthines

The methylxanthines are purine derivatives. Three plant-based methylxanthines provide the stimulant effects of three common beverages: **caffeine** (in coffee), **theophylline** (in tea), and **theobromine** (in cocoa). Theophylline is the only clinically important member of this group. The compound is commonly formulated as aminophylline, the soluble salt complex theophylline-ethylenediamine. Theophylline and its analogs are available in both prompt-release and slow-release oral forms that are eliminated by cytochrome P450 drug-metabolizing enzymes in the liver. Clearance varies with age (highest in young adolescents), smoking status (higher in smokers), and concurrent use of other drugs that inhibit or induce hepatic enzymes.

The methylxanthines inhibit phosphodiesterase (PDE), the enzyme that degrades cAMP to AMP (Figure 35-6), thus increasing cAMP levels. Methylxanthines inhibit several forms of PDE. Inhibition of PDE3 in airway smooth muscle is thought to mediate the bronchodilation effect, while inhibition of PDE4 in inflammatory cells is thought to mediate the anti-inflammatory effect by decreasing release of inflammatory mediators. Methylxanthines also block adenosine receptors in the CNS and isolated airway smooth muscle, but a relationship between this action and the bronchodilating effect has not been clearly established. A proposed additional anti-inflammatory effect of theophylline is increased histone deacetylation of inflammatory genes. Acetylation of these histones is a prerequisite for inflammatory gene transcription. Whether the clinical efficacy of methylxanthines like aminophylline is due to their bronchodilation or anti-inflammatory mechanism of action, or both, is currently still debated.

Although originally developed for both asthma treatment and prophylaxis, theophylline has been replaced by newer drugs for this condition. Accelerating the drug's decline has been the narrow therapeutic index and severe toxicities. However, theophylline is still used clinically in the treatment of COPD. Methylxanthines improve contractility of skeletal muscles, which may decrease fatigue of the diaphragm. These drugs decrease blood viscosity, though the mechanism of action is unknown. Another methylxanthine derivative, **pentoxifylline**, is used in the treatment of intermittent claudication.

Methylxanthines have a narrow therapeutic index. Therapeutic plasma concentrations range from 5 to 20 mg/L, whereas adverse effects begin to occur in some patients when plasma concentrations reach 15-20 mg/L. Common ADRs include GI distress, tremor, and insomnia. Severe nausea and vomiting, hypotension, cardiac arrhythmias, and convulsions may result from overdose. Very large overdoses (eg, in suicide attempts) are potentially lethal because of arrhythmias and convulsions.

ANTI-INFLAMMATORY DRUGS

Phosphodiesterase Type-4 Inhibitors

In an attempt to reduce toxicity while maintaining therapeutic efficacy, many nonmethylxanthine PDE inhibitors were investigated. **Roflumilast** is a selective PDE-4 inhibitor that increases inflammatory cell intracellular cAMP levels, which reduces cytokine release, and the subsequent infiltration of inflammatory cells into bronchial tissues. Roflumilast also attenuates bronchial tissue fibrotic remodeling and decreases mucociliary dysfunction. Roflumilast is approved for treatment of COPD, but not for asthma. The drug has been shown

to improve pulmonary function and decrease the frequency of moderate or severe exacerbations. Roflumilast has a wider therapeutic index than theophylline and monitoring is not required. Significant ADRs include diarrhea, nausea, headache, and dizziness. Some individuals have noted weight loss while using the drug.

Glucocorticoids

For an expanded discussion of the mechanism of action, clinical uses, and systemic toxicities of glucocorticoids, see Chapter 23.

All glucocorticoids are potentially beneficial in severe asthma. However, because of their toxicity, systemic (oral) glucocorticoids are used chronically only if other drug delivery options are unsuccessful. However inhaled administration of glucocorticoids (eg, **beclomethasone, budesonide, flunisolide, fluticasone, mometasone, ciclesonide**) is relatively safe because systemic absorption is limited. Ciclesonide is a prodrug activated by bronchial esterases that is comparably effective to other inhaled glucocorticoids. When systemically absorbed, ciclesonide binds tightly to plasma proteins until metabolism, which further limits systemic ADRs when this drug is administered via inhalation.

Inhaled glucocorticoids have become common first-line therapy for individuals with moderate to severe asthma. Inhaled glucocorticoids are now considered appropriate (even for children) in most cases of moderate asthma that are not fully responsive to inhaled β_2 agonists. Research suggests that early use of glucocorticoids may prevent the severe, progressive inflammatory changes characteristic of long-standing asthma. This is a shift from earlier beliefs that glucocorticoids should be used only in severe refractory asthma. In such cases of severe asthma, patients are usually hospitalized and stabilized on daily systemic **prednisone** and then switched to inhaled or alternate-day oral therapy before discharge. In status asthmaticus (acute severe bronchospasm unresponsive to usual bronchodilator medications), intravenous glucocorticoids include **prednisolone** (the active metabolite of prednisone) and **hydrocortisone**. These parenteral steroids are lifesaving and apparently act more promptly than in ordinary asthma. Their mechanism of action in this condition is not fully understood.

Figure 35-7 illustrates part of the anti-inflammatory mechanism of action for glucocorticoids. Glucocorticoids inhibit phospholipase A_2, reducing the release of arachidonic acid, and inhibiting the expression of the inducible form of cyclooxygenase—COX-2 (Chapter 34). Ultimately, there is a decreased production of several inflammatory metabolites: leukotrienes, prostaglandins, and thromboxane. Excessive activity of phospholipase A_2 is thought to be particularly important in asthma because leukotrienes are extremely potent bronchoconstrictors, and also participate in the late inflammatory response. Research also suggests that glucocorticoids increase the responsiveness and prevent tachyphylaxis of β_2 adrenoceptors in the airway.

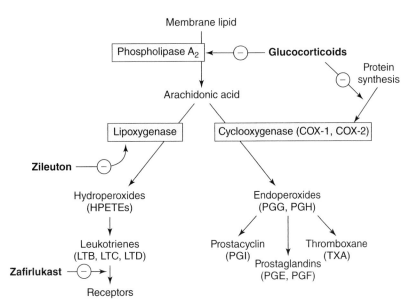

FIGURE 35-7 **Flow diagram of the eicosanoid cascade and the mechanisms of action of different anti-inflammatory drugs.** Glucocorticoids inhibit the release of arachidonic acid, the substrate for lipoxygenase and cyclooxygenase, both types 1 and 2 (COX-1 and COX-2). Other leukotriene pathway antagonists either inhibit the lipoxygenase enzyme directly, or inhibit lipoxygenase products (leukotrienes D_4 or E_4) from activating their receptors.

Glucocorticoids bind intracellular receptors and activate glucocorticoid response elements in the nucleus, resulting in synthesis of substances that prevent the full expression of inflammation and allergy.

The risk of systemic toxicities from inhaled glucocorticoids is negligible, but may occur. Changes in oropharyngeal flora can result in candidiasis; this risk may be reduced by rinsing the mouth and pharynx with water following each inhaled treatment. Inhaled administration can occasionally result in a very small degree of adrenal suppression, but this is rarely significant. If oral (systemic) glucocorticoid therapy is required, adrenal suppression can be reduced by using alternate-day therapy (ie, giving the drug in slightly higher dosage every other day rather than smaller doses every day). Major systemic ADRs are much more likely to occur if systemic treatment is required for more than 2 weeks, as in severe refractory asthma. In children, regular use of inhaled steroids causes mild growth retardation over the first year of therapy, but these children eventually reach predicted adult stature.

LEUKOTRIENE PATHWAY INHIBITORS

Because of the role leukotrienes play in many inflammatory diseases, drugs that interfere with leukotriene synthesis or their receptor interactions have been developed. These drugs are not as effective as glucocorticoids in severe asthma, although a subset of patients have particularly favorable responses. Unfortunately, at present no clinical features allow identification of responders prior to therapy.

Lipoxygenase Inhibitors

Zileuton is an orally active drug that selectively inhibits 5-lipoxygenase, a key enzyme in the conversion of arachidonic acid to leukotrienes. The drug is effective in preventing both exercise- and antigen-induced bronchospasm. Zileuton is also effective against "aspirin allergy," the bronchospasm that results from aspirin ingestion by individuals who apparently divert all eicosanoid production to leukotrienes when the cyclooxygenase pathway is inhibited. The toxicity of zileuton includes occasional elevation of liver enzymes. Therefore, this drug is less popular than the leukotriene receptor antagonists.

Leukotriene Receptor Antagonists

Zafirlukast and **montelukast** are antagonists at the LTD_4 as well as LTE_4 leukotriene receptors. These drugs are orally active and have been shown to be effective in preventing exercise-, antigen-, and aspirin-induced bronchospastic attacks. Thus, they are recommended therapy for asthma maintenance, but not for treatment of acute episodes of asthma. Toxicity is generally low for these drugs with only headaches occurring in more than 2% of the patients.

TARGETED THERAPY

Anti-IgE Monoclonal Antibodies

Because of the pivotal role IgE plays in response to allergens, targeted therapy against this immunoglobulin has been developed. **Omalizumab** is a humanized monoclonal antibody targeted against the portion of IgE that binds to cell surface receptors (Fcε-R1 and Fcε-R2) on mast cells, basophils and other cells that release inflammatory mediators. Omalizumab inhibits IgE binding to its cell surface receptor, but does not activate the already receptor-bound IgE. Thus, in the presence of an allergen, IgE-mediated cell activation with subsequent release of inflammatory mediators is inhibited. Omalizumab's use is restricted to treating severe asthma. In this population, the drug decreases the frequency and severity of exacerbations, especially those severe enough to require hospitalizations. The drug has also been proven effective in the treatment for chronic recurrent urticaria, and for peanut allergy. Like all antibodies, omalizumab cannot be administered orally because as proteins, they will be readily degraded in the digestive system. The drug is given by subcutaneous injection every 2-4 weeks. Omalizumab carries a small risk for anaphylaxis, and a period of observation following infusion is recommended.

Anti-(IL-5) Pathway Monoclonal Antibodies

T_H2 cells secrete IL-5, resulting in bronchial tissue recruitment of eosinophils and eosinophilia. A substantial proportion of patients with severe asthma have airway and peripheral eosinophilia driven by the upregulation of IL-5-secreting T_H2 lymphocytes. Two humanized monoclonal antibodies targeting IL-5, **mepolizumab** and **reslizumab**, and another targeting the IL-5 receptor, **benralizumab**, have recently been developed for the treatment of eosinophilic asthma. Like omalizumab, reslizumab carries a small (0.3%) risk of anaphylaxis. Mepolizumab, although not associated with anaphylaxis, has resulted in reports of hypersensitivity. Some patients who received mepolizumab have reported reactivation of herpes zoster.

REHABILITATION RELEVANCE

For some patients, asthmatic attacks may be precipitated by exercise—called exercise-induced asthma or exercise-induced bronchospasm (EIB). The latter term is preferable, as it reflects that EIB usually does not involve the inflammation and mucus formation that accompanies asthma in other cases. One strategy of pre-exercise prevention of EIB includes the use of short-acting bronchodilators taken approximately 20 minutes prior to activity to allow for maximal bronchial airway dilation.

Treatment of upper and lower respiratory tract disorders often includes both prescription and OTC medications. As such, it is imperative that therapists remember to ask about use of all medications and adjust therapy assessments and goals accordingly. ADRs relative to physical therapy depend on the drug class as well as method of delivery. Risks of particular

drug classes or drugs as well as strategies to optimize rehabilitation are highlighted below.

- **Decreased respiratory drive** may occur during aerobic activities in patients taking opioid antitussives. Monitor respiratory rate and blood oxygen saturation with pulse oximeter.
- **Increased blood pressure** may occur when nasal decongestants are taken systemically because these α_1 agonists cause vasoconstriction. A potential consequence of increased blood pressure is angina, especially during exercise, which also increases cardiac workload. Monitor vital signs and relative perceived exertion to keep workload below the anginal threshold.
- **Orthostatic hypotension** may occur in patients taking oxymetazoline (in high doses, acts as agonist at α_{2A} receptors), some antihistamines (those that are α_1 receptor antagonists), or opioid antitussives. Caution may be required when patients are transitioning from recumbent to upright postures. These drugs may also cause headaches.
- **Sedation** may increase fall risk when patients are taking antihistamines or opioid antitussives. Sedation may decrease cognitive function. Providing simple step-by-step therapy instructions may improve patient comprehension.
- **Cardiac arrhythmias** and **convulsions** may occur in patients taking theophylline due to the drug's narrow therapeutic window. If patients present with signs/symptoms, check whether the documented plasma drug level is current.
- **Tachycardia** may occur in COPD patients taking β_2 agonists by inhalation, especially if patients do not rinse their mouth after administration. In patients with heart disease, angina or arrhythmias may occur at high doses because β_2 agonists also stimulate cardiac β_1 receptors. Monitor vital signs during therapy sessions, especially during exercise.
- **Hyperglycemia** as a result of insulin resistance may occur even with inhalation of glucocorticoids if patients fail to rinse their mouth following administration. Increased plasma glucose can be exacerbated by aerobic activities in therapy (exercise-induced hyperglycemia). In diabetic patients, monitor plasma glucose levels prior to exercise. Chronic use of glucocorticoids may also result in **osteoporosis** (Chapter 23).
- **Asthmatic attacks** may be precipitated by exercise in some patients. Prevention of exercise-induced bronchospasm includes the use of short-acting bronchodilators taken approximately 20 minutes *prior* to activity to allow for maximal bronchial airway dilation.
- In individuals with respiratory dysfunction, **dyspnea** may occur during lumbar traction or aquatherapy due to reduced ventilatory capacity. Patients may require administration of short-acting bronchodilators prior to activity to facilitate maximal bronchial airway dilation.

CASE CONCLUSION

During the aerobic part of the aquatherapy designed to increase pain-free function, L.B. developed exertional dyspnea due to a combination of factors. Although L.B. was not diagnosed with COPD, the patient currently smokes, has a significant smoking history, had asthma in childhood, and uses prescribed bronchodilators as needed (ipratropium and albuterol). This information strongly suggests a diminished pulmonary reserve. Nadolol in his combination antihypertensive medication (nadolol and bendroflumethiazide) is a nonspecific β-receptor antagonist. Therefore, this drug would block both β_1 receptors on the heart and β_2 receptors on the smooth muscle of the bronchioles. The latter blockade would cause bronchoconstriction, making breathing more difficult. With L.B. in the pool up to his neck, the hydrostatic pressure on the thorax increases. This increased external pressure diminishes ventilation and thus reduces gas exchange. Weights on the lower extremities would also diminish elevation of the rib cage during inspiration. The combination of these factors exceeded the patient's pulmonary reserve during the aerobic portion of therapy, and he became dyspneic. Finally, smoking a cigarette prior to the therapy session decreased the oxygen-carrying capacity of the red blood cells. Incomplete combustion of organic matter (smoking) results in the formation of carbon monoxide. Carbon monoxide binds to hemoglobin in red blood cells to form carboxyhemoglobin. Carboxyhemoglobin prevents the binding of oxygen to hemoglobin, leading to hypoxemia and peripheral tissue hypoxia. Patients should be strongly advised not to smoke prior to performing aerobic activities, because the oxygen-carrying potential of the blood is diminished.

CHAPTER 35 QUESTIONS

1. Which of the following statements is untrue?

   a. Expectorants thin and liquefy respiratory secretions.
   b. Alpha-1 adrenoceptor antagonists act as decongestants.
   c. Histamine-1 receptor antagonists decrease symptoms of allergic reactions.
   d. Antitussives suppress coughing.

2. Which of the following drugs is an agonist at both α_1 and β receptors?

   a. Phenylephrine
   b. Pseudoephedrine
   c. Oxymetazoline
   d. Diphenhydramine

3. Which of the following drugs may cause hypotension when taken in large doses due to an effect at α_2 adrenoceptors?

   a. Pseudoephedrine
   b. Diphenhydramine
   c. Oxymetazoline
   d. Guaifenesin

4. Which of the following drugs is an opioid derivative?

   a. Pseudoephedrine
   b. Diphenhydramine
   c. Oxymetazoline
   d. Dextromethorphan

5. In asthma, what is the inflammatory phase?

   a. Early phase
   b. Delayed phase
   c. Acute phase
   d. Late phase

6. Which of the following is *not* a mechanism of bronchodilation?

   a. Stimulation of β_1-adrenergic receptors
   b. Inhibition of phosphodiesterase
   c. Inhibition of muscarinic receptors
   d. Inhibition of adenosine receptors

7. Which of the following drugs is considered a methylxanthine?

   a. Roflumolist
   b. Aminophylline
   c. Ipratropium
   d. Salmeterol

8. Which of the following drug classes' major mechanism of action is *not* anti-inflammatory?

   a. Glucocorticoids
   b. Leukotriene inhibitors
   c. β_2-Adrenergic agonists
   d. Phosphodiesterase type-4 (PDE-4) inhibitors

9. Which of the following monoclonal antibodies inhibits the interleukin-5 (IL-5) receptor?

   a. Mepolizumab
   b. Reslizumab
   c. Omalizumab
   d. Benralizumab

10. Which of the following drugs is effective as first-line treatment in short-term relief of acute asthma attacks?

   a. Albuterol
   b. Cromolyn
   c. Omalizumab
   d. Montelukast

Drugs Used in Gastrointestinal Disorders

CASE STUDY

R.J. is a 63-year-old woman with a 20-year history of type 2 diabetes mellitus. The patient has hyperglycemia, hypertension, and hyperlipidemia for which she is taking metformin, amlodipine, benazepril, and atorvastatin. She has a history of neuropathic ulcers at the first metatarsal head on the plantar surfaces of both feet. The most recent ulcer achieved full wound closure 5 months ago. Two weeks ago, R.J. was diagnosed with gastroparesis and prescribed metoclopramide as a prokinetic. Last week, the healed neuropathic ulcer on the first left metatarsal head reulcerated. R.J. was referred to physical therapy for wound evaluation and possible foot orthotics to prevent further breakdown.

REHABILITATION FOCUS

Drugs that are swallowed pass through the gastrointestinal (GI) system prior to reaching the systemic circulation. Thus, drugs used to treat GI conditions have the potential to interfere with all other orally administered drugs leading to drug-drug interactions. These interactions may result in a decreased therapeutic effect due to decreased absorption of non-GI drugs, or adverse effects from higher drug plasma concentration due to decreased metabolism of non-GI drugs. Many drugs used to treat GI disorders may be obtained over-the-counter (OTC). Use of OTC drugs complicates accurate assessment of the drug history because it is not unusual for patients to forget to include OTC drugs when asked by the healthcare provider about medications. A classic example is the very common use of antihistamines used in acid-peptic disease.

NEURONAL CONTROL OF THE GI SYSTEM

The various components of the GI tract serve several functions, including digestive, excretory, endocrine, and exocrine. Control of these functions requires neuronal activity from both local and higher centers. The digestive system is innervated through connections with the central nervous system (CNS) and by a collection of highly organized neurons called the enteric nervous system (ENS) located within the intestinal walls. The ENS is often considered a third division of the autonomic nervous system. The ENS contains hundreds of millions of neurons, the majority of which are contained in the myenteric and submucosal plexuses. The ENS receives preganglionic fibers from the parasympathetic system as well as postganglionic sympathetic axons. There is bidirectional communication between the CNS and ENS and between the ENS and sympathetic prevertebral ganglia. Fibers from the cell bodies in these plexuses travel to the smooth muscle of the gut to control motility. Other motor fibers go to the secretory cells. The ENS also receives sensory input from within the wall of the gut. Sensory fibers transmit information from the mucosa and from stretch receptors to motor neurons in the plexuses and to postganglionic neurons in the sympathetic ganglia. The parasympathetic and sympathetic fibers that synapse on enteric plexus neurons appear to play a modulatory role.

Multiple neurotransmitters, neuromodulators, and autocoids are present in the GI system and control many functions. Because autocoids are typically produced and act locally, they do not fall into traditional neurotransmitter or hormonal classifications. The GI system contains numerous peptide autacoids and at least two important amine autacoids—histamine and serotonin (5-HT). (Histamine was previously discussed in its role in the respiratory system [Chapter 35] and 5-HT was discussed in its role in the CNS [Chapters 12 and 19].) Enterochromaffin-like (ECL) cells release histamine and stimulate H_2 receptors, which results in gastric acid secretion into the stomach. 5-HT is produced from tryptophan and stored in vesicles in the enterochromaffin (EC) cells of the gut as well as neurons in the ENS. 5-HT serves not only as a neurotransmitter in the ENS, but also as a local hormone that modulates GI smooth muscle activity. After release, both histamine and 5-HT may be metabolized by monoamine oxidase. Dopamine (Chapters 4, 12, 17, and 18) is an amine that

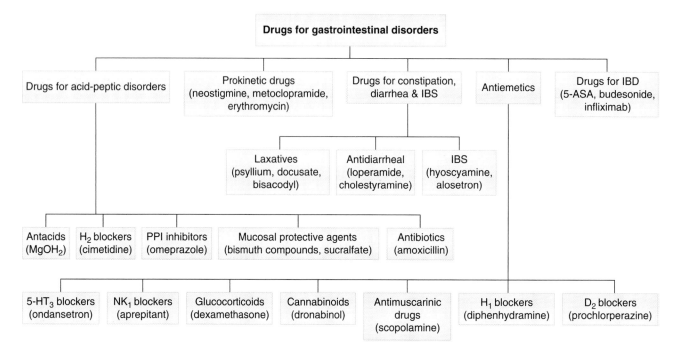

FIGURE 36-1 **Drug classes used in the treatment of gastrointestinal disorders.** These include: drugs for treating acid-peptic dysfunction, prokinetic drugs, drugs for constipation (laxatives), diarrhea (antidiarrheals), drugs to treat irritable bowel syndrome (IBS), antiemetics, and drugs to treat inflammatory bowel disease (IBD). Prototype drugs are in parentheses. 5-ASA, 5-aminosalicylic acid; 5-HT₃, serotonin type 3 receptor; D_2, dopamine type 2 receptor; H_1, histamine type 1 receptor; H_2, histamine type 2 receptor; NK_1, neurokinin type 1 receptor; PPI, proton pump inhibitor.

indirectly modulates gastric motility. Stimulation of D_2 receptors on cholinergic neurons in the ENS inhibits acetylcholine release onto the smooth muscle. These amines and additional transmitters also play a role in regulating emesis. Other GI autacoids include cytokines and prostaglandins (Chapters 32 and 34).

These transmitters, modulators, and their receptors provide numerous important drug targets. Many drugs used in GI disease have been discussed in earlier chapters and those drugs are briefly reviewed in this chapter. Other drugs that have not been presented previously are discussed in more detail. Figure 36-1 outlines the drugs used to treat GI disorders into major classes.

PHYSIOLOGY OF STOMACH ACID SECRETION

Erosion and ulceration of the lining of the GI tract are common problems that arise when the caustic effects of pepsin, acid, and/or bile overwhelm defenses such as mucus, prostaglandins, and bicarbonate. Cells lining the stomach include mucus-producing cells, parietal cells, and gastrin-containing cells. Parietal cells have receptors for gastrin, histamine, and acetylcholine (Figure 36-2). When gastrin or acetylcholine binds to their respective receptors, they increase cytosolic calcium, which activates protein kinases that stimulate acid secretion from H^+/K^+ ATPase (proton pump) on the epithelial surface of the parietal cell. By exchanging intracellular H^+ for

K^+ present in the lumen of the stomach, the proton pumps in the parietal cells effectively acidify the stomach. Near to the parietal cells are gut endocrine cells called enterochromaffin-like cells (ECL). These cells, which also have receptors for gastrin and acetylcholine, are the major source for histamine. After release, histamine binds to the H_2 receptor on the parietal cell, resulting in activation of adenylate cyclase and increased intracellular cyclic adenosine monophosphate (cAMP). The cAMP activates protein kinases that stimulate H^+ secretion by the proton pump. In humans, research suggests that the major effect of gastrin upon acid secretion is mediated indirectly through the release of histamine rather than directly through parietal cell stimulation. Finally, the parasympathetic system stimulates stomach acid secretion. Efferent fibers of the vagus nerve release acetylcholine that binds to M_3 receptors on parietal cells, directly stimulating stomach acid secretion. Vagal fibers also innervate ECL cells. Activation of M_3 receptors on ECL cells indirectly increases acid secretion via histamine release onto the parietal cells.

DRUGS USED IN ACID-PEPTIC DISORDERS

Acid-peptic diseases include gastroesophageal reflux disease (GERD), gastric and duodenal ulcers, and stress-related mucosal injuries. In all of these conditions, mucosal erosion or ulcerations occur. Most of the drug classes used to treat acid-peptic ulcer disorders reduce intragastric acidity by modifying

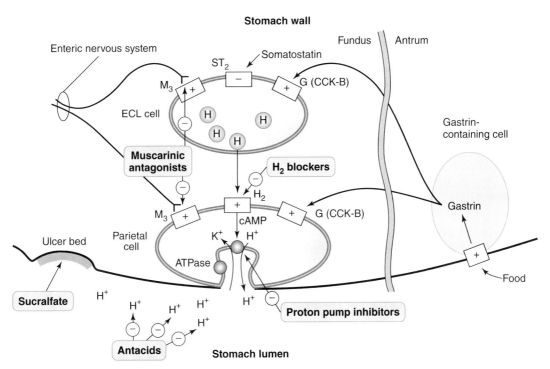

FIGURE 36-2 **Sites of action of some drugs used in acid-peptic ulcer disease.** Receptor types involved include muscarinic M_3, which binds acetylcholine, and histamine H_2. Antacids bind free protons (H^+). Proton pump inhibitors prevent secretion of protons into the stomach lumen. Sucralfate binds to erosions on the epithelial lining of the stomach. The site of action of bismuth compounds is not presented, but these agents coat the epithelial lining similar to sucralfate, and possibly stimulate mucus and bicarbonate secretion. CCK, cholecystokinin; ECL, enterochromaffin-like.

the systems that control acid secretion into the stomach lumen (Figure 36-2). These include antacids, H_2 receptor blockers, proton pump inhibitors (PPIs), and antimuscarinic drugs (Chapter 5). Other drugs promote mucosal defense against acidic erosion of the lining of the stomach (bismuth compounds, sucralfate) or eradicate the bacterium *Helicobacter pylori* (antibiotics).

Antacids

Antacids are physical agents that react with protons (H^+) in the lumen of the gut (Figure 36-2). Antacids differ mainly in their absorption and effects on stool consistency. The most popular antacids are **magnesium hydroxide (Mg[OH]$_2$)** and **aluminum hydroxide (Al[OH]$_3$)** and **calcium carbonate** (eg, TUMS). Neither of these weak bases is significantly absorbed from the bowel after oral administration. Magnesium hydroxide has a strong laxative effect, whereas aluminum hydroxide has a constipating effect. Although these agents are available as single-ingredient products, combined formulations are usually preferred because they balance the laxative and constipating effects. Calcium carbonate and **sodium bicarbonate** are also weak bases, but they differ from aluminum and magnesium hydroxides in that they are absorbed from the gut lumen and thus have more systemic effects. In individuals with renal insufficiency or when given in high doses, the unreacted alkali may be absorbed, resulting in metabolic alkalosis.

H$_2$ Receptor Antagonists

Four H_2 receptor antagonists are available: **cimetidine** (the prototype), **ranitidine**, **famotidine**, and **nizatidine**. The latter three differ only in having fewer drug interactions than cimetidine. These antihistamines produce reversible and relatively selective blockade at H_2 receptors. They have no significant blocking actions at H_1 or autonomic receptors and the only therapeutic effect of clinical importance is the reduction of gastric acid secretion.

H_2 blockers are available OTC and by prescription. They are orally active, with half-lives of 1-3 hours. Because they are relatively nontoxic, they can be given in large doses, so that the duration of action of a single dose may be from 12 to 24 hours. In acid-peptic disorders, especially duodenal and gastric ulcers, the H_2 blockers reduce symptoms, accelerate healing, and prevent recurrences. Although H_2 blockers are still clinically used (especially OTC formulations), PPIs (see below) are more commonly prescribed for most clinical indications.

In general, H_2 antagonists are very safe drugs, with adverse drug reactions (ADRs) such as diarrhea, headache, fatigue, myalgia, and constipation occurring in less than 3% of patients. Cimetidine is a potent inhibitor of some hepatic drug-metabolizing enzymes and may also reduce hepatic blood flow. When used chronically or in high doses, cimetidine also has significant antiandrogen effects. Ranitidine has a weaker inhibitory effect on hepatic drug metabolism; neither it nor the other H_2 blockers appear to have any endocrine effects. Mental status changes (confusion, hallucinations, agitation) may occur with administration of *intravenous* H_2 antagonists, especially in patients in the intensive care unit who are elderly or who have renal or hepatic dysfunction. These events may be more common with cimetidine. Mental status changes rarely occur in ambulatory patients.

Proton Pump Inhibitors

Proton pump inhibitors (PPIs) were introduced in the late 1980s. Due to their effective reduction of stomach acid secretion and relatively safe profile, PPIs are now among the most widely prescribed drugs worldwide for acid-peptic disorders. Six PPIs are clinically available: **omeprazole** (prototype), **esomeprazole, lansoprazole, dexlansoprazole, pantoprazole,** and **rabeprazole**. To prevent acid inactivation in the stomach and allow absorption in the small intestine, oral preparations are formulated for delayed-release as acid-resistant enteric-coated tablets or capsules. PPIs are rapidly metabolized in the liver, with half-lives of 1-2 hours. However, their durations of action are approximately 24 hours, and they may require 3-4 days of treatment to achieve their full effectiveness. Their bioavailability is decreased by as much as 50% when taken with food. Hence, PPIs should be taken on an empty stomach.

PPIs are lipophilic weak bases that diffuse from the blood into the parietal cell canaliculi (deep infoldings that extend the secretory surface area) where they become protonated and concentrated more than 1000-fold. There they convert to compounds that irreversibly inactivate the proton pump (H^+/K^+ ATPase).

PPIs are the most effective agents for treating erosive reflux disease and esophageal complications of GERD. PPIs are used increasingly as first-line therapy for GERD, though initial treatment with H_2 blockers should be considered due to recent safety concerns (see below). Within 6 months after discontinuation of PPI use, GERD symptoms recur in over 80% of individuals. In peptic ulcer disease, PPIs afford more rapid symptom relief and faster ulcer healing for duodenal ulcers (and gastric ulcers to a lesser extent) compared with H_2 antagonists. All the PPIs heal more than 90% of duodenal ulcers within 4 weeks and a similar percentage of gastric ulcers within 6-8 weeks.

In roughly 10-20% of people that frequently take nonsteroidal anti-inflammatory drugs (NSAIDs), *asymptomatic* peptic ulceration occurs. A smaller percentage of these individuals develop ulcer-related complications such as bleeding and perforation. For people with ulcers caused by NSAIDs, therapy with either H_2 antagonists or PPIs provides rapid ulcer healing only if the NSAID is discontinued. Continued use of the NSAID impairs ulcer healing. In people with NSAID-induced ulcers who *require* continued NSAID therapy, treatment with a PPI more reliably promotes ulcer healing.

PPIs are also very effective in peptic ulcer disease associated with the bacterium *H pylori*. For *H pylori*–associated ulcers, there are two therapeutic goals: to heal the ulcer and to eradicate the organism. After completion of antibiotic therapy (see below), the PPI should be continued once daily for a total of 4-6 weeks to ensure complete ulcer healing.

In critically ill patients, PPIs may be given via a nasogastric tube, or by intravenous infusions, to reduce the risk of clinically significant stress-related mucosal bleeding. Immediate-release omeprazole is the only PPI approved by the United States Food and Drug Administration (FDA) for this indication. PPIs are also useful in the treatment of Zollinger-Ellison syndrome, which is a condition usually associated with a gastrin-secreting tumor.

Minor adverse effects of PPIs occur infrequently and include diarrhea, abdominal pain, and headache. Although PPIs have been considered extremely safe, several recent safety concerns highlight the principle of prescribing the lowest effective dose and evaluating the risks versus benefits of chronic treatment. PPIs may decrease the oral bioavailability of vitamin B_{12} and certain drugs (eg, digoxin, ketoconazole) that require acidity for effective GI absorption. Because gastric acid is a major barrier to the colonization and infection of the gut, PPI users have an increased risk of hospital- and community-acquired *Clostridium difficile* infection and a smaller risk of other enteric infections. Acid suppression also alters normal feedback inhibition so hypergastrinemia may occur in some people taking PPIs. PPIs can also cause allergic interstitial nephritis. Last, though casuality has not been established, some studies (but not all) have shown that chronic PPI use is associated with an increased risk of dementia and a modest increase in hip fracture risk. Due to the latter, the FDA requires all PPIs to carry a warning of a possible increased risk of spine, hip, and wrist fractures.

Bismuth Compounds

Two bismuth compounds are available. **Bismuth subsalicylate** (eg, Pepto-Bismol) is a nonprescription formulation that is widely used for nonspecific treatment of dyspepsia and acute diarrhea. In the United States, **bismuth subcitrate potassium** is available only as a combination prescription product that also contains metronidazole and tetracycline for the treatment of *H pylori*. Bismuth subsalicylate undergoes rapid dissociation within the stomach, allowing absorption of salicylate. Salicylate (like aspirin) is readily absorbed and excreted in the urine. Over 99% of the bismuth appears in the stool.

Several mechanisms have been proposed for the protective effect of bismuth. Bismuth coats gastric and duodenal ulcers and erosions, creating a protective layer against acid and pepsin. The drug may also stimulate mucus and bicarbonate secretion. Bismuth subsalicylate reduces stool frequency and liquidity in acute infectious diarrhea, due to salicylate inhibition of intestinal prostaglandin production and chloride secretion. Bismuth has direct antimicrobial effects and binds enterotoxins, accounting for its benefit in preventing and treating traveler's diarrhea. Bismuth compounds have direct antimicrobial activity against *H pylori* and are used in four-drug regimens for the eradication of *H pylori* infection (see below).

Bismuth formulations have excellent safety profiles. Bismuth causes harmless blackening of the stool, which may be mistaken as the black, tarry stools associated with upper GI bleeding (melena). Liquid bismuth formulations may also cause harmless darkening of the tongue. Bismuth agents should be used for short periods only and should be avoided in individuals with renal insufficiency. High dosages of bismuth subsalicylate may lead to salicylate toxicity.

Sucralfate

Sucralfate is a salt of sucrose bound to sulfated aluminum hydroxide. Sucralfate is a small, poorly soluble molecule that polymerizes in the acid environment of the stomach. This polymer binds to injured tissue and forms a protective coating over ulcer beds. The drug accelerates healing of peptic ulcers and reduces the recurrence rate. Unfortunately, sucralfate must be taken four times daily on an empty stomach. Sucralfate is too insoluble to have significant systemic effects. Constipation occurs in 2% of patients due to the aluminum salt. Topical sucralfate is occasionally used in a wide variety of open integumentary wounds as a protective barrier and to minimize excessive exudate.

Antibiotics

Chronic infection with *H pylori* occurs in the majority of individuals with recurrent non-NSAID-induced peptic ulcers. Eradication of this bacterium greatly reduces the recurrence rate of ulcers in these patients. Antibiotics are required in all effective regimens for *H pylori* eradication. Until recently, the most commonly recommended treatment consisted of a 14-day regimen of "triple therapy" that included a PPI (twice daily), the antibiotic **clarithromycin** (twice daily), and either **amoxicillin** or **metronidazole** (also twice daily). Due to increasing treatment failures attributable to rising clarithromycin resistance, "quadruple therapy" is now recommended as first-line treatment for patients who likely have clarithromycin resistance. Quadruple therapy is a 14-day treatment regimen, with two options. Both treatment regimens include a PPI. PPIs promote eradication of *H pylori* directly by a minor antimicrobial effect and indirectly by raising intragastric pH, which lowers the minimal inhibitory concentrations of antibiotics required to eliminate *H pylori*. Each treatment option includes a PPI twice daily with either: (1) bismuth subsalicylate, metronidazole, and tetracycline, all given four times daily; or (2) amoxicillin, clarithromycin, and metronidazole, all given twice daily. After completion of antibiotic therapy, the PPI should be continued once daily for a total of 4-6 weeks to ensure complete ulcer healing.

PHYSIOLOGIC REGULATION OF GASTROINTESTINAL MOTILITY

The enteric nervous system is composed of interconnected networks of ganglion cells and nerve fibers mainly located in the submucosa (submucosal plexus) and between the circular and longitudinal muscle layers (myenteric plexus). These networks give rise to nerve fibers that connect with the mucosa and smooth muscle. Although extrinsic sympathetic and parasympathetic nerves project onto the submucosal and myenteric plexuses, the ENS can independently regulate GI motility and secretion. Extrinsic primary afferent neurons project via the dorsal root ganglia or vagus nerve to the CNS (Figure 36-3). Release of 5-HT from intestinal mucosa EC cells stimulates 5-HT$_3$ receptors on the extrinsic afferent nerves, stimulating nausea, vomiting, or abdominal pain. Serotonin also stimulates submucosal 5-HT$_{1P}$ receptors of the intrinsic primary afferent nerves (IPANs), which contain calcitonin gene-related peptide (CGRP) and acetylcholine and project to myenteric plexus interneurons. The myenteric interneurons are important in controlling the peristaltic reflex, promoting release of excitatory mediators proximally and inhibitory mediators distally. Serotonin 5-HT$_4$ receptors on the presynaptic terminals of the IPANs appear to enhance release of CGRP or acetylcholine. Both 5-HT$_3$-receptor antagonists and 5-HT$_4$-receptor agonists have effects on GI motility and visceral afferent sensation.

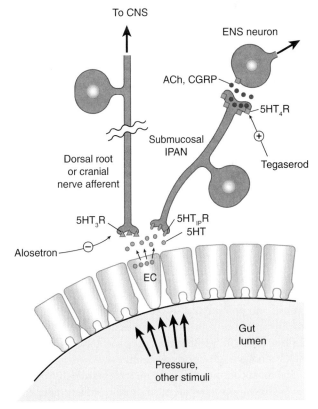

FIGURE 36-3 **Role of serotonin (5-HT) in GI motility.** Release of 5-HT by enterochromaffin (EC) cells from gut distention or other stimuli stimulates submucosal intrinsic primary afferent neurons (IPANs) via 5-HT$_{1P}$ receptors (5-HT$_{1P}$R) and extrinsic primary afferent neurons via 5-HT$_3$ receptors (5-HT$_3$R). Submucosal IPANs activate the enteric neurons responsible for peristaltic and secretory reflex activity. Stimulation of 5-HT$_4$ receptors (5-HT$_4$R) on presynaptic terminals of IPANs enhances release of acetylcholine (ACh) and calcitonin gene-related peptide (CGRP), promoting reflex activity. CNS, central nervous system; ENS, enteric nervous system.

PROKINETIC DRUGS

Drugs that stimulate the motor function of the gut (prokinetic agents) have significant potential clinical applications. For example, drugs that increase lower esophageal sphincter pressure may be useful in GERD. Drugs that improve gastric emptying help gastroparesis. Drugs that stimulate the small intestine help postoperative ileus. Last, drugs that accelerate colonic transit help constipation. However, only a few agents that stimulate gut motor function are clinically available and none of them are able to selectively stimulate only *one* region of the GI tract.

Cholinomimetic Drugs

Drugs affecting the cholinergic system have been previously discussed (Chapter 5). **Neostigmine** is an acetylcholinesterase inhibitor that enhances gastric, small intestine, and colonic emptying. Intravenous neostigmine is used in the treatment of hospitalized patients with acute large bowel distention. Administration results in prompt colonic evacuation of flatus and feces in the majority of patients. Cholinergic ADRs include excessive salivation, nausea, vomiting, diarrhea, and bradycardia.

Metoclopramide

Activation of dopamine receptors in the GI tract inhibits cholinergic-mediated smooth muscle stimulation. Thus, inhibition of dopamine in the gut produces prokinetic effects. **Metoclopramide** is a D_2-receptor antagonist that increases esophageal peristaltic amplitude, increases lower esophageal sphincter pressure, and enhances gastric emptying. The drug has no effect on small intestine or colonic motility.

Metoclopramide is available for use in GERD. However, because of the superior efficacy and safety of antisecretory drugs, metoclopramide is used mainly in combination with antisecretory drugs in individuals with regurgitation or refractory heartburn. Metoclopramide also produces symptomatic improvement in a small number of individuals with chronic dyspepsia. Metoclopramide is used in the treatment of patients with delayed gastric emptying due to diabetic gastroparesis and postsurgical disorders (vagotomy, antrectomy). Metoclopramide is sometimes administered to hospitalized patients to promote advancement of nasoenteric feeding tubes from the stomach into the duodenum.

The most common ADRs of metoclopramide involve the CNS. Restlessness, drowsiness, insomnia, anxiety, and agitation occur in 10-20% of patients, especially older adults. Extrapyramidal effects (dystonia, akathisia, parkinsonian features) due to central dopamine receptor blockade occur acutely in 25% of patients given high doses, and in 5% of patients receiving long-term therapy. Chronic metoclopramide treatment can produce tardive dyskinesia that may be irreversible. Unless absolutely necessary, long-term use should be avoided, especially in older adults. Metoclopramide may elevate prolactin levels, causing galactorrhea, gynecomastia, impotence, and menstrual disorders.

Macrolide Antibiotics

Motilin is a peptide secreted by cells in the proximal small intestine that regulates smooth muscle contraction patterns in the upper GI tract. Macrolide antibiotics such as **erythromycin** directly stimulate motilin receptors on GI smooth muscle and promote the onset of a cephalic to caudal propulsion in the stomach and small intestine. Intravenous erythromycin is beneficial in some patients with gastroparesis, though tolerance develops rapidly. Erythromycin is used in patients with acute upper GI hemorrhage to promote gastric emptying of blood before endoscopy.

DRUGS USED IN CONSTIPATION, DIARRHEA, AND IRRITABLE BOWEL SYNDROME

Both constipation and diarrhea are common and uncomfortable GI dysfunctions. Constipation is characterized by infrequent bowel movements, usually associated with hardened feces and difficulty when movements occur. Constipation may be due to lack of sufficient fiber in the diet or a decreased urge to defecate (which may occur in older adults), or the result of damage to the enteric nerve plexus (such as in diabetes mellitus). There are also many drugs such as opioid analgesics (Chapter 20) that cause constipation. In contrast, diarrhea is characterized by unusually frequent and loose or liquid bowel movements. Diarrhea is also defined by volume of feces (large versus small) and by duration (acute versus chronic). Diarrhea may originate from inflammatory causes, such as in inflammatory bowel disease (IBD), enteric infections, lactose intolerance, or secretory mechanisms that occur when enterotoxins are released during some GI bacterial or viral infections. Irritable bowel syndrome (IBS) is an idiopathic chronic, relapsing disorder associated with recurrent episodes of abdominal pain, bloating, distention, or cramps plus diarrhea, constipation, or both. With episodes of abdominal discomfort, IBS sufferers note a change in the frequency or consistency of their bowel movements.

Pharmacologic therapies for these GI dysfunctions include laxatives for constipation and antidiarrheal drugs for diarrhea. In individuals with IBS, GI distress may be treated with antispasmodic drugs along with low doses of tricyclic antidepressants (Chapter 19) that have no effect on mood, but may alter central processing of visceral afferent information. The anticholinergic properties of these drugs may affect GI motility and secretion, reducing stool frequency and liquidity. Finally, tricyclic antidepressants may alter receptors for enteric neurotransmitters such as 5-HT, affecting visceral afferent sensation.

Laxatives

Laxatives increase the probability of a bowel movement by one or more mechanisms. These agents are available OTC and by prescription. Although laxatives are self-prescribed by a large

TABLE 36-1 Major laxative mechanisms and representative laxative drugs.

Mechanism	Examples
Bulk-forming	Polycarbophil, psyllium
Chloride secretion activator	Lubiprostone, linaclotide
Lubricating	Mineral oil, glycerin
Opioid receptor antagonist	Methylnaltrexone, alvimopan
Osmotic	Magnesium hydroxide or citrate, polyethylene glycol, lactulose
Stimulant (cathartic)	Bisacodyl, cascara, senna
Stool-softening	Docusate, mineral oil

portion of the population, the overwhelming majority of people do not need laxatives. For most people, intermittent constipation is best prevented with a high-fiber diet, adequate fluid intake, regular exercise, and the heeding of nature's call. Individuals that do not respond as expected to dietary changes or fiber supplements should undergo medical evaluation before self-initiating long-term laxative treatment. Laxatives may be classified by their major mechanism of action, but many work through more than one mechanism. Table 36-1 presents the mechanisms of action for laxatives with examples from each classification.

Oral bulk-forming laxatives are indigestible hydrophilic colloids that absorb water and form a bulky mass that distends the colon, causing a reflexive contraction of the bowel. These formulations are derived from plant products (**psyllium**) and synthetic fibers (**polycarbophil**). Bacterial digestion of plant fibers within the colon may lead to increased bloating and flatus.

Stool softeners may be administered orally or rectally. **Docusate** allows water to penetrate into the stool, resulting in expansion and bowel contraction. In contrast, **mineral oil** softens stool by retarding water absorption from the stool and also lubricates its passage through the bowel and rectum. Mineral oil is helpful to prevent and treat fecal impaction in young children and debilitated adults. Aspiration of mineral oil may result in a severe lipid pneumonitis. Long-term use may impair absorption of fat-soluble vitamins (A, D, E, K).

Because the large intestine can neither concentrate nor dilute fecal fluid, fecal water is isotonic throughout the colon. *Osmotic laxatives* exploit this property of the colon. Osmotic laxatives include nonabsorbable but soluble sugars (**lactulose**) or salts (**magnesium hydroxide**, **magnesium citrate**) that result in increased stool liquidity due to an obligate increase in fecal fluid. The rapid movement of water into the distal small bowel and colon leads to a high volume of liquid stool followed by bowel evacuation. High doses of osmotically active agents produce prompt bowel evacuation within 1-3 hours. When the osmotic laxative sugars are used, they are metabolized by colonic bacteria and produce severe flatus and cramps. Lavage solutions containing **polyethylene glycol (PEG)** are commonly used for complete colonic cleansing before GI endoscopic procedures. In contrast to the osmotic sugars, PEG does not produce significant cramps or flatus.

Cathartics are stimulant laxatives that are either naturally derived (**cascara**, **senna**) or synthetic (**bisacodyl**). These drugs induce bowel movements potentially by direct stimulation of the ENS and colonic electrolyte and fluid secretion. The naturally occurring laxatives are poorly absorbed. After hydrolysis in the colon, they produce a bowel movement in 6-12 hours when given orally and within 2 hours when given rectally. Synthetic bisacodyl has minimal systemic absorption and induces a bowel movement within 6-10 hours when given orally or 30-60 minutes when taken rectally. Long-term use of cathartic laxatives may be required in individuals with neurologic impairment and people who are bed-bound in long-term care facilities. No ADRs have been documented with chronic use of these drugs.

Chloride secretion activators represent the newest class of laxatives that are only available by prescription. These drugs have their effect by increasing chloride-rich fluid secretion into the intestine, which stimulates intestinal motility and shortens intestinal transit time. **Lubiprostone** is a prostanoic acid derivative that activates the type 2 chloride channel (ClC-2) in the small intestine. **Linaclotide** and **plecanatide** stimulate guanylate cyclase-C on the luminal surface of intestinal cells. This stimulation leads to increased intracellular and extracellular cyclic guanosine monophosphate (cGMP), activating the cystic fibrosis transmembrane conductance regulator (CFTR) channel. Clinical uses of these drugs include constipation associated with IBS and chronic idiopathic constipation. Chloride secretion activators are effective laxatives. In 50% of patients, lubiprostone induces a bowel movement within 24 hours of a single dose. For linaclotide and plecanatide, 1 week of treatment results in an average increase of 1-2 bowel movements per week. These drugs have diarrhea as a common ADR, and lubiprostone may cause nausea in up to 30% of patients due to delayed gastric emptying. Compared to older and less expensive laxatives, the efficacy and safety of chloride secretion activators have not been validated by clinical trials.

A common and well-recognized ADR associated with acute and chronic opioid use (Chapter 20) is constipation that results from decreased intestinal motility, which prolongs transit time and increases absorption of fecal water. These effects are mainly mediated through intestinal mu (μ)-opioid receptors. *Selective antagonists of the μ-opioid receptor* (**methylnaltrexone** and **alvimopan**) promote laxation. Because these opiates do not readily cross the blood-brain barrier, they inhibit peripheral μ-opioid receptors without impacting analgesic effects within the CNS. Because of possible cardiovascular toxicity, alvimopan is restricted to short-term use in hospitalized patients only. For opioid-induced constipaton, docusate is typically used.

Antidiarrheal Drugs

Antidiarrheal agents may be used safely in individuals with mild to moderate acute diarrhea, and in people with IBS with associated diarrhea. Antidiarrheal drugs should not be used in

TABLE 36-2 Major antidiarrheal mechanisms and representative drugs.

Mechanism	Examples
Binds bile salts	Cholestyramine, colestipol
Binds enterotoxins	Colloidal bismuth
CFTR inhibitor	Crofelemer
Opioid receptor agonist	Loperamide, diphenoxylate

CFTR, cystic fibrosis transmembrane conductance regulator.

individuals with bloody diarrhea, high fever, or systemic toxicity because of the risk of worsening the underlying condition. These drugs should be discontinued if diarrhea is worsening despite therapy. The mechanisms of action and prototypical drugs are presented in Table 36-2.

As previously discussed under laxatives, *opioid agonists* have significant constipating effects through μ receptors. Although all opioids are constipating, those that enter the CNS have central effects and carry potential for addiction, which limit their usefulness as antidiarrheal agents. **Loperamide** is a nonprescription opioid that does not cross the blood-brain barrier and has no analgesic properties or potential for addiction. Tolerance to long-term use has not been reported. In 2018, the FDA issued a safety alert to healthcare professionals warning that higher than recommended doses of loperamide may result in serious cardiac dysfunction resulting in death. **Diphenoxylate** is a prescription opioid that has no analgesic properties in standard doses. At higher doses, the drug has CNS effects, and prolonged use can lead to opioid dependence. To discourage overdosage, preparations of diphenoxylate commonly contain small amounts of **atropine**. The anticholinergic properties of atropine may also contribute to the antidiarrheal action (Chapter 5). Although there are no significant ADRs associated with diphenoxylate, the added atropine may increase fall risk in older adults due to anticholinergic effects. **Eluxadoline** is a prescription opioid approved for the treatment of IBS-associated diarrhea. Eluxadoline should not be used in people with a history of pancreatitis, alcoholism, or sphincter of Oddi dysfunction. Liver enzymes may also be elevated. Constipation occurs in approximately 8% of those taking the drug.

Bile salt-binding resins (**cholestyramine, colestipol, colesevelam**) may be used to prevent diarrhea in disorders that affect the terminal ileum. Normally, bile salts are absorbed in the terminal ileum. Conditions affecting the terminal ileum (surgical resection, Crohn's disease) cause bile salts to remain in the intestinal lumen, which can result in secretory diarrhea. Chapter 26 discusses the mechanism of action and ADRs for the bile salt-binding resins.

Whereas the CFTR channel activators linaclotide and plecanatide are used to alleviate constipation, the *CFTR inhibitor* **crofelemer** decreases chloride secretion to alleviate diarrhea. Crofelemer is used to treat antiretroviral drug-associated diarrhea (Chapter 28). Last, the use of *bismuth compounds*

as antidiarrheal agents was discussed previously under drugs used in acid-peptic disease.

DRUGS USED IN IRRITABLE BOWEL SYNDROME

In addition to the laxative and antidiarrheal drugs discussed above, antispasmodics (anticholinergics) and 5-HT$_3$ receptor antagonists are clinically used in the treatment of IBS. **Dicyclomine** and **hyoscyamine** are both anticholinergic drugs promoted as providing relief of abdominal pain or discomfort through antispasmodic actions. However, the efficacy of antispasmodics for relief of abdominal symptoms has never been convincingly demonstrated and these drugs have significant anticholinergic ADRs (Chapter 5). The latter effect contraindicates their use in older adults. For these reasons, antispasmodics are infrequently used.

Activation of 5-HT$_3$ receptors in the GI tract stimulates visceral afferent pain sensation via extrinsic sensory neurons from the gut to the spinal cord and CNS (Figure 36-3). Inhibition of afferent GI 5-HT$_3$ receptors may reduce unpleasant visceral afferent sensation, including nausea, bloating, and pain. Blockade of central 5-HT$_3$ receptors also reduces the central response to visceral afferent stimulation. In addition, 5-HT$_3$-receptor blockade on the terminals of enteric cholinergic neurons inhibits colonic motility, especially in the descending colon, increasing total colonic transit time. **Alosetron** is a highly potent 5-HT$_3$-receptor antagonist that has been approved for treating women with severe IBS that have diarrhea as the chief problem and who have not responded to more conservative treatments. Alosetron's efficacy in men has not been established. The drug is rapidly absorbed from the GI tract with a bioavailability of 50-60%. The plasma half-life is 1.5 hours, but alosetron has a much longer duration of effect due to slow dissociation from the receptor once bound. Constipation occurs in up to 30% of patients with diarrhea-predominant IBS, requiring discontinuation of the drug in 10%. Alosetron is associated with rare but serious ischemic colitis (sometimes fatal) in 0.3% of patients.

PHYSIOLOGY OF VOMITING

The brainstem "vomiting center" is a loosely organized neuronal region within the lateral medullary reticular formation. This center coordinates the complex act of vomiting through interactions with cranial nerves VIII and X and neural networks in the nucleus tractus solitarius that control respiratory, salivatory, and vasomotor centers (Figure 36-4). Multiple receptor types have been identified in the vomiting center. There are four important sources of afferent input to the vomiting center. The "chemoreceptor trigger zone" or area postrema is accessible to emetogenic stimuli in the blood or cerebrospinal fluid because of its location at the caudal end of the fourth ventricle. This zone is rich in dopamine D$_2$ receptors and opioid receptors, and possibly serotonin 5-HT$_3$

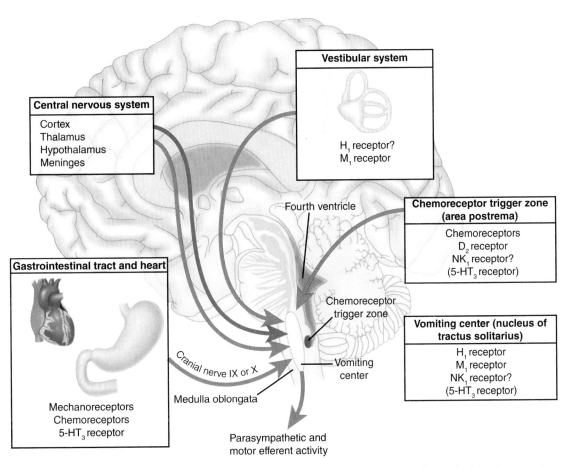

FIGURE 36-4 **Neurologic pathways involved in the genesis of nausea and vomiting.** Antagonists to the following receptors are used to prevent or treat nausea and vomiting: histamine type 1 (H_1), muscarinic type 1 (M_1), neurokinin type 1 (NK_1), serotonin type 3 (5-HT_3), and dopamine type 2 (D_2). Cannabinoid receptor agonists are also used (not shown).

receptors and neurokinin (NK_1) receptors. Afferent input from the vestibular system via cranial nerve VIII is important in motion sickness. It is rich in muscarinic M_1 and histamine H_1 receptors. Afferent input from vagal and spinal nerves from the GI tract are rich in 5-HT_3 receptors. Irritation of the GI mucosa from a variety of stimuli (eg, chemotherapy, distention) leads to release of mucosal 5-HT. Activation of 5-HT_3 receptors stimulates vagal afferent input to the vomiting center and chemoreceptor trigger zone. The last important input to the vomiting center is the CNS, which plays a key role in vomiting due to psychiatric disorders and as well as psychologic and physiologic stress.

ANTIEMETIC DRUGS

Nausea and vomiting may be manifestations of a wide variety of conditions including ADRs from medications, pregnancy, systemic diseases, vestibular disorders, CNS infection or increased intracranial pressure, radiation or chemotherapy, and GI disorders. Identification of the neurotransmitters involved with vomiting has allowed development of a diverse group of antiemetic drugs that have affinity for various receptors. Combinations of antiemetic drugs with different

mechanisms of action are often used, especially in individuals with vomiting due to chemotherapeutic drugs. Drug classes subsequently discussed include many presented in previous chapters and new drug classes. For the former, only the clinical uses of the drugs will be highlighted with references to previous chapters for pharmacokinetics, pharmacodynamics, and ADRs.

Serotonin 5-HT_3 Receptor Antagonists

Selective 5-HT_3 receptor antagonists have potent antiemetic properties that are mediated in part through central 5-HT_3-receptor blockade in the vomiting center and chemoreceptor trigger zone (Figure 36-4), but mainly through blockade of peripheral 5-HT_3 receptors located on extrinsic intestinal vagal and spinal afferent nerves (Figure 36-3). The clinical uses of these drugs are restricted to postoperative and postradiation nausea and vomiting and chemotherapy-induced nausea and vomiting (CINV). In the United States, four selective 5-HT_3 receptor antagonists are available: **ondansetron**, **granisetron**, **dolasetron**, and **palonosetron**. The first three drugs have a serum half-life of 4-9 hours and may be administered once daily by oral or intravenous routes. All three drugs have comparable efficacy and tolerability when administered at equipotent doses. Palonosetron is a newer intravenous drug that has greater affinity for the 5-HT$_3$ receptor subtype and a long serum half-life of 40 hours. All four drugs undergo extensive hepatic metabolism and are eliminated by renal and hepatic excretion. Although 5-HT$_3$ receptor antagonists are effective as single drugs for the prevention of CINV, their efficacy is enhanced by combination therapy with a glucocorticoid (**dexamethasone**), NK$_1$ receptor antagonist, or a dopamine D$_2$ antagonist also discussed within this section. The 5-HT$_3$ receptor antagonists are well-tolerated drugs. The most common ADRs are headache, dizziness, and constipation. All four drugs cause a small but statistically significant prolonged QT interval, but this is most pronounced with dolasetron. Serotonin syndrome has been reported in individuals taking 5-HT$_3$ receptor antagonists in combination with other drugs that increase CNS serotonergic activity (Chapter 19).

Neurokinin NK$_1$ Receptor Antagonists

Aprepitant, **netupitant**, and **rolapitant** are oral formulations. **Fosaprepitant** is a prodrug of aprepitant and administered intravenously. These drugs cross the blood-brain barrier and mediate their antiemetic properties through highly selective NK$_1$-receptor blockade in the area postrema (Figure 36-4). The half-lives of aprepitant, netupitant, and rolapitant are 12, 90, and 180 hours, respectively. All three drugs are metabolized by the liver. NK$_1$-receptor antagonists are used in combination with 5-HT$_3$-receptor antagonists and/or glucocorticoids for the prevention of acute and delayed nausea and vomiting from highly emetogenic chemotherapeutic regimens. For individuals unable to tolerate oral therapy, fosaprepitant may be given as a single intravenous dose. The addition of the antipsychotic drug **olanzapine** (Chapter 18) further decreases the incidence of acute and delayed nausea and vomiting. The NK$_1$-receptor antagonists are well tolerated with a low incidence of fatigue and dizziness. The drugs are metabolized by CYP3A4 and may inhibit the metabolism of other drugs metabolized by the CYP3A4 pathway. Aprepitant decreases the international normalized ratio (INR) in patients taking the anticoagulant warfarin (Chapter 11).

Cannabinoids

Dronabinol is Δ^9-tetrahydrocannabinol (THC), the major psychoactive chemical in marijuana (Chapter 21). Dronabinol is almost completely absorbed in the GI system, but undergoes significant first-pass hepatic metabolism. The metabolites are excreted slowly over days to weeks in the feces and urine. The drug's appetite stimulant and antiemetic mechanisms are not understood. Combination therapy with phenothiazines (Chapter 18) provides synergistic antiemetic action and appears to attenuate the adverse effects of both drugs. Dronabinol has some autonomic effects that may result in tachycardia and orthostatic hypotension. Dronabinol has no significant drug-drug interactions, but may potentiate the clinical effects of other psychoactive drugs.

Other Drugs

The glucocorticoids (Chapter 23) dexamethasone and **methylprednisolone** both have antiemetic properties, but the basis for these effects is unknown. These drugs appear to enhance the efficacy of 5-HT$_3$-receptor antagonists for prevention of acute and delayed nausea and vomiting in patients receiving moderately to highly emetogenic chemotherapy regimens. Benzodiazepines (Chapter 13) such as **lorazepam** or **diazepam** are used before the initiation of chemotherapy to reduce anticipatory vomiting or vomiting caused by anxiety. H$_1$ blockers (Chapter 35) and antimuscarinic drugs (Chapter 5) have weak antiemetic activity alone, although they are particularly useful for the prevention or treatment of motion sickness. **Diphenhydramine** is a first-generation H$_1$ blocker that is commonly used in conjunction with other antiemetic drugs for treatment of chemotherapy-induced emesis due to its sedating properties. **Meclizine** is an H$_1$ receptor antagonist with minimal sedation that is used for the prevention of motion sickness and the treatment of vertigo. **Hyoscine** (scopolamine) is a prototypical antimuscarinic drug and one of the best drugs for preventing motion sickness. Due to high incidence of anticholinergic effects when given orally, scopolamine is better tolerated as a transdermal patch. Substituted benzamides include **metoclopramide** (discussed previously) and **trimethobenzamide**. The primary antiemetic mechanism of trimethobenzamide is believed to be due to antagonism of dopamine receptors, but the drug also has weak antihistaminergic activity. For prevention and treatment of nausea and vomiting, metoclopramide may be given orally or intravenously every 6 hours. Trimethobenzamide may be given orally or intramuscularly. Several classes of antipsychotic drugs can also be used for their antiemetic and sedative properties (Chapter 18). Their antiemetic properties are mediated through inhibition of dopamine and muscarinic receptors, while their sedative properties are due to their antihistamine activity. The antipsychotic drugs most commonly used as antiemetics are **droperidol, prochlorperazine, promethazine**, and **thiethylperazine**. The antiemetic properties of olanzapine may be attributable to inhibition of dopamine D$_2$ and serotonin 5-HT$_{1c}$ and 5-HT$_3$ receptors. Droperidol is extremely sedating when given intravenously or intramuscularly in antiemetic dosages.

DRUGS USED IN INFLAMMATORY BOWEL DISEASE

Inflammatory bowel disease (IBD) comprises two distinct disorders: ulcerative colitis (UC) and Crohn's disease. The etiology and pathogenesis of these autoimmune disorders remain poorly defined. For this reason, pharmacologic treatment of inflammatory bowel disorders often involves drugs that belong to different therapeutic classes with different mechanisms of action and ADR profiles. The drug classes and individual drugs used to treat IBD include aminosalicylates, anti-integrin agents, glucocorticoids, methotrexate, purine analogs (azathioprine and 6-mercaptopurine), and anti-TNF agents.

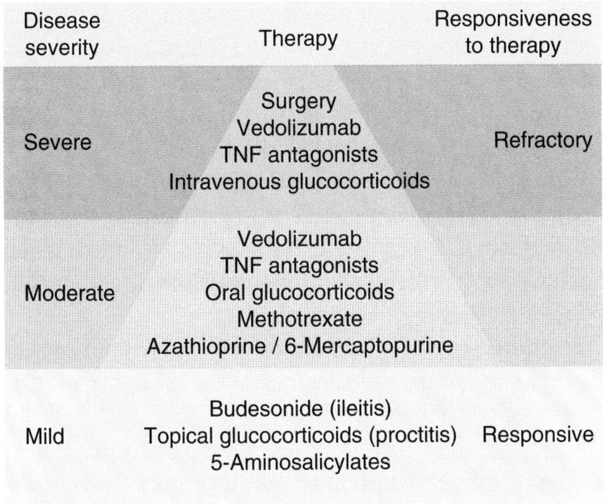

Disease severity	Therapy	Responsiveness to therapy
Severe	Surgery Vedolizumab TNF antagonists Intravenous glucocorticoids	Refractory
Moderate	Vedolizumab TNF antagonists Oral glucocorticoids Methotrexate Azathioprine / 6-Mercaptopurine	
Mild	Budesonide (ileitis) Topical glucocorticoids (proctitis) 5-Aminosalicylates	Responsive

FIGURE 36-5 Therapeutic pyramid approach to inflammatory bowel disease. Treatment choice is predicated on both severity of illness and responsiveness to therapy. Agents at the bottom of the pyramid are less efficacious, but carry a lower risk of serious adverse effects. Drugs may be used alone or in various combinations. Patients with mild disease may be treated with 5-aminosalicylates (with ulcerative colitis or Crohn's colitis), topical (suppository or enema) glucocorticoids (ulcerative colitis), or oral budesonide (Crohn's ileitis). Patients with moderate disease or patients who fail initial therapy for mild disease may be treated with the following to promote disease remission: oral glucocorticoids, immunomodulators (azathioprine/mercaptopurine or methotrexate), anti-TNF antibodies, or vedolizumab. Patients with moderate disease who fail other therapies or patients with severe disease may require intravenous glucocorticoids, anti-TNF antibodies, vedolizumab, or surgery. TNF, tumor necrosis factor.

Figure 36-5 illustrates the therapeutic approach to choosing drug regimens based on disease severity, responsiveness, and drug toxicity. Many of these drugs have been discussed in previous chapters; only their clinical use in IBD will be discussed here. References to previous chapters for pharmacokinetics, pharmacodynamics, and ADRs are provided.

Aminosalicylates

Drugs that contain **5-aminosalicylic acid (5-ASA)** have been used successfully for decades in the treatment of IBD. 5-ASA differs from salicylic acid only by the addition of an amino group. In IBD, aminosalicylates are believed to work topically in areas of diseased GI mucosa. In the context of *bowel disease*, the term "topical" does not refer to medication applied to the skin. Instead, the term refers to medication that is taken enterally, but does not significantly penetrate the wall of the gut mucosa to enter the systemic circulation. Unfortunately in the case of *unformulated aqueous* 5-ASA, up to 80% is absorbed from the proximal small intestine and thus does not reach the distal small bowel or colon in appreciable quantities. To overcome the rapid absorption of 5-ASA from the proximal small intestine, special formulations (**sulfasalazine, olsalazine, balsalazide**) have been designed to deliver 5-ASA to various distal segments of the small bowel or the colon. The formulations

bind two molecules of 5-ASA to each other, or 5-ASA to an alternative molecule. These formulations prevent absorption in the proximal bowel, yet are metabolized by resident bacteria in the terminal ileum and colon to release 5-ASA. Consequently, high concentrations of active drug are made available in the terminal ileum or colon. Alternatively, 5-ASA is formulated into various forms of **mesalamine**. This class of medications includes proprietary formulations (known generically as mesalamine) that package 5-ASA in various ways to deliver it to different segments of the small or large bowel.

Although unformulated 5-ASA is readily absorbed from the small intestine, absorption of 5-ASA from the colon is extremely low. The absorbed 5-ASA is metabolized in the gut and liver and excreted by the kidney. The metabolite is devoid of anti-inflammatory activity. In sulfasalazine (composed of 5-ASA and sulfapyridine), the sulfapyridine is absorbed and has a role in the treatment of rheumatic disorders (Chapter 34). The mechanism of action of 5-ASA is not certain. Evidence suggests that 5-ASA modulates inflammatory mediators derived from both the cyclooxygenase and lipoxygenase pathways. Other potential mechanisms of action of the 5-ASA drugs relate to their ability to interfere with the production of inflammatory cytokines. 5-ASA inhibits the activity of nuclear factor-κB (NF-κB), an important transcription factor for proinflammatory cytokines. 5-ASA may also inhibit cellular functions of natural killer cells, mucosal lymphocytes, and macrophages. Finally, the drug may act as a scavenger of reactive oxygen metabolites.

The formulations of 5-ASA are considered to be first-line agents for treatment of mild to moderate active ulcerative colitis and are effective at inducing and maintaining remission. Their efficacy in Crohn's disease is unproven, although many clinicians use 5-ASA agents as first-line therapy for mild to moderate disease involving the colon or distal ileum. The effectiveness of 5-ASA therapy depends in part on achieving high drug concentration at the site of active disease. Suppositories or enemas containing 5-ASA are useful in individuals with ulcerative colitis or Crohn's disease confined to the rectum or distal colon. In those with disease that extends to the proximal colon, all of the above formulations may be useful. For the treatment of Crohn's disease involving the small bowel, mesalamine compounds that release 5-ASA in the small intestine have a theoretical advantage over the other drugs.

Sulfasalazine has a high incidence of adverse effects, most of which are attributable to systemic effects of the sulfapyridine molecule. Up to 40% of individuals cannot tolerate therapeutic doses of sulfasalazine. The most common ADRs are dose-related and include GI upset, headaches, arthralgia, myalgia, bone marrow suppression, and malaise. Hypersensitivity to sulfapyridine, and rarely 5-ASA, are also possible. Sulfasalazine impairs folate absorption and processing; hence, dietary supplementation with 1 mg/day folic acid is recommended. In contrast, other 5-ASA formulations are well tolerated. In most clinical trials with 5-ASA formulations, the frequency of ADRs is similar to that in patients treated with placebo. For unclear reasons, olsalazine may stimulate a secretory diarrhea in 10% of patients. This diarrhea should not be confused with active IBD. Rare cases of interstitial nephritis are reported, particularly with high doses of mesalamine formulations. This ADR may be attributable to the higher serum 5-ASA levels attained with these drugs.

Anti-Integrin Therapy

Integrins are a family of adhesion molecules on the surface of leukocytes that may interact with selectins, another class of adhesion molecules on the surface of the vascular endothelial cells. Interaction between these adhesion molecules allows circulating leukocytes to adhere to the vascular endothelium and subsequently exit the vessel wall to get into the tissues. Integrins are heterodimers that contain α and β subunits.

Two monoclonal antibodies directed against integrins are available for the treatment of IBD: **natalizumab** and **vedolizumab**. Both are administered intravenously. Natalizumab was previously discussed for its use in the treatment of multiple sclerosis (Chapter 32). Natalizumab inhibits immune cell migration into the bowel and the CNS. Because of the latter effect, natalizumab increases the risk of progressive multifocal leukoencephalopathy (PML) due to reactivation of a human polyomavirus (JC virus). Vedolizumab is a monoclonal antibody with activity specifically directed against the α4/β7 integrin, which blocks interaction of leukocytes only with vascular endothelial cell adhesion molecules in the gut in order to prevent their migration into the bowel. Because vedolizumab does not affect lymphocyte migration into the CNS, the risk of PML is believed to be extremely low. With the advent of vedolizumab, natalizumab is almost never used for the treatment of IBD. Vedolizumab is increasingly used as a second-line treatment for individuals with moderate to severe ulcerative colitis or Crohn's disease who cannot take agents directed against tumor necrosis factor (TNF) due to adverse effects, lack of efficacy, or loss of response. After intravenous induction therapy, patients with a clinical response are treated with intravenous maintenance therapy every 8 weeks. Vedolizumab appears to have a low incidence of serious adverse effects. Neutralizing antibodies may develop in 2-10% of patients.

Other Drugs

Several other medications that dampen the immune system may be used in the treatment of IBD. These drug classes and individual drugs include glucocorticoids (Chapter 23), methotrexate (Chapters 31, 32, and 34), azathioprine and 6-mercaptopurine (Chapters 32 and 34), and anti-TNF agents (Chapters 32 and 34).

Both topical and systemic glucocorticoids are used in the treatment of IBD. **Hydrocortisone** enemas, foam, or suppositories are used to maximize colonic tissue effects and minimize systemic absorption when treating active IBD in the rectum and sigmoid colon. Absorption of hydrocortisone is reduced with rectal administration, although 15-30% of the administered dosage is still absorbed. **Budesonide** is a potent synthetic analog of prednisolone that has high affinity for the glucocorticoid receptor but is subject to rapid first-pass hepatic metabolism. Two pH-controlled delayed-release oral formulations of budesonide are available that release the drug either in the distal ileum or colon. **Prednisone** and **prednisolone** are the most commonly used oral glucocorticoids. These drugs have an intermediate duration of biologic activity allowing once-daily dosing.

Methotrexate has both anticancer and immunosuppressive properties. Methotrexate is used to induce and maintain remission in individuals with Crohn's disease, but its efficacy in UC is uncertain. Induction is initiated by once weekly subcutaneous injection. If a satisfactory response is achieved within 8-12 weeks, the weekly dose is reduced.

Azathioprine is a purine antimetabolite. The active form of the drug is **6-mercaptopurine**. Azathioprine has immunosuppressive properties and is clinically used for induction and maintenance of remission of ulcerative colitis and Crohn's disease. After 3-6 months of treatment, 50-60% of patients with active disease achieve remission. These agents help maintain remission in up to 80% of patients. For individuals that depend on long-term glucocorticoid therapy to control active disease, these purine analogs allow dose reduction or elimination of steroids in the majority.

In people with IBD (especially Crohn's disease), there is a dysregulation of the helper T cell type 1 (TH1) response and regulatory T cells. One of the key proinflammatory cytokines in IBD is TNF. Four monoclonal antibodies to human TNF-α are approved for the treatment of IBD: **infliximab**, **adalimumab**, **golimumab**, and **certolizumab**. Infliximab, adalimumab, and certolizumab are approved for the acute and chronic treatment of individuals with moderate to severe Crohn's disease that have had an inadequate response to conventional therapies. Infliximab, adalimumab, and golimumab are approved for the acute and chronic treatment of moderate to severe ulcerative colitis. With induction therapy, these agents lead to symptomatic improvement in 60%, and disease remission in 30% of people with moderate to severe Crohn's disease. The median time to clinical response is 2 weeks. With chronic, regularly scheduled therapy, clinical response is maintained in more than 60% of patients and disease remission in 40%. However, one-third of patients eventually lose response despite higher doses or more frequent injections. Loss of response may be due to the development of antibodies to the anti-TNF biologic agents, or to other mechanisms. Infliximab is approved for the treatment of individuals with moderate to severe ulcerative colitis that have had inadequate previous therapeutic responses. After induction therapy, 70% of patients have a clinical response and one-third achieve a clinical remission. With continued maintenance infusions every 8 weeks, approximately 50% of patients have continued clinical response. Adalimumab and golimumab are also approved for moderate to severe ulcerative colitis, but they appear to be less effective.

REHABILITATION RELEVANCE

Every physical therapist is aware of how GI dysfunction (nausea, vomiting, diarrhea) can negatively affect the ability of individuals to participate in rehabilitation. In addition, therapy sessions involving vertical orientation, vestibular challenges, and gait training may provoke or exacerbate nausea and vomiting. Therapists may also be involved in providing interventions and modalities to *mitigate* nausea and vomiting. For example, the use of certain modes of transcutaneous electrical nerve stimulation (TENS) on acupuncture points combined with antiemetic drugs can help prevent emesis following chemotherapy and surgical procedures. A working knowledge of the mechanisms of action, pharmacokinetics, and clinical efficacy of drugs affecting the GI system may benefit daily physical therapy practice. Highlighted below are ADRs that have a significant effect on physical therapy practice. For the ADRs associated with glucocorticoids, see Chapter 23. For those associated with anti-TNF biologic agents, see Chapters 32 and 34.

- **Fall risk** is increased with several drug classes used to treat different GI dysfunctions, though the underlying mechanisms may be different. **Sedation** and **drowsiness** are common with benzodiazepines, some antipsychotics, dronabinol, NK_1-receptor antagonists, metoclopramide, H_1 blockers, and M_1 blockers used in the treatment of nausea and vomiting. Dronabinol may also increase fall risk due to **orthostatic hypotension**. When treating patients taking these drugs, especially in the acute care setting, fall-risk prevention should be a major focus.

- **Cardiac arrhythmias** (long QT syndrome) are associated with dolasetron and the other $5\text{-}HT_3$-receptor antagonists, though to a lesser extent. Heart rate monitoring should be included in aerobic programs with patients taking these drugs. If an arrhythmia is detected or suspected during therapy, appropriate medical services should be contacted immediately. Therapists should also recognize that supratherapeutic doses of loperamide (opioid) are associated with long QT syndrome and cardiac death.

- **Myalgia** and **arthralgia** are associated with sulfasalazine therapy. If this is suspected, exercise interventions and goals should be reduced and the prescribing healthcare provider contacted.

- **Dystonia, akathisia,** and **parkinsonian manifestations** may be important ADRs when metoclopramide is used. Physical therapists may notice these extrapyramidal motor dysfunctions prior to other healthcare professionals. If drug-induced extrapyramidal dysfunction is suspected, the prescribing healthcare provider should be contacted immediately because prolonged use of the drug may result in a higher risk of permanent dysfunction.

- Chronic use of proton pump inhibitors may be associated with **increase in hip fracture risk**. There is not yet a correlation between length of PPI administration and increased risk of fracture and the potential mechanism for increased fracture risk has not been identified. However, because PPI use is so common, integration of weightbearing and resistance training would likely be beneficial to bone health.

CASE CONCLUSION

The physical therapist knew R.J. from previous encounters for evaluation and treatment of the neuropathic ulcers. R.J. arrived today as scheduled for evaluation. The therapist greeted the patient in the waiting room and noted that she had difficulty initiating sit-to-stand activity, requiring her husband's assistance. When R.J. finally stood, she had a wide base of support, suggesting initial instability in standing. R.J. demonstrated notable difficulty initiating gait and was once again assisted by her spouse. During ambulation, she had decreased step length that resulted in a slow shuffling gait. When R.J. was finally seated on a treatment table, she and her husband confirmed that the functional changes observed since the therapist last saw her were recent, though they could not provide a specific timeframe. The physical therapist reviewed R.J.'s medication list with her, noting that multiple antihypertensive and cardiovascular medications may cause orthostatic hypotension, which presents upon initial standing. However, R.J.'s instability during standing, difficulty initiating gait, and slow shuffling pattern were more consistent with extrapyramidal motor dysfunction. These manifestations were recent and appeared to coincide with the newer prescription for metoclopramide to treat her gastroparesis. Metoclopramide's prokinetic mechanism of action is via inhibition of dopaminergic receptors in the GI system. However, an ADR is drug-associated parkinsonism due to inhibition of central dopamine receptors in the extrapyramidal system. The physical therapist immediately alerted the healthcare professional prescribing the metoclopramide of R.J.'s recent functional impairments.

CHAPTER 36 QUESTIONS

1. Which of the following drugs is clinically used for acid-peptic disease, but also has the potential to treat diarrhea by binding enterotoxins?

   a. Bismuth
   b. Cimetidine
   c. Omeprazole
   d. Misoprostol

2. Which of the following drugs used in irritable bowel syndrome has its antispasmodic action via inhibition of muscarinic receptors in the gastrointestinal system?

   a. Crofelemer
   b. Hyoscyamine
   c. Linaclotide
   d. Lubiprostone

3. Which of the following drugs is a mu opioid receptor antagonist that is used to treat constipation?

   a. Docusate
   b. Magnesium citrate
   c. Methylnaltrexone
   d. Polyethylene glycol

4. Which of the following drugs increases gastrointestinal motility by stimulating motilin receptors?

   a. Metoclopramide
   b. Dronabinol
   c. Plecanatide
   d. Erythromycin

5. Which of the following drugs inhibits the cystic fibrosis transmembrane conductance regulator channel?

   a. Crofelemer
   b. Linaclotide
   c. Lubiprostone
   d. Psyllium

6. Which of the following drugs used to treat diarrhea associated with irritable bowel syndrome inhibits serotonin type 3 receptors in the gastrointestinal system?

   a. Ondansetron
   b. Alosetron
   c. Granisetron
   d. Palonosetron

7. Which of the following drugs produces its antiemetic action by inhibiting neurokinin receptors?

   a. Ondansetron
   b. Dexamethasone
   c. Aprepitant
   d. Scopolamine

8. Which of the following drugs used in the treatment of inflammatory bowel disease acts via 5-aminosalicylic acid (5-ASA)?

   a. Azathioprine
   b. Vedolizumab
   c. Sulfasalazine
   d. Methotrexate

9. Which of the following is a monoclonal antibody that binds to the α4/β7 integrin receptor on leukocytes and inhibits their migration from the vasculature?

   a. Vedolizumab
   b. Infliximab
   c. Adalimumab
   d. Certolizumab

10. Which of the following is an antiemetic that may also increase appetite?

   a. Loperamide
   b. Dronabinol
   c. Eluxadoline
   d. Methylnaltrexone

Index

Note: Page numbers followed by *f* and *t* indicate figures and tables.